Bailey & Love's
Essential Operations in Oral and Maxillofacial Surgery

T0293160

Bailey & Love's
Other Titles

Bailey & Love's Short Practice of Surgery, 28th Edition (2023)
Edited by P. Ronan O'Connell, Andrew W. McCaskie, Robert D. Sayers

Bailey & Love's Essential Clinical Anatomy (2019)
John Lumley, John Craven, Peter Abrahams, Richard Tunstall

Bailey & Love's
Essential Operations in Oral and Maxillofacial Surgery

Edited by

Peter A. Brennan

MD, PhD, FRCS, FRCSI, Hon FRCS(Glasg), FFST, FDSRCS

Consultant Oral and Maxillofacial Surgeon

Honorary Professor of Surgery

Portsmouth Hospitals University NHS Trust

Portsmouth, UK

Rabindra P. Singh

MBChB(Hons), BDS, MFDSRCS, MRCSEd, PG Cert Clin Ed, FHEA, FRCS(Eng)

Consultant Maxillofacial/Head and Neck Surgeon

University Hospital Southampton NHS Foundation Trust

Southampton, UK

Kaveh Shakib

PhD, FRCS(OMFS), MRCS, FDSRCPS(Glas), FDSRCS(Eng), MBBS, BDS

Consultant Oral and Maxillofacial Surgeon

Division of Surgery & Interventional Sciences, University College London

London, UK

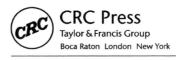

CRC Press
Taylor & Francis Group
Boca Raton London New York

CRC Press is an imprint of the
Taylor & Francis Group, an **informa** business

First edition published 2024
by CRC Press
4 Park Square, Milton Park, Abingdon, Oxon, OX14 4RN

and by CRC Press
2385 NW Executive Center Drive, Suite 320, Boca Raton, FL 33431

ISBN: 9781032030562 (hbk)
ISBN: 9780367772581 (pbk)
ISBN: 9781003186458 (ebk)

DOI: 10.1201/9781003186458

Typeset in Baskerville MT Std
by Evolution Design & Digital Ltd (Kent), UK

Contents

Bailey & Love's Essential Operations Bailey & Love's Essential Operations
Bailey & Love's Essential Operations Bailey & Love's Essential Operations
Bailey & Love's Essential Operations Bailey & Love's Essential Operations

Foreword

By P. Ronan O'Connell

It is a great pleasure to introduce the first edition of *Bailey & Love's Essential Operations in Oral and Maxillofacial Surgery* and to congratulate editors Professor Peter Brennan, Mr Rabindra Singh and Professor Kaveh Shakib, their contributing authors and our B&L publishers on this excellent book.

Bailey & Love's Short Practice of Surgery, first published in 1932, has been venerated by generations of medical students and surgeons as a repository of the core knowledge needed for safe surgical practice. However, the editors understand that in the modern era, a parent textbook can only cover knowledge essential for early surgical training and recognise the need for a compendium of texts to take B&L readership to the next level of speciality knowledge.

Bailey & Love's Essential Operations in Oral and Maxillofacial Surgery is the first in a planned compendium of operative texts designed to support trainees in higher surgical and sub-specialty training. The current text remains true to the heritage and traditions of the parent textbook. The most up-to-date content in Oral and Maxillofacial Surgery is presented in a familiar format and style. The text, written by a series of internationally renowned authors, is clear and concise throughout. Each chapter is richly illustrated with operative photographs and accompanying line diagrams where needed.

A particular feature of each chapter is a section on 'Top Tips and Hazards' gleaned from years of expert practice. Such pearls of wisdom are a valuable addition to the text in keeping with the great traditions of Hamilton Bailey and McNeal Love.

I am sure readers will enjoy *Bailey & Love's Essential Operations in Oral and Maxillofacial Surgery* and trust that it will be a useful adjunct to their study and clinical practice.

P. Ronan O'Connell
MD FRCSI FRCSGlas (Hon) FRCSEdin (Hon)
RCSEng (Hon) FCSHK (Hon) FRCPSC (Hon)

Editor in Chief, *Bailey & Love's Short Practice of Surgery*

Bailey & Love's Essential Operations Bailey & Love's Essential Operations
Bailey & Love's Essential Operations Bailey & Love's Essential Operations
Bailey & Love's Essential Operations Bailey & Love's Essential Operations

Foreword

By Mike McKirdy

I am delighted to introduce this new first edition of *Bailey & Love's Essential Operations in Oral and Maxillofacial Surgery*. The original *Bailey & Love's Short Practice of Surgery* (now on its 28th Edition), has been used by generations of surgeons around the world. The addition of a new series of surgical sub-speciality operative textbooks by the publishers, and with the same ethos as Bailey and Love's itself, has been long awaited.

Bailey & Love's Essential Operations in Oral and Maxillofacial Surgery (OMFS) is a collection of comprehensive and contemporary practical resources designed to provide students, trainees, and specialist surgeons with a deep understanding of the principles, techniques, and innovations that define this specialised branch of surgery. It should be of interest to any surgeon who operates in the head and neck area including OMFS, Ear, Nose and Throat, Plastic, Reconstructive, and General Surgery.

This practical textbook has been meticulously compiled by a team of well-respected senior editors from the United Kingdom and is beautifully illustrated with operative images, supplemented by easy-to-follow diagrams as appropriate. It provides a step-by-step approach for the different operations across the whole remit of OMFS, and most chapters have references for further reading.

The editors have brought together respected experts from around the world for all the OMFS sub-specialties. The book also includes innovative chapters on human factors and improving safety in the operating theatre, medico-legal aspects of OMFS practice, head and neck imaging and the latest developments in tissue engineering.

There is no currently up-to-date textbook of operative OMFS available to rival this new title. Therefore, it should be the first point of reference for both trainees and established surgeons who have an interest in this rapidly expanding and fascinating specialty.

Mike McKirdy
MBChB FRCS FRCS (General Surgery)

President
Royal College of Physicians and Surgeons of Glasgow

Bailey & Love's Essential Operations Bailey & Love's Essential Operations
Bailey & Love's Essential Operations Bailey & Love's Essential Operations
Bailey & Love's Essential Operations Bailey & Love's Essential Operations

Preface

Oral and maxillofacial surgery (OMFS) continues to advance at a great pace, which is testament to the skills that the specialty brings to benefit patient care. As with any surgical discipline, it is important that trainees grasp the basic principles of operative surgical practice before developing skills and competence in the various OMFS procedures. To prepare for these varied and often complex procedures, prior knowledge and understanding is important, and it enhances both performance and enjoyment in the operating theatre.

In this new book, developed from the renowned Bailey & Love series, we have aimed to cover the essential surgical techniques across the remit of the specialty and have enlisted the help of respected colleagues and trainers from around the world.

We believe that prior to performing any operative surgery, colleagues should understand human factors and how to minimise error in the operating theatre, so have included a chapter on this important subject at the beginning of this book. Following consideration of other relevant broader areas for safe surgical practice, the book has 10 further sections, taking readers through all the major OMFS sub-specialties. While we respect that some colleagues may not specialise in cleft, skull base, aesthetic or thyroid surgery, these have been included for completeness. To maintain consistency throughout, each chapter has been written and formatted in a similar manner, with (where relevant), essential surgical anatomy, operative steps, top tips and recommended further reading. Chapters have been illustrated with both operative images and/or drawings as necessary to aid understanding. The book concludes with a section on advances in OMFS including robotic surgery, interventional radiology and tissue engineering.

For a new project of this size, we respect that there may be areas that we have omitted or not covered in as much depth, given the publishing constraints. We would be delighted to hear from colleagues with suggestions for additional content or material that they would like to be included in any future editions.

We acknowledge that this new book title had its origins from *Operative Oral and Maxillofacial Surgery* edited by John Langdon, Mohan Patel, Robert Ord and Peter Brennan. We take this opportunity to thank John, Mo and Bob for their contribution over many years. We are also grateful to contributors from that book who have written chapters here, and to those who kindly allowed their chapters to be updated and revised for this new title.

Finally, we hope that this new book will not only help colleagues in their understanding of technical surgery in our complex and varied discipline, but that it will also benefit patient safety.

Primum non nocere

Peter A. Brennan
Rabindra P. Singh
Kaveh Shakib

We dedicate this edition to our trainees – past, present and future.

Bailey & Love's Essential Operations Bailey & Love's Essential Operations
Bailey & Love's Essential Operations Bailey & Love's Essential Operations
Bailey & Love's Essential Operations Bailey & Love's Essential Operations

Acknowledgements

Authors from *Operative Oral and Maxillofacial Surgery*, Third Edition edited by John Langdon, Mohan Patel, Robert Ord and Peter Brennan.

In this day and age, it is impossible to produce a book like this without the contribution of numerous individuals. Although it would be impractical to mention all those who have played a part in producing *Bailey & Love's Essential Operations in Oral and Maxillofacial Surgery*, we would be remiss not to mention those whose chapters from *Operative Oral and Maxillofacial Surgery*, Third Edition informed the basis of many new chapters.

John Langdon
Mohan Patel
Robert Ord

Konrad P. Aguila
Christopher M. Avery
Andrew W. Baker
Abhishake Banda
Jaime Brahim
Robert P. Bentley
Greg Boyes-Varley
Jacqueline Brown
James S. Brown
Catherine Bryant
John F. Caccamese
Luke Cascarini
John Cawood
Luc Cesteleyn
Domenick P. Coletti
Corazon Collantes-Jose
Steve Connor
Joseph R. Deatherage
Risal Djohan
Stephanie J. Drew
Donita Dyalram
Barrie T. Evans

Rhodri Evans
Tirbod Fattahi
Stephen E. Feinberg
Tim Flood
G. E. Ghali
Bahar Bassiri Gharb
Clare Gleeson
Gillian L. Hall
Ahmed M. Hashem
Ian Holland
Colin Hopper
Bruce Horswell
Christoph T. Huppa
Kenji Izumi
Paul A. Johnson
Leonard B. Kaban
Eugene E. Keller
King Kim
Elizabeth A. Kutcipal
Dorothy A. Lang
Janice S. Lee
Andrew Lyons
David W. MacPherson
E. Antonio Mangubat
Joe McManners
John S. Millar

George Obeid
Maria E. Papadaki
Phil Pirgousis
Clive A. Pratt
N. Ravindranathan
Alexander D. Rapidis
Salvatore L. Ruggiero
Nabil Samman
Henning Schliephake
Alexander Schramm
Kishore Shekar
Miller H. Smith
Helen Spencer
Leo F. A. Stassen
Paul J. W. Stoelinga
Adrian Sugar
Navin Vig
Peter D. Waite
David A. Walker
Gary Warburton
Frank Wilde
Jennifer E. Woerner
Eduardo C. Yap
David M. Yates
Jacob Yetzer

Chapter 3, *Imaging Techniques in Maxillofacial Surgery* may contain material from *Imaging Techniques, Including Tomography-Guided Biopsy and Flurodeoxyglucose-Positron Emission Tomography* by Steve Connor, and *Ultrasound Imaging, Including Ultrasound-Guided Biopsy* by Rachel S. Oeppen and Rhodri Evans which have been revised and updated by the current authors.

Chapter 4, *Histopathological Assessment of Resection Specimens* may contain material from *Oral and Oropharyngeal Squamous Cell Carcinoma: Pathological Assessment of Resection Specimens and Neck Dissections* by Gillian L. Hall which has been revised and updated by the current author.

Chapter 5, *Minor Oral Surgery* may contain material from *Tooth Extraction* by Catherine Bryant, *Removal of Unerupted Teeth* by Catherine Bryant and Clare Gleeson, and *Surgical Endodontics* by Helen Spencer which have been revised and updated by the current author.

Chapter 9, *Principles of Dental Implant Surgery* may contain material from *Basic Implantology – An American Perspective* by Jaime Brahim, and *Basic and Advanced Implantology – A European Perspective* by John Cawood and Mohan Francis Patel which have been revised and updated by the current authors.

Chapter 10 *Bone Augmentation Techniques in Oral Implantology* may contain material from *Adjunctive Office-Based Techniques for Bone Augmentation in Oral Implantology* by Gary Warburton and Abhishake Banda which has been revised and updated by the current authors.

Chapter 12, *Facial Trauma Assessment and Emergency Procedures* may contain material from *Emergency Procedures* by David W. MacPherson and Clive A. Pratt which has been revised and updated by the current authors.

Chapter 14, *Contemporary Maxillofacial Fixation Techniques* may contain material from *Contemporary Maxillofacial Fixation Techniques* by Domenick P. Coletti which has been revised and updated by the current authors.

Chapter 17, *Zygomatic Fractures* may contain material from *Middle Third Fractures* by Joe McManners, Jeremy McMahon and Ian Holland which has been revised and updated by the current authors.

Chapter 24, *Access Surgery* may contain material from *Access Surgery* by Madangopolan Ethunandan, Barrie T. Evans and Dorothy A. Lang which has been revised and updated by the current author.

Chapter 25, *Resection of the Mandible and Maxilla* may contain material from *Jaw Resection* by James S. Brown which has been revised and updated by the current author.

Chapter 26, *Skull Base and Orbital Tumour Resection* may contain material from *Excision of Skin Lesions and Orbital and Nasal Reconstruction* by Bruce Horswell, and *Tumours of the Skull Base* by Madangopolan Ethunandan, Barrie T. Evans and Dorothy A. Lang which have been revised and updated by the current authors.

Chapter 28, *Management of Benign and Malignant Skin Lesions* may contain material from *Excision of Skin Lesions and Orbital and Nasal Reconstruction* by Bruce Horswell which has been revised and updated by the current authors.

Chapter 31, *Local and Pedicled Orofacial Flaps* may contain material from *Reconstructive Surgery – Local and Pedicled Orofacial Flaps* by Nabil Samman which has been revised and updated by the current authors.

Chapter 32, *Lip Reconstruction* may contain material from *Local Resection and Reconstruction of Oral Carcinomas and Lip Cancer* by Robert A. Ord and Donita Dyalram which has been revised and updated by the current authors.

Chapter 33, *Pectoralis Major Flap* may contain material from *Pectoralis Major* by Andrew Lyons which has been revised and updated by the current authors.

Chapter 36, *Radial Forearm Flap* may contain material from *Radial Forearm Flap* by Christopher M. Avery which has been revised and updated by the current authors.

Chapter 38, *Anterolateral Thigh Flap* may contain material from *Anterolateral Thigh Flap* by Andrew Lyons which has been revised and updated by the current author.

Chapter 39, *Deep Circumflex Iliac Artery (DCIA) Flap* may contain material from *Vascularized Iliac Crest Grafts* by Andrew Lyons which has been revised and updated by the current author.

Chapter 42, *Latissimus Dorsi Flap* may contain material from *Latissumus Dorsi Flap* by Andrew W. Baker which has been revised and updated by the current authors.

Chapter 43, *Acute and Delayed Dynamic Facial Reanimation* may contain material from *Facial Reanimation* by Henning Schliephake which has been revised and updated by the current authors.

Chapter 44, *Submandibular, Sublingual and Minor Salivary Gland Surgery* may contain material from *Submandibular, Sublingual, and Minor Salivary Gland Surgery* by John D. Langdon which has been revised and updated by the current authors.

Chapter 46, *Surgery of the Parotid Gland* may contain material from *Facial Nerve Dissection and Formal Parotid Surgery* by John D. Langdon which has been revised and updated by the current authors.

Chapter 48, *Thyroid and Parathyroid Surgery* may contain material from *Thyroidectomy* by Rui Fernandes and Jacob Yetzer which has been revised and updated by the current authors.

Chapter 50, *Temporomandibular Joint Arthroscopy: Diagnostic and Operative Technique* may contain material from *Temporomandibular Joint Arthroscopy: Diagnostic and Operative Technique* by Joseph P. McCain and King Kim which has been revised and updated by the current authors.

Chapter 52, *Treatment of Temporomandibular Joint Ankylosis* may contain material from *Treatment of Temporomandibular Joint Ankylosis* by Andrew J. Sidebottom which has been revised and updated by the current authors.

Chapter 54, *Orthognathic Surgery of the Mandible* may contain material from *Orthognathic Surgery of the Mandible* by Paul A. Johnson which has been revised and updated by the current authors.

Chapter 55, *Orthognathic Surgery of the Maxilla* may contain material from *Orthognathic Surgery – Maxilla (Le Fort I, II and III)* by George Obeid which has been revised and updated by the current author.

Chapter 56, *Genioplasty* may contain material from *Orthognathic Surgery of the Mandible* by Paul A. Johnson which has been revised and updated by the current author.

Chapter 57, *Mandibular and Maxillary Distraction Osteogenesis* may contain material from *Mandibular Distraction Osteogenesis by Intraoral and Extraoral Techniques* and *Maxillary Distraction Osteogenesis by Intra-oral and Extra-Oral Techniques* by David A. Walker which has been revised and updated by the current authors.

Chapter 58, *Surgical Management of Craniosynostosis* may contain material from *Surgical Management of Craniosynostosis* by David M. Yates, Jennifer E. Woerner and G. E. Ghali which has been revised and updated by the current author.

Chapter 59, *Surgical Management of Obstructive Sleep Apnoea* may contain material from *Sleep Apnoea and Snoring, Including Non-Surgical Techniques* by Joseph R. Deatherage and Peter D. Waite which has been revised and updated by the current authors.

Chapter 62, *Primary Repair of Cleft Palate* may contain material from *Primary Repair of Cleft Palate* by Christoph T. Huppa which has been revised and updated by the current author.

Chapter 63, *Alveolar Bone Grafting* may contain material from *Alveolar Bone Grafting in Cleft Patients* by Serryth Colbert, Adrian Sugar and Tim Flood which has been revised and updated by the current author.

Chapter 64, *Cleft Rhinoplasty* may contain material from *Cleft Rhinoplasty* by V. Ilankovan and Tian Ee Seah which has been revised and updated by the current authors.

Chapter 65, *Face, Neck and Brow Lift Surgery* may contain material from *Brow Lift and Facelift, Including Endoscopic Surgery* by Tirbod Fattahi which has been revised and updated by the current author.

Chapter 67, *Otoplasty* may contain material from *Aesthetic Otoplasty* by Leo F. A. Stassen which has been revised and updated by the current authors.

Chapter 68, *Septorhinoplasty and Nasal Reconstruction* may contain material from *Rhinoplasty and Septoplasty: Closed and Open Rhinoplastic Techniques* by Luc Cesteleyn, N. Ravindranathan and Corazon Collantes-Jose, *Rhinoplasty for Southeast Asian Noses: Open and Closed Approaches* by Corazon Collantes-Jose, Eduardo C. Yap and Konrad P. Aguila, and *Post-Traumatic Rhinoplasty* by Luc Cesteleyn which have been revised and updated by the current authors.

Chapter 69, *Autologous Fat Grafting for Facial Rejuvenation and Asymmetry Correction* may contain material from *Laser Skin Resurfacing* by Navin Vig which has been revised and updated by the current authors.

Chapter 70, *Tissue Engineering* may contain material from *Tissue Engineering* by Miller H. Smith, Kenji Izumi and Stephen E. Feinberg which has been revised and updated by the current authors.

Chapter 71, *Principles of Laser Surgery* may contain material from *Laser: General Principles* by Madangopolan Ethunandan and Colin Hopper which has been revised and updated by the current author.

Chapter 72, *Interventional Radiology of the Head and Neck* may contain material from *Treatment Techniques, Surgery and Sclerosants* by Maria E. Papadaki and Leonard B. Kaban, and *Interventional Radiology of the Head and Neck* by John S. Millar which have been revised and updated by the current author.

Chapter 73, *Transoral Robotic Surgery* may contain material from *Transoral Robotic Surgery* by Joshua E. Lubek which has been revised and updated by the current author.

Associate Editors

PART 3
TRAUMA
Edited by Simon Holmes

PART 7
TEMPOROMANDIBULAR JOINT
DISORDERS AND SURGERY
Edited by Andrew J. Sidebottom

PART 8
ORTHOGNATHIC AND CRANIOFACIAL
SURGERY
Edited by Tom Aldridge

PART 9
CLEFT LIP AND PALATE
Edited by Simon van Eeden

Contributors

Nabeela Ahmed
Queens Medical Centre
Nottingham, UK

Peyman Alam
University Hospitals Sussex NHS Foundation Trust
West Sussex, UK

Tom Aldridge
Portsmouth Hospitals University NHS Trust
Portsmouth, UK

Mohammed Al-Gholmy
Portsmouth Hospitals University NHS Trust
Portsmouth, UK

Mohammed A. Al-Muharraqi
Bahrain Defence Force Hospital
Riffa, Bahrain

Haytham al-Rawi
Solihull Hospital
Solihull, UK

Duaa Al-Sayed
St George's University Hospital
London, UK

Jasper Bekker
Portsmouth Hospitals University NHS Trust
Portsmouth, UK

R. Bryan Bell
Providence Cancer Institute
Portland, OR, USA

Robert P. Bentley
King's College Hospital
London, UK

Rishi Bhandari
Barts Health, Queen Mary University
London, UK

Brian Bisase
Queen Victoria Hospital
East Grinstead, UK

Anna Bock
Uniklinik RWTH
Aachen, Germany

Greg Boyes-Varley
University of Witwatersrand
Johannesburg, South Africa

Dominic Bray
Dominic Bray Facial Plastic Surgery
London, UK

Peter A. Brennan
Portsmouth Hospitals University NHS Trust
Portsmouth, UK

Jocelyn Brookes
UCL Institute of Cardiovascular Sciences
London, UK

Jacqueline Brown
Guy's and St Thomas' Hospital
London, UK

Neil W. Bulstrode
Great Ormond Street Hospital
London, UK

Briana J. Burris
Massachusetts General Hospital
Boston, MA, USA

Eric R. Carlson
University of Tennessee Graduate School of Medicine
Knoxville, TN, USA

Serryth Colbert
Royal United Hospitals
Bath, UK

Roger Currie
Crosshouse Hospital
Crosshouse, UK

Rhodri Davies
The Royal London Dental Hospital
London, UK

Mark Devlin
National Cleft Surgical Service for Scotland
Glasgow, UK

Giovanni Diana
Queen Elizabeth University Hospital
Glasgow, UK

Ioanna Dimasi
Barts Health NHS Trust
London, UK

George Dimitroulis
Epworth-Freemasons Hospital
Melbourne, Australia

David Drake
Royal Hospital for Children
Glasgow, UK

Martin Duplantier
Oral Facial Surgery Center
Houma, LA, USA

Siavash Siv Eftekhari
Methodist Richardson Medical Center
Frisco, TX, USA

Ross O. C. Elledge
University Hospitals Birmingham NHS Foundation
Trust
Birmingham, UK

Jan S. Enzler
University Hospital
Bern, Switzerland

Michael P. Escudier
King's College
London, UK

Madan G. Ethunandan
University Hospital Southampton
Southampton, UK

Martin Evans
Children's Hospital Birmingham
Birmingham, UK

Rebecca Exley
University College Hospitals
London, UK

Kunmi Fasanmade
Oxford University Hospitals NHS Foundation Trust
Oxford, UK

Rui Fernandes
University of Florida College of Medicine
Jacksonville, FL, USA

Maria Florez-Martin
University College London
London, UK

Kandasamy Ganesan
Southend University Hospital
Southend, UK

Montey Garg
Oxford University Hospitals NHS Foundation Trust
Oxford, UK

Ralph W. Gilbert
Toronto General Hospital
Toronto, Canada

Adriaan O. Grobbelaar
Inselspital University Hospital
Bern, Switzerland

Ben Gurney
Royal Surrey County Hospital
Guilford, UK

Simon C. Harvey
University College London Hospital
London, UK

Nathalie Higgs
University Hospitals Sussex NHS Foundation Trust
West Sussex, UK

Simon Holmes
Barts Health NHS Trust
London, UK

Frank Hölzle
RWTH University of Aachen
Aachen, Germany

Dale Howes
University of Sydney
Sydney, Australia

Velupillai Ilankovan
Poole Hospital NHS Foundation Trust
Dorset, UK

Robert Isaac
University Hospital Southampton
Southampton, UK

Steve Jarvis
Jarvis Bagshaw Ltd
Somerset, UK

Jean-Pierre Jeannon
Guy's and St Thomas' Hospital
London, UK

Gavin Jell
University College London
London, UK

Darin Johnston
David Grant Medical Center (USAF)
Fairfield, CA, USA

Deepak Kalaskar
Royal Free Hospital
London, UK

Cyrus J. Kerawala
The Royal Marsden Hospital
London, UK

Baber Khatib
Head and Neck Institute
Portland, OR, USA

Moni Abraham Kuriakose
Shanku Medical Centre
Kerala, India

Panayiotis A. Kyzas
Royal Blackburn Teaching Hospital
Blackburn, UK

David Laraway
Queen Elizabeth University Hospital
Glasgow, UK

Vickie Lee
Imperial College Healthcare NHS Trust
London, UK

Joshua E. Lubek
University of Maryland Medical Center
Baltimore, MD, USA

Colin MacIver
Mayo Clinic Abu Dhabi
Abu Dhabi, UAE

Nijaguna Mathad
University Hospital Southampton
Southampton, UK

Ahmed S. Mazeed
Sohag University Hospital
Sohag, Egypt

Joseph P. McCain
Harvard School of Dental Medicine
Boston, MA, USA

Mark McGurk
University College London Hospitals
London, UK

Jeremy McMahon
Queen Elizabeth University Hospital
Glasgow, UK

Ashraf Messiha
St George's Hospital
London, UK

Caroline Mills
Great Ormond Street Hospital
London, UK

Konstantinos Mitsimponas
James Cook University Hospital
Middlesborough, UK

Florencio Monje
Extremadura University
Badajoz, Spain

Afshin Mosahebi
University College London
London, UK

Annakan V. Navaratnam
Charing Cross Hospital
London, UK

Carrie Newlands
University of Surrey
Guildford, UK

Laurence Newman
The Queen Victoria Hospital
East Grinstead, UK

Rachel Oeppen
University Hospital Southampton NHS
Foundation Trust
Southampton, UK

James Padgett
University Hospitals Sussex NHS Foundation Trust
Sussex, UK

Michael Perry
Northwick Park Hospital
Harrow, UK

Sirisha Ponduri
Queen Alexandra Hospital
Portsmouth, UK

Jay Ponto
Portland Providence Medical Center
Portland, OR, USA

David Powers
Duke University Medical Center
Durham, NC, USA

Siavash Rahimi
Instituto Dermopatico dell'Immacolata
Rome, Italy

Krishna Shama Rao
Inga Health Foundation
Bangalore, India

Azadeh Rezaei
University College Hospital
London, UK

Majid Rezaei
University of Florida
Gainesville, FL, USA

Francesco M. G. Riva
The Royal Marsden NHS Foundation Trust
London, UK

Clare Rivers
Queen Elizabeth University Hospital
Glasgow, UK

Will Rodgers
Great Ormond Street Hospital
London, UK

Ajoy Roychoudhury
All India Institute of Medical Sciences
New Delhi, India

Craig Russell
Queen Elizabeth University Hospital
Glasgow, UK

Nadeem Saeed
Great Ormond Street Hospital
London, UK

Hesham A. Saleh
Charing Cross Hospital
London, UK

Tian Ee Seah
TES Clinic for Face and Jaw
Singapore

Kaveh Shakib
University College London
London, UK

Andrew J. Sidebottom
Park and Spire Hospitals
Nottingham, UK

Mark Singh
Bristol Royal Infirmary
Bristol, UK

Rabindra P. Singh
University Hospital Southampton NHS
Foundation Trust
Southampton, UK

James Sloane
Royal Surrey County Hospital
Guildford, UK

Graham Smith
St George's Hospital
London, UK

Alistair Smyth
Leeds General Infirmary
Leeds, UK

Kyung Tae
Hanyang University
Seoul, South Korea

Andrew B. G. Tay
National Dental Centre
Singapore

Ewen Thomson
Forth Valley Royal Hospital
Larbert, UK

Peter Thomson
James Cook University
Cairns, Australia

Nirav Pravin Trivedi
SMC Hospital
Mehsana, India

Simon van Eeden
Alder Hey Children's Hospital
Liverpool, UK

Daniel van Gijn
Chris O'Brien Lifehouse
Sydney, Australia

Leandros-Vassilios Vassiliou
Royal Blackburn Teaching Hospital
Blackburn, UK

Christopher Vinall
Leicester Royal Infirmary
Leicester, UK

Craig Wales
Queen Elizabeth University Hospital
Glasgow, UK

Ashleigh Weyh
University of Illinois at Chicago
Chicago, IL, USA

Michael Williams
East Sussex Healthcare NHS Trust
East Sussex, UK

Michael L. Winstead
University of Tennessee Medical Center
Knoxville, TN, USA

Poonam Yadav
All India Institute of Medical Sciences
New Delhi, India

Alexander Zargaran
Royal Free Hospital
London, UK

David Zargaran
Royal Free Hospital
London, UK

John Zuniga
University of Texas Southwestern Medical Center
Dallas, TX, USA

Bailey & Love's Essential Operations Bailey & Love's Essential Operations
Bailey & Love's Essential Operations Bailey & Love's Essential Operations
Bailey & Love's Essential Operations Bailey & Love's Essential Operations

PART 1 | Broader considerations in operative maxillofacial surgery

Chapter 1

Human Factors to Improve Patient Safety and Teamworking

Peter A. Brennan, Rachel Oeppen, Steve Jarvis

INTRODUCTION

Error is a part of being human and can almost be considered as 'normal'. We make, on average, five to seven mistakes every day. When we go to work and particularly to the operating theatre, we do not deliberately intend to cause medical error, but sadly some sort of error occurs with 1 in 20 hospital admissions, and of these another 1 in 20 (so 1 in 400) is serious, often resulting in patient harm.

In this chapter, human factors and their application, including various methods to help reduce error and promote better team working and morale, will be discussed. Factors that affect individual performance including hunger, hydration, emotional state and tiredness will be considered. Effective communication, situational awareness (SA) and ways to improve team working will then be discussed. By making changes to practice, patient safety can be improved and working experiences enhanced.

WHAT ARE HUMAN FACTORS?

There are many definitions of this term, but a simple one to remember is how we interact with each other (in teams), the systems in which we work, our variability and the factors that affect our performance and those of team members. Human factors (HF) application in healthcare can lead to improved patient safety, better team working and improved staff morale.

We all make mistakes, with an average of five to seven simple errors affecting each of us every day. We accept annoying errors such as forgetting a wallet or mobile phone as an inevitable part of day-to-day life, but often fail to appreciate that highly consequential errors in our work (causing patient harm and mortality) happen for the very same reasons. Just as we cannot prevent all day-to-day errors, we can never completely eliminate error in our professional work. Hence, the term 'never event', which includes wrong site surgery, retained instruments and swabs and incorrect nasogastric tube placement, is something of a misnomer.

The Roman philosopher Cicero (106–43 BC) wrote, "anyone is liable to err (make a mistake), but only a fool persists in error". Learning from mistakes and sharing lessons widely with others is one of the most important elements to improving patient safety across healthcare.

ERROR IN HEALTHCARE

The interplay of human error and HF in clinical incidents (including the many factors that have their origins in the hospitals and organisations where we work) is becoming more widely understood. It is often more than one issue (or layer) that leads to error, and this is readily represented by the well-known Swiss cheese model (*Figure 1.1*). Often factors are multifactorial and take place simultaneously – recognising this fact is the first step to understanding HF application in surgery. These multifactorial issues include ones that affect us as individuals such as tiredness, repetition, stress, the effects of distraction and multitasking. Other factors can occur as part of team working and these include poor communication or leadership, loss of SA and steep (or flat) authority gradients. The introduction of the World Health Organization (WHO) surgical checklist has improved attitudes toward pre-surgery briefing and patient safety and the benefits of recognising and applying these HF principles in surgery is well known.

One in 20 hospital admissions results in some form of error, and of these 1 in 20 (so 1 in 400 admissions) is serious. The operating theatre is known to be one of the most dangerous places in the hospital as a result of high patient turnover, site-specific treatments, many heterogeneous surgical procedures, staff limitations and unfamiliar teams.

What are the different types of error and failure?

The Human Factors Analysis and Classification System (HFACS) categorises failure across four broad domains in line with Reason's Swiss cheese theory (*Figure 1.1*). These are (1) organisational influences; (2) unsafe supervision; (3) preconditions to unsafe acts; (4) unsafe acts. The theory is that in ideal environments, single errors (unsafe acts) rarely happen, and even when they do, they are mitigated or captured such that no harm results from them. However, occasionally, a combination of problems at each level interacts or accumulates and a

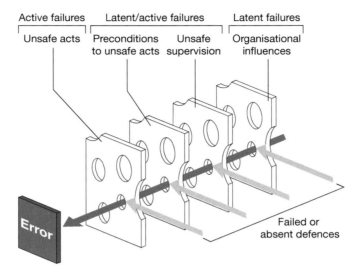

Figure 1.1 The Swiss cheese model of human error. Each 'slice of the cheese' can act as a barrier to prevent error or can facilitate occurrence of an error.

'perfect storm' of conditions results in which an error or accident occurs.

In the cheese metaphor, such a combination is represented by a hole in each cheese slice aligning to allow the accident through (*Figure 1.1*). This would be a result of a mix of organisational issues (such as demoralised workforce), poor supervision (such as unsupported staff), error-promoting conditions (such as poor lighting or poor equipment design) and, once the error occurs, no barriers to stop it causing damage (such as no alerting system when the wrong switch is selected).

Following this theory, in preventing accidents caused by human error, it is important to look at all levels of the organisation rather than simply the individuals. Examples of failures in the clinical setting that can have their origin in the employing organisation include pressures of overbooked clinics or operating theatre sessions, meeting clinical and hospital targets and prolonged working hours without breaks. Medical error may therefore begin to develop well before the actual event itself (such as wrong site surgery) as a result of institutional failure.

WHAT HUMAN FACTORS SHOULD WE BE CONSIDERING FOR SURGERY?

Table 1.1 summarises some important HF that can contribute to and ultimately lead to surgical error as categorised by the HFACS. These include factors that affect us as individuals such as tiredness and fatigue,

nutritional status, emotional states including anger and stress, multitasking and loss of SA. These will now be considered further.

Tiredness and fatigue

Both commercial and military aviation recognise how tiredness and fatigue can influence personal performance and increase the likelihood of accidents and as a result, there are rules in place for maximum work hours. Tiredness (a state that can only be reversed by sleep) and fatigue (more complex in its aetiology and can be the result of chronic tiredness, physical or mental exhaustion) are both found in surgical team members. Both can reduce complex cognitive tasks, decision making and SA as well as impairing our technical and physical performance. The value of taking regular short breaks, for example during a long and complex 8-hour operation, is not only beneficial for individuals and teams but may also prevent error from occurring. Most would not drive for 8 hours non-stop so why can it be deemed safe to do so for surgery? One useful fact to remember is that our cognitive function after being awake for 18 hours is comparable with being twice over the UK legal alcohol limit for driving. Increasingly, employers recognise that tired clinicians are much more likely to make a mistake, not to mention the effects on mood and general wellbeing. No one else knows how an individual feels, and if they have been operating throughout the night and are expected to work the following day, the few words "I don't feel safe" can be very powerful when discussing with managers or other colleagues.

TABLE 1.1 Simplified Human Factors Analysis and Classification System (HFACS) relevant to surgery. The different levels are analogous to the holes in the Swiss cheese model lining up to cause an error

Organisational influences within the hospital

Hospital targets and pressures to deliver results (either perceived or real)

Climate, process and resource management within the hospital

Communication, training and recognition by the senior management of human factors responsible for possible error

Unsafe supervision

Inadequate supervision of trainees or other healthcare staff

Failure of briefings/complacency with WHO checklist

Failure of the team to know what to do when things go wrong

Loss of situational awareness, especially if not recognised by the theatre team

Preconditions to unsafe acts

Fatigue, hunger and nutritional status

Emotional influences (anger, personal issues), running late

Tiredness, boredom, communication issues, remember HALT

Environmental factors: background noise, distractions, lighting, ambient temperature, humidity

Panic

Unsafe acts (less likely)

Unfamiliar with changes from what is seen as a 'normal event'

Distracting and multitasking

Operating outside of one's area of expertise, or following a long period of no operating (surgical currency)

Abbreviation: HALT, Hungry, Anxious/Angry, Late (or Lonely), Tired.

Hydration and nutritional status

Hydration, nutrition and individual recovery are often overlooked areas of HF but are crucial in the operating theatre to maintain performance. Even small deficits in total body water can have a significant impact on cognitive function, resulting in poorer decision making, causing sleepiness, headaches, impatience and apathy. For example, a 1–2 kg loss of body water from an individual of average build reduces cognitive function by 15–20%. This tends to happen slowly so that the individual is unaware of their deteriorating performance. Sufficient hydration is particularly important if personal protective equipment (PPE) is being worn, as this can increase the rate of perspiration and loss of body water. Water requirements are unique to individuals and, while a multitude of factors including body mass, ambient temperature, pregnancy and diet play a role, the minimal requirement is approximately 2 litres per day.

Good, balanced nutrition distributed over a sensible time period also helps to optimise personal performance and supports complex mental and physical tasks over a sustained period, for example, consumption of a well-balanced, small-portioned meal every 3–4 hours consisting of complex carbohydrates, protein and healthy fats. In contrast, large meals eaten over erratic time periods consisting of simple sugars or processed foods are more likely to produce fluctuating energy levels, which can have a detrimental effect on work. One only needs to consider athletes to realise how effective good nutrition can be at improving performance. Planned breaks during long operating lists, clinics and on-call periods also ensure enough opportunity can be afforded for all team members to recover.

Emotion and stress

Mental perspective and its impact on work performance needs to be recognised. Powerful emotions such as anger or upset can easily interfere with decision making, especially when trying to perform a task that requires intense concentration. The operating theatre can itself be a stressful environment for the surgical team – many will have heard colleagues raise their voices, which can be a result of stress or other factors aligning. In such situations, error is far more likely, not to mention the potential effect of loss of civility on the wider team, which can lead to respect being lost, among other negative effects.

Pausing during an operation (if it is safe to so do) to address any underlying issues may reduce the likelihood of error. We recommend taking a short break, again if it is safe to do so. Bringing the above factors together,

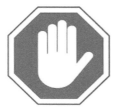

Hungry

Angry

Late or lonely

Tired

Figure 1.2 HALT is a simple mnemonic to prompt us to stop, if safe to do so, when any of these factors arise. Each can raise the risk of error.

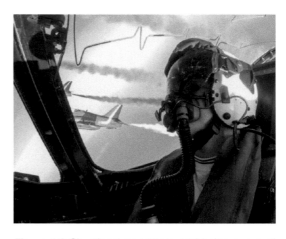

Figure 1.3 Situational awareness and being aware of what is going on around us is demonstrated clearly in this cockpit photo taken by one of the pilots of the UK Royal Air Force Aerobatic Team, The Red Arrows.

the easy-to-remember mnemonic HALT – Hungry, Anxious/Angry, Late (or Lonely), Tired – is a powerful reminder of the factors that can lead to surgical error, as well as recommending the value of stopping when one or more of these arise (*Figure 1.2*). Recognising the impact of stress and emotion not only helps reduce risk of error but also benefits surgical training and leads to more effective and happier team working, all of which ultimately improve overall patient management. 'Lonely' is included in the mnemonic as this introduces the idea of remembering the value of involving colleagues for complex cases or after a prolonged period of not operating (during COVID, for example). Dual surgeon operating can be very useful in this regard. Not only can this give surgeons confidence, but it can also improve patient outcomes.

Situational awareness

A simple definition of SA is being aware of what is going on around us (*Figure 1.3*). Awareness and appreciation of factors that raise the risk of medical error (summarised in *Table 1.2*) can be used to improve SA for both individuals and the whole team. However, it is important to note that SA is dynamic and can change quickly, and we must consider our ability (or not) to adapt to such changes. For example, a surgeon can become fixated on a task, develop tunnel vision and become blind to other factors that readily occur, thus losing wider SA. This can be exacerbated by confirmation bias in which the surgeon over-weighs cues or information that confirms the direction they are already following. This could include convincing themself of an anatomical structure or location when it is something quite different. Many errors have occurred as a result including, for example, cut bile ducts, ureters and important nerves.

Recognising the value of SA alongside a well-briefed team, all of whom feel safe and able to voice their concerns, provides the best environment in which to reduce the risk of medical error. In this way, team members are looking out for each other, thereby improving safety and working more effectively. By

TABLE 1.2 Situations that might raise the chance of error in the operating theatre environment. Being aware of these can help improve situational awareness

High physical or mental workloads

Interruptions and distractions during key parts of an operation

Tasks requiring an 'out of normal' response and/or unanticipated new tasks

Multitasking

Changes in physical environment

actively thinking ahead (having the best SA), errors can be avoided. Consider that the best drivers are those who anticipate problems early, thereby avoiding potentially hazardous situations. Similarly, thinking about and discussing with the team any potential 'what if?' scenarios before an operation commences can reduce the likelihood of a startle reaction, and ensure the team is best prepared.

The concept of PPP – Patient, Procedure, People (team) – has recently been introduced. This is a useful way of prompting oneself to regain wider SA when something does not seem quite right. In some circumstances, it may be the procedure that needs re-discussing first to help regain SA. In most instances, stepping back from the acute situation (if safe to do so) and discussing with the team is the best way to understand the problem and decide the best course of action. This tool has been adapted from the aviation mnemonic ANC – Aviate, Navigate, Communicate.

TEAM BRIEF AND DEBRIEF, LOWERING AUTHORITY GRADIENTS AND ENHANCING COMMUNICATION

Patient care is rarely, if ever, performed in isolation from other team members. The introduction of the WHO checklist and team brief has resulted in significant improvements to patient safety in theatre. Enhancing team working, understanding, value and reduced hierarchy all contribute toward safer patient outcomes. The way in which a briefing is conducted is important. It should not be rushed and, from the outset, all team members should feel valued equally and empowered to speak up if they have any concerns, without fear of retribution. *Table 1.3* provides a summary of items that may be included in both briefing and debriefing sessions. The team brief should also stress the importance of looking out for each other to reduce the likelihood of losing SA and highlighting when factors such as tiredness and stress can be seen in others. During periods of intense concentration, surgeons can experience attentional tunnelling, and quickly lose track of time. Several hours can pass, and the reliance on others to keep an eye on the clock and suggest a short break perhaps after 3 hours is good practice.

Similarly, distraction of attention away from the primary task can be detrimental to performance at safety-critical times during the operation when full concentration is required. Any potential distractions should be discussed at the team brief and predictable distractions kept to a minimum. The sterile cockpit approach (where pilots focus only on flying below 10 000 ft with no distractions) is a valuable technique to apply in theatre. A simple distraction such as a telephone call asking for advice during a complex part of an operation significantly raises the risk of error. It is far better to either limit predictable distractions (including noise) during these times or stop and focus on one task at a time rather than trying to multitask.

At the end of the operating list, it is good practice to conduct a short debrief. This does not necessarily have to be formal, but it gives an opportunity to discuss what went well, and what could be improved for next time. The power of saying "Thank you" to the team cannot be overemphasised. Gaining feedback from other team members on our own performance is also valuable and builds practice and non-technical skills.

In aviation, the most junior airline pilot is actively encouraged to question the most senior captain without fear. Similarly, empowering all surgical team members including medical students, trainees, nurses and non-clinical staff to voice their concerns ensures a safe working environment for everyone. Of course, this has to be managed within reason by each individual, and the leader recognised as such, as they have the ultimate responsibility for the decisions made. A flat hierarchy is as dangerous as a steep one, as this can lead to situations such as no one knowing who is doing what, or the

TABLE 1.3 Items to consider during a team briefing. A debrief is a powerful way to develop and enhance team working for future operating sessions
A well-prepared team is advantageous in that every member knows their role and looks out for their colleagues. It can also help team members to feel valued.
Briefing
Introductions, open culture, "Please speak up if concerned"
Leadership, team working and decision making
Think about the 'what if?' scenarios that might occur during a procedure
Identify the major steps and who will be doing what
Ask "What am I expected to do if and when something goes wrong?"
Situational awareness – how to intervene when something does not seem right
Debriefing
Consider debriefing for learning
What went well?
What should we do differently next time?
What do you think about my performance today?
Saying "Thank you" to the team!

leader being unable to discharge their responsibilities. However, what is most important is to be clear that any team member can speak up if concerned without fear, and that their concern will be listened to.

Effective communication between team members is an essential element to good team working and interaction. Regular use of open questions such as "What do you think we should do? What would you suggest here?" is a good tool to bring the team together. The use of pronouns (e.g. "Pass me it/that") should be avoided, especially at safety-critical times; instead, use of proper nouns (e.g. the name of a required instrument) will ensure clear instructions. Finally, 'repeat back' is a useful tool to confirm that a message has been heard and understood by the receiver. Just because a team member has said something, does not automatically mean that others have heard and understood the message or instruction.

In summary, HF application is essential to ensure both individuals and teams are best optimised to care for patients. Some elements are simply common sense, stopping for a short break regularly just as we would do while driving a long distance. However, it can be all too easy to leave common sense at the front door of the hospital when we come to work.

FURTHER READING

Brennan PA, Davidson M. Improving patient safety: we need to reduce hierarchy and empower junior doctors to speak up. *BMJ* 2019;**366**:l4461.

Brennan PA, Holden C, Shaw G, Morris S, Oeppen RS. Leading article: What can we do to improve individual and team situational awareness to benefit patient safety? *Br J Oral Maxillofac Surg* 2020;**58**:404–8.

Brennan PA, Oeppen R, Knighton J, Davidson M. Looking after ourselves at work: the importance of being hydrated and fed. *BMJ* 2019;**364**:l528.

Hardie J, Brennan PA. Patient, Procedure, People (PPP): recognising and responding to intra-operative critical events. *Ann R Coll Surg Eng* 2022;**104**:409–13.

Panagioti M, Khan K, Keers RN et al. Prevalence, severity, and nature of preventable patient harm across medical care settings: systematic review and meta-analysis. *BMJ* 2019;**366**:l4185.

<table>
<tr><td>

Chapter

2

</td><td>

Medico-Legal Issues in Surgery

Laurence Newman

</td></tr>
</table>

INTRODUCTION

The purpose of this chapter is to offer maxillofacial surgeons an insight into the legal principles and processes surrounding issues of clinical negligence. This reflects practice in England, which varies across the devolved nations and worldwide.

LITIGATION

The annual cost of harm arising from clinical activity in the UK during 2019/2020 covered by the Clinical Negligence Scheme for Trusts was £8.3 billion, approximating 4% of the NHS annual budget. Clinical negligence claims must be made within 3 years of either the date that the negligence occurred or of the date that the claimant became aware of injury. This is a lengthy and costly process frequently run on a Conditional Funding Agreement, known as 'no-win, no-fee'.

Expert witness

An expert witness is a person with a specialised skill or knowledge called upon by a Court of Law to express an opinion. Medical expert witness work encompasses writing Condition & Prognosis reports, which require examination of the claimant who typically has suffered trauma. The expert's role is to give an opinion and impartially advise the court on the claimant's current condition, and to advise on any future treatment costs (priced as if performed privately) that would be required to put the claimant back into the position they would have been had the injury not occurred. An everyday example would be the cost of scar revision.

Clinical negligence claims involve the expert writing a report on matters relating to Breach of Duty & Causation. It is not the role of the expert witness to decide whether or not negligence has occurred. That is a matter for the court. It is the role of the expert witness to advise how a responsible body of reasonably competent surgeons would have managed the case based on contemporary clinical practice at that point in time. Modern surgical techniques, for example, cannot be considered retrospectively.

Court structure

The structure of the court system is shown in *Figure 2.1.*

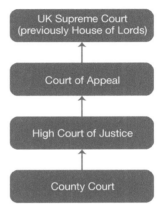

Figure 2.1 Hierarchy of the court system in the UK.

CLINICAL NEGLIGENCE

Surgeons principally face two allegations when faced with a claim brought in negligence. These are "This only happened because the surgery you performed was below acceptable standards", and/or "You never told me that this complication could have happened, and had you done so I would not have consented".

To succeed, the claimant must prove that the surgeon owed them a duty of care, that the doctor breached that duty of care and that causation flowed such that the injury complained of arose as a direct and foreseeable consequence of the act or omission. To establish clinical negligence, each of these three facets must be met.

The 'but for' test

This is the standard test used to establish causation: "But for the negligence, the injury would not have occurred". A patient attended A&E in the early hours with abdominal pain and vomiting. The doctor did not attend, advising him to contact his GP in the morning. The patient died 5 hours later. The case was 'but for' the doctor's failure to examine, the patient would have survived. Breach of Duty was admitted in that the doctor should have seen the patient; however, the case failed on causation. The court held that, even if he had been examined, the patient would have died as a result of arsenic poisoning.

The Bolam test

Bolam underwent electroconvulsive therapy (ECT) during which he sustained an acetabular fracture. His case was that he had not been warned of the risk of fracture; he had not been given muscle relaxation or any form of restraint. At the time medical opinion was divided. In evidence, one expert stated that he had only seen such a fracture once in 50 000 patients treated with ECT.

Thus, the *Bolam principle* was established in 1957, stating that

> A doctor is not guilty of negligence if he has acted in accordance with the practice accepted as proper by a responsible body of medical men skilled in that particular art … a doctor is not negligent if he is acting in accordance with such a practice merely because there is a body of opinion that takes a contrary view.[1]

The Bolitho modification

A 2-year-old boy admitted with croup developed respiratory embarrassment. The nurse called for help. The Senior Registrar, who was in clinic, did not attend as requested but claimed to have arranged for a Senior House Officer (SHO) to attend. The SHO's bleep was faulty and was thus unaware. The child later arrested and subsequently died.

A case brought in negligence alleged that had the doctor attended she would have intubated, preventing cardiopulmonary arrest. Five experts testified that they would have intubated, three expressing the opposite view that intubation was a dangerous procedure in a 2 year old and should be avoided. The case failed.

The *Bolam principle* was thus modified such that "a doctor is not negligent if he or she acts in accordance with a responsible body of medical opinion, provided that the court finds such an opinion to be logical".[2]

Breach of duty of care

A duty of care starts once a clinical decision is made, for example by triaging referral letters. A breach of duty would be deemed to have occurred if the treatment fell outside that which a responsible body of reasonably competent doctors would or would not have done. This is a standard *Bolam* defence. A day 1 Consultant will be judged to the same standard as a Consultant of 25 years.

Causation

This is the biggest hurdle a claimant needs to clear if they are to win. It has to be shown on the balance of probability that the harm flowed from the breach.

What is consent?

This is the patient's continuing and voluntary permission to receive a particular treatment based on an adequate knowledge of the nature, purpose and likely risks of the treatment, including the likelihood of its success and any alternatives to it.

Mental Capacity Act (MCA) 2005 and Mental Health Act (MHA) 2007

The MCA states that a competent patient will understand and retain the information relevant to the decision, use and weigh that information in the balance and communicate his/her decision by any means. The MHA defines capacity such that a patient should understand the nature, purpose and likely effects of the treatment.

Does a patient detained under the MHA have capacity to refuse treatment? This was considered in the case of *Re C*, a paranoid schizophrenic detained in Broadmoor who developed a gangrenous leg. Amputation was recommended. *C*'s position was that he was a world expert in the management of gangrene and refused amputation. The fact he was deluded did not mean that he lacked capacity. His refusal was held to be valid in that he sufficiently understood the nature, purpose and effects of the proposed amputation and that he retained capacity to consent to, or refuse, medical treatment laying out the criteria for capacity. Adult patients with capacity may refuse treatment even if such a decision appears incorrect to the doctor, even if the refusal may place the patient's health or indeed their life at risk.

Consent and the disclosure of risk

Since 1957, *Bolam* has led sway in consent. It was accepted that it was reasonable not to warn of a particular risk if other surgeons would do the same. This was upheld in the 1974 case of *Sidaway*, who was rendered paralysed following spinal surgery. It was alleged that there had been an inadequate warning of a 1% risk of paralysis. It was accepted that a responsible body of neurosurgeons would not have warned of the risk of paralysis following spinal surgery. *Bolam* prevailed and the case failed.

Pearce involved a pregnant woman 14 days past her delivery date. She asked about being induced or having a caesarean section. The consultant advised waiting for a natural delivery. The baby was stillborn. Suing in negligence, it was argued that the consultant should have advised that there was an increased risk of stillbirth if there was a significant delay. The claimant's argument was that had she known this fact, she would have insisted on a caesarean. The court ruled that "if there is a significant risk which would affect the judgement of a reasonable patient, then in the normal course it is the responsibility of a doctor to inform the patient of that significant risk, if the information is needed so that the patient can determine for him or herself as to what course he or she should adopt".

The case *Chester v Afshar* considered a patient who underwent microdiscectomy, developed cauda equina syndrome and was left paraplegic. It was contested that at no stage had the surgeon warned of the risk of paralysis. The House of Lords held that "the doctor in question had been under a duty to warn the patient of a 1–2% risk that the proposed operation might lead to a seriously adverse result". This put paid to the often-quoted statement "You do not have to warn if the risk is 1% or less". Warnings should be given regarding all significant risks.

Montgomery

A 5-foot tall diabetic woman delivered her son vaginally. The birth took 12 minutes from the head crowning. Complications from shoulder dystocia resulted in hypoxic brain injury to the baby, with resultant cerebral palsy and a brachial plexus injury. The obstetrician had not discussed this increased risk with the mother. Suing in negligence, it was alleged that had the mother been warned, she would have requested a caesarean section. Damages of £5.25 million were awarded.

This case defined what is considered a material risk:

> The doctor is therefore under a duty to take reasonable care to ensure that the patient is aware of any material risks involved in any recommended treatment and of any reasonable alternative or variant treatments. The test of materiality is whether, in the circumstances of the particular case, a reasonable person in the patient's position would be likely to attach significance to the risk, or the doctor is or should reasonably be aware that the particular patient would be likely to attach significance to it.[3]

Ramifications of Montgomery

This ruling promotes shared decision-making between doctor and patient; the provision of evidence-based information about alternatives and outcomes. A doctor must provide information in a comprehensible way and ensure it is properly understood and should not bombard a patient with technical information or simply obtain a signature on a consent form. The Supreme Court noted "even those doctors who have less skill or inclination for communication, or who are hurried, are obliged to pause and engage in the discussion that the law requires". *Bolam* no longer applies to consent.

The burden of proof is on the doctor to show that they have warned of a particular risk. Not infrequently, the records fail to show this. Additionally, and not infrequently, records fail to document there has been a discussion about any alternative procedures, including doing nothing.

Who should seek consent?

In everyday maxillofacial practice, can an inexperienced specialty registrar (StR) seek consent for a bimaxillary osteotomy, a parotidectomy or an oncology case? Royal College of Surgeons (RCS) guidance advises "The surgeon discussing treatment with the patient should be suitably trained and qualified to provide the treatment in question and have sufficient knowledge of the associated risks and complications, as well as any alternative treatments available for the patient's condition".[4] Can this be applied to an inexperienced trainee?

Cases brought in negligence

The Sommelier

A Sommelier, warned of lingual nerve injury, developed said complication following removal of an impacted wisdom tooth. On review at 2 weeks, he complained of a numb tongue with compromised taste. He had not been warned regarding the possibility of taste impairment. The dental core trainee (DCT) advised "It should improve within 18 months, but come back then if it is not better". No improvement ensued.

A case was brought in negligence alleging had the claimant been fully warned, he would not have agreed to have his wisdom tooth removed. Additionally at no time was the possibility of lingual nerve repair discussed. He would have explored this option had he been given the opportunity.

The claimant won substantial damages. The defence conceded that impairment of taste was a material risk and he should have been warned. Also, there should have been a discussion of the potential benefits of lingual nerve exploration and/or repair. A failure to do so denied the claimant of the opportunity to explore this option.

Untreated displaced condyle

Consider a case of displaced right mandibular angle and left condylar fractures. The surgeon elected to perform an open reduction and internal fixation (ORIF) to the angle fracture only, resulting in a lateral open bite. The case brought argued that it was negligent not to perform ORIF to the condyle. But for this omission, the malocclusion would not have eventuated. The case settled out of court, with the defence accepting that the claimant should have been offered condylar ORIF and but for this omission, harm would not have occurred.

Epithelial dysplasia undergoing malignant transformation

A 46-year-old man had biopsy-proven moderate epithelial dysplasia on the left lateral tongue. He was reassured by an StR that this was benign and discharged. Fifteen months later, he re-presented with a cT2N0M0 biopsy-proven squamous cell carcinoma (SCC) at the same site. He underwent partial glossectomy, selective neck dissection and free-flap reconstruction. As a result of a close 2-mm margin and adverse histopathological features, he underwent adjuvant radiotherapy.

It was alleged that it was unreasonable to discharge him; that he was not given the option to have the dysplastic area removed; that had the dysplasia been removed, he would not have developed a SCC; that had he been kept under outpatient review and had a

SCC developed, it would have been staged cT1N0M0 for which he would have undergone wide local excision with sentinel lymph node biopsy. Additionally, he would have avoided radiotherapy.

Was it reasonable to discharge him with a diagnosis of moderate dysplasia? It was agreed that a responsible body of reasonably competent maxillofacial surgeons would have excised the entire dysplastic area and that the failure to do so was a breach of duty. It was conceded that there was no evidence of field change disease and that, on the balance of probability, a SCC would not have developed had the dysplasia been completely excised. The claimant would most likely have been kept under outpatient review and had a SCC developed, it would have been picked up at an earlier stage. He would then have avoided a neck dissection, a free flap and radiotherapy. A substantial out-of-court settlement was agreed.

REFERENCES

1 *Bolam v Friern Hospital Management Company* [1957] 2 All ER 118, 12.
2 *Bolitho v City of Hackney Health Authority* [1999] 39 BMLR 1, HL.
3 *Montgomery v Lanarkshire Health Board* [2015] UKSC 11.
4 Royal College of Surgeons. *Consent: Supported decision making. A guide to good practice*. Royal College of Surgeons; 2018.

Chapter 3

Imaging Techniques in Maxillofacial Surgery

Rachel Oeppen, Jasper Bekker

INTRODUCTION

Maxillofacial imaging has evolved with the development of newer imaging technologies. Conventional plain radiography and dental imaging is now commonly supplemented by cross-sectional modalities such as computed tomography (CT), magnetic resonance imaging (MRI) and ultrasound, together with functional imaging with positron emission tomography (PET). It is important to be aware of the benefits and limitations of imaging techniques to determine the most appropriate approach for each clinical scenario (*Tables 3.1–3.3*). In particular, the risk of biological damage from ionising radiation must be considered for higher-dose examinations such as PET/CT. The Ionizing Radiation (Medical Exposure) Regulations 2000 (IRMER) lay down basic measures required for protection of patients and workers from the harmful effects of medical radiation exposure.

PLAIN RADIOGRAPHS

The x-rays are produced by a point source and, after passing through the body part of interest, are detected by non-screen (dental radiography) or intensifying screen/film combinations (extraoral radiography). Tomography refers to a technique whereby the x-ray source and film move during the exposure providing a 'section' that is in focus and blurring of structures outside the area of interest. Applications include conventional dental panoramic tomography, tomograms of the temporomandibular joints (TMJs) and mandibular tomograms for implant planning. Digital radiography units (using digital receptors to intercept the x-ray beam rather than intensifying screens) are now replacing conventional units. This allows transmission of data to image processing and storage devices as well as communications networks.

CONTRAST STUDIES

Contrast media may be introduced into a vessel, lumen or cavity to render it radio-opaque and allow radiological visualisation in 'real time' with fluoroscopic imaging or with serial radiographs. Contrast media used for this purpose are mainly non-ionic iodinated contrast agents. These carry a small risk of adverse reaction including anaphylaxis and renal impairment when given intravenously, which must be balanced against the benefits of the procedure. Before contrast injection, information is required from the patient including details of any prior history of contrast reaction, asthma, renal problems, diabetes and metformin therapy. If intravenous contrast is contraindicated, other imaging techniques may be recommended. For example, MRI-angio time of flight (TOF) is a good alternative to contrast for vessel imaging (*Figure 3.1a–c*). Interventional radiology uses digital subtraction angiography (DSA), both for diagnostic vessel imaging and intervention or treatment (*Figure 3.1d–h*).

ULTRASOUND

Ultrasound imaging does not require ionising radiation, is readily available, non-invasive and inexpensive. It is useful for examining superficial structures, producing high-quality images in multiple planes. Ultrasound

TABLE 3.1 Imaging of facial and neck infection		
Imaging modality	Imaging issues	Comment
Radiographs		Radiographs to assess for dental disease
CT (contrast-enhanced) MRI (gadolinium-enhanced)	Distinguishing abscess from phlegmon	Contrast-enhanced CT and gadolinium-enhanced MRI equivalent for assessing phlegmon versus abscess
	Disease extent, vascular compromise and infection source	CT superior for assessing associated mandibular cortical erosion and salivary gland calculi

TABLE 3.2 Imaging of mandibular osteomyelitis/ORN

Imaging modality	Imaging issues	Comment
Radiography	Confirm diagnosis and exclude other lesions	Oral pantomogram helpful for assessing dentition and predisposing conditions such as fractures or systemic bone disease
	Response to treatment	Appropriate for follow-up
MRI (thin section)	Low T1-w with gadolinium enhancement and increased short TI inversion recovery (STIR) signal corresponds to active infection in the medullary cavity	MRI should be primary cross-sectional imaging for acute and chronic osteomyelitis
CT	Osteolysis in the acute phase with subsequent periosteal reaction	CT superior for detecting the degree of cortical destruction, presence of sequestra and the degree of cortical removal that would be required
	Sclerosis sequestration in subacute/chronic osteomyelitis	

TABLE 3.3 Imaging of maxillofacial malignancy

Key imaging issues	• Primary tumour extent and submucosal extension (to correlate with mucosal inspection) • Evidence of bone invasion (e.g. mandible), neurovascular involvement, midline extension, perineural extension, orbital and skull base infiltration (subsite dependent) • Identification of nodal metastases (especially if outside area of intended neck dissection and for radiotherapy planning) • Detection of distant metastases or synchronous primary tumours
Imaging modality	**Comment**
CT (contrast-enhanced)	CT preferred: • If CT chest also required • In very unwell or elderly patients • If MRI contraindications or • If obscuring dental amalgam
MRI (gadolinium-enhanced)	MRI preferred: • For salivary gland tumours • Any potential skull base or intracranial involvement (e.g. nasopharynx) • To attempt better definition of poorly defined primary lesion on CT, particularly for radiotherapy planning MR and CT complementary for paranasal sinuses tumours and mandibular invasion (CT initially preferred)
CT, CXR (chest staging)	CT chest (usually including upper abdomen) most often indicated but depends on local protocols Note high incidence of non-specific small lung nodules that will be detected
PET CT	PET CT may be used: 1. In the setting of symptomatic recurrent disease: • If suspicion of recurrence but biopsy negative • Conventional (CT/MRI) assessment has not fully delineated recurrence (because of scar tissue) • Occasionally before undergoing treatment with curative intent to exclude other synchronous primaries/metastases

(Continued)

TABLE 3.3 (Continued) Imaging of maxillofacial malignancy	
	2. Surveillance imaging: • Persistent primary/nodal disease post-chemoradiotherapy • Surveillance of primary tumour with high risk of recurrence
	3. In the setting of an unknown primary tumour ideally prior to panendoscopy and biopsy
	4. Rarely for assessment of primary or nodal disease for primary staging
Ultrasound	• There are advantages of ultrasound (relative to MRI/CT) for nodal assessment • Ultrasound uses additional criteria to detect smaller pathological nodes and may also be used to guide FNA • Utility is guided by local expertise • Particular scenarios in which ultrasound ± FNA may be required include indeterminate contralateral nodes in the N0 neck using CT/MRI

can be combined with fine needle aspiration (FNA) for cytology or core biopsy for histopathology, making it a highly specific diagnostic tool.

The choice of where to start scanning will depend on the clinical scenario. For example, for a patient with a lipoma of the posterior triangle, a detailed assessment of both sides of the neck is not required, whereas a patient with a squamous cell carcinoma (SCC) primary who is undergoing a staging scan of the neck needs a bilateral assessment of all the major lymph node territories in the neck.

The following indications will be considered:

- Lymph node assessment
- Salivary glands
- Imaging lumps and bumps
- Ultrasound-guided FNA and percutaneous core biopsy

Lymph nodes

Normal nodes have a well-defined ellipsoid shape, with an intermediate to low reflectivity homogeneous cortex and highly reflective central hilus. Overall length is irrelevant, with normal cervical nodes frequently measuring 3–4 cm in maximum longitudinal (L) dimension. However, short-axis (S) measurements should not normally exceed 10 mm. The more rounded a node, the more likely it is to contain metastatic disease (*Figure 3.2*).

Abnormal nodes display reduced reflectivity (i.e. tend to be hypo-echoic or 'black') with a tendency to lose the central echogenic hilus. Vascularity may increase and have a disordered pattern. Peripheral or subcapsular vessels are a particularly strong sign of malignancy.

Lymphomatous lymph nodes characteristically appear rounded, often retaining a central echogenic hilus, and possess a homogenous, hypo-echoic (pseudo-cystic) cortex. Colour flow imaging often reveals plethoric hilar vascularity. Identification of these characteristics should prompt the operator into carrying out a core biopsy or recommending excision

biopsy depending on local preference to allow rapid diagnosis.

Salivary glands

The most common problems encountered include sialolithiasis, inflammatory conditions and tumours.

Sialolithiasis

Intraglandular calculi are easier to identify than ductal stones. Frank duct dilatation (*Figure 3.3a–d*) or sialectasis may be seen, and ultrasound will also demonstrate the complications of calculi, including abscess formation and sialocele.

Ultrasound cannot definitively exclude calculi. If there is a strong clinical suggestion of salivary duct obstruction and ultrasound examination is negative, sialography will be required to exclude a stone/stricture (*Figure 3.4*).

Inflammation

Acute salivary gland inflammation occurs in response to suppurative sialadenitis and viral infection. Inflammation causes gland hypertrophy and hypo-echogenicity, that is, the salivary glands lose their normal bright echotexture. The association of Sjögren's disease with lymphoma needs to be recognised and if a hypo-echoic mass is seen within an affected salivary gland, lymphoma must be considered.

Tumours

Approximately 80% of salivary tumours are benign, 80% occurring within the parotid with 80% of these being pleomorphic adenoma. The vast majority of parotid tumours lie within the superficial portion of the gland, allowing easy assessment with ultrasound. However, in the case of large or deep masses, the deep extent of a lesion can be difficult to assess (necessitating CT or MRI). Ultrasound cannot always predict whether salivary gland lesions are benign or malignant (although irregularity, abnormal vascularity and the presence of enlarged or suspicious nodes aid accuracy) and is

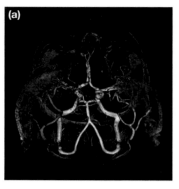
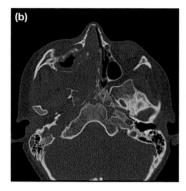
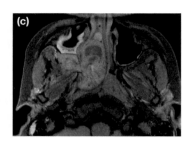
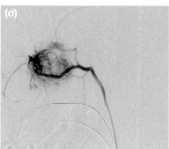
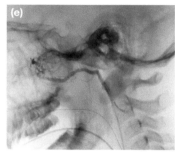
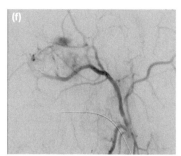
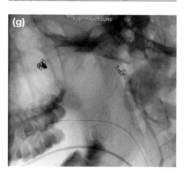

Figure 3.1 (a) 3D projection magnetic resonance imaging (MRI)-angio time of flight (TOF) in the arterial phase of a common/external carotid angiogram demonstrates a hypertrophic maxillary artery and vascular blush (in blue) secondary to a juvenile angiofibroma (JAF) in a 10-year-old boy. (b) Computed tomography (CT) shows widening of the right sphenopalatine foramen. (c) MRI axial T1WI fat saturated with contrast confirms large infiltrating JAF centred on the right sphenopalatine foramen and nasal cavity with classic punctate and serpentine flow voids. (d) Digital subtraction angiography (DSA) of same patient pre-embolisation showing arterial tumour parenchymal blush of the JAF after selective contrast injection into the right maxillary artery in lateral projection. (e) Unsubtracted image prior to embolisation. (f) DSA again in lateral projection post-embolisation prior to surgical intervention showing coils at level of arterial pedicle JAF and absence of arterial tumour parenchymal blush. (g) Unsubtracted image post-embolisation. (h) Post-treatment MRI T2WI without evidence of residual disease.

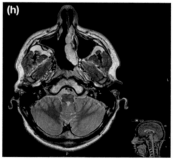

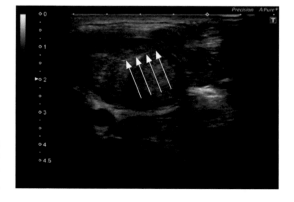

Figure 3.2 Node with greater than normal short/long ratio with needle for ultrasound-guided fine needle aspiration – a metastatic squamous cell carcinoma node.

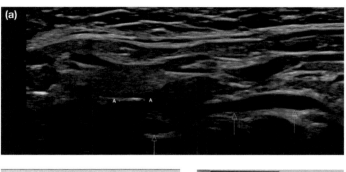

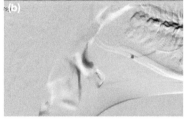

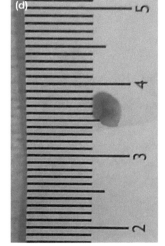

Figure 3.3 (a) Dilated main subman-dibular duct (arrows), typical of mobile ductal stone (marked between A's) on ultrasound. (b, c) Sialogram confirmed mobile stone on digital subtraction sialography. (d) 4-mm stone after ultra-sound-guided basket retrieval.

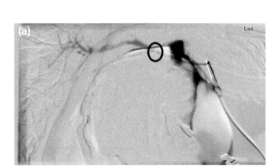

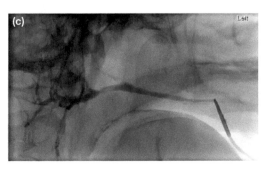

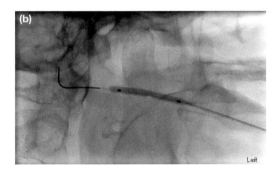

Figure 3.4 (a) High-grade short stenosis (circle) main parotid duct with contrast flowing back into the oral cavity because of stricture. (b) Sialoplasty with balloon at level of stricture. (c) Post-sialoplasty without stenosis and free-flowing contrast.

usually used in conjunction with fine-needle sampling. The smaller the salivary gland the more likely that any tumour detected will be malignant, that is, a tumour in the sublingual gland has a far higher likelihood of malignancy compared with a mass in the parotid gland.

Other malignant salivary gland tumours (muco-epidermoid, adenoid cystic and acinic cell carcinomas) occur more frequently in the sublingual and submandibular glands than in the parotid glands. Features suggestive of malignancy include poor definition with heterogeneous echotexture, disorganised colour flow and the presence of associated nodes. Using these criteria, malignancy can be predicted in around 80% of cases using ultrasound alone.

Lipomas

Lipomas are benign encapsulated subcutaneous lesions, which are frequently encountered in the neck. Typical sonographic features include hyper-echogenicity, linear internal echoes perpendicular to the ultrasound beam, compressibility and a lack of internal vascularity on colour flow or colour Doppler imaging. Intramuscular lipomas can mimic muscle and can be difficult to define with ultrasound.

Branchial cleft cyst

Most branchial cysts arise from the second branchial arch remnants, and present as a mass at the angle of the mandible, often following an infection. The typical location is abutting the posterior aspect of the submandibular gland, lying lateral to the carotid bifurcation and immediately anterior to the anterior border of the sternomastoid. On ultrasound, these lesions are typically cystic. It may be impossible to distinguish between a second branchial cleft cyst and a necrotic lymph node metastasis due to SCC.

Thyroglossal duct cyst

Thyroglossal duct cysts can arise at any position along the course of the thyroglossal duct remnant but the majority are related to the hyoid bone, with most occurring at the level of or inferior to the hyoid.

On ultrasound, thyroglossal duct cysts may appear cystic, heterogeneous or pseudo-solid due to varying content of debris, haemorrhage or infection. Classically, they are embedded in the strap muscles, often 'splitting' the strap muscles. Malignant degeneration of the epithelial lining occurs rarely and any solid component that appears to contain micro-calcification (i.e. suggestive of papillary carcinoma) should undergo sampling.

Thyroid gland

As the thyroid gland is situated in a superficial location in the anterior neck, it is readily imaged with ultrasound. A detailed description of thyroid ultrasound is beyond the scope of this text; however, thyroid disorders, including generalised gland enlargement and focal nodules, are relatively commonly encountered in clinical practice. In the one-stop clinic environment, thyroid nodules are likely to represent the second most common presenting mass, after lymph nodes. The increasing use of ultrasound means that incidental thyroid nodules are frequently detected in between 50% and 70% of females over the age of 50. Although thyroid nodules are very common, thyroid cancer is extremely rare.

Ultrasound-guided FNA and core biopsy

Ultrasound is a very useful adjunct in percutaneous sampling procedures, allowing direct visualisation of the needle and structures to be avoided.

For many conditions, for example SCC lymph node metastases, FNA will be the initial sampling technique. Core biopsy may be reserved as a second-line test when cytology is unable to provide the answer. However, where lymphoma is considered as a possible diagnosis, core biopsy undoubtedly has a superior role.

COMPUTED TOMOGRAPHY

Computed tomography (CT) is a modality with rapid image acquisition which is widely available. A CT scanner consists of an x-ray tube which generates and directs a fan of x-rays towards the body part of interest, and the attenuation of the x-rays by the patient's tissues is detected. The process is repeated as the tube and detectors rotate and the patient is advanced through the scanner. The degree of x-ray absorption by each volume of tissue (voxel) is displayed as a pixel, which is allocated a number (Hounsfield unit). This information may be digitally manipulated to optimise visualisation of the tissues of interest (e.g. by changing the range of 'numbers' in the grey scale or 'window width' or by using algorithms to alter the 'sharpness' of the image). The same information may be used to provide multiplanar reformats or rendering of three-dimensional (3D) objects to facilitate visual assessment. Imaging of soft tissues generally requires the administration of iodinated contrast medium to demonstrate enhancing pathological tissues and delineate vascular structures from adjacent soft tissues such as lymph nodes. Artefact from metallic materials such as dental restoration may markedly degrade images of the face due to 'beam-hardening artefact'; however, there are methods to reduce this, such as angling of the scan plane or the use of specific image reconstruction techniques. The availability of CT fluoroscopy and 'in room' CT controls/monitors has improved the safety and efficacy of CT-guided biopsies of deep facial and skull base lesions (*Figure 3.5*).

Multislice computed tomography (MSCT) acquires multiple slices per tube rotation. Current scanners

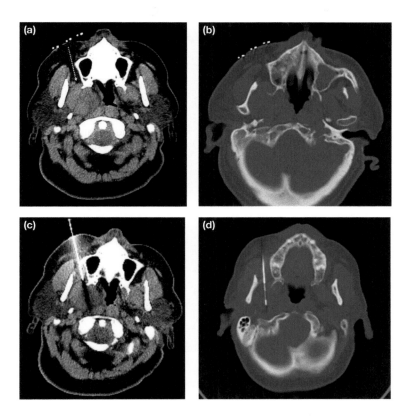

Figure 3.5 (a) Non-contrast soft tissue window axial computed tomography (CT) demonstrating skin markers overlying the right cheek with pathway through the buccal fat space (dashed arrow) to the right parapharyngeal tumour. (b) Bone window CT demonstrating skin markers, the right buccal space and remodelling of the right lateral pterygoid plate secondary to local mass effect from the right parapharyngeal tumour. (c) Coaxial needle passing through the right buccal fat space to the superficial margin of the right parapharyngeal tumour. (d) Core biopsy needle within the right parapharyngeal tumour with deployment of the cutting needle.

typically acquire 256 or 320 slices for some applications. MSCT has the potential to scan standard volumes with shorter acquisition times, so reducing movement artefact (e.g. due to swallowing) or requirement for sedation and optimising vascular opacification (e.g. for CT angiographic studies). MSCT also allows the scanning of larger volumes or the use of narrower section thickness (as low as 0.1–0.5 mm) so optimising the 3D dataset for post-processing and interactive 3D image-guided surgery.

The benefits of CT should always be weighed against the risks of ionising radiation exposure.

Cone beam computed tomography (CBCT) has developed as a technique that provides high-resolution 3D data at low-radiation doses (equivalent to 2–8 orthopantomograms (OPTs)). The equipment may resemble that of a conventional dental panoramic tomography unit (patient erect) or may mimic a conventional CT scanner (patient supine). A cylinder- or sphere-shaped volume of data is rapidly acquired with a single tube rotation. Some CBCT equipment is designed to simulate intraoral radiographs by imaging small volumes (e.g. two to three teeth) at high resolution, while other equipment is designed to image the whole maxillofacial region (e.g. 15 cm³ spheres). The low tube currents utilised to reduce the radiation dose unfortunately preclude adequate imaging of soft tissue structures.

Evidence-based guidelines for the use of CBCT in dental and maxillofacial radiology have been produced by the SEDENTEXCT project (www.sedentexct.eu/files/guidelines_final.pdf).

MAGNETIC RESONANCE IMAGING

Magnetic resonance imaging (MRI) does not require ionising radiation and is therefore recommended in cases where it would provide the same information as CT unless contraindicated. Advantages relative to CT are higher soft tissue resolution and less dental artefact but MRI scans take significantly longer, up to 30–45 minutes. Contraindications to the use of MRI include metallic foreign bodies including most cardiac pacemakers (see www.MRIsafety.com).

MRI delivers radiofrequency pulses within a high magnetic field, with the signals generated dependent on the behaviour of protons within the tissues. Signals can be resolved into two main components T1 and T2 (*Figure 3.6*). The benefits of MRI regarding soft tissue imaging become particularly apparent when imaging the meniscus of the TMJ (*Figure 3.7*). MRI contrast enhancement may be achieved with gadolinium-based agents. Patients requiring gadolinium are evaluated for the presence of severe renal insufficiency as there is a rare association with nephrogenic systemic

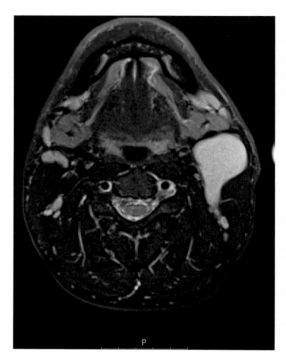

Figure 3.6 Axial T2-w fat-saturated magnetic resonance image shows a T2 hyperintense left second branchial cleft cyst.

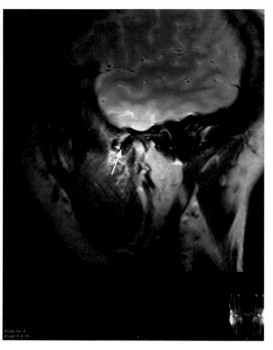

Figure 3.7 Sagittal T2 image of temporomandibular joint showing a small joint space effusion and partial anterior disc displacement (arrow) in open mouth position oblique parasagittal.

fibrosis (NSF). Pre- and post-gadolinium (contrast medium) T1-w sequences should be performed. T1-w sequences may also be combined with fat saturation post-gadolinium, such that increased signal due to enhancement is not masked by high T1 fat signal (see *Figure 3.1c*). Gadolinium is used to characterise pathological lesions that exhibit variable signal and patterns of enhancement.

Typical imaging sequences for a study of the face and neck would include T1-w axial, T2-w axial, T1-w post-gadolinium axial, STIR coronal and T1 fat saturated post-gadolinium coronal images. Diffusion weighted imaging (DWI) is also a routine sequence in many centres, and has a developing role, being particularly useful in assessment of residual tumour following treatment with chemoradiotherapy.

POSITRON EMISSION TOMOGRAPHY AND OTHER RADIOISOTOPE IMAGING

PET differs from the previously mentioned anatomical techniques in that it provides functional imaging of metabolic activity. This has proved very useful in the setting of maxillofacial malignancy, with improved diagnostic accuracy relative to CT and MRI. Most PET imaging studies of the head and neck use the short-lived radiotracer 18-fluorodeoxyglucose ([18]FDG), which allows examination of altered glucose metabolism as a marker of tumour activity. PET alone does not provide the same anatomical detail as CT or MRI. Functional and anatomical CT images (PET-CT), and MRI images (PET-MR) are therefore obtained on the same scanner.

PET must be interpreted with an awareness of the limitations in detecting small volume (particularly <3–4 mm) disease, including superficial mucosal lesions, lymph node micro-metastases and necrotic lymph nodes. Some tumours (such as salivary gland tumours) are not [18]FDG avid. Some centres use an objective measure of FDG uptake (SUV) to increase diagnostic specificity for malignant lesions. There are also pitfalls due to false-positive findings resulting from normal tracer distribution (e.g. salivary and thyroid gland, muscle activity and Waldeyer's ring) and inflammatory tissue (e.g. lymph nodes, early stages post-tumour treatment and healing bone).

ACKNOWLEDGEMENTS

We acknowledge the contributions of Roma Dave, Portsmouth Hospitals NHS Trust, and Dr Rhodri Evans.

FURTHER READING

Ahuja AT, Evans RM (eds.). *Practical Head and Neck Ultrasound*. New York, NY: Greenwich Medical Media Limited; 2000.

Couzins M, Ali R, Mitchell OR *et al.* Computed tomography-guided transfacial buccal space core biopsy of deep head and neck space lesions: our experience. *Br J Oral Maxillofac Surg* 2021;**59**:1238–42.

Koch BL, Harnsberger HR (eds.). *Diagnostic Imaging: Head and Neck*. Philadelphia, PA: Elsevier; 2017.

The Royal College of Radiologists. *iRefer: Making the Best Use of Clinical Radiology*. Version 8.0.1. The Royal College of Radiologists; 2017.

Weller A, Sharif B, Qarib MH *et al.* (2019). British Thyroid Association 2014 classification ultrasound scoring of thyroid nodules in predicting malignancy: diagnostic performance and inter-observer agreement. *Ultrasound* 2020;**28**:4–13.

Chapter 4

Histopathological Assessment of Resection Specimens

Siavash Rahimi

INTRODUCTION

Head and neck specimens submitted to the histopathology laboratory consist of biopsies and resection specimens, which can include different structures and tissue in a small-sized specimen, and by definition, are anatomically complicated. Most of the malignant mucosal neoplastic tissue in resection specimens is squamous cell carcinoma (SCC). The key features to be highlighted in a pathology report are not simply the histopathological diagnosis, frequently known by head and neck surgeons and oncologists, but histological subtype, differentiation, thickness, extension, status of surgical margins, etc.

This chapter briefly discusses the histopathological assessment of head and neck biopsies and resection specimens, including the neck dissection (ND) with particular reference to the histopathology of the sentinel node biopsy.

SPECIMEN SUBMISSION

Specimens should be received in buffered formalin, positioned in the correct anatomical locations and laid on a relatively solid support such as cork, foam/polystyrene or heavy card. The dimensions of the specimens should be measured in mm. Photographing large specimens may be useful to resolve any possible discrepancy between the macroscopic appearance and histopathological examination. Furthermore, any photographs can be recorded permanently in the patient record.

Sutures or pins are used to secure the specimens but the critical areas essential for the diagnosis, such as tumour, papillary foci, white/red patches, erosive areas suspicious for dysplasia and surgical margins, should be avoided.

With regard to biopsies from vesiculobullous diseases, which require direct immunofluorescence examination, fresh sample tissue carried in an appropriate transport medium should be submitted.

MACROSCOPIC EXAMINATION

Resection/dissection specimens

The surgical resection/dissection specimens should be carefully measured. Macroscopic characteristics and the extent of the tumour should be described in detail, and possibly, accompanied by photography. The surgical margins should be inked.

The specimen should be cut into slices of thickness ~2–3 mm. Resections from the lateral tongue and, generally, lateral parts of the oral cavity should be performed using a coronal plane. Conversely, for specimens from the anterior part of the mouth, cutting on a sagittal plane is advised.

For processing, the most representative slices, possibly without necrosis, should be used. The slide(s) should show the maximum extent of the neoplasm, in terms of dimension and thickness, and should include the nearest closest resection margins. It is good practice to process more than one tissue slice.

Biopsies

These should be measured in three dimensions, and colour and consistency should be described. For incisional biopsies, any detectable lesion such as white/red foci, ulceration, irregularity of surface and polypoid areas should be reported and measured. To indicate the orientation and for embedding purposes, the incisional biopsies may be marked by ink. The large incisional biopsies should be bisected through the long axis, the closest margins of excision specimens should be sampled transversely (along the short axis).

Neck dissection

The histopathology laboratory can receive the ND en bloc or divided into separate anatomical levels. The specimens should be immersed in a sufficient volume of formalin to cover the full specimen. The en bloc resection specimens, as for excision specimens, should be pinned on a solid support and each anatomical nodal level should be marked. Any additional nodal groups should be submitted in separate labelled containers.

When ND is already divided by the surgeon into the different anatomical levels, each level should be submitted in a separate labelled container. It is important to check the status of fixation of the specimen; the lymph nodes are better identified in fixed tissue. Lymph nodes >3–4 mm in maximum dimension are searched by palpation and observation. Within each level, each lymph node with adjacent adipose tissue is harvested and placed in labelled cassettes. Larger lymph nodes must be bisected and consequently each half, in turn, is sliced in a perpendicular plane.

Sentinel lymph node biopsy

Sentinel lymph node biopsy is performed by some in the management of clinically N0 neck, early (T1–2) SCC of the oral cavity. It is worth mentioning that many institutions have not adopted the sentinel node biopsy technique, and there is still no international standardised consensus laboratory guideline for processing and interpretation of sentinel lymph nodes.

Specimens are received in 10% buffered formal saline solution. Usually, the radioactivity counts are provided for each node sample but there is no risk from radioactivity. For sampling, the adjacent adipose tissue should be removed and submitted for embedding in a separate block. However, the adipose tissue should not be removed completely because extranodal neoplastic spread is a common finding in metastatic sentinel lymph node. The node should be sliced longitudinally along the hilum. Small lymph nodes (<3 mm in thickness) should be embedded in toto; for larger nodes (>6 mm in thickness), three or more slices are required to reduce the workload of serial sections.

SECTIONING AND STAINING

It is good practice to cut the samples at 100 μm intervals. This is particularly useful for suspected dysplastic lesions. However, careful examination of the block is necessary to ensure that there is sufficient tissue available.

Haematoxylin and eosin (H&E) stain is routinely used for all cases. For non-neoplastic cases, it is good practice to use Periodic acid–Schiff (PAS) staining, which helps to identify the fungal organisms.

Special stains are used for rare disease (e.g. Congo Red for amyloidosis; chloroacetate esterase for granulocytic sarcoma). Immunocytochemistry is needed for rare neoplasms (e.g. lymphomas, melanomas, granular cell tumour) or unusual cases of squamous carcinoma when a clear squamous differentiation is not detected (p40 and p63).

For vesiculobullous disorders, immunofluorescence for IgG, IgA, IgM, C3 and fibrinogen is carried out on fresh samples.

Procedure for sentinel lymph node biopsy

With regard to cutting blocks, there should be minimum trimming. Four serial sections should be done. A second serial section is picked up on a standard slide and 1, 3 and 4 sections are usually chosen for treated slides.

Level 1 and serial 2 slides are stained with H&E and sent for reporting. If carcinoma is detected in a Level 1-Series 2 H&E stained slide, to exclude extranodal spread, deeper levels should be performed. If a Level 1-Series 2 H&E stained slide is negative for carcinoma, then the block should be cut at 5×125 μm curls and consequently another four serial sections at 5 μm each

should be performed. Cutting should be continued with alternate sets of 130 μm curls followed by four per 5 μm section until the whole tissue has been cut out.

The serial section 2 on standard slides and serial sections 1, 3 and 4 on treated slides should be picked up. It is good practice to label the slides as Level 2-Series 1–4, Level 3-Series 1–4, Level 4-Series 1–4, etc., for each 150 μm set. All serial 2 slides from all levels should be stained with H&E and sent for reporting and the remaining slides should be stored.

If all H&E sections are negative for SCC, then serial 3 slides should be stained with pan-cytokeratin (AE1/3) immunohistochemistry. Notably, the neck nodes may contain benign residual tissue (e.g. thyroid parenchyma) or benign melanocytic naevus. Therefore, further immunohistochemistry (e.g. thyroglobulin, TTF-1 or S100) may be necessary.

Note that single cytokeratin-positive cells should be considered as isolated tumour cells (ITCs).

HISTOPATHOLOGY
Resection specimens

It is well known that during fixation and processing tissue shrinkage occurs; however, no compensation should be made for this. In addition to the macroscopic measurement of the tumour, the maximum diameter and depth of the neoplasm should be measured using an optical micrometer.

Accurate histological analysis of the main tumour and invasive front of the tumour should be carried out. The distance of all surgical resection margins should be measured in detail with an optical micrometer.

If the neoplasm involves bone or is very close to it, the soft tissue margins should be examined as a preliminary, prior to decalcification.

Some histopathological findings are related to prognosis in terms of local recurrence, lymph node, distant metastasis and survival. The histopathology report should include all necessary data that are essential for prediction of the clinical outcome.

In case of the occurrence of multiple SCCs, if tumours are separated by non-dysplastic epithelium, each neoplasm should be described separately. The degree of keratinisation, nuclear pleomorphism and mitotic activity determine the histological degree of differentiation. The histological subtypes of SCC are conventional, verrucous, cuniculatum, papillary, acantholytic, adenosquamous, basaloid, spindle cell, giant cell and undifferentiated.

Nerve/perineural invasion shall be considered as such only if is detected at the advancing front of the tumour. A margin is considered clear at >5 mm; close if it lies between 1 and 5 mm; and involved at <1 mm.

Ideally, the report should include the site and subsite, maximum dimension of the neoplasm (mm), maximum thickness and depth of invasion (mm) (*Figure 4.1a,b*), histological type (for squamous cell carcinoma

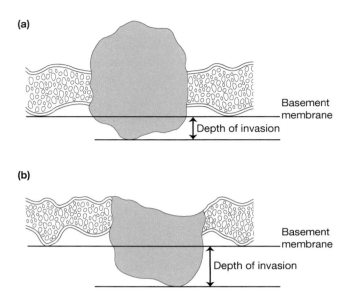

(a)

Basement membrane

Depth of invasion

(b)

Basement membrane

Depth of invasion

Figure 4.1 Depth of invasion in (a) exophytic and (b) ulcerated tumour.

(SCC) the subtype, e.g. conventional, acantholytic, etc., and degree of differentiation should be reported), invasive front (cohesive or infiltrative), lymphovascular and neural invasion, and bone and/or cartilage invasion. It is essential to specify the distance (mm) of invasive tumour to all margins (mucosal, deep). Any severe epithelial dysplasia present should be mentioned in the report and also whether or not the dysplasia involves the resection margins.

As for oropharyngeal squamous cell carcinoma, the degree of differentiation should not be reported. It is mandatory to report the status of the human papilloma virus (HPV) infection that can be assessed by immunohistochemistry with p16, which is an excellent surrogate of HPV infection, or by molecular methods (PCR and RNA-ISH) when available.

Lymph nodes

The side (left or right), type of ND (standard radical/modified, comprehensive/selective), anatomical level, size and number, and presence of the extracapsular spread of metastases should be stated.

With the size of metastasis, the dimension of the metastatic deposit itself is considered and not the dimension of the lymph node. In the case of conglomerated metastatic lymph nodes, calculating the exact number of involved lymph nodes is arduous and, therefore, the overall maximum dimension of the largest matted mass together with an estimate of the number of the nodes is yielded.

Metastatic deposits of 0.2–2.0 mm are considered micro-metastases, while deposits of <0.2 mm are regarded as ITCs. In head and neck pathology, lymph nodes containing ITCs are considered as positive nodes and, consequently, a completion ND is recommended.

FURTHER READING

Elsheikh MN, Rinaldo A, Hamakawa H, Mahfouz ME, Rodrigo JP, Brennan J et al. Importance of molecular analysis in detecting cervical lymph node metastasis in head and neck squamous cell carcinoma. *Head Neck* 2006;**28**:842–9.

Gurney BAS, Schilling C, Putcha V et al. Sentinel European Node Trial (SENT): 3-year results of sentinel node biopsy in oral cancer. *Eur J Cancer* 2015;**51**:2777–84.

Rahimi S. HPV-related squamous cell carcinoma of oropharynx: a review. *J Clin Pathol* 2020;**73**:624–9.

Woolgar JA. Histopathological prognosticators in oral and oropharyngeal squamous cell carcinoma. *Oral Oncol* 2006;**42**:229–39.

Woolgar JA. The topography of cervical lymph node metastases revisited: the histological findings in 526 sides of neck dissection from 439 previously untreated patients. *Int J Oral Maxillofac Surg* 2007;**36**:219–25.

Bailey & Love's Essential Operations Bailey & Love's Essential Operations
Bailey & Love's Essential Operations Bailey & Love's Essential Operations
Bailey & Love's Essential Operations Bailey & Love's Essential Operations

PART 2 | Oral surgery and implantology

Chapter

5

Minor Oral Surgery

Kandasamy Ganesan

INTRODUCTION

Minor oral surgical procedures can be an unpleasant experience if not planned and carried out over an appropriate time period. Any unpleasantness can leave patients with long-term negative feelings towards dentistry. In planning for surgery, it is imperative to acknowledge any challenges for patients, considering anatomical, physiological and behavioural factors.

Each patient should be evaluated through appropriate history, clinical examination and imaging. A customised surgical plan is required for each patient to ensure a predictable surgical outcome and minimise any complications.

Although basic minor oral surgical principles are similar, the required level of surgical skill varies according to the difficulty of the surgical procedure. Hence, appropriate case selection is important.

PATIENT ASSESSMENT FOR A SURGICAL PROCEDURE INCLUDING AN EXTRACTION

Prolonged mouth opening for more than 30 minutes can be tiring for patients. Predictable planning is required to maximise patient cooperation for a successful procedure.

Clinical assessment

Clinical parameters to be considered:

- Posteriorly positioned teeth have reduced surgical access
- Any restrictions to mouth opening will reduce access. Opening of the mouth should be assessed prior to the procedure
- The skeletal relationship:
  - Class II: difficult access for mandible, particularly when there are over-erupted lower anterior teeth reducing inter-incisal distance
  - Class III: difficult access for the maxillary posterior teeth but easier for mandibular posterior teeth
- Mandibular tori/buccal bony exostoses increase the thickness of buccal or lingual cortices or both,

thus, challenging extractions should be anticipated in such cases
- The position of the tooth, that is, lingual or palatal tilt tend to have a thick buccal cortex, hence, there may be resistance to buccal movement while removing
- With crowded/imbricated teeth, there can be a danger of subluxating the adjacent teeth

Radiographic assessment: Plain image

A general evaluation to assess the difficulty of dental extraction should consider the following:

- Length of the roots
- Divergent roots
- Increased number of roots
- Curved apical thirds/dilaceration
- Bulbous roots due to increased cemental deposition
- Root-treated teeth
- Root fractures
- Resorption of the root below the bone level
- Over-hanging restorations including tightly fitted adjacent crowns
- Density of the bone
- Lack of periodontal ligament space

In addition, when evaluating mandibular teeth:

- Location of inferior alveolar canal
- Location of mental foramen especially when elevating the flap and application point for the elevators
- Depth of impaction
- Angulation of the impacted teeth. As a rule of thumb, a tooth with an occlusal surface toward the operator is easier to extract compared with one where the occlusal surface is facing away

Specific to the maxillary sinus:

- Lone standing molar
- Pneumatised sinus in between the divergent roots
- Periapical infection/granuloma breaching the sinus floor

Additional assessment needs for third molar extraction

Principal factors to consider are:

Angulation of the impacted tooth

This can be determined by drawing a vertical line parallel to the perpendicular/long axis of the fully functional lower second molar in complete occlusion with upper teeth and the impacted tooth. *Figure 5.1* shows 'mesio-angular and horizontal' angulation, where a vertical line drawn through the impacted tooth crosses the vertical line drawn through second molar, compared with *Figure 5.2* in which the lines move away from each other (above the occlusal plane), known as 'disto-angular'. If the lines are parallel, as shown in *Figure 5.3*, this is 'vertical' angulation.

In addition, teeth can be tilted buccal or lingual too.

Depth of impaction

Level of impaction can be assessed by drawing lines at different levels on a radiograph, ideally an ortho-pantomogram (OPT). A useful guide to adopt is a line along the occlusal surfaces of fully erupted teeth in occlusion, taking the curve of Spee into consideration. The location of the occlusal surface of an impacted tooth in relation to this line (*Figure 5.4*) will indicate the depth of impaction and the level of challenge to anticipate in removal. Generally, impacted teeth closer to this line are easier to extract and those further away from the line are met with increasing difficulty. Any difficulty may be exacerbated by factors such as patient age (more difficult with older age), restricted mouth opening, root shape, and number and the angulation of the roots.

Relation to mandibular ramus

The position of the ascending ramus should be considered in relation to the mesio-distal width of the impacted tooth (*Figure 5.5*). As the ramus overlaps the crown of the impacted tooth, this increases the difficulty of extraction. This may also mean that the flap raised is anatomically closer to the lower end of the buccinator muscle and is in close proximity to the long buccal neurovascular bundle, which increases the risk of damage to the long buccal neurovascular structures

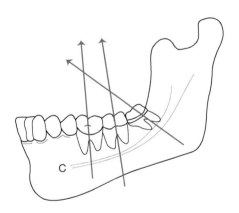

Figure 5.1 Angulation of an impacted tooth: mesio-angular.

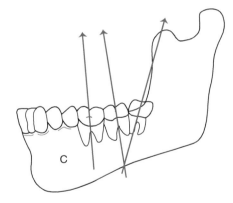

Figure 5.2 Angulation of an impacted tooth: disto-angular.

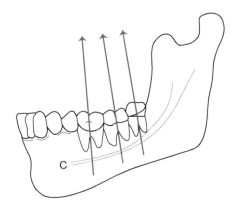

Figure 5.3 Angulation of an impacted tooth: vertical.

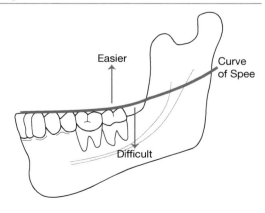

Figure 5.4 Assessing level of impaction. The downward arrow highlights increasing difficulty with increasing depth.

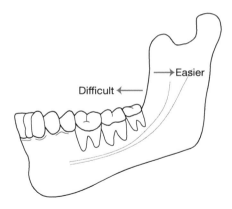

Figure 5.5 Position of the ascending ramus in relation to wisdom tooth.

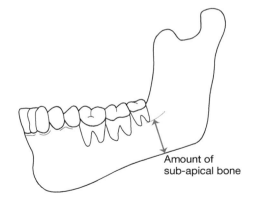

Figure 5.6 Assessing the amount of sub-apical bone.

with bleeding from the vessel and the possibility of sensory disturbance to buccal mucosa.

Height of the basal bone

A reduced amount of sub-apical bone below the apex of the wisdom teeth (*Figure 5.6*) is a risk for sustaining a mandible fracture during or immediately after removal of the impacted tooth.

SURGICAL REMOVAL
Removal of fractured molars: Upper and lower

If a tooth crown is fractured, the clinician requires access to remove the remaining tooth substance. Raising a flap is often necessary to visualise the remaining tooth and to allow necessary bone and root removal.

General principles for raising a flap

Prior to raising a flap, there are several important factors to consider. The flap design should ensure vascular supply to the entire length of the flap, protect adjacent anatomical structures, such as mental nerve, and allow the flap to rest on underlying bone to prevent soft tissue collapse. An ideal flap:

● Has a wide base and avoids transection of the gingival papilla
● Includes mucosa, submucosa and periosteum as a single layer
● Has adequate direct visual access to avoid unnecessary tension on the flap margins, which may lead to iatrogenic tear
● Allows for tension-free closure to prevent wound dehiscence postoperatively

Raising the flap

To raise a good full-thickness mucoperiosteal flap, it is important to incise down to the underlying surface

of the bone. Care must be taken to avoid any slippage of the blade when met with underlying uneven bone. An intact full-thickness mucoperiosteal unit is vital for good bone healing, prevention of soft tissue collapse and avoidance of bleeding from the mucosal tear. To facilitate raising the flap as a single unit, a good periosteal elevator should be used, such as a Molt Elevator No 9, Buser Spear Head Elevator or a Prichard Elevator.

To prevent blunting of the interdental papilla, the incision must include the whole of the inter-dental papilla. Also, releasing incisions must avoid all the vital structures, particularly the mental and long buccal neurovascular bundles. Releasing incisions should not be made on the palatal or lingual aspects.

Flap designs for non-third molar teeth

Figure 5.7 illustrates three flap designs. The choice of which to use is at the clinician's discretion. A three-sided flap may allow a relatively inexperienced surgeon a wide access in which to perform the surgery. A two-sided flap may be preferred by an intermediate-level user, while experienced surgeons may prefer flapless minimal periosteal release with which to divide the roots and elevate them.

Bone removal

Bone removal is undertaken using a rose head bur with a high-speed electrical handpiece of minimum 35 000–40 000 rpm, with a saline coolant. There are two important reasons for performing bone removal:

● To expose the root and gain further hold on the tooth substance to facilitate extraction
● To remove inflexible cortical bone. With increasing age, the cortical bone becomes rigid and resistant to any elevation of the roots, therefore removal of the cortical bone is required. This process includes creation of a gutter by initially removing non-bleeding cortical bone around the roots, and then bleeding bone which confirms exposure of

(a) Three-sided flap (rare users)

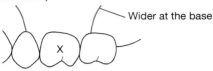

Wider at the base

(b) Two-sided flap once experienced (moderate users)

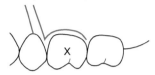

c) Envelope flap with no releasing incisions (frequent operators)

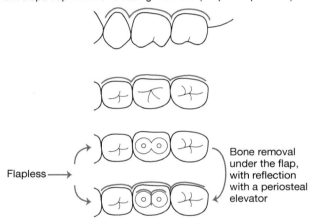

Flapless ⟶

Bone removal under the flap, with reflection with a periosteal elevator

Figure 5.7 Flap designs for non-third molar teeth. (a) Three-sided flap for beginners, enables visualisation of the entire buccal bone to root relationship. (b) Two-sided flap. (c) Flapless/ envelope flap without a releasing incision. Bone removal done around the roots to create a narrow gutter to mobilise the roots. x indicates planned extraction.

the underlying softer medullary bone (see *Figure 5.16*). Softer medullary bone allows for easy root elevation

Lower molar surgical extraction

Figure 5.8 provides a diagrammatic representation of lower molar surgical extraction.

Upper molar extraction

Figure 5.9 illustrates upper molar extraction. An upper molar with three roots is divided into three sections: mesio- and disto-buccal roots and palatal root. Once divided, a luxator is inserted to individually elevate the root.

Suturing

A figure-of-8 suture is placed on the socket to assist with haemostasis (*Figure 5.9e*). The needle is passed through the mesio-buccal papilla to diagonally disto-palatal papilla, then re-entered to mesio-palatal papilla and then diagonally to disto-buccal. A knot is tied on the buccal aspect.

When to leave the roots behind

A root tip of <2–4 mm with no evidence of surrounding periapical pathology can usually be left behind. At times it may be difficult to visualise the root remnant and there may be a danger of displacing the root remnant into adjacent anatomical space such as maxillary sinus. In such circumstances, a decision may be required on whether to leave the root *in situ*. Occasionally, brisk bleeding or patient's ill health may support leaving the root tip and arranging any further removal as a second stage if indicated.

Maxillary tuberosity fracture

The incidence of maxillary tuberosity fracture while removing the last standing upper molars is around 0.6%. This section discusses prevention and management of this complication.

Prevention. Clinical: Surgical access depends on palatal or buccal inclination of the tooth. A fully erupted tooth will have less of a tuberosity in comparison with a partially or unerupted upper third molar tooth. This becomes even more challenging when the patient opens the mouth wide. Placing an elevator or

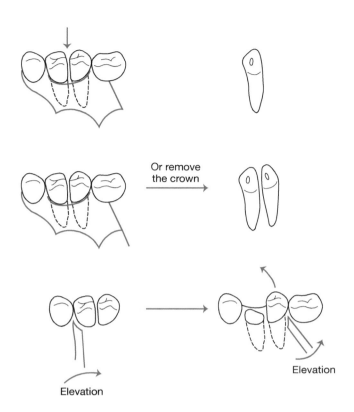

Or remove the crown

Elevation

Elevation

Figure 5.8 Lower molar surgical extraction. Similar to Figure 5.7, three different flaps can be used to gain access to remove the roots. Here, a two-sided flap with a distal relieving incision has been used to create a bony gutter to allow elevation of the roots.

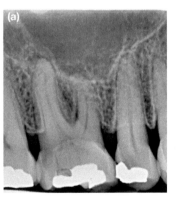

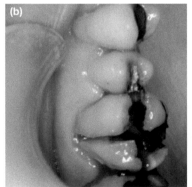

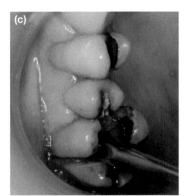

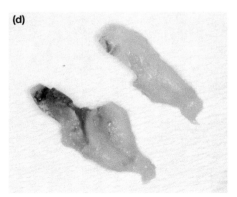

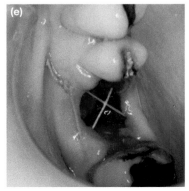

Figure 5.9 (a) Upper molar with three roots. (b) Divided into mesio- and disto-buccal roots and palatal root. (c) Insertion of luxator. (d) Extracted roots. (e) Suturing.

forceps on the tooth and advising the patient to close the mouth allows the coronoid process to move backwards to increase the access and allows buccal movement of the tooth. If and when a flap is raised and bone removal needed, a Laster retractor is ideal to improve the access and also to prevent iatrogenic displacement of the tooth into the infratemporal fossa. Finally, as the tooth is being elevated out of the socket, the palatal mucosa must be carefully monitored. If there is mucosal blanching, then the tissue is likely to tear. To avoid this tear, mucoperiosteum must be separated away from the tooth/bone.

Radiological: A single-rooted tooth is generally easier to extract than a multiple-rooted tooth which has increased surface area. Curve of the roots parallel to the path of exit makes it easier to elevate/extract. The amount of tuberosity posterior to the crown also determines the possibility of fracture of the tuberosity; the less the amount of bone, the less likely is a fracture. With increasing age, ankylosis, hypercementosis and pneumatisation of the sinus around the roots of the posterior teeth, especially posterior to the thick zygomatic buttress, the bone becomes anatomically weaker and is prone to fracture, possibly resulting in oroantral communication.

After fracture: If significant tuberosity fracture has occurred and the clinician is not experienced in dealing with such complication, it may be advisable to abandon the procedure and seek help. If the tooth is symptomatic or infected, then the best action is to proceed to remove the tooth and carefully peel the entire mucoperiosteum of the bone without a tear to achieve a primary closure. If the tooth is asymptomatic, then it may be advisable to temporise the tooth with occlusal surface being relieved of the occlusion. Wiring the tooth to the adjacent teeth with composite to immobilise the fracture will facilitate bone healing. After 6 weeks or more, a further attempt may be made to extract the tooth.

Oroantral communication (OAC) and its management

The incidence of OAC ranges between 0.31% and 4.7% following the extraction of upper teeth. OAC up to 2 mm with a preserved alveolar bone, coupled with strict postoperative advice not to blow the nose, will often allow spontaneous healing. Larger communications can be closed with a buccal advancement flap, which involves raising a full-thickness mucoperiosteal flap with a distal and a mesial releasing incision with the aim of achieving a wide base flap. Once raised, periosteal scoring parallel to the sulcus can be undertaken to allow lengthening of the flap to achieve a tension-free primary closure.

Surgical removal of lower third molars

In addition to the knowledge gained from removal of the roots of the fractured teeth for other teeth, further challenges are expected in third molar removal due to naturally reduced surgical access as identified as part of the clinical assessment.

Raising a flap

Flaps must provide an adequate access to visualise the impacted tooth and its surrounding bone and protect the soft tissue from being traumatised or excessively stretched. A distal releasing incision is common to any flap design for lower third molar removal and this incision should be placed buccally. Often, retraction of tissues while performing a distal releasing incision results in pulling of lingual tissues over the retromolar ridge and any releasing incisions made over the ridge risk damaging the lingual nerve.

Envelope and three-sided flaps are used for wisdom teeth. The envelope flap (*Figure 5.10*) is essentially a safe basic flap, which provides a wide access and flexibility to convert into a three-sided flap. It can be extended anteriorly to the first molar if necessary.

The three-sided flap (*Figure 5.11*) is usually used for pre-planned surgery and by experienced surgeons who do not anticipate any need for further access to soft tissue elevation and expect bone removal to be well within the flap boundaries.

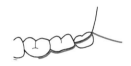

Figure 5.10 An envelope flap.

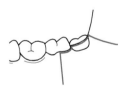

Figure 5.11 A three-sided flap.

Surgical planning for removal of lower third molar

Using the clinical and radiological information available, some pre-surgical planning can be done to predict the flow of the surgery.

- Option 1 (*Figure 5.12*)
  - Vertical sectioning to divide the crown and the root as one unit (yellow line)
  - Remove the distal part first (red line 1) to create space for the second mesial half to be elevated. Note this is also elevated along the curve of the root (red line 2)

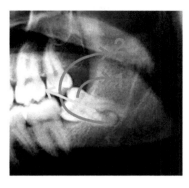

Figure 5.12 Planning for a two-rooted mesio-angular tooth, option 1.

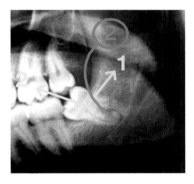

Figure 5.13 Planning for a two-rooted mesio-angular tooth, option 2.

- Option 2 (*Figure 5.13*)
  - Horizontal sectioning of the crown to separate it from the roots (yellow line 1). First cut (yellow line 1) must be executed to create a smaller mesial and larger distal half to ensure the crown does not wedge itself. This cut is often challenging to perform due to reduced access on mesio-angular or horizontally impacted wisdom teeth

A similar plan can be applied to both mesio-angular and horizontally impacted teeth. In a disto-angularly impacted tooth, there is a lack of elevation point in the mesial aspect due to lack of bone in between the second and third molars. Secondly, the distal and cervical bone is embedded underneath the distal part of the crown. Hence, the distal part of the crown must be removed to access this bone (*Figure 5.14*) and subsequently, guttering of this bone allows elevation of the tooth (*Figures 5.15* and *5.16*).

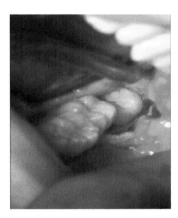

Figure 5.15 Envelope flap with a distal releasing incision.

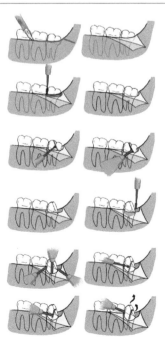

Figure 5.14 Surgical planning for a two-rooted disto-angular wisdom tooth.

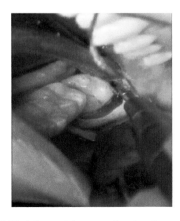

Figure 5.16 A buccal bony gutter to show adequate cortical bone has been removed.

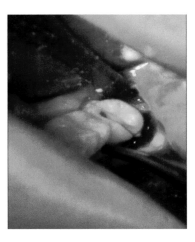

Figure 5.17 Vertical splitting of the crown to divide the wisdom tooth into mesial and distal halves for easier removal.

When there are two roots, often a separate vertical sectioning may be needed to separate the roots (*Figure 5.17*). If the crown is sectioned entirely, careful buccal bone removal can be done distal and buccal to the second molar to visualise and achieve an elevation point.

Ankylosed deciduous teeth

The prevalence of ankylosis and infra-occlusion in primary molars is between 8% and 14% in children aged 6–11 years. Distal tipping of the premolar and mesial tipping of the first molar often occurs when the deciduous tooth submerges under the oral mucosa, resulting in reduced surgical access.

As these teeth are ankylosed to the bone without any periodontal ligament space, often the root fractures at the junction of root/bone interface. This either can be left alone for spontaneous resorption or a rose head bur can be used to remove the root/non-bleeding bone. Gentle oozing confirms that the root has been removed. If the ankylosed root has been left behind, it is important to communicate this with the orthodontist as they are likely to see a radiopaque material on any radiographic images close to root of the teeth which are planned to be mobilised orthodontically.

SURGICAL EXPOSURES OF TEETH/ CANINES

An impacted tooth can be defined as a tooth whose eruption is considerably delayed, and clinically or radiologically they are located away from the expected final position. With the exception of the third molars, upper canines are the most commonly impacted teeth, with a reported frequency of between 0.8% and 3%. Other commonly impacted teeth include upper central incisors and second premolars.

Surgical exposure for palatally impacted teeth

If an exposure of a palatally impacted tooth is indicated, there are three common surgical approaches: closed exposure with bracket and chain, open exposure without bracket and chain and open exposure with bracket and chain.

Closed exposure

A mucoperiosteal flap is raised and the tissues (thin bone and follicle) overlying the impacted tooth are removed. A low-profile orthodontic bracket with a gold chain is bonded to the crown of the tooth, preferably with a light cured composite. Placement of the bracket should be done on the most accessible surface of the tooth. Every effort should be made to avoid placing the bracket on the labial aspect to avoid fenestration of the labial cortical bone and the labial attached gingiva on orthodontic alignment of the tooth.

Figure 5.18a shows a palatal bulge prior to exposure of an impacted palatal canine, and in *Figure 5.18b* a mucoperiosteal flap has been raised. A 3-mm chisel has been used to carve the surrounding bone to expose the tooth. Care must be taken not to remove the bone below the cemento-enamel junction of the tooth as this may cause periodontal attachment problems in the long term. Also, as follicle aids formation of healthy junctional epithelium, care must be taken not to remove follicle on mesial and distal aspects of the canine. Excessive curettage of the follicle may result in recession of the exposed tooth or the adjacent tooth. Once the bracket is bonded to the tooth with a light cure composite, the chain needs to be immobilised to the arch wire with a suture (*Figure 5.18c*). The wound is then closed with resorbable sutures (*Figure 5.18d*).

Open exposure

The overlying mucosa and bone are removed to expose the underlying crown of the tooth. This can be done by excising the mucosa immediately overlying the impacted tooth (gingival-sparing procedure) and the bone without raising a flap (*Figure 5.18e*). Or, alternatively, a flap can be raised as described for a closed exposure and the overlying mucosa excised (*Figure 5.18f*). A straight artery clip is used to hold the mucosa and a blade used to excise the mucosa. A wedge of tissue can then be excised to the width of the size of the tooth (*Figure 5.18g*). Bipolar diathermy is used to achieve haemostasis.

A summary of the advantages and disadvantages of open versus closed exposure of the canines is given in *Table 5.1*.

Labially impacted teeth: apically repositioned flap

Unlike palatally impacted teeth where the mucosal surface is entirely lined by keratinised epithelium, labial

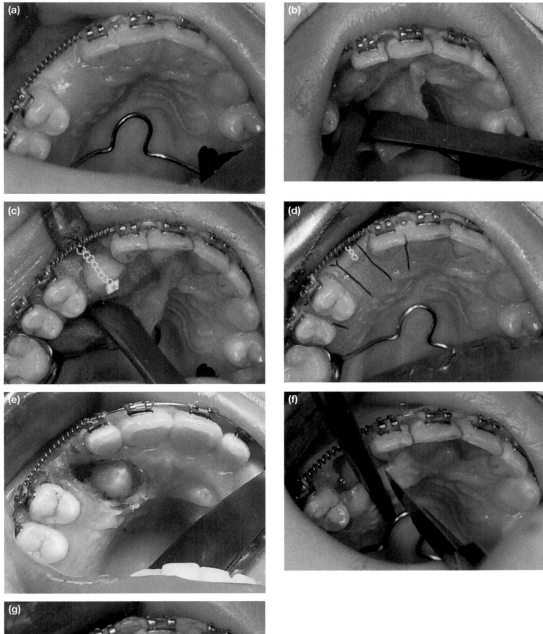

Figure 5.18 Surgical exposure of palatally impacted teeth. (a–d) Closed exposure. (e–g) Open exposure. (a) Palatal bulge. (b) Raised mucoperiosteal flap. (c) Chain immobilised to the arch wire. (d) Wound closure. (e) Excising the mucosa immediately overlying the impacted tooth. (f) Alternatively, a flap is raised and overlying mucosa excised. (g) Wedge of tissue excised.

TABLE 5.1 Open exposure versus closed exposure of impacted canines

Postoperative factors	Open exposure	Closed exposure
Patient factors	No significant difference clinically	
Comfort (postop pain/discomfort)		
Patient perception of recovery (healing)	Longer healing time	Morbidity is lower
Periodontal health	No clinically significant difference	
Clinical factors	No clinically significant difference	
Surgical time	Closed exposure requires more time compared with open exposure	
Ankylosis-related root resorption	3.5%	14.5%
Duration of orthodontic treatment	No clinically significant difference	
Aesthetics	No clinically significant difference	
Risk of re-exposure	9-15% Gingival regrowth is the main reason for re-exposure	3-30% Bond failure is the main reason for re-exposure

mucosa has only 3–4 mm keratinised attached gingiva. Removal of this resistant tissue is likely to result in periodontal complications in the long term. Hence, all labial exposures are modified to preserve this minimally available keratinised tissue.

Figure 5.19a shows a palpable and a visible bulge created by the labially positioned ectopic canine. An envelope flap is raised to confirm the presence of the canine (*Figure 5.19b,c*). A distal incision is made parallel to the vertical axis of the tooth and along the distal aspect of the canine (*Figure 5.19d*). The bone is chiselled around the exposed canine (*Figure 5.19e*), while avoiding leaving any bone exposed throughout the tooth exposure. *Figure 5.19f* shows a mesial releasing incision but slightly altered to avoid uncovering the gingival covering from the lateral incisor. Flap is apically repositioned to achieve tooth exposure (*Figure 5.19g*).

EXTRACTION OF SUPERNUMERARY TEETH

Supernumerary teeth can occur in any area but are more common in the anterior maxilla. A supernumerary tooth can cause a failure or delayed eruption of a permanent tooth, diastemas, displacement causing abnormal occlusal position of a tooth and root resorption. They can also cause dentigerous cysts.

The most common form is mesiodens, occurring between maxillary central incisors. More rarely, they can be located in the premolar and disto-molar region. The most common supernumerary teeth are conical type. Mesiodens may cause diastema but often does not cause impaction. Cone beam computed tomography (CBCT)-aided pre-surgical planning may be useful in removal of these impacted teeth to minimise the risk of poor postoperative outcomes such as damage to the roots of the adjacent teeth, unnecessary flaps and bone

removal, and devitalising the adjacent teeth. A parallax technique to locate the ectopic supernumerary tooth using a periapical and an OPG where the impacted tooth is close to the apices of fully erupted teeth is often found to be inadequate. CBCT is helpful to locate these ectopic impacted teeth three-dimensionally.

Often, the conical supernumerary type is inverted with the crown facing the nasal floor. This warrants surgical removal only when it is likely to interfere with the orthodontic movement of the teeth.

A normal erupting tooth creates an eruption trough, which reduces the blood supply, thins out the bone and creates a bony bulge, which can be seen on raising the flap. A gentle scrape away of the bone reveals the underlying follicle and enamel of the tooth. But in an inverted tooth, none of these visual aids are available, therefore approximate bone removal is often done to expose the underlying root. It may be difficult to differentiate between cementum and the bone. Often, bleeding from the medullary bone provides further visual assistance to reach the impacted tooth.

Challenges associated with supplemental teeth

Surgical errors, such as incorrect tooth extraction, can be minimised with use of CBCT for three-dimensional visualisation to accurately assess the location of the supernumerary teeth. *Figure 5.20a* is a CBCT image highlighting the presence of an additional structure at the apices of the anterior teeth. *Figure 5.20b* is a panoramic view showing a retained upper right A and unerupted incisors associated with supplemental teeth. *Figure 5.20c* is a CBCT assessment allowing identification of supplemental teeth based on their level of development and three-dimensional assessment of the teeth shapes.

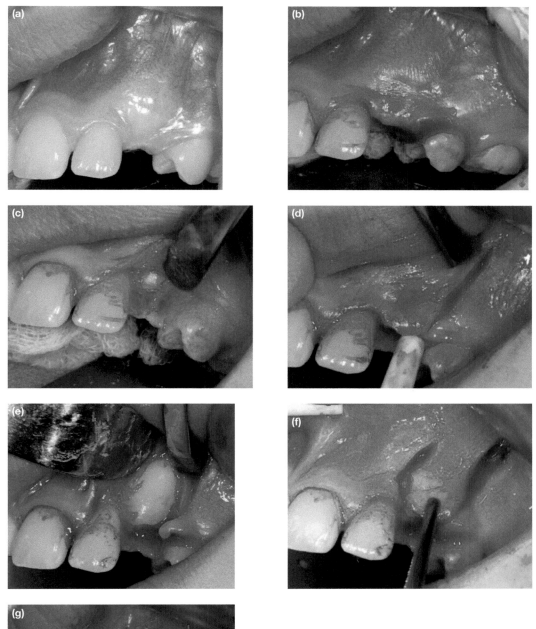

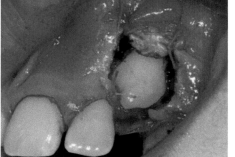

Figure 5.19 Surgical exposure of labially impacted teeth. (a) Palpable, visible bulge created by the labially positioned ectopic canine. (b) Envelope flap raised. (c) Tip of the canine is visible. (d) Distal incision. (e) Chiselling of bone around the exposed canine. (f) Mesial releasing incision. (g) Flap is apically repositioned to achieve tooth exposure.

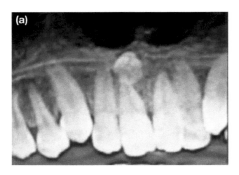

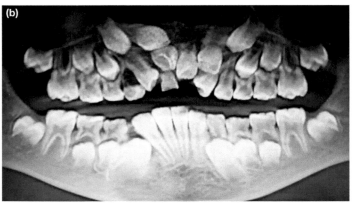

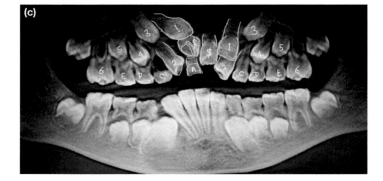

Figure 5.20 Cone beam computed tomography (CBCT) images of supernumerary teeth. (a) An additional structure at the apices of the anterior teeth. (b) Panoramic view of a retained upper right A and unerupted incisors. (c) CBCT assessment of supplemental teeth.

SURGICAL ENDODONTICS

Surgical endodontics encompasses apicectomy (root-end resection), lateral perforation repair, root resection and hemisection. Only apicectomy is discussed in detail here, but the surgical principles applied in the other procedures are essentially similar.

Indications

Apicectomy may be considered in cases of:

- Failed orthograde endodontic treatment even after repeat root canal treatment
- Failure to instrument root canals fully using an orthograde approach, for anatomical (inaccessible

acute curved root tips), developmental (calcified root canals) or iatrogenic reasons (perforations, retrieval of broken instruments)
- Excessive leakage of the root canal material with persistent prolonged symptoms
- A granuloma or a cyst requiring removal for histo-pathology
- Repairable apical fractures as identified on a CBCT scan

Assessment

Ideally, cases will be assessed using a periapical radiograph showing the whole extent of the lesion. CBCT may be helpful if there are vital anatomical structures around the root end such as neurovascular bundle, sinus etc., to visualise the full extent of the cystic lesion and also to identify the exact location of perforations.

Surgery

Preoperative analgesia is recommended, including a nonsteroidal anti-inflammatory drug (if safe to use). Also, rather than using prophylactic antibiotics, a pre-surgical mouth rinse with chlorhexidine gluconate (0.12%) will reduce the salivary bacteria load. Local/regional anaesthesia will be sufficient in many cases unless there is a large associated cystic lesion.

Flap design depends on the size, location in relation to the roots of the teeth and extent of the associated lesion. Based on these factors, flaps can be designed with or without involvement of the gingival margin: flaps involving the gingival margin may result in gingival recession, whereas flaps that do not include the gingival margin are semilunar, horizontal sulcus incision and Luebke–Oschenbein flaps.

A submarginal incision aims for papillary preservation with a horizontal incision made 2–4 mm above the cervical margin and within the attached gingiva to avoid any papillary necrosis. A two-sided flap is ideal for repairing lateral perforation, especially in the upper anterior region, whereas a three-sided flap (*Figure 5.21a*) is ideal for accessing the full length of the root, therefore suited for perforation repair, especially when lesions extend towards the cervical margin of the root.

Luebke–Oschenbein surgical access is ideal when the granuloma or cyst involves the apical third of the source tooth. This flap also avoids raising the attached gingiva (*Figure 5.21b*), therefore minimising the chances of scar contraction-related gingival recession.

Regarding bone removal, when there are no obvious visible defects, care should be taken to locate the apex to create a bony window to gain access for instrumentation, apicectomy and also the root-end restoration.

Curettage is performed to remove the granulation tissue or cyst around the affected root ends.

Root-end resection is carried out by removing the diseased root ends to allow regeneration of bone and repair of the periodontal ligament in relation to the apex and cementum. Root-end resection of up to 3 mm will eliminate 78% of apical ramifications and 93% of lateral canal. It also aims to remove the anatomical obstruction and any broken instruments. Perforations can be repaired, and orthograde root canal sealing applied. In addition, it allows preparation of a root-end cavity and placement of a restoration of choice. If mineral trioxide aggregate (MTA) has been used for the orthograde filling, often a no root-end preparation is necessary as this provides good sealant properties with minimal leakage. The root-end cavity can be prepared using a contra-angled micro handpiece or ultrasonic tips.

A flat resected surface is an ideal finish for an apicected root tip. This allows the clinician to examine for any cracks, anatomical variations and orthograde obturating material, and can be further aided by use of an operating microscope at high power magnification and methylene blue staining. Conventionally, a 30–45' bevel was placed, but the advent of the microscope has enabled resection perpendicular to the long axis of the tooth, which substantially decreases the number of exposed dentinal tubules.

For apical seal, the retrograde filling material of choice is MTA. Other options are modified zinc oxide eugenol cements (IRM), which include polymethacrylate and Super EBA (ethoxy benzoic acid) (*Table 5.2*); however, only MTA stimulates hard-tissue deposition in direct contact with the tooth material.

The wound is closed appropriately with resorbable sutures.

(a)

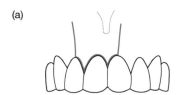

(b)

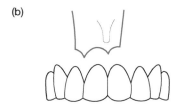

Figure 5.21 (a) A three-sided flap including the attached gingiva. (b) This flap spares the attached gingiva.

TOP TIPS AND HAZARDS

- Do not blindly apply elevation without visualising the roots.
- Avoid apical pressure when removing the broken root apices of upper teeth to prevent pushing the roots into the antrum.
- Beware of distally inclined and impacted teeth as they are a lot more challenging than mesially inclined teeth.
- Avoid excessive force while elevating a distally impacted lower third molar, especially when there is a reduced sub-apical bone, to avoid iatrogenic mandibular fracture.
- Request a CBCT for poorly localised impacted teeth on plain radiographs, for example, supernumerary teeth.

TABLE 5.2 Root-end materials

Material	Content	
Zinc oxide eugenol	Eugenol and zinc oxide powder	Important to manage the powder:liquid ratio to make adequate filling material Eugenol inhibits prostaglandins and fibroblastic activity
IRM, intermediate restorative material	Powder: zinc oxide and polymethyl methacrylate Liquid: eugenol and acetic acid	No evidence of cementogenesis
MTA, mineral trioxide aggregate	Calcium silicate, calcium carbonate, bismuth sulphate, calcium sulphate and calcium aluminate	Evidence of cementogenesis Long setting time and unaffected by moisture, least microleakage

FURTHER READING

Alkadhimi AF, Ganesan K, Al-Awadhi EA. Open or closed exposure for palatally impacted maxillary canines? A review. *Ortho Update* 2017;**10**:102–10.

Chong B, Rhodes J. Endodontic surgery. *Br Dent J* 2014;**216**:281–90.

Kurol J, Koch G. The effect of extraction of infra-occluded deciduous molars: a longitudinal study. *Am J Orthod* 1985;**87**:46–55.

Parrish J, Gohel-Andrews K, Ganesan K. Management of palatally ectopic canines part 1: Importance of histological developmental understanding in improving outcomes. *Adv Oral Maxillofacial Surg* 2022;**8**:100348.

Varghese G. Management of impacted third molars. In: Bonanthaya K, Panneerselvam E, Manuel S, Kumar VV, Rai A. (eds). *Oral and Maxillofacial Surgery for the Clinician*. Springer; 2021.

Bailey & Love's Essential Operations Bailey & Love's Essential Operations
Bailey & Love's Essential Operations Bailey & Love's Essential Operations
Bailey & Love's Essential Operations Bailey & Love's Essential Operations

PART 2 | Oral surgery and implantology

<table>
<tr><td>Chapter

6</td><td># Cysts and Benign
Tumors of the Jaws

Eric R. Carlson, Michael L. Winstead</td></tr>
</table>

INTRODUCTION AND OVERVIEW

Cysts and benign tumors of the jaws are intriguing pathologic entities that can be aggressive, destructive and prone to persistence if not properly removed. Their workup must be performed in a precise and methodical fashion to provide effective first-line surgical treatment.

The assignment of a benign versus a malignant designation to a neoplastic pathologic process of the jaws is established based on well-accepted and time-honored histologic criteria, such as the presence or absence of necrosis, invasion and mitotic figures, as well as the observed natural history of the pathologic entity, such as the ability of the lesion to recur and metastasize to distant sites. In addition, the adjective aggressive has been routinely applied to malignant neoplasms due to their ability to grow rapidly while indiscriminately and recklessly invading surrounding structures, known as anatomic barriers. Clinical features of skin invasion and histologic features of perineural invasion are, in fact, defining elements of the aggressive character of malignant tumors of the head and neck. By contrast, non-aggressive pathologic processes are more likely to grow slowly while respecting the integrity of surrounding soft tissues including skin, and not threatening the patient's life, thereby connoting a benign designation. Some benign tumors of the jaws might be misconstrued in terms of their true, aggressive biologic behavior due to their benign designation with an underestimation of their destructive and life-threatening character. Under these circumstances, it is possible that conservative therapy for such benign tumors might be non-justifiably offered to patients with observed recurrence of the neoplasm. When benign tumors are removed with the realization of negative histologic margins, their reappearance is generally considered to be unlikely; however, with a cure effectively predicted and most commonly realized. Strictly speaking, when benign jaw tumors reappear following surgical extirpation, they are often incorrectly described as recurrent when, in fact, they truly represent persistent disease due to prior incomplete removal.

Some malignant tumors might be distinctly non-aggressive in terms of their relative indolent biologic behavior and relative slow growth compared to the more typical aggressive malignant tumors. Under these circumstances, unnecessarily radical therapy could be carried out for such malignant tumors with excessive removal of tissue that need not be removed. Therein, the astute clinician recognizes the paradox inherent in the expressions 'aggressive malignant tumors' and 'non-aggressive benign tumors', can distinguish those tumors that do not fall into these pretentious categories and can primarily provide evidence-based tumor surgery with curative intent, and with form and function maintained as important secondary objectives.

CLASSIFICATION OF CYSTS AND BENIGN TUMORS OF THE JAWS

The World Health Organization (WHO) classification of head and neck tumors represents an attempt to achieve uniform nomenclature for international conversation. The uniformity is intended to standardize epidemiological investigation with precise comparisons of lesion incidence worldwide. The classification's fifth edition published in 2022 offers reclassifications and additions that reflect an improved comprehension of the behavioral and morphological range of odontogenic cysts and tumors. The 2022 benign odontogenic tumor classification (*Table 6.1*) reflects numerous changes from its 2005 classification. Of importance is the nomenclature change of the ameloblastomas, now designated as ameloblastoma, conventional; ameloblastoma, unicystic; and ameloblastoma, peripheral/extraosseous. The 2005 designated solid/multicystic ameloblastoma was replaced by ameloblastoma without further elaboration in the 2017 classification, yet some pathologists and surgeons continue to use the solid/multicystic terminology to differentiate the ameloblastoma from the unicystic ameloblastoma. Clearly, differentiation of the conventional ameloblastoma from the unicystic ameloblastoma is paramount due to the different requirements for surgical cure. The ameloblastic fibrodentinoma and the ameloblastic fibro-odontoma do not appear in the 2017 or the 2022 classifications due to being considered developing odontomas, a controversial change that is viewed by some surgeons and pathologists with skepticism.

The 2022 odontogenic cyst classification (*Table 6.2*) represents a renewed inclusion of these entities that were eliminated from the second edition published in 1992 to the third edition published in 2005. Odontogenic cysts, similar in radiographic appearance to some

TABLE 6.1 2022 World Health Organization classification of benign odontogenic tumors

Ameloblastoma, conventional

Adenoid ameloblastoma

Ameloblastoma, unicystic

Ameloblastoma, extraosseous/peripheral

Metastasizing ameloblastoma

Squamous odontogenic tumor

Calcifying epithelial odontogenic tumor

Adenomatoid odontogenic tumor

Ameloblastic fibroma

Primordial odontogenic tumor

Odontoma

Dentinogenic ghost cell tumor

Odontogenic fibroma

Odontogenic myxoma

Cementoblastoma

Cemento-ossifying fibroma

From: Vered M, Wright JM. Update from the 5th Edition of the World Health Organization Classification of Head and Neck Tumors: Odontogenic and Maxillofacial Bone Tumours. *Head and Neck Pathol* 2022;**16**:63–75.

TABLE 6.2 2022 World Health Organization classification of odontogenic cysts

Radicular cyst

Inflammatory collateral cyst

Post-surgical ciliated cyst

Dentigerous cyst

Odontogenic keratocyst

Lateral periodontal and botryoid cyst

Gingival cyst

Glandular odontogenic cyst

Calcifying odontogenic cyst

Orthokeratinized odontogenic cyst

Nasopalatine duct cyst

From: Vered M, Wright JM. Update from the 5th Edition of the World Health Organization Classification of Head and Neck Tumors: Odontogenic and Maxillofacial Bone Tumours. *Head and Neck Pathol* 2022;**16**:63–75.

odontogenic tumors that can be cystic, clearly require inclusion in a classification of jaw pathology.

Surgery for benign processes of the jaws is a function of the aggressive versus non-aggressive biologic behavior of the lesion with the proper recognition and execution of required linear and anatomic barrier margin

principles. Linear margin principles refer to the quantitative inclusion of uninvolved soft and hard tissues surrounding the tumor. Their inclusion is planned and required due to the understanding that tumors are not seamlessly demarcated entities. Rather, tumors extend beyond their clinical and/or radiographic margins, such that inclusion of seemingly normal tissue increases the likelihood of complete tumor removal. Anatomic barriers are soft and hard tissues that surround a pathologic process and attempt to forestall its growth and infiltration of uninvolved tissues. The quintessential example is a capsule that surrounds some, but not all benign tumors. Unencapsulated benign neoplasms include the ameloblastoma and the pleomorphic adenoma, which are pseudoencapsulated. Some benign tumors produce a capsule while unencapsulated benign tumors result in the host producing a pseudocapsule, both serving as effective anatomic barriers. Malignant tumors do not produce capsules, and are rarely, if ever, pseudoencapsulated. Other anatomic barriers include cortical bone, periosteum, muscle, mucosa, dermis and skin.

PREOPERATIVE COMMON PATHWAYS FOR WORKUP OF JAW PATHOLOGY

Jaw lesions in general, and odontogenic cysts and tumors specifically, collectively represent an abstruse and often elusive group of diagnoses to surgeons not intimately familiar with their clinical and radiographic presentations. It becomes incumbent on clinicians to obtain a comprehensive history to initiate the diagnostic process while also identifying important information to permit establishment of a differential diagnosis. Patients presenting or referred for workup and treatment of jaw pathology must be asked questions regarding the chronicity of the lesion, the rapidity of growth, associated pain or lack thereof, the perception of mobile teeth and neurosensory disturbances, among others. A focused physical examination follows that serves, in part, to assess the anatomic barriers that surround the lesion under investigation. The proximity of the tumor to overlying dermis, palpable cortical perforation by the cyst or tumor, and possible violation of the oral mucosa should be determined and recorded.

Plain film (panoramic radiograph) and sophisticated imaging with computed tomography (CT) or magnetic resonance imaging (MRI) are routinely required for the workup of suspected cysts and benign tumors in preparation for surgical ablation. The clinician's personal preference will dictate the sequence of performing an incisional biopsy of the lesion and obtaining the contrast-enhanced CT scans. A critical review of the CT scan will not only permit refinement of the differential diagnosis, but also enable a more accurate assessment of involved anatomic barriers, while also assessing the pre-test probability of a vascular lesion. Evaluation of CT scans also permits planning of the

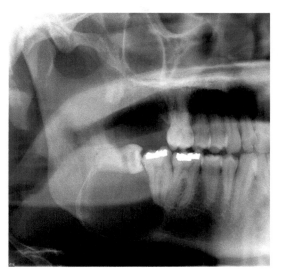

Figure 6.1 Unilocular radiolucency of the right mandible that represents an orthokeratinized odontogenic cyst. The differential diagnosis for this lesion includes entities that are treated identically. The lesion was therefore removed without an incisional biopsy, whereupon the diagnosis was first established following complete removal of the cyst.

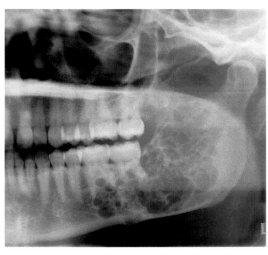

Figure 6.2 Multilocular radiolucency of the left mandible. The differential diagnosis for this lesion includes entities that are treated vastly differently. As such, the multilocular radiolucency typically undergoes incisional biopsy before providing definitive therapy to guide the surgeon in terms of specific operative treatment such as segmental resection versus enucleation and curettage. The incisional biopsy of this lesion established a diagnosis of conventional ameloblastoma such that this patient underwent segmental resection with immediate reconstruction of the mandible.

surgical approach to the lesion, specifically regarding an intraoral versus a combined intraoral and extraoral approach to ablation. Finally, the CT appearance of the lesion might persuade the clinician to proceed directly with excision of the lesion without first obtaining an incisional biopsy. For example, the surgeon might be inclined to perform an enucleation and curettage surgery for a unilocular radiolucency of the jaws without first obtaining an incisional biopsy (*Figure 6.1*), while learning of the precise microscopic diagnosis only after providing definitive surgical management of that lesion. By contrast, that surgeon will most commonly obtain an incisional biopsy of a multilocular radiolucency (*Figure 6.2*) to first establish the lesion's microscopic diagnosis prior to performing definitive surgical management of that lesion.

Jaw pathology can present microscopic nuances on incisional biopsies that might create interpretive challenges for pathologists not intimately familiar with these entities, thereby possibly resulting in incomplete or incorrect microscopic diagnoses. Clearly, a failure to properly diagnose the lesion could result in a failure to properly treat the patient's pathology. When an incisional biopsy is submitted for histologic diagnosis therefore, it is valuable for a highly specialized pathologist to review the biopsy and offer a reliable tissue diagnosis to permit the surgeon to perform appropriate surgery. When cases have been diagnosed by those not routinely

familiar with odontogenic pathology, for example, a review by an experienced pathologist is essential to this end. Further, a biopsy performed by a referring surgeon in which the tissue diagnosis was offered by a pathologist who does not work with the accepting surgeon is best accessioned and interpreted by a pathologist at the hospital where the surgeon accepting responsibility for the patient will be providing definitive surgical management. Such a review could either confirm the existing microscopic diagnosis of the incisional biopsy or result in a change in diagnosis. The change in the incisional biopsy diagnosis will potentially lead to a change in surgical management.

OPERATIVE MANAGEMENT OF CYSTS AND BENIGN ODONTOGENIC JAW TUMORS

Odontogenic cysts

The odontogenic cysts most commonly encountered in oral and maxillofacial surgery practice include dentigerous cysts and odontogenic keratocysts. In general terms, dentigerous cysts are typically unilocular radiolucencies, while many odontogenic keratocysts are multilocular radiolucencies in the experience of these authors. Certainly, some odontogenic keratocysts are unilocular radiolucent lesions, but dentigerous

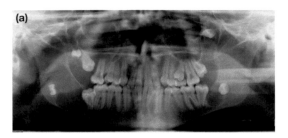

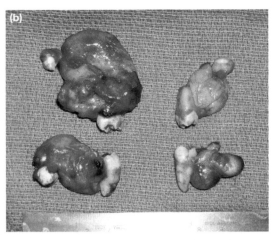

Figure 6.3 Panoramic radiograph (a) of an 11-year-old patient with unilocular radiolucencies of the bilateral maxilla and mandible. The multifocal nature of these radiolucencies allows the surgeon to place odontogenic keratocysts high on the differential diagnosis, with a high likelihood of nevoid basal cell carcinoma syndrome. The patient underwent enucleation and curettage of the four lesions (b) and four odontogenic keratocysts were confirmed on microscopic evaluation.

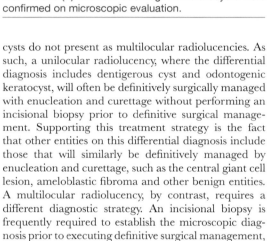

cysts do not present as multilocular radiolucencies. As such, a unilocular radiolucency, where the differential diagnosis includes dentigerous cyst and odontogenic keratocyst, will often be definitively surgically managed with enucleation and curettage without performing an incisional biopsy prior to definitive surgical management. Supporting this treatment strategy is the fact that other entities on this differential diagnosis include those that will similarly be definitively managed by enucleation and curettage, such as the central giant cell lesion, ameloblastic fibroma and other benign entities. A multilocular radiolucency, by contrast, requires a different diagnostic strategy. An incisional biopsy is frequently required to establish the microscopic diagnosis prior to executing definitive surgical management, primarily to distinguish the odontogenic keratocyst from the ameloblastoma that can often appear similar radiographically.

- Odontogenic cysts are not managed with attention to linear margin and anatomic barrier principles
- The enucleation procedure should be executed with an attempt to remove the cyst in one piece whenever possible
- Wide surgical access, bright lights and a generally anesthetized patient permit complete removal of the cyst
- The removal of etiologic and associated teeth increases the likelihood of complete removal of the cyst
- The curettage is performed with a sharp Molt curette and may be assisted with adjunctive procedures such as the application of Carnoy's solution, methylene blue or 5-fluorouracil to the resultant cyst cavity in bone

Of great importance in diagnosis and management of the odontogenic keratocyst is detecting the presence of nevoid basal cell carcinoma syndrome. The diagnosis need not include elaborate genetic testing of patients. Rather, recognizing the phenotype and the radiographic features of this syndrome readily permits identification of affected patients, particularly the existence of one or more radiolucent lesions of the jaws (*Figure 6.3*). Under such circumstances, the biopsy of a jaw lesion will confirm the presence of a syndromic odontogenic keratocyst.

Benign odontogenic tumors

Many of the benign odontogenic neoplasms exemplify prototypical principles for benign tumor surgery of the jaws. These include the ameloblastoma, odontogenic myxoma, Pindborg tumor and the radio-opaque cemento-ossifying fibroma. They are true neoplasms that require attention to detail to the principles of bony linear margins and the surrounding anatomic barriers when performing extirpative tumor surgery. These tumors also emphasize the observed paradox of aggressive local, albeit slow, growth.

When a benign neoplastic process exists on the top of the differential diagnosis of a pathologic entity of the jaws, an incisional biopsy is valuable to establish the precise microscopic diagnosis. Its expressed purpose is to permit the surgeon to tailor a surgical procedure in the best interests of cure of the neoplasm, specifically resection versus enucleation and curettage. Finally, the incisional biopsy will rule out the presence of a very rare malignant odontogenic tumor that would require a vastly different surgical treatment plan, specifically regarding the performance of a neck dissection.

The approach to resection of the conventional ameloblastoma, odontogenic myxoma, Pindborg tumor and radio-opaque cemento-ossifying fibroma remains at the discretion of the surgeon, whether transoral or transcutaneous/transoral. In general, the size of the tumor and its superior extent will dictate the specific ablative approach (*Figure 6.4*).

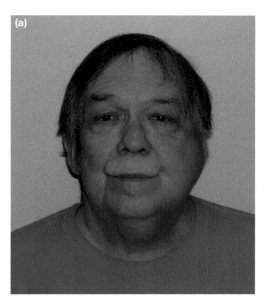

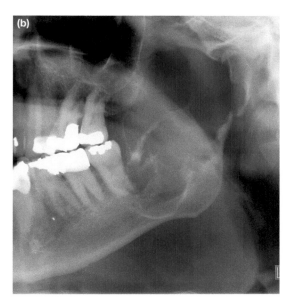

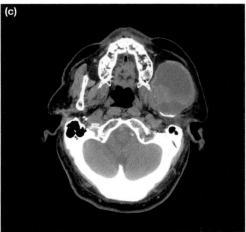

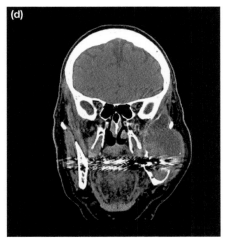

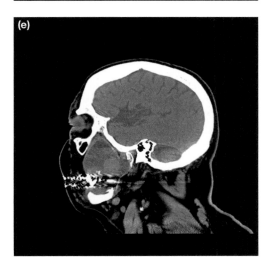

Figure 6.4 An obvious swelling of the left side of the patient's face is noted (a) in association with a panoramic radiograph that identifies a destructive radiolucent process of the left mandible (b). This lesion of the left mandible underwent incisional biopsy that established a diagnosis of conventional ameloblastoma. The patient underwent CT scans (c, d and e) that provided an appreciation for the tumor's extension into the temporal region. Preoperative embolization of the left maxillary artery was performed to reduce intraoperative blood loss. (*Continued*)

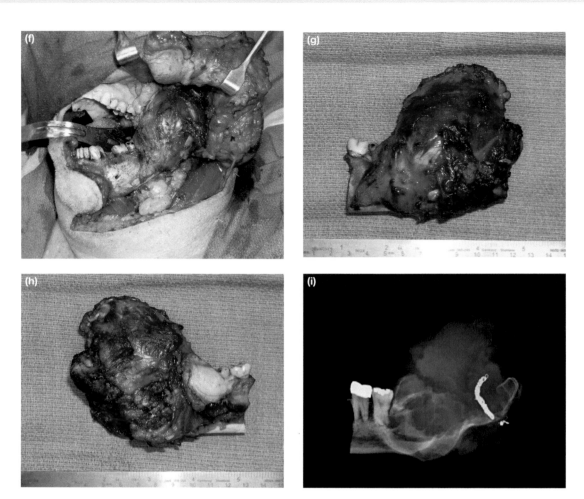

Figure 6.4 (*Continued*) The patient required extended access through a lip-split approach that provided exceptional access to the region superior to the zygomatic arch **(f)**. The tumor specimen was easily resected **(g and h)** and a specimen radiograph was obtained **(i)**. The patient underwent immediate reconstruction with a fibular osteocutaneous free flap.

Based on the physical examination of the patient and assessment of preoperative CT scans, the surgery begins with a dissection and pre-planned sacrifice of anatomic barriers on the tumor specimen. One-centimeter linear bony margins are planned and executed for the conventional ameloblastoma, odontogenic myxoma and Pindborg tumor, while a 5-mm bony margin suffices for the resection of the radio-opaque cemento-ossifying fibroma.

Ideally, a specimen radiograph is obtained to assess the adequacy of the resection in terms of included linear margins. The surgeon will establish a preoperative decision regarding planned reconstruction of the ablative defect of the mandible, with an immediate microvascular bone flap, non-vascularized graft or a reconstruction bone plate and an early delayed bone graft.

The luminal and intraluminal subtypes of the unicystic ameloblastoma, odontoma, ameloblastic fibroma, squamous odontogenic tumor, adenomatoid odontogenic tumor, odontogenic fibroma and the radiolucent cemento-ossifying fibroma are properly managed by enucleation and curettage procedures.

The mural subtype of the unicystic ameloblastoma represents a conundrum in terms of effective treatment. The mural variant of the unicystic ameloblastoma is truly a locally aggressive benign neoplasm of the jaws whose biologic behavior parallels that of the conventional ameloblastoma. As such, the surgeon might opt to manage the mural subtype of the unicystic ameloblastoma with resection with 1-cm bony margins. A definitive diagnosis of the mural subtype of the unicystic ameloblastoma may occasionally be made following an enucleation and curettage surgery, under which

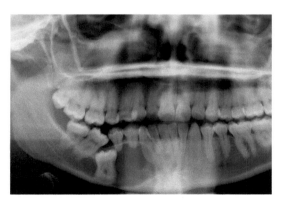

Figure 6.5 Unilocular radiolucent lesion of the right mandible. Primary enucleation and curettage of the lesion resulted in a diagnosis of unicystic ameloblastoma, primarily luminal subtype, but with the initiation of mural disease. Long-term follow-up is required for this diagnosis.

circumstances the surgeon may wish to adopt close clinical and radiographic follow-up rather than committing the patient to a return to the operating room for resection (*Figure 6.5*).

Serial panoramic radiographs should be obtained at regular intervals to promptly diagnose the presence of persistent disease with the subsequent performance of resection. If the diagnosis of a mural subtype of the unicystic ameloblastoma is made based on incisional biopsy, we recommend consideration of primary operative management with resection.

A similar approach to the juvenile ossifying fibroma (JOF) is recommended. The recurrence rate for JOF treated with local excision or curettage is variable such that if this treatment is selected, careful longitudinal follow-up is imperative. Surgical resection with 1-cm bony margins is associated with a lower rate of persistent disease and should be considered as primary surgical therapy.

POSTOPERATIVE FOLLOW-UP OF PATIENTS

The postoperative follow-up of patients with odontogenic cysts and benign tumors depends on the microscopic diagnosis of the lesion, the pathology report's margin status in the case of tumors and the natural history of the lesion. Due to their frequently aggressive biologic behavior, long-term clinical and radiographic follow-up is beneficial to ensure effective cure of patients. This statement is particularly valid for the ameloblastoma; ameloblastoma, mural subtype; odontogenic myxoma; Pindborg tumor; and odontogenic keratocyst.

TOP TIPS AND HAZARDS

- Cysts and benign odontogenic tumors of the jaws may present radiographic similarities such that the surgeon should consider incisional biopsy prior to performing definitive surgical management, particularly when multilocular radiolucencies are noted.
- The odontogenic keratocyst stands alone as a cyst that has the propensity for persistent disease at variable times postoperatively. As such, long-term follow-up is required. In fact, the surgeon might wish to follow up these patients indefinitely.
- Although typically slow-growing, benign odontogenic tumors of the jaws can be as aggressive, destructive and life-threatening as the more rapidly growing malignant tumors of the jaws. The biologic behavior of benign odontogenic tumors should therefore not be underestimated and curative intent surgery with resection should be planned accordingly.
- Long-term, and possibly indefinite, follow-up should occur for patients following resection for conventional ameloblastoma; ameloblastoma, mural subtype; odontogenic myxoma; and Pindborg tumor.
- Some odontogenic tumors in fact represent hamartomas that are approached with enucleation and curettage surgeries with curative intent.
- The resection of a benign odontogenic tumor of the mandible presents the unique opportunity for immediate reconstruction, most commonly with a fibular free flap.

FURTHER READING

Carlson ER, Schlieve T. Odontogenic cysts and tumors. In: Miloro M, Ghali GE, Larsen PE, Waite P (eds). *Peterson's Principles of Oral and Maxillofacial Surgery*, 4th edition, Springer Nature, 2022, chapter 31, pp. 891–933.

Carlson ER, Ghali GE. Benign aggressive jaw tumors. In: Har-El G, Day TA, Nathan CAO, Nguyen SA (eds). *Head and Neck Surgery*, Thieme Medical and Scientific Publishers Private Limited; 2013, chapter 24, pp. 263–83.

Carlson ER, Oreadi D, McCoy JM. Nevoid basal cell carcinoma syndrome and the keratocystic odontogenic tumor. *J Oral Maxillofac Surg* 2015;**73**:S77–86.

Kennedy RA. WHO is in and WHO is out of the mouth, salivary glands, and jaws section of the 4th edition of the WHO classification of head and neck tumours. *Br J Oral Maxillofac Surg* 2018;**56**:90–5.

Vered M, Wright JM. Update from the 5th Edition of the World Health Organization Classification of Head and Neck Tumors: Odontogenic and Maxillofacial Bone Tumours. *Head and Neck Pathol* 2022;**16**:63–75.

Chapter 7

Head and Neck Infections

Rishi Bhandari, Simon Holmes, Rhodri Davies

INTRODUCTION

"Never let the sun set on undrained pus…"

Many surgical maxims are taught, arguably none more so than this, and it still holds true in current oral and maxillofacial surgery practice. When treating head and neck space infections, the operative management should be expedited over less urgent cases in the emergency theatre setting due to the risk of airway compromise.

The introduction of antibiotics has vastly reduced the prevalence of, and morbidity and mortality associated with cervicofacial abscesses but swift surgical decompression still represents the standard of care for all space-occupying infections. Unfortunately, antibiotic therapy can provide false reassurance or prolonged reliance on medical treatment, thus risking a delay in the provision of definitive surgical management.

Head and neck space infections have many causes (*Figure 7.1*), but the old adage of 'common things

occur commonly' is very true and infections in this area should be considered odontogenic unless otherwise proven. Less common aetiologies (*Figure 7.2*) prompt a systematic approach to investigation, diagnosis and formulation of an appropriate medical and surgical treatment plan.

The general physiological response of patients to severe infections is well documented in the medical literature. Most high-volume centres and medical organisations share developed guidelines for immediate treatment of patients presenting with sepsis. This has led to a very aggressive management of infections from the moment they present to the emergency department.

When assessing these patients, it should be highlighted that they can be time-critical as infections can compromise the airway and add significant complexity to their management. The patients presenting will invariably require surgical intervention, many of whom will be admitted to facilitate expeditious treatment on an emergency operating list. As a result, severe neck

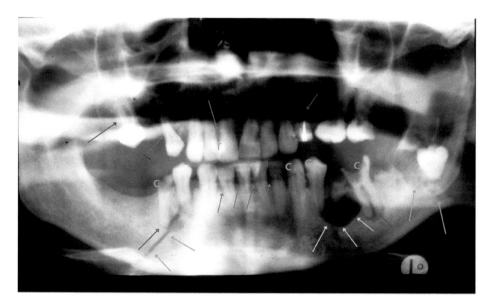

Figure 7.1 Dental pathologies. The most common pathologies causing space infections in the head and neck are demonstrated here. The list is not exhaustive. Note root filled teeth (blue arrow), periodontal bone loss (red arrow), caries (c), the odontogenic cyst (yellow arrow), the apical lesion (purple arrow), mandibular fractures (green arrow) and the heavily restored teeth.

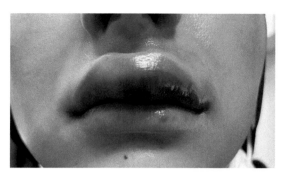

Figure 7.2 Infected lip filler. This is by no means an uncommon presentation. Increasing numbers of well-meaning but not trained practitioners are in practice. Other foreign bodies traumatically inserted, particularly organic material, have a similar clinical course.

cervicofacial abscesses are commonly treated out-of-hours, and require conscientious serial review and active monitoring.

This chapter will concentrate on the major head and neck space infections, which are usually a mixed flora of facultative anaerobic Gram positive and negative bacteria.

PATHOPHYSIOLOGY OF HEAD AND NECK SPACE INFECTIONS

Appreciation of the host response to infection is vital in the acute management of patients presenting with head and neck space infections. The initial response can often be subtle but gradually overwhelm the host.

Clinical manifestations of infection are often based around the acute response to inflammation:

- Swelling
- Redness
- Temperature
- Pain
- Loss of function

The above can often present in a variable manner and should inform the clinician to look at the nature of the infection, together with the source. Should the cause of the infection not be identified and managed, then the infection will both recur and worsen with subsequent presentation.

The acute infective picture can progress to involve adjacent anatomical structures, some initially occult, and provoke a generalised acute systemic reaction or systemic inflammatory response syndrome (SIRS). As with all acute infections, there is potential for the infection to progress to sepsis and influence host response, resulting in septic shock. These clinical syndromes can be life-threatening reactions to an infection and are essentially the activation of hosts' immune and coagulation systems causing systemic deterioration and

physiological instability. Reactions are characterised by tachycardia, hypotension (often not responsive to intravenous fluid boluses) and reduced end organ perfusion with subsequent dysfunction. Close liaison with intensive care professionals is mandatory and supportive physiological interventions should be implemented immediately.

Of note, it is worth remembering that head and neck infections can present more chronically with suppuration, progressive bone involvement and loss of sections of alveolar bone and adjacent teeth.

AETIOLOGY

Causation involves initiation by a septic focus, which is usually odontogenic (*Figure 7.3*). The common dental pathologies such as advanced caries causing pulpal necrosis, periodontal bone loss and inflamed pericoronal tissues should all be sought and excluded prior to consideration of other causes (*Figure 7.4*). Uncommonly odontogenic cysts, particularly inflammatory, dentigerous and primordial can be implicated. Other causes include salivary stones, sialadenitis, tonsilitis, osteomyelitis, osteoradionecrosis and chemonecrosis. Rarer causes can be suspected according to the individual case. Infection post trauma could implicate a foreign body, particularly organic material, for example wood, or a non-healing fracture. Causation can also be iatrogenic secondary to fillers used in cosmetic procedures (*Figure 7.2*). Rarer causes include a neoplastic process.

SURGICAL ANATOMY

The head and neck is compartmentalised by arrangement of fascia, both superficial and deep, which supports the somatic and visceral anatomical structures. The individual compartments are often poorly separated and are potential spaces for tracking of infection. These spaces are susceptible to spread of infection and can act as poorly draining reservoirs, which prolong the clinical course of a process, and their proximity to the airway is of considerable surgical concern. The space around the soft and hard tissues of the mandible and maxilla is termed the masticator space, and therefore the tracking of infection is influenced by the muscle insertions. Detailed knowledge of this anatomy is vital to effectively and safely accessing these spaces.

PREOPERATIVE CONSIDERATIONS
Initial assessment

Odontogenic space infections can present with the patient in extremis; from airway compromise, hypovolaemia or septic shock. Initial triage in the acute setting should be targeted at excluding the severely ill patient. Patients may need to be transferred to high-dependency areas and immediate referral for senior anaesthetic opinion should be sought. Consideration of referral to

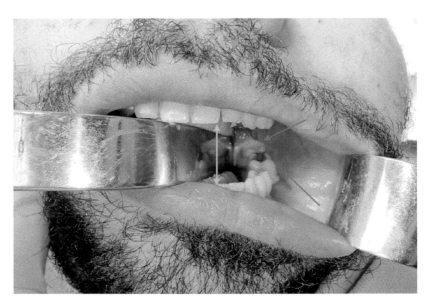

Figure 7.3 A patient with odontogenic infection associated with the lower left third molar. Note the purulent discharge from around the tooth (blue arrow), the fullness in the left buccal sulcus implying a collection (red arrow) and the throat pack placed to prevent aspiration of purulent material or antiseptic prep or irrigation (green arrow). Despite being under general anaesthetic with muscle relaxant, the mouth opening remains limited (yellow arrow).

intensive care should also be considered. Should acute surgical intervention be required, then the theatre coordinator should be alerted, and other surgical teams alerted as to the potential need to expedite care.

Red flags are:

- Difficulty in breathing and speaking
- Sitting upright or resistant to lay flat

- Drooling
- Inability to swallow saliva
- Raised floor of mouth
- Tachypnoea
- Stridor
- Use of accessory muscles of respiration

The patient's vital signs should be assessed and a general physical examination performed to exclude the signs of sepsis.

Surgical airway

Although a surgical airway can be considered, this should only be in extremis, as it represents a significant risk and surgical instrumentation can spread infection inferiorly to the mediastinum. If required, however, front of neck access typically involves a cricothyroidotomy in preference to a tracheotomy. Invariably a skilled anaesthetist with head and neck experience can avoid this and may use an awake fibreoptic intubation technique.

Investigations

The investigations for suspected odontogenic infections will be dictated by the clinical examination.

Bedside

Point of care tests can be performed rapidly; for example, in instances where the patient is physiologically unstable, a venous or arterial blood gas may be

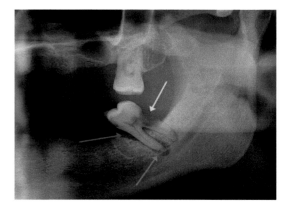

Figure 7.4 A mandibular molar with three separate dental disease processes. The blue arrow indicates the periodontal loss of attachment, in addition note the furcation involvement. The yellow arrow denotes dental decay, and the red arrow apical disease. It is by no means unusual to have this degree of dental neglect in the community.

performed. Finger-prick blood glucose can be helpful diagnostically or used as a screening tool for undiagnosed diabetes mellitus.

Laboratory

Routine blood tests would typically include a full blood count, providing relevant information on leukocyte number and subtypes, and platelet count. Moderate leukocytosis can indicate an immune response to infection, with a neutrophilia typically suggesting a bacterial aetiology (*Figure 7.5*). Leukopenia or neutropenia may indicate a degree of immunosuppression, both relevant for treatment and further investigation. Leukocytes within normal range or an increase in an alternative subtype may point towards a walled-off or sterile collection or an alternative diagnosis, for example, tender neck swelling due to the lymphadenopathy of infection mononucleosis. Thrombocytopenia is relevant information prior to surgical intervention. A renal and electrolyte panel is recommended both from a preoperative point of view, but also to provide information on volaemic status and to guide intravenous fluid therapy. C-reactive protein (CRP) is typically measured as an indicator of acute inflammation; CRP is commonly raised in severe odontogenic infections (*Figure 7.5*). Other routine laboratory tests that may be indicated include coagulation panel to assess for bleeding diatheses, liver function tests as a baseline for high-dose antibiotic effects and HbA1C to measure longer-term diabetic control. In some centres, HIV testing has become common as odontogenic infections can be seen as a first presenting symptom.

Imaging

In suspected odontogenic infections, it is commonplace to investigate the cause with a periapical or orthopantomogram plain radiograph (*Figure 7.6a*). Signs of significant decay, pulp exposure or periapical lesions might indicate a causative tooth. Upper standard occlusal films can be useful for impacted palatal teeth and lower standard occlusal for buccal or lingual orientation, or for assessing for submandibular duct stones.

Should a space infection be suspected then cross-sectional imaging should be strongly considered.

A contrast-enhanced computed tomography scan is the most useful modality (*Figure 7.6b–g*), which enables surgical planning by ensuring abscess pattern, loculation and space involvement are appreciated preoperatively. Furthermore, the resolution facilitates detailed three-dimensional dental assessment of root morphology, and the relationship with the inferior dentoalveolar nerve and bone perforation or sequestra (*Figure 7.6h–j*). Additional information such as signs of submandibular gland infection, sialoliths and vascular anatomy can also inform the surgeon.

Typical radiological features of an odontogenic abscess might include a peripherally enhancing hypodense loculated lesion, localised fat stranding, mass effect on adjacent structures (e.g. airway), an adjacent carious tooth with periapical radiolucency and cortical bone dehiscence (*Figure 7.6b–j*).

Other imaging modalities such as ultrasound can be valuable radiological tools to aid diagnosis of neck swelling and guide needle aspiration. In the subacute setting, uses include mapping residual collections, identifying sinus tracts or determining echotexture indicating inflammatory phlegmon rather than abscess. It also has the benefit of guiding fine-needle aspiration (FNA) of tissue for cytology or pus for microbiological assessment.

Magnetic resonance imaging (MRI) is rarely used in the acute setting, but can be useful postoperatively or in subacute cases with more unusual features. Indications for odontogenic infections might include osteomyelitis, sinus tracts or chronic or recurrent collections. MRI with contrast or MR venography is also a useful modality in investigating cavernous sinus thrombosis or orbital compartment syndrome – rare complications of severe odontogenic infections discussed below.

Specialist investigations

Samples of pus, soft tissue and bone may be swabbed, aspirated or biopsied prior to surgery or intraoperatively. These samples may be sent for microbiological assessment including gram stain, culture and antibiotic sensitivities. In cases of unclear diagnosis or macroscopically abnormal tissue, biopsies may be sent for histopathological analysis. Lastly, neck lumps that have undergone FNA, often ultrasound-guided, can be sent for cytology.

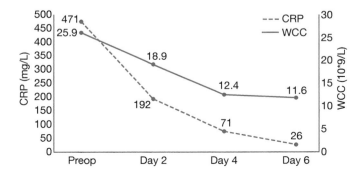

Figure 7.5 Downtrending results of total white cell count (WCC) and C-reactive protein (CRP) in a severe odontogenic multispace infection after surgical management. The x-axis shows the preoperative blood results and the subsequent postoperative results. Note the consistent downward trend – this is a key component of determining recovery postoperatively.

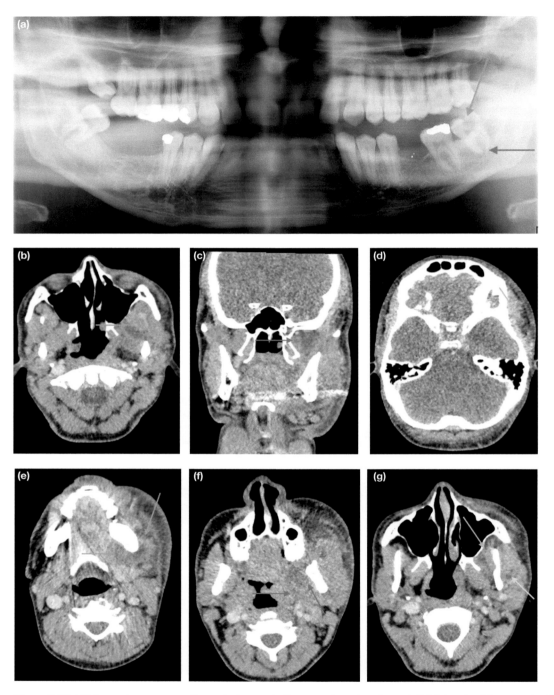

Figure 7.6 (a) Orthopantomogram radiograph demonstrating grossly carious lower left third molar (blue arrow) with associated periapical bone radiolucency (red arrow). (b–d) Computed tomography (CT) images of a complex multi-spatial odontogenic cranio-cervicofacial abscess. Extension of the hypodense area in the temporalis, infratemporal space and adjacent to the lateral pterygoid (blue arrow). Collection lateral to the lateral pterygoid plate and up to the skull base (red arrow). Collection within the temporal space and temporalis muscle itself (green arrow). (e–g) Further CT images. Note the hypotenuse area at the lower border of the mandible in the submandibular region and both buccally and lingually (blue arrows), the hypotenuse area in the pterygomandibular and parapharyngeal spaces (red arrows), the abscess extension medial to the coronoid and lateral to the lateral pterygoid plate (green arrow) and the collection in the submasseteric space and also within the masseter muscle itself (yellow arrow).

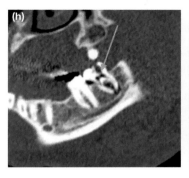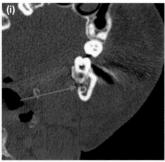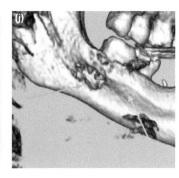

Figure 7.6 (h–j) Three CT images showing the causative tooth. Note the gross coronal decay, pulp exposure and periapical bone loss (blue arrow), the relationship with the inferior dento-alveolar nerve canal and the associated lingual bone loss (red arrow). Due to the proximity this may cause neuritic symptoms. On the 3D render, the bony lingual perforation can be seen and visible root apices (green arrow). Note the location in reference to the mylohyoid ridge and free edge (yellow arrow); this relationship will often dictate the spread of infection.

Diagnosis

Prior to surgery it is mandatory that the odontogenic pathological cause, or other aetiological factor is identified and documented, together with the spaces that are affected. A treatment plan involving exactly which tooth is to be removed, and which drainage points used is fully documented. An open consent form with extraction of teeth as necessary is not standard of care.

Cellulitis

Without collection is commonly seen, particularly in the maxilla. This may be managed by broad spectrum antibiotics. It is important to mark the margins of the cellulitis with a permanent marker, so that subsequently the response to medical management may be assessed (*Figure 7.7*).

OPERATIVE TECHNIQUE

The principles of treatment are to remove the source of infection, incise into the abscess and establish drainage. This is typically performed under a naso- or orotracheal airway with a throat pack. The presence of a pack is recorded on the theatre white board, which also details which teeth to be removed.

Surgical access

As a principle, the incision is cited in the most dependent part of the abscess space to allow as much free drainage as possible. Any incision through skin is placed in the most cosmetic position possible. The surgical incision must also take into account the requirement for removal of the causative tooth. Often, considerable decompression can be achieved by removing the tooth (important to have a pus swab ready), which if the tooth comes out easily, will inform the incision required to drain the spaces.

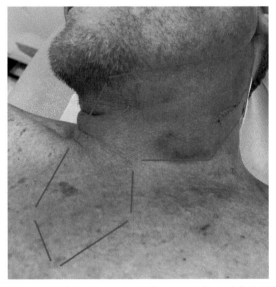

Figure 7.7 Cellulitis marked. The cause is an infected fractured mandible. The patient was systemically unwell and treated with a combination of co-amoxiclav and metronidazole. Consider the causative organism and culture of wound site, and blood must be followed to check progress.

Maxilla

Most maxillary infections are drained through intraoral incisions in the free mucous membrane local to the affected tooth.

Mandible

Mandibular infections are usually drained through a combination of intra- and extraoral incisions. The decision to use extraoral incisions depends on the extent and position of the spaces affected. Any swelling below the lower border of the mandible usually requires an external incision. Intraoral incisions are made in the free mucous membrane adjacent to the tooth anteriorly, and laterally in the premolar region. The mental nerve is quite safe if only the mucous membrane is incised. Usually, any pus will readily find its way through.

Extraoral incision: Submandibular

The patient is positioned supine on the table in a neutral position, and a small sandbag is placed under the shoulder. The lower border is marked (*Figure 7.8*), and the chin is then lifted away from the affected side, exposing the side of the neck.

A small incision is made two fingerbreadths below the drawn line and dissection is continued through the platysma muscle, with the subplatysmal plane confirmed and fascia identified. Note, to avoid iatrogenic damage, attempts should be made to identify to the submandibular gland. A pair of McIndoe scissors or a clip is placed into the wound and 'punched through' the fascia, aiming at the lower border inferior to the roots of the offending tooth. The opening may be deepened by inserting a small finger into the hole (*Figure 7.9*). At this point pus is normally released, so it is advisable to have a 'pus swab' ready. Exploration and de-loculation can then proceed depending on the spaces involved. A surgical drain – either corrugated or Yates is typically left *in situ*.

Intraoral incision: Submasseteric

This space is approached using a third molar incision. In the case of a submasseteric infection, the anterior edge of masseter is readily identified and the muscle easily lifted up using a Howarth periosteal elevator.

Pus is normally readily obtained; however, if no pus is identified, then the masseter is dissected off the mandible and the surgeon places a finger of the opposite hand externally on the lower and posterior border to check the extent of the dissection. Intraoral drains can be used, but an elegant alternative is to insert a medium-sized clip into the oral incision to the skin at the lower border, incise through the skin, punch the clip through, and then grasp the drain externally and pull it through into the mouth (*Figure 7.10*).

Intraoral incision: Lingual, pterygomandibular and lateral pharyngeal

These are approached via the third molar incision, extending into a lingual dissection. The key is to ensure that subperiosteal dissection is achieved when passing over into the lingual space. A wide and gentle subperiosteal approach will ensure a tension-free dissection.

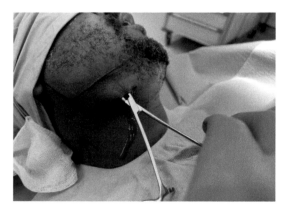

Figure 7.9 Submandibular incision. Ideally, the incision should be made 'two finger breadths' below the mandible, and sited at the most fluctuant part. If the skin is affected, in the nearest part that is 'most normal'. If the abscess is pointing into affected skin, then on opening the clip, the skin will tear. This may be unavoidable.

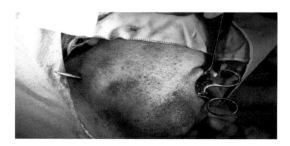

Figure 7.10 The clip is passed through the oral incision and advanced to just under the skin. A small incision allows the clip to be pushed through. The surgical drain is then grasped by the clip and pulled inside the wound. In this way, a dependent drainage is achieved.

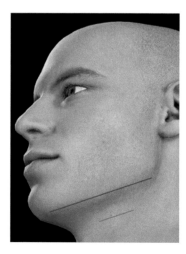

Figure 7.8 The mandible is marked in the chin-forward neutral position at the lower border (blue line). The head is turned away from the operator and the chin lifted. The incision is sited two finger breadths below the lower border (red line), ideally within a skin crease.

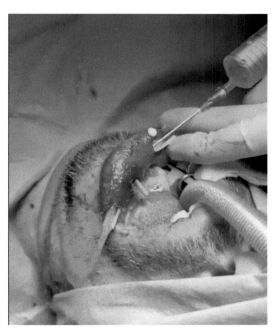

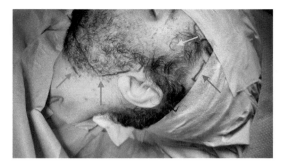

Figure 7.12 Patient preoperatively prepped, draped and marked. The arrows indicate the temporal incision (blue arrow), the dotted area of temporal fluctuance (yellow arrow), the root of the zygomatic arch (orange arrow), the posterior and inferior border of the mandible (red arrow) and the cervical incision (green arrow).

Figure 7.11 Through-and-through drainage with irrigation of a lip abscess. The drains were removed at 48 hours, and 1 week later the scars were imperceptible. Ignore the lip abscess at your peril!

Incision for lip abscess

This condition is serious and unless managed appropriately can lead to loss of lip tissue. The lip is incised along the mucosal creases of the lip, that is, perpendicular to the vermilion border and drained with a 'through-and-through' drain. The wound is irrigated through the drains every 2 hours until the wound is clean (*Figure 7.11*).

Complex mixed odontogenic space infections

Surgical management of the case with the preoperative radiology in *Figure 7.6* is illustrated in *Figures 7.12–7.21*. Note the anatomical definition and sequential and logical surgical access and labelling of the surgical drains.

POSTOPERATIVE CARE

Surgical drains should be monitored closely twice a day, observing the drainage achieved. The amount of discharge usually reduces over 12–48 hours, and drains may be serially shortened and subsequently removed. For complex collections using multiple drains, careful management and recording of clinical progress in the notes on each drain site is crucial. Serial blood tests charting progress with CRP and white cell count (WCC) will inform clinical progress (*Figure 7.5*).

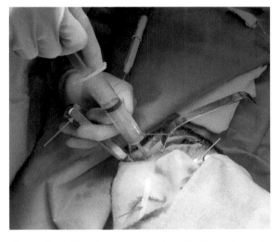

Figure 7.13 Blood-stained purulent discharge is aspirated from a dental abscess (blue arrow). A Coupland's is used to simultaneously elevate the tooth to release the pus and facilitate uncontaminated sampling (red arrow). A Steri strip has been placed on the exposed upper eyelid to ensure the exposed cornea is protected (green arrow). Note the nasal tube in the right nostril – the pyrexia-related sweating caused non-adherence of the tape, requiring securing of the tube to the nasal septum.

A combination of slow clinical resolution and static or deteriorating blood markers may indicate repeat ultrasound or contrast CT imaging and the need for second-look surgery.

COMPLICATIONS

In addition to extension into the defined anatomical spaces, pus can track beyond these into the retropharynx, pre-vertebral space, skull base and superiorly

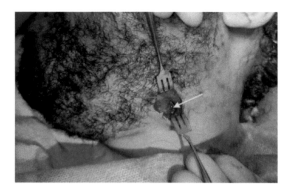

Figure 7.14 The dissected and retracted cervical incision. Note the assistant's use of the cat's paws retractors to both expose and lift the tissues (blue arrows). Red arrows indicate the anatomical layers of skin, subcutaneous tissue and platysma muscle, while the green arrow indicates the deep cervical fascia below through which dissection must pass through to enter the submandibular space (yellow arrow), directed towards the lower border of the mandible and the collection.

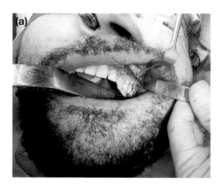
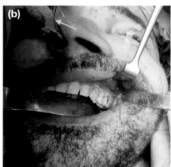

Figure 7.15 The upper left sulcus incision used to initially access the posterior maxillary or superior portion of the buccal space. (a) Note the incision placed just above the superior border of the attached gingiva leaving a cuff of unattached tissue to suture to (blue arrow). The dissection is deep to periosteum onto bone (red arrow). (b) With dissection superiorly, pus is encountered (green arrow). Of note, in this case, dissection was continued to the pterygomaxillary junction with retraction provided by a small Lack's retractor. The pterygoid space was entered and further pus was encountered. The tape on the nasal tube is now sutured to the septum to prevent inadvertent extubation when manoeuvring the head (yellow arrow).

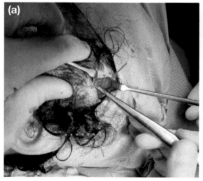
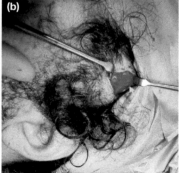

Figure 7.16 The superior temporal space and infratemporal fossa were accessed through a Gillies incision. (a) The position of the incision in relation to the helix of the ear is indicated by the blue arrow. The incision is placed 2–3 cm superior and anterior over temporalis muscle to avoid the superficial temporal vessels and the frontal branch of the facial nerve. Note the dissection is through skin, subcutaneous tissue, temporo-parietal fascia, loose areola tissue and the superficial fascia of the temporalis muscle (red arrow). Blunt dissection then continues on the temporalis muscle in a subfascial plane (green arrow). (b) The yellow arrow indicates the pus encountered. In this case dissection was required to continue down to the zygomatic arch and the infratemporal fossa.

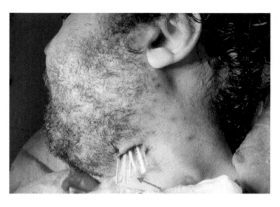

Figure 7.17 The submandibular drains. There are multiple drains individually sutured *in situ* (blue arrow), with the ends cut in different ways to aid identification of the space they are placed in (red arrow). This is particularly useful when deciding on removal of particular drains. In this case they were Rounded: submandibular -> buccal -> infratemporal -> temporal; Notched: submasseteric -> retromandibular; Slanted: sublingual -> pterygomandibular. Note the surface contour of the external jugular vein (green arrow). It is a useful reminder to avoid this when making the incision.

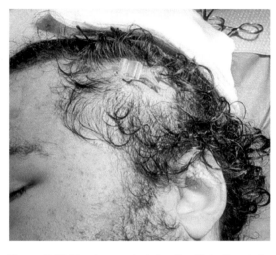

Figure 7.19 The temporal drain site. Note the drain is half-width to facilitate easier placement and less discomfort on shortening and removal (blue arrow). A suture is left untied to allow pain-free closure once the drain has been shortened or irrigation is no longer required (red arrow).

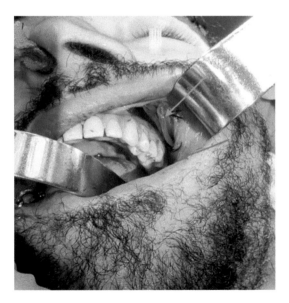

Figure 7.18 Two drains were placed in an upper buccal sulcus incision (blue arrow). In this case one drain passed lateral to the pterygoid plates and into the pre-styloid space. The second passed into the buccal space. Note the raised area of mucosa with an opening representing the parotid duct orifice (red arrow).

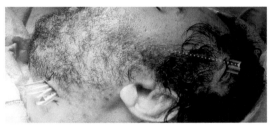

Figure 7.20 The temporal and cervical drains. Note the temporal drain is 'through and through' and connects to the neck.

into the temporal space. Cellulitis and pus can extend inferiorly into the mediastinum. This has a high mortality rate and can result in empyema, pneumonia, arrhythmias and erosion of the great vessels.

Cellulitis (*Figure 7.7*) is commonly seen with or without collection of pus in odontogenic spaces. The patient is usually pyrexial and the overlying skin red and hyperaemic. It is essential to mark the margins of the infection with an indelible marker. That way progress can be followed while the patient is on intravenous antibiotics. The colour will fade and the margins of the inflammation will recede.

Odontogenic infections of the maxilla can involve both the paranasal sinuses and the orbit. Abscess formation in the post-septal or intraconal spaces can result in orbital compartment syndrome with resultant ophthalmoplegia and blindness. Posterior progression of

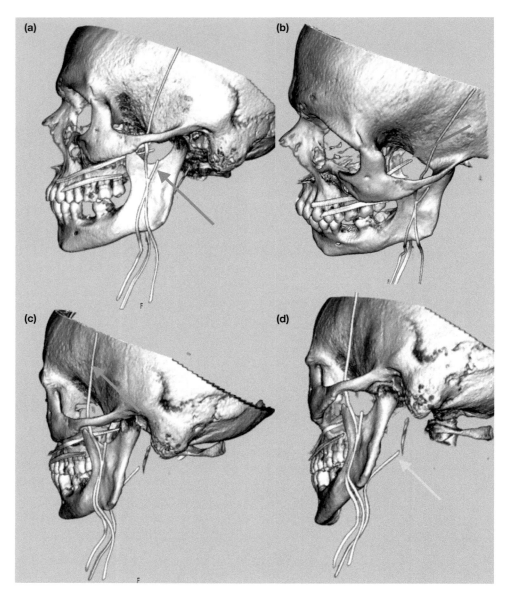

Figure 7.21 Three-dimensional computed tomography rendered images showing the drain placement. The radio-dense strip is visible. (a) The submasseteric drain tip is placed up to the sigmoid notch and condylar neck (blue arrow). (b) The upper buccal drain tip is sited posterior to the lateral pterygoid plate in the pre-styloid parapharyngeal space (red arrow). (c) The temporal drain lying medial to the zygomatic arch in the infratemporal fossa, traversing the lateral aspect of the coronoid and continuing to the neck (green arrow). (d) The tip of the lingual/pterygomandibular drain is adjacent to the inferior aspect of the styloid process (yellow arrow). In cases such as these, careful understanding of drain position facilitates aftercare.

infection and subsequent septic emboli can, due to the valveless venous drainage in the pterygoid plexus and ophthalmic veins, travel to the cavernous sinus, forming thromboses. Cavernous sinus thrombosis can result in ophthalmoplegia and blindness, and additionally cause dural sinus thrombosis and raised intracranial pressure.

Dependent on the microorganism involved, neck space infections can progress to necrotising fasciitis and spread rapidly, devitalising overlying tissues. However, untreated odontogenic cervicofacial abscess can alternatively discharge either intraorally or extraorally and spontaneously decompress.

Chronic complications usually revolve around inadequately treated or residual infection (*Figure 7.22*). Occult or undrained locules of pus may result in recalcitrant signs of infection or ongoing purulent discharge from drain sites or dental sockets. Advanced infection involving the alveolar bone of the offending tooth can progress to osteomyelitis, manifesting as intra-oral mucosal dehiscence, bony sequestra or extraoral sinuses. In the long term, patients may be left with tris-mus due to muscle fibrosis, particularly significant with submasseteric or pterygomandibular space infections.

Chronic low-grade infections, particularly with multiple sinuses and scarring, should raise the possi-bility of actinomycosis (*Figures 7.22* and *7.23*), and require long courses of antibiotic therapy to manage. On drainage, the appearance of 'sulphur granules' representing macroscopic colonies are pathognomonic.

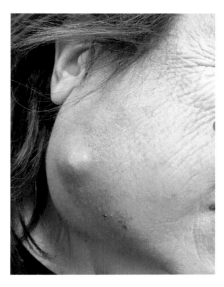

Figure 7.23 Actinomycosis – this chronically swollen right facial swelling was caused by a neglected man-dibular fracture and was quite painless. Incision and drainage demonstrated 'sulphur granules'. The labora-tory should be informed if actinomycosis is suspected prior to sending the culture swab.

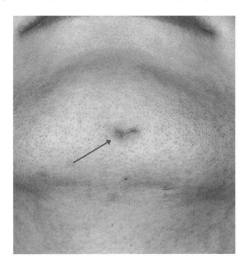

Figure 7.22 Chronic sinus (blue arrow). Inevitably, the patient had undergone attempted excision of the lesion by a dermatologist who failed to observe the non-vital discoloured lower left incisor.

FURTHER READING

Gibson D, Offiah C. Tissue spaces of the head and neck. In: Brennan PA, Mahadevan V, Evans BT (eds). *Clinical Head and Neck Anatomy for Surgeons.* London: CRC Press; 2015, chapter 20.

Jevon P, Abdelrahman A, Pigadas N. Management of odontogenic infections and sepsis: an update. *Br Dent J* 2020;**229**:363–70.

Stathopoulos P, Igoumenakis D, Shuttleworth J, Smith W, Ameerallly P. Predictive factors of hospital stay in patients with odontogenic maxillofacial infections: the role of C reactive protein. *Br J Oral Maxillofac Surg* 2017;**55**:367–70.

TOP TIPS AND HAZARDS

- If there are concerns with the airway, a skilled anaesthetist with head and neck experience may use an awake fibre optic intubation technique, which may prevent a surgical airway procedure.
- Early intervention is key to a successful outcome. Do not delay incision and drainage for imaging unless this is absolutely necessary.
- Ensure that all loculations of abscess are broken down and washed out during drainage.
- Do not rush to remove the drains too early. If needed, the patient can be discharged home with a drain and brought back to clinic for its removal.

Chapter
8

Trigeminal Nerve Injuries and Repair

John Zuniga, Andrew B. G. Tay

INTRODUCTION

Trigeminal nerve injuries may occur from third molar surgery, local anesthetic injections, orthognathic surgery, maxillofacial trauma, implant surgery, pathology surgery or salivary gland surgery, and most often involve the inferior alveolar nerve (IAN), the lingual nerve (LN) and the infraorbital nerve (ION). Nerve repair is indicated where the nerve injury is significant (Sunderland IV or V degree injury), evidenced either by direct visual inspection or by clinical neurosensory testing or adjunctive testing (i.e. magnetic resonance neurography, trigeminal nerve conduction, chemosensory testing, etc.). Repair should be carried out at the earliest opportunity under microscopic magnification.

INDICATIONS

- Witnessed nerve injury from third molar surgery, orthognathic surgery (e.g. sagittal split osteotomy), implant surgery or mandibular or maxillary trauma
- Non-witnessed nerve injury with persistent severe or complete sensory impairment for approximately 3–6 months after third molar surgery, orthognathic surgery (e.g. sagittal split osteotomy), implant surgery or mandibular or maxillary trauma
- Planned nerve resection during mandibular tumor ablative surgery and reconstruction
- Chemical nerve injury (e.g. endodontic irrigation accident)
- Neuropathic pain

PREOPERATIVE EXAMINATION AND INVESTIGATIONS

Evaluation of a patient with a nerve injury begins with the primary complaint, history, a complete examination of the head and neck, including an intraoral examination, clinical neurosensory testing and imaging. The extent of altered sensation should be mapped. The intraoral examination includes palpation of the lingual aspect of the mandibular molar region for LN injuries, then mental foramen for IAN injuries and below the orbital rim for ION injuries.

Clinical neurosensory testing

This consists of a three-level dropout algorithm that grades the extent of nerve injury into five categories. Level A consists of two-point discrimination and directional brushstroke, Level B consists of contact detection assessed with Semmes Weinstein monofilaments and Level C consists of pain threshold and tolerance assessed with a sharp instrument or an algometer. Nerve injury is graded as having no sensory impairment (Level A normal), mild (Level A abnormal), moderate (Level A and B abnormal), severe (Level A and B abnormal with Level C increased) or complete sensory impairment (Levels A and B abnormal with Level C no response).

The presence of neuropathic pain may be assessed with neuropathic pain testing (NPT), which includes Level A (brushstroke) for allodynia, Level B (repetitive stimulus with a supra-threshold Semmes Weinstein monofilament) for hyperpathia and Level C for hyperalgesia. A diagnostic nerve block with local anesthesia can indicate if nerve pain is likely to be peripheral versus central in etiology.

Imaging

Imaging includes panoramic radiography, computed tomography (multi-slice CT or cone beam CT), and magnetic resonance neurography (MRN). CT imaging can be useful for assessing damage to structures adjacent to the IAN or LN such as extraction sockets for IAN injuries and lingual plate damage for LN injuries. MRN is a promising modality that can provide information about the extent of peripheral nerve damage and formation of neuromas.

OPERATIVE TECHNIQUE

The patient is laid supine on the operating table, and turned to keep the anesthetic machine at about the waist level of the patient. The patient should be positioned to allow two surgeons to sit on either side of the patient's head with an operating microscope over the patient's head.

The operation is performed under general anesthesia with nasoendotracheal intubation. The throat is packed with moist ribbon gauze and the endotracheal tube secured.

For lingual nerve repair, a sandbag is placed under the patient's shoulders to prop up the mandible.

If a nerve graft site has been identified prior to surgery, the selected location is prepared and draped for access.

An operating microscope with two operator eyepieces should be available; the microscope focal distance is set at 250 mm with the zoom at mid-range. The operator eyepieces should be adjusted to suit the surgeons, and draped. If available, video camera feed from the operating microscope is useful for recording and allowing other team members to see the procedure.

Microsurgery in the oral cavity requires longer microsurgical instruments, usually around 18 cm in length, and preferably of the bayonet design. Bipolar diathermy and two separate suction tubings should be available.

Local anesthetic with epinephrine (adrenaline) is given as an inferior alveolar nerve block and infiltrated around the operative site.

Lingual nerve repair

Access

The operating surgeon sits on the same side as the operation site. The patient's head is kept central and a modified Dingman mouth gag is inserted to position the mouth open, using the tongue blade to keep the tongue from the operative site. Penny towels are used to prop up the Dingman handle (*Figure 8.1*).

An intraoral mucosal incision is made with a No. 15 Bard-Parker (B-P) scalpel over the ascending ramus to the distal of the mandibular second molar. A buccal extension is made from the distal of the molar to the buccal sulcus, and a lingual extension is made to the lingual sulcus curving forward up to the mandibular first molar (*Figure 8.2*).

The buccal and lingual mucosal flaps are raised supraperiosteally using a periosteal elevator and Metzenbaum curved dissecting scissors, and secured to the modified Dingman frame with 3/O or 4/O black silk sutures (*Figure 8.3*). Suction of the operative site is provided using a fine Frazier suction.

Preparation

The lingual nerve is located and exposed beginning at healthy nerve proximal and distal to the injury site; the lingual nerve is often found in a pouch of fat. The exposed proximal and distal nerve segments are carefully retracted with vessel loops, one proximal and one distal to the injury site (*Figure 8.4*). The injury site is often adherent to the lingual aspect of the mandible, and is released with careful microdissection using curved micro scissors.

A modified background is placed beneath the released nerve. The background is made by sharply cutting the luer-lock end of the small gauge butterfly venipuncture system, then advancing this cut end through

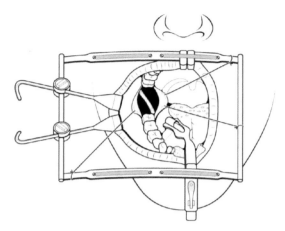

Figure 8.1 Modified Dingman retractor for lingual nerve microsurgical repair access.

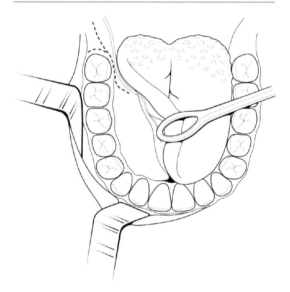

Figure 8.2 Incision to access the lingual nerve.

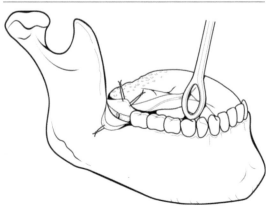

Figure 8.3 Flaps are reflected and secured to the Dingman retractor.

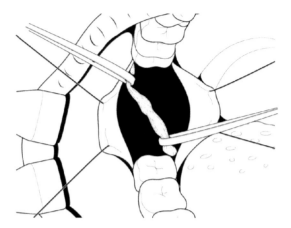

Figure 8.4 Retraction of proximal and distal lingual nerve with vessel loops.

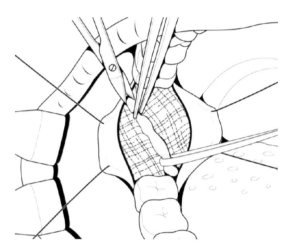

Figure 8.5 Lingual nerve on modified background in preparation for neuroma resection.

a 'tunnel' created in a 1×1 inch neuropatty and securing the tubing within the neuropatty with silk suture. The neuropatty is then placed beneath the nerve at the injury site, and the needle end of the modified butterfly venipuncture system is inserted into the lumen of an active suction tubing.

The nerve is examined under microscopic magnification (25×). The injury may be a complete transection with a neuroma at the end of each nerve segment, or a partial transection with a neuroma in continuity. The neuroma is carefully excised with straight micro scissors and the nerve ends trimmed to expose the fascicular surfaces with periodic irrigation with heparin-saline (*Figure 8.5*).

A 6/O or 7/O monofilament suture passed in the epineurium of each segment to adjacent muscle and used to approximate the nerve segments together to facilitate repair without undue tension. If the nerve segments cannot be coapted without tension (approximately 0.5 cm or more of nerve gap ischemia occurs with 5% elongation and impaired axon regeneration occurs with 7.4% elongation), a nerve graft will be necessary.

Microsuture

The trimmed nerve endings are coapted, using the vasa nervorum as a guide aligning the nerve segments. Using an 8/O or 9/O monofilament on a cutting needle, the first suture is placed at the 12 o'clock position; a longer strand is left. Further sutures are placed in similar manner at the 4 and 8 o'clock positions (*Figure 8.6*). The nerve may be 'flipped over' holding the suture strands with micro forceps.

The intervening gaps in the coaptation site are closed with circumferential sutures placed at regular intervals around the nerve; usually six to eight sutures are required. The repaired nerve is examined and any excess suture is trimmed. The approximating suture and then the background are carefully removed.

Connector-Assisted Repair: If the surgeon chooses to apply the Connector-Assisted Repair® (CAR) technique, a 4 × 10 Axoguard® Connector (Axogen Inc., Alachua, FL, USA) is used on the proximal and distal ends of the autograft or allograft assembled off the operating table using the surgical microscope or loupes (clinician preference) to be efficient with time and to ensure proper technique is maintained before insertion under tension-free conditions, based on the measured gap size. The construct is then brought into the field for insertion.

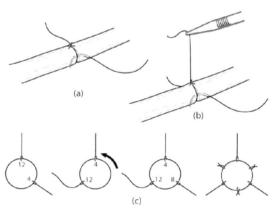

Figure 8.6 Microsuture sequence of neurorrhaphy. The first suture is placed at the 12 o'clock position, followed by the second suture at the 4 o'clock position (a). These sutures are left long to provide a holding point. The nerve is rotated to expose the underside surface, where the third suture is placed at the 8 o'clock position (b). The nerve repair is completed by placing other sutures in between the first three sutures (c, right).

The native LN stumps are inserted into the pre-prepared constructs and the CAR is accomplished using only two 8-0 sutures via the parachute technique or traditional method so that the graft and native nerve are touching or within 3 mm of each other within the connector to complete the CAR technique (*Figures 8.7* and *8.8*).

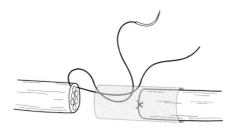

Figure 8.7 Connector-assisted repair (CAR).

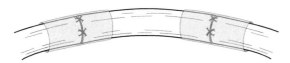

Figure 8.8 Nerve graft using connector-assisted repair (CAR).

Once the nerve repair is completed, a commercially available nerve wrap 5 × 20 mm Axoguard® Protector (Axogen Inc.) is wrapped around the allograft to isolate it from the traumatized wound bed.

Inferior alveolar nerve repair

Access

The operating surgeon sits on the opposite side from the operation. The patient's head may be turned to the side opposite the operation site. An incision is made just above the mandibular buccal sulcus from the midline of the lower lip posteriorly to the ascending ramus, using a No. 15 B-P scalpel. A subperiosteal flap is raised exposing the mandible from the alveolus to the inferior border, including the mental foramen, taking care to preserve the mental nerve.

A small round bur is used to create grooves radiating outwards from the mental foramen, then joined to form windows in the buccal cortical bone. The bone windows are carefully fractured with either a Coupland or Warwick-James elevator, taking care to avoid the mental nerve. Windows are created in a similar manner over the course of the inferior alveolar nerve from anterior to posterior, bearing in mind the upward and backward turn made by the nerve before it exits the mental foramen (*Figure 8.9*).

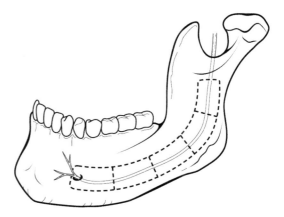

Figure 8.9 Lateral decortication to expose the inferior alveolar nerve.

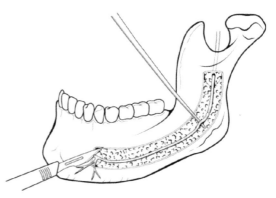

Figure 8.10 Incisive nerve division with a scalpel, lateralization of inferior alveolar nerve and preparation of nerve injury (nerve hook).

The inferior alveolar nerve is exposed to 1 cm beyond the site of injury; the incisive branch is sharply divided with a scalpel and the inferior alveolar nerve is carefully dissected free from its bed (*Figure 8.10*).

Preparation

The proximal and distal nerve segments are lifted from the mandibular bone with a nerve hook, and a modified neuropatty background is placed beneath the nerve segments. The nerve is examined under microscopic magnification. The injury may be a complete transection or a partial transection with a neuroma in continuity. The neuroma is carefully excised with straight micro scissors and the nerve ends trimmed to expose the fascicular surfaces with periodic irrigation with heparin-saline.

If necessary, a 6/O or 7/O monofilament suture is passed through the epineurium of each segment and used to approximate the nerve segments together to facilitate repair without undue tension. As the distal

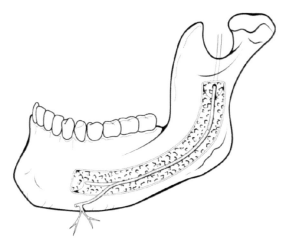

Figure 8.11 Transposition of the mental nerve posteriorly for completion of nerve repair.

nerve is transposed towards the proximal, a nerve graft will usually not be necessary.

Microsuture

The trimmed nerve endings are coapted, using 8/O or 9/O monofilament in the same manner as described for lingual nerve repair. The distal nerve segment with the mental nerve is positioned posteriorly to the original foramen to avoid a nerve graft (*Figure 8.11*). CAR may be used (see section under *Lingual Nerve Repair*).

Infraorbital nerve repair

Access

The operating surgeon sits on the opposite side to the operation. Two approaches are used for microneurosurgical repair of the infraorbital nerve: a cutaneous approach is used when the site of injury is proximal to the infraorbital foramen; an intraoral approach is used when the site of the injury is close to or distal to the infraorbital foramen.

Cutaneous approach: The globe is protected with a temporary tarsorrhaphy using 4/O silk suture or a scleral shell. The subciliary incision line is drawn with a skin marker approximately 2 mm inferior to the eyelashes along the length of the lower eyelid. The incision may be extended laterally to 2 cm beyond the lateral canthus, curving inferiolaterally following a natural skin crease. The incision line is infiltrated with local anesthetic with epinephrine. The subciliary incision is made with a No. 15 B-P scalpel to the subcutaneous layer, until the underlying orbicularis oculi muscle is visible.

Sharp curved scissors are used for subcutaneous dissection for a few millimeters inferiorly toward the inferior orbital rim. Scissors are used to dissect through the orbicularis oculi muscle to the periosteum overlying

the inferior orbital rim, reaching the plane between the muscle and septum orbitale.

The skin-muscle flap of tissue is elevated from the lower eyelid and retracted inferiorly. The periosteum over the inferior orbital rim is incised with a No. 15 B-P scalpel a few millimeters below the edge of the rim. The periosteum is elevated with a periosteal elevator until the infraorbital foramen is reached, usually located 7–9 mm inferior to the inferior orbital rim.

A groove around the infraorbital foramen is made with a small round bur. The bone around the foramen is carefully removed with Rongeur forceps. The ION is exposed by unroofing the infraorbital canal to 1 cm beyond the nerve injury site.

Intraoral approach: An intraoral vestibular incision is made in the unattached mucosa of the maxillary vestibule from the midline to the zygomatic process. The ION and infraorbital foramen are exposed via a subperiosteal dissection. The ION immediately branches into up to 10 branches at the foramen.

A small round bur is used to create a groove around the infraorbital foramen. The bone around the foramen is carefully removed with a Rongeur forceps. The infraorbital canal is carefully unroofed exposing the infraorbital nerve until 1 cm beyond the injury site, and may reach the orbital floor (*Figure 8.12*).

Preparation

The proximal and distal nerve segments are lifted from the bone with a nerve hook, and a modified neuropatty background is placed beneath the nerve segments. The nerve is examined under microscopic magnification. The injury may be a complete transection or a partial

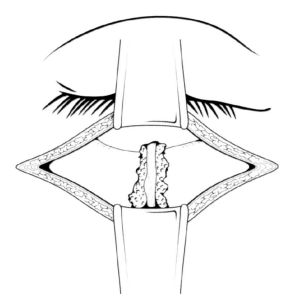

Figure 8.12 Transcutaneous approach to infraorbital nerve injury.

transection with a neuroma in continuity. The neuroma is carefully excised with straight micro scissors and the nerve ends trimmed to expose the fascicular surfaces with periodic irrigation with heparin-saline.

An approximating suture using 6/O or 7/O monofilament is passed through the epineurium of each segment and used to approximate the nerve segments together to facilitate repair without undue tension.

Microsuture

The trimmed nerve endings are coapted, using 8/O or 9/O monofilament in the same manner as described for lingual nerve repair.

CAR may be used (see section under *Lingual Nerve Repair*).

Wound closure

The microscope is moved out of the operative field. The operative site is irrigated with saline, and the wound is closed in layers with resorbable and non-resorbable sutures as appropriate for mucosa or skin. The patient is reversed and extubated by the anesthetist.

Sural nerve graft

The sural nerve remains the 'workhorse' of autogenous nerve graft applications in trigeminal nerve repair. Alternative autogenous nerve graft locations are the greater auricular and medial antebrachial cutaneous nerves.

The sural nerve is easily harvested by a 2-cm curvilinear incision one finger breadth distal and superior to the lateral malleolus of the ankle. The sural nerve, the small saphenous vein and artery are within the subcutaneous tissues of the lateral leg and are superior to the fascia of the posterior tibialis muscle.

The nerve is isolated from the vein and artery using vessel loops and dissected as far distally and proximally as possible (*Figure 8.13*). The most distal end is transected sharply and the sural nerve exteriorized to determine the length required for adequate grafting of the lingual or inferior alveolar nerve (*Figure 8.14*).

If greater length is required, a second incision above and parallel to the first is made until the adequate length of nerve is obtained. At least 1 cm of proximal nerve is spared so that after harvesting, the proximal stump can be repositioned into the muscle to avoid painful neuroma formation. This is accomplished by creating a small 'trapdoor' access through the posterior tibialis fascia to expose the muscle and then suturing the proximal stump of the sural nerve against muscle using resorbable suture, closing the fascia over the stump and completing the skin closure (*Figure 8.15*).

The wound is then dressed and supported with an elastic gauze bandage (Ace bandage). Non-weight-bearing crutches are provided. The patient is instructed to change the bandage daily to avoid compression for 1 week. Non-weight-bearing activity is enforced for 2 weeks, after which sutures are removed.

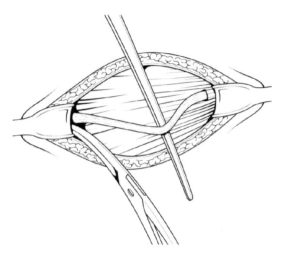

Figure 8.13 Sural nerve is lateralized.

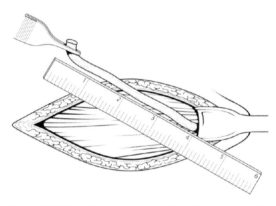

Figure 8.14 Sural nerve is exteriorized to determine its length.

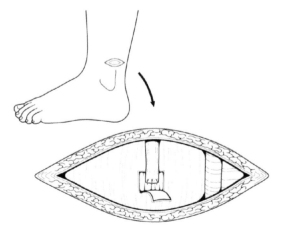

Figure 8.15 Sural nerve stump buried in muscle under fascial trapdoor.

Alternatives

Autogenous nerve grafting may not be possible or may be refused by the patient. Autogenous vein grafts or autogenous frozen-thawed muscle grafts may be considered for intermediate length nerve gaps.

The Avance® nerve allograft (Axogen Inc.) is a proprietarily processed, chondroitinase-treated, decellularized donor human nerve tissue. It contains laminin, which is neurotropic. The allograft is available in a variety of sizes in length and diameter. The most useful size for restoring the IAN in mandibular resection and reconstruction is 70 mm length at 2–3 mm or 3–4 mm diameter; shorter lengths (15 mm) are used for LN repair with gaps of more than 5 mm. The Avance nerve allograft has to be ordered prior to surgery, is supplied sterile and must be kept frozen (at or below −40°C) until it is thawed for use.

IAN restoration in mandibular resection and reconstruction

Immediate reconstruction of the IAN in cases of mandibular resection involves a four-step process:

1 Identification of the mental nerve as it exits the mental foramen on the side of the pathology
2 Ablation of the pathology according to oncologic principles, with preservation of the proximal and distal nerve stumps marked by visible sutures
3 For large defects that involve the IAN proximal to the mandibular foramen or distal to the mental foramen, immediate reconstruction of the resected IAN using the processed nerve allograft is performed
4 For smaller defects, insertion of vascularized or non-vascularized bone graft and soft tissue flap is performed first. This is followed by reconstruction of the IAN using the processed nerve allograft, which is placed lateral or inferior to the bone graft, reconstruction plate or both. Microclips are used to attach the nerve allograft to the lateral soft tissue flap, which allows localization of the nerve to be avoided during implant surgery later

POSTOPERATIVE CARE AND RECOVERY

A gauze pack may be placed over the operative site intraorally. The patient is transferred to the Postoperative Anesthesia Care Unit and may either be allowed home or admitted to the ward overnight. Analgesia and chlorhexidine mouth rinse are prescribed; postoperative wound care instructions are provided. Adjunctive medication for neuropathic pain should be continued if this has been in use preoperatively. The patient is followed up 7–10 days later and may be given instructions for sensory retraining to be continued for up to 1 year after surgery. Mandibular range of motion should be normal by 1 month. Clinical neurosensory testing is performed at 3, 6 and 12 months postoperatively. Sensory regeneration should be complete by 1 year in the majority of patients so that discharge should occur after 1 year. Exceptions to this rule occur due to age, location and degree of injury. Older patients, more distal injuries (mental nerve versus IAN) and complete transaction injuries requiring nerve grafts are expected to reach maximum regeneration over longer times (beyond 1 year).

COMPLICATIONS

- *Intraoperative bleeding:* usually arrested with diathermy or packing Gelfoam
- *Infection:* treated with antibiotics and chlorhexidine rinse
- *Wound dehiscence:* treated with regular irrigation or rinsing with chlorhexidine
- *Pathological fracture of the mandible:* may be treated with antibiotics and non-chew diet, or closed/open reduction and fixation
- *Trismus:* may be a sequela of surgery, likely self-limiting; analgesics, soft diet and passive jaw opening exercises may be helpful
- *Inability to locate one nerve segment:* if the proximal segment cannot be found, the distal segment may be connected to another nerve (nerve share). If the distal segment cannot be found, the proximal nerve should be repositioned (nerve end buried in adjacent muscle to avoid neuroma formation)
- *Neuropathic pain:* development of neuropathic pain after nerve repair is rare when there is no neuropathic pain before surgery
- *Neuroma formation in nerve graft donor site:* may leave alone or surgically resect the neuroma

TOP TIPS AND HAZARDS

- Position the patient appropriately before commencing surgery so that the microsurgeons are comfortable throughout the procedure.
- Demagnetize the microsurgical instruments before surgery.
- Use an operating microscope that has two viewing ports and a video feed.
- Use a neuropatty with suction via a butterfly cannula as background.
- Irrigate the nerve repair site with heparin-saline during neurorrhaphy.

FURTHER READING

Epker BN, Gregg JM. Surgical management of maxillary nerve injuries. *Oral Maxillofac Surg Clin North Am* 1992;**4**:439–45.

Gregg JM. Surgical management of lingual nerve injuries. *Oral Maxillofac Surg Clin North Am* 1992;**4**:417–24.

LaBanc JP, Van Boven RW. Surgical management of inferior alveolar nerve injuries. *Oral Maxillofac Surg Clin North Am* 1992;**4**:425–37.

Zuniga JR, Essick GK. A contemporary approach to the clinical evaluation of trigeminal nerve injuries. *Oral Maxillofac Surg Clin North Am* 1992;**4**:353–67.

Zuniga JR, Mistry C, Tikhonov I, et al. Magnetic resonance neurography of traumatic and nontraumatic peripheral trigeminal neuropathies. *J Oral Maxillofac Surg* 2018;**76**:725–36.

Bailey & Love's Essential Operations Bailey & Love's Essential Operations
Bailey & Love's Essential Operations Bailey & Love's Essential Operations
Bailey & Love's Essential Operations Bailey & Love's Essential Operations

PART 2 | Oral surgery and implantology

Chapter
9

Principles of Dental Implant Surgery

Kaveh Shakib, Konstantinos Mitsimponas

INTRODUCTION

The pioneering work on osseointegration in the 1970s paved the way for a successful introduction of dental implants as a mainstream means of dental rehabilitation. An implant is considered osseointegrated when it is in direct contact with the bone and there is no relative movement between the two.

Although the relationship between the bone and the dental implant appears to be similar to that of bone and the root of a tooth, the fundamental difference of the absence of a suspension mechanism in the form of the periodontal ligament, significantly alters the mechanical behaviour of the system.

Continued improvement of implant surface properties, design and surgical techniques has resulted in persistently high success rates. The definition of success varies between studies, ranging from the survival of the implant to absence of implant mobility to the radiological absence of bone loss around the implant over a variable period. It is generally accepted that dental implants represent a gold standard option of restoration of lost teeth.

ESSENTIAL SURGICAL ANATOMY

An understanding of the relevant surgical anatomy is of vital significance for the success of the procedure. In the case of dental implants, it is also important to understand how the anatomy of the mandible and the maxilla change following the loss of teeth.

In the maxilla, the surgeon needs to be aware of the position of the maxillary sinus, the floor of the nasal cavity, the nasopalatine canal and the greater palatine foramen. It is important also to appreciate the direction of bone resorption for the maxilla; this is centripetal and thus, results in the buccal/labial placement of the edentulous crest.

In the mandible, the lingual bony undercut in the posterior molar area, the inferior dental canal and the mental foramina are the structures of which to be aware. Following an initial antero-inferior course below the mandibular foramen, the canal runs horizontally and laterally just under the roots of the mandibular molars. To avoid inadvertent injury to the contents of the mandibular canal, a distance of 2 mm from this should be allowed for in implant placement. The

mental nerve prior to its exit from the foramen forms a loop that runs anterior and inferior to the foramen by a few millimetres.

Availability of both satisfactory bone volume and quality is a prerequisite for implant surgery. There is no universally accepted classification; however, as an example, the Lekholm and Zarb classification has been used to describe the quantity and quality of the available mandibular or maxillary bone. For bone quantity, five classes are identified: (1) most of the alveolar bone is present; (2) moderate residual ridge resorption has occurred; (3) advanced residual ridge resorption has occurred and only basal bone remains; (4) some resorption of the basal bone has taken place; and (5) extreme resorption of the basal bone has taken place. For bone quality, four classes have been described: (1) almost the entire jaw comprises homogenous compact bone; (2) a thick layer of compact bone surrounds a core of dense trabecular bone; (3) a thin layer of cortical bone surrounds a core of dense trabecular bone of favourable strength; and (4) a thin layer of cortical bone surrounds a core of low-density trabecular bone.

PREOPERATIVE CONSIDERATIONS, INDICATIONS AND INVESTIGATIONS

Careful evaluation of the patient's medical history and appropriate patient selection are crucial to success in implant surgery, as a direct correlation of general medical status and implant failure rate has been clearly documented. The need for implants increases with age; it is only to be expected that the comorbidities of the patients will increase as well.

A particular concern has been raised for patients on bisphosphonate treatment (or similar antiresorptive agents). Some consider the use of intravenous bisphosphonates as an absolute contraindication for implant placement due to the high risk of medication-related osteonecrosis of the jaw (MRONJ). Oral bisphosphonates are considered less hazardous, and several studies report good results of implant placement for these patients. In any case, additional caution is required when managing patients on bisphosphonates.

Following detailed discussion with patients including risk of jaw necrosis, the authors do regularly place dental implants in patients who have received intravenous and oral bisphosphonates under antibiotic prophylaxis for up to 10 days post-surgery.

Recent studies have shown increased risk of implant failure in patients who are allergic to penicillin. The reason for this increased risk is not clear.

Planning of implant surgery, as part of the overall dental health, is perhaps the most important step in the dental rehabilitation process. Joint consultation with a restorative specialist for planning, sequencing of treatment (extractions, bone graft, etc.), temporary restorations and fabrication of surgical stents are all included in the initial planning step. Surgical stents can help surgical planning and aid communication between the implant surgeon and prosthodontist.

A thorough examination, completed with an appropriate radiographic examination is required prior to proceeding to treatment planning. For straightforward cases, orthopantomogram and dental periapical radiographs might be sufficient for planning. Nevertheless, the use of a cone beam computed tomography (CBCT) scan has become standard practice.

Instrumentation

In addition to routine oral surgical instruments, placement of dental implants may be facilitated with the use of socket dilators. Rotary instruments must be used with the correct speed (650–1000 RPM) and torque (16–20 N).

Drilling of bone results in significant heat generation. Utilisation of single-use drills, operated at low speed with copious irrigation with cooled saline will minimise damage to osteoblasts and aid the osseointegration process.

General notes about dental implant surgery

Implant surgery is typically performed under a combination of short- and long-acting local anaesthetics with vasoconstrictors. Addition of intravenous sedation enhances patient experience and improves tolerance. The infiltration buccally and lingually provides adequate anaesthesia for lower molar implant surgery.

Perioperative antibiotic such as amoxycillin, co-amoxiclav or clindamycin, should be administered enterally or parenterally. Local preparation includes chlorhexidine mouth rinse preoperatively.

Postoperative management

Most surgeons continue antibiotic therapy for up to 5 days. Application of an ice pack immediately post-surgery provides comfort and reduces swelling. Patients should maintain meticulous oral hygiene care and in addition to soft brushing, use saline, hydrogen peroxide or chlorhexidine mouthwash for a week after meals.

Implant site selection

Selection of the appropriate position for implant placement is key to a successful result. The ideal position of the implant must be balanced with availability of bone. Primary stability is a prerequisite for osseointegration, and is typically achieved when bone with sufficient thickness (1.5 mm) and quality surrounds the implant in all directions.

Following placement, the implant should ideally be completely embedded in bone. If we were to imagine that the implant is positioned in an osseous 'box', small defects in one of the four box sides could in some cases be tolerated, although a form of grafting should ideally be used. The prognosis without grafting is worse for defects extending to two of the four sides. If defects in more than one side are expected, the case should be planned with grafting in mind.

To maintain vital bone, implants should not be placed closer than 1.5 mm to a nearby tooth or closer than 3 mm to a nearby implant. These considerations particularly apply for implant surgery in the premolar and lower incisor areas. These parameters should be incorporated into the treatment plan so that an implant of an appropriate diameter is chosen and placed at the desired position.

STEPWISE OPERATIVE TECHNIQUE

Conventional approach

For the placement of a single implant, an isolated crestal incision with minimal releasing incisions resulting in a triangular or a trapezoid flap respectively are usually utilised. Vertical release incisions are rarely required for implant surgery. The mucoperiosteum is gently elevated to provide sufficient view of the buccal and the lingual/palatal aspect of the crest. Reflection of the flap over the labial cortical bone for a 1–2 dental implant surgery is unnecessary and further strips the blood supply to the labial bone.

The exact sequence of drills and surgical steps is governed by each specific manufacturer. In practice, the point of implantation is then marked with the use of a round burr followed by a pilot drill. The general principle is the use of progressively wider drills, so that an implant socket of appropriate dimensions for the chosen implant is prepared.

Following each pilot drilling step, placement of a direction guide pin can be used to check the axis of implant placement. If more than one implant is placed, the guide pins allow for parallel placement of the implants. When using surgical guides, care must be taken to allow unrestricted flow of the coolant fluids to the drills.

When the surrounding bone is not dense enough, a condensing drill or socket dilators can be used, in part, to prepare the implant recipient site. Several systems require the use of some shaping drills in the end, to change, for example, the implant socket shape from cylindrical to conical.

Once the implant socket has been sufficiently prepared, the implant can be transferred in the bone. Most systems allow placement of the implants either using the implant drill or a handheld ratchet. A common practice is to utilise the drill up to the final few millimetres of placement, subsequently using the ratchet to finetune the placement but also to get a feel for the stability of the implant.

The next step depends on the treatment plan; if a direct or early loading protocol is to be used, a healing abutment is used, and the wound is closed around this abutment. If the surgeon has elected to allow the implant to heal and integrate before loading, a healing screw is placed and the mucoperiosteal flap is brought back and sutured to its original place. In the case that a healing screw is used, this needs to be removed and exchanged with a healing abutment once the healing period has completed and the implant is ready to be loaded. Usually, a crestal incision suffices in this instance; the mucoperiosteum is deflected and once the implant is localised, the screws are exchanged, and the wound is closed around the healing abutment.

Wound closure is achieved using resorbable sutures with emphasis on achieving a soft tissue seal around transmucosal healing abutments when in one-stage surgery cases.

Guided surgery/flapless surgery

The advent of guided surgery has considerably changed the practice of implant surgery by offering unprecedented capabilities of precise design and planning and outcome predictability. A more prosthesis-driven approach was made feasible by computer-aided design and manufacturing techniques. Moreover, the exact pre-surgical localisation of dental implants allowed for the option of a more conservative surgical approach, that is, flapless surgery.

For guided surgery, a combination of CBCT scan, digital impressions and appropriate planning software with an implant library are used to locate exactly the implant position in the maxilla or the mandible, so that the desired prosthesis can be appropriately supported. This surgical planning can be transferred to the patient with the aid of a computer-aided designed surgical splint that contains all the information for implant placement such as the exact location, direction of placement and depth of implantation. A CAD/CAM surgical splint can be used for placement of implants with the previously discussed technique.

However, as all these details are predetermined, this voids the necessity of raising a flap for implant placement, making flapless surgery feasible. Thus, once the surgical splint is secured in the correct position (something that can be confirmed utilising several reference points), biopsy punches can be used to remove the gingiva from the location in which the implants are to be positioned.

Possible complications and how to deal with them

A number of intraoperative complications can compromise successful implant placement. The presence of bacteria at the site of placement puts the implant at risk. This is usually observed in cases of immediate implant placement when the preoperative evaluation of the surgical site is inadequate but can also be seen in cases of implant placement in sites with previous infection. In any case, ensuring infection control prior to placement is vital.

A similar complication, also observed mostly in direct implantation cases, is the presence of root remnants in the implant site and the placement of the implants in direct contact with them, thus increasing the chances of infection and implant failure. Atraumatic extraction techniques when implants are to be placed and careful evaluation of the extraction site prior to implant placement can help prevent this complication; however, should this occur, close follow-up is warranted.

In cases of drilling in hard bone, the implant drill can become 'stuck' and difficult to disengage. Should this occur, the burr can be disengaged from the drill and removed from the bone with careful anticlockwise rotation.

The implant placement protocol needs to be adjusted according to the available bone quality. In general, less dense bone requires more careful osteotomy and implant insertion. The removal and reinsertion of implants is not ideal but particularly should be avoided in less dense bone cases. Depending on the intraoperative findings, an implant might need to be countersunk or increased healing time might be required.

Several implant systems utilise a final drill to shape the implant socket as a last step prior to implant placement. Occasionally, use of a final drill in a bone that is not sufficiently dense can result in overpreparation and compromise the implant's primary stability. Therefore, the decision to use a final drill must be made after taking into consideration the quality of the available bone. Should overpreparation occur, grafting might become necessary.

Inadequate planning or intraoperative errors can lead to buccal plate dehiscence after implant placement, with less than 1.5 mm of bone remaining around the implant. This problem occurs in cases of thin alveolar ridge. Ideally, preoperative planning would identify the problem, indicating the need for use of an appropriate technique to widen the ridge before implant placement. However, should the problem become apparent during surgery, grafting must be considered. The loss of the whole buccal plate during placement should prompt the surgeon to remove the implant and graft the site, allowing the site to heal before re-attempting placement of the implant.

Implant pressure necrosis is a rare complication that can occur as a result of over-compression of the crestal bone by over-tightening of the implant. This can lead to bone loss and implant failure. The appropriate torque should be used for implant placement. Observation of higher torque during placement might be an indication of a dense bone that requires the use of a threader.

Incorrect positioning of implants is a common problem and can result in failure of the treatment. In principle, the previously mentioned rules for the minimal distance between implants, and between implants and adjacent teeth, should be used. Similarly, placing the implants too far away from teeth or adjacent implants can become a prosthetic problem. Incorrect implant angulation can also create difficulties for the prosthodontist. Small discrepancies and deviations can, in some cases, be tolerated and corrected (e.g. use of angled abutments and ridge rapping). When the deviation from the desired position is considerable, either a localised osteotomy of the implant bed or removal of the implant and attempted replacement after healing might be necessary.

Misplaced implants in the maxillary antrum or, less frequently, in the nasal cavity, have been described as a complication that requires surgical retrieval. In the mandible, placing the implant too close to, or in, the mandibular canal and injuring the inferior alveolar nerve with resulting sensory deficit is a well-documented complication. If a sensory deficit occurs following implant placement, the site should be clinically and radiologically evaluated. Retracting the implant and relieving the compression may result in improvement, and in some cases resolution. Permanent inferior dental nerve injury is uncommon but suitable cases can be considered for nerve repair.

TOP TIPS AND HAZARDS

- A detailed treatment plan in collaboration with a prosthodontist is vital for successful dental implant surgery.
- The position of dental implant placement must be planned with consideration of aesthetic and restorative needs balanced with anatomical availability of bone.
- Gentle handling of soft tissues, and sufficient cooling of rotary instruments is vital for satisfactory healing and osseointegration.
- Incorrect angulation during implant bed preparation is difficult to correct and attempts at correction can lead to increasing diameter of the implant preparation site and inadequate primary stability.

Chapter 10 Bone Augmentation Techniques in Oral Implantology

Kaveh Shakib, Graham Smith

GENERAL PRINCIPLES

Sufficient bone volume is essential for initial primary stability, leading to successful osseointegration and long-term survival of dental implants. Bone volume is typically restricted by the presence of the maxillary sinus, inferior alveolar nerve and physiological resorption of alveolar height following loss of teeth.

Numerous materials and techniques have been described for reconstruction of implant recipient sites. The selection is governed by the volume, location and morphology of the defect. This chapter focuses on alveolar bone augmentation techniques that can be performed in the office (outpatient) environment.

Classification of grafting materials

- Autogenous bone is harvested from the patient
- Allogenic bone is typically harvested from cadavers
- Xenogenic bone is harvested from a different species (bovine)
- Alloplastic describes inert or synthetic materials

Autogenous bone remains the gold standard graft material. It possesses osteogenic, osteoinductive and osteoconductive properties, whereas allografts have only osteoconductive and possibly inductive properties. Alloplasts are merely osteoconductive.

Bone graft materials may be used either individually or in combination with autogenous bone. Addition of biologically active materials such as platelet-rich plasma and bone morphogenic proteins (BMPs) have been reported. Their use adds to the costs and complexity of the treatment, with no sufficient data to support superior outcomes.

Bone donor sites for office use

Intraoral bone donor sites are suitable for augmentation of up to two implant sites. Larger defects require use of other sites such as iliac crest. *Table 10.1* outlines the potential bone stock of different donor sites.

Suitable intraoral donor sites in maxilla and mandible are shown in *Figure 10.1*. Office-based, harvest of bone shavings from the calvarium and proximal tibia are reported but not widely practiced.

Selection of the appropriate donor site is determined by many factors including bone volume required, type of bone required (cancellous or cortico-cancellous)

TABLE 10.1 Potential bone volume available from various donor sites

Site	Potential bone volume (mL)
Cortical shavings from maxilla/mandible	2–5
Bony exostoses/tori	Variable
Suction-line bone traps	Variable
Mandibular symphysis	5
Mandibular ramus	5–10

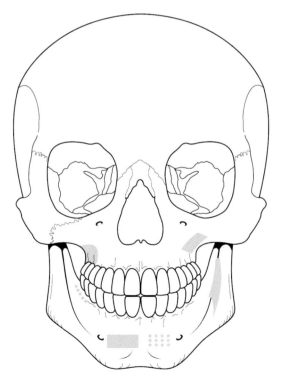

Figure 10.1 Donor sites in the maxilla and mandible.

and the proximity of the donor and reconstruction sites. Harvesting from a donor site in the proximity of the recipient sites reduces the number of surgical sites and postoperative symptoms.

Instrumentation

Harvest of the autogenous graft may be performed using traditional burs, saws, discs, trephines, scrapers, socket dilators, osteotomes and piezosurgery. Titanium microscrews are required to secure onlay grafts.

Bone scrapers are available as single-use or as surgical steel instruments. Single-use bone scrapers are increasingly popular, with the advantage of collection and storage of 2.5 cc of harvested bone.

Rotary trephines can be used to assist with accurate determination of the depth and diameter of the cortical bone harvest.

Piezosurgery uses a range of tips that oscillate at ultrasonic frequencies, cutting bone while preserving soft tissue. The reported advantages of piezosurgery over traditional rotary instruments include lack of thermal injury or bone necrosis and that osteocytes remain viable at the osteotomy site.

General note about bone grafting procedures

Intraoral bone grafting procedures are performed under a combination of short- and long-acting local anaesthetics with vasoconstrictors. Addition of intravenous sedation enhances the patient experience and improves tolerance of involved procedures.

Perioperative antibiotics such as amoxycillin, co-amoxiclav or clindamycin should be administered enterally or parenterally. Local preparation includes chlorhexidine mouth rinse preoperatively.

Postoperative management

Most surgeons continue antibiotic therapy for 5–7 days. The donor sites can remain painful for several days and generous analgesia is recommended. Application of an ice pack immediately post-surgery provides comfort and reduces swelling. Patients should maintain meticulous oral hygiene care and in addition to brushing, use saline, hydrogen peroxide or chlorhexidine mouthwash for 2 weeks after meals. The diet should be restricted to soft consistency for 24 hours and advanced to normal over time to minimise the risk of wound dehiscence.

DONOR SITES

Mandibular symphysis

There is a limited supply of cancellous bone in this region, but there is adequate cortical bone stock to augment up to 1.5–2 cm in length, 1 cm in height and 4–7 mm in thickness. Some reports suggest superior bone quality at the grafted site when the bone is

harvested from the symphysis compared with other sites including the iliac crest.

Preoperative assessment

Cone beam computed tomography (CBCT) provides assessment of volume of bone, and allows identification of residual pathology (retained roots, cysts), delayed healing of sockets, indication of the quality of the bone and the anatomic constraints (bony undercuts, deficiencies).

Procedure

Access to the symphysis can be achieved by a vestibular/labial incision 5–7 mm below the mucogingival junction (*Figure 10.2*). Alternatively, a sulcular/crestal incision can be used but this has the potential disadvantage of possibly resulting in bone resorption at the crest if the labial bone is thin, and therefore is reliant on the overlying periosteum for its blood supply.

In common with genioplasty (see *Chapter 56*), a vestibular/labial mucosal incision is made from canine to canine. The bellies of mentalis muscle may need to be divided depending on the level of the mentalis origin. Soft tissues are elevated inferiorly down to the inferior border of the mandible in the subperiosteal plane. The required length of the bone graft dictates the lateral extension of the dissection.

With the anterior mandible exposed, there are some important anatomical constraints that should be outlined prior to performing the osteotomies (*Figure 10.3*). The superior horizontal osteotomy should remain at least 5 mm inferior to the incisor and canine apices. The inferior horizontal osteotomy should maintain at least 5 mm of intact cortical bone at the inferior border. If the lateral osteotomies need to be placed close to the mental foramina for larger grafts, 5 mm of bone should remain anterior to the foramen, as the mental nerve may course anteriorly prior to exiting the mental foramen.

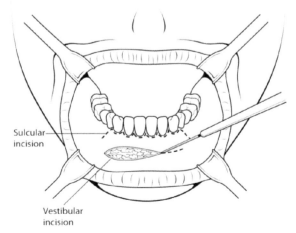

Sulcular incision

Vestibular incision

Figure 10.2 Access incisions for the mandibular symphysis.

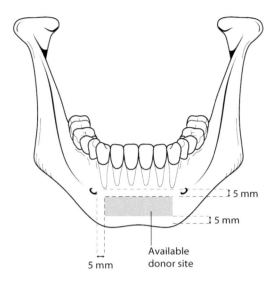

5 mm

5 mm

Available
donor site

5 mm

Figure 10.3 Mandibular symphysis donor site.

Bone may be harvested from the anterior mandible within these anatomic boundaries either using trephines to obtain multiple cores of cortico-cancellous bone (maintaining the integrity of the lingual cortex), or using small fissure burs, saws or piezosurgery tips to outline a block of cortico-cancellous bone. A midline vertical osteotomy may also be made to facilitate removal of two blocks of bone. The bone graft is then removed by completing the osteotomies with curved osteotomes. Small amounts of additional cancellous bone can be harvested up to the lingual cortical plate using curettes.

The soft tissues are closed in layered fashion, resuspending the bellies of the mentalis muscles prior to closure of the mucosal incision with sutures.

There are advocates for augmenting the donor site with allogenic bone or collagen soaked in BMP and covered with a resorbable membrane. The rationale is to minimise the bony defect after the healing phase compared with simply closing the soft tissues. The disadvantage includes additional cost of BMPs and risk of infection of the resorbable membranes.

Complications

Possible complications include bleeding, haematoma, infection, wound dehiscence, mental nerve injury, incisor/canine devitalisation and mandible fracture. The donor site can remain painful for a number of weeks. In common with genioplasty, altered muscle attachment and soft tissue chin profile is a risk of this procedure.

Mandibular ramus

The dimensions of the external oblique ridge (EOR) determine the potential size of the graft. Typically, a cortico-cancellous block of bone measuring up to 3 cm in length and 1 cm in height may be obtained from

the ramus, although the thickness of bone is limited to approximately 4 mm due to the underlying inferior alveolar nerve.

Preoperative assessment

Panoramic radiographs are adequate to assess the volume of bone available and the location of the inferior alveolar nerve. CBCT scans add more information, as discussed above.

Procedure

The EOR is accessed through a linear mucosal incision starting at the level of the occlusal plane and extending down into the buccal vestibule as far forward as the first molar region. Traumatic or supra-periosteal lingual flap elevation may cause lingual nerve injury. The osteotomies may be created with burs, microsaws or piezosurgery tips. The posterior vertical osteotomy is made through the outer cortex perpendicular to the external oblique ridge at the level of the occlusal plane, or at a point of adequate thickness. The anterior vertical osteotomy is also made through the outer cortex. The distance between the posterior and anterior cut is determined by the desired graft length and may extend as far forward as the distal aspect of the first molar tooth. The height of these cuts corresponds to the height of the desired graft. The posterior and anterior osteotomies are then connected superiorly with a horizontal osteotomy 3–4 mm in depth. The depth of all these cuts is monocortical. The inferior connecting cuts are made with a round bur or an angled piezosurgery tip. The inferior cut simply scores the cortex, enabling fracture along this line during subsequent luxation of the graft with osteotomes. Thin osteotomes are used to complete the osteotomies staying along the buccal cortical plate to avoid potential injury to the inferior alveolar nerve. Larger osteotomes are then used to free the block of bone (*Figure 10.4*). Caution is needed to ensure the inferior alveolar nerve is not tethered to the graft prior to removal. The bed of the osteotomy is then inspected where the inferior alveolar nerve may be visualised. Small amounts of cancellous bone may be removed with curettes while being mindful of the location of the nerve. It is not usually necessary to graft the donor site as bony regeneration is adequate.

Complications

Complications include haematoma, infection, wound dehiscence and inferior alveolar or lingual nerve injury. The incidence of sensory deficit following ramus harvest is reported to be lower than that at symphyseal harvest, at 8% and 16%, respectively.

Maxillary tuberosity and zygomaticomaxillary buttress

The volume of bone available from these sites is limited but may be mixed with allogenic material for added

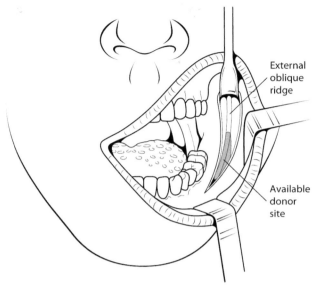

Figure 10.4 Mandibular ramus donor site.

volume. There is evidence of increased graft resistance to resorption with addition of artificial hydroxy appetite material. Once a standard mucoperiosteal flap is elevated, bone shavings can be harvested from these sites using shaving devices to remove bone from the tuberosity area taking care not to enter the maxillary antrum. There is also the option of removing a small and thin window of bone from the anterior maxillary wall in the buttress region. This window is typically only 2–3 mm thick and 1 cm × 1 cm in dimension.

RECIPIENT SITE TECHNIQUES

Onlay graft

Vertical augmentation is challenging. Onlay grafts may be used to augment the width and/or the height of the alveolus. Harvested bone should be kept moist until grafting. The success of onlay grafts relies on recipient bed vascularity, close approximation and contact between graft and the recipient site, and immobilisation.

The incision for the recipient site may be made at the crest of the ridge or in the vestibule. Incisions on the crest give easy access but they are often directly over the graft and are at risk of dehiscence with subsequent graft failure and loss. Incisions placed in the vestibule are away from the graft, but the flap relies on perfusion from the lingual or palatal side and is therefore at risk for breakdown, especially if the crest is composed of dense fibrous tissue.

The recipient bed should be prepared to allow close approximation between the recipient bed and the onlay graft, as well as improved immobilisation of the graft. This is often achieved by reduction of convexities and mortising the bed to receive the graft. A small bur may

be used to perforate the recipient site as well as the graft itself. The recipient site perforations are monocortical. This is performed to encourage capillary ingrowth and vascularisation. The block is then stabilised using two 1.2-mm diameter screws to avoid rotation (*Figure 10.5*). The screws should be positioned at accessible sites to aid future removal. If greater width is desired than the thickness of the graft will allow, the graft may be placed as two layers, or secured using positioning screws leaving space under the graft that can be filled with cancellous bone or allogenic bone (*Figure 10.6*). Any sharp edges of the graft are smoothed to reduce the chance of mucosal breakdown. Cancellous bone or allogenic bone may be placed around the periphery to further augment the site and anticipate some postoperative resorption. This particulate bone graft may also be placed as an interpositional graft between the block

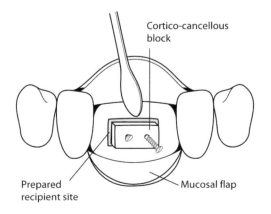

Figure 10.5 Mortised onlay graft.

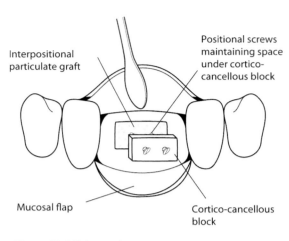

Figure 10.6 Onlay graft.

graft and recipient site for contour discrepancies that may create unfavourable surgical dead space and soft tissue ingrowth. Membranes may be overlaid onto the graft, although many surgeons feel that this increases the risk of wound dehiscence and infection. However, if the periosteum is to be released and additional particulate bone graft is used around the margins of the block graft, a membrane should be considered. Loose and unstable particulate bone graft should not be introduced into tissue planes deep to the periosteum.

Augmentation of the height of alveolar bone does not restore the soft tissue deficiency and soft tissue coverage can be challenging. Tension-free closure over the site is vital to minimise the risk of wound dehiscence, which may result in graft failure. Prior to closure, the buccal periosteum may need to be incised and undermined to allow advancement of the flap. The grafted site should be allowed to heal and consolidate for 4–6 months prior to implant placement.

Maxillary sinus grafting

The edentulous posterior maxilla is often occupied by a large pneumatised antrum, resulting in vertical bone deficiency. Grafting the floor of the sinus increases the vertical dimension of bone available for successful implant placement. Until recently, this has been performed with simultaneous placement of the implants if there was at least 3 mm of native bone height to provide primary stability. With less than 3 mm of bone height, implant placement was deferred to a second procedure 4–6 months following the sinus graft. Recent literature reports successful implant placement in as little as 1 mm of native bone height, provided there is adequate width (>8 mm). It may be that the quality (density) of the recipient bone is more important than height. Undersized drilling of implant osteotomy site provides additional primary stability.

Preoperative preparation

CBCT scans provide detailed three-dimensional visualisation of the sinus floor and surrounding walls, including the presence of septae within the sinus. In addition, scans allow visualisation of the sinus mucosa. Patients with sinusitis or sinus disease should be managed before grafting.

Procedure

Access to the sinus is performed through a window in the lateral wall. A crestal or sulcular incision is made away from the bony window. Once a full-thickness mucoperiosteal flap is elevated and the lateral wall of the maxilla and sinus is exposed, a 1 cm × 1.5 cm bony window is created anterior to the zygomaticomaxillary buttress (*Figure 10.7*).

The superior osteotomy is placed inferior to the infraorbital nerve at the level of the planned graft height, while the inferior osteotomy should lie approximately 3 mm above the floor of the sinus to avoid the multiple septations and recesses often encountered along the sinus floor, which make completing the osteotomy and infracturing the bony window problematic. The bony window is created using a diamond bur or a piezosurgery tip to minimise the chance of Schneiderian membrane perforation. Alternatively, the bony outline of the osteotomy can be thinned using a narrow

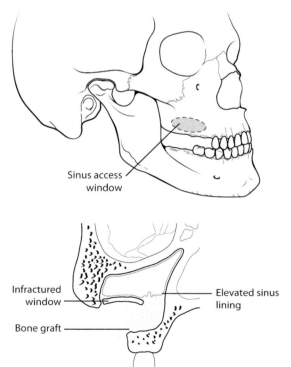

Figure 10.7 Sinus lift/augmentation.

bone scraper device. Small Schneiderian membrane perforations (<3 mm) are inconsequential, but larger perforations should be covered with a resorbable membrane after elevation of the lining and prior to insertion of the graft. Once the bony window is created and the sinus lining is visible around the periphery, sinus curettes are used to carefully mobilise and elevate the Schneiderian membrane with the cortical window still attached. Once mobilised, the membrane and bony window are turned into the sinus such that the bony segment now becomes the new elevated sinus floor. The space beneath the elevated bony segment and the lining is filled with bone or substitute graft material (*Figure 10.7*). The volume of the graft placed should allow for 20% resorption prior to implant placement. The average volume of graft material required to augment the sinus is 1–2 cc. Autogenous bone remains the gold standard, but this may be mixed with or even substituted with allogenic bone with good success.

To close the site, a resorbable membrane is placed over the bony window and the mucoperiosteal flap is sutured with resorbable sutures.

Postoperative management

In addition to the usual postoperative management of intraoral graft sites, patients should be instructed in sinus precautions. These are especially important if the sinus lining was perforated, and should include no nose blowing for at least 3 weeks and use of nasal decongestants and saline nasal spray.

Complications

Potential complications include infection, acute maxillary sinusitis, wound breakdown and subsequent failure of the graft, injury to the infraorbital nerve, injury to adjacent teeth and oro-antral fistula. Patients with a history of chronic sinusitis are at higher risk of developing infection and loss of bone grafts.

Alveolar bone splitting/spreading

Osteotomies along the alveolar crest may be performed to increase the width of the alveolus (*Figure 10.8*). To maintain blood supply to the osteotomised inner and outer segments, the periosteum is left attached to the bone. This is achieved by a crestal or vestibular incision, and a supraperiosteal dissection of the labial or buccal mucosal flap. The crestal osteotomy may be made with a saw, a small fissure bur or a piezosurgery tip. The vertical osteotomies may be carried through both inner and outer cortical plates. The vertical osteotomies are usually 1 cm in height. Once the osteotomies are made, osteotomes are driven into the crestal cut and the cortical plate(s) are pedicled on the overlying periosteum. The intervening space may then be implanted or grafted with bone graft materials. The segments and intervening graft may be stabilised using screws for immobilisation during the healing phase. Some surgeons prefer covering the site with a resorbable membrane prior to suturing.

Segmental alveolar bone distraction osteogenesis

Distraction osteogenesis is an emerging method for alveolar tissue reconstruction. This technique avoids the need for bone grafts and restores both hard and soft tissue deficiencies resulting in superior aesthetic and functional outcome.

A vestibular mucosal incision is made and a buccal mucoperiosteal flap elevated, exposing the lateral cortex, without elevation of the crestal mucosa. The segmental osteotomy is planned immediately adjacent to neighbouring teeth to gain full defect coverage but avoiding damage to periodontium.

The vertical distractor is placed into the desired position and the microplates are bent carefully to the mandibular shape. The vector of the distraction should be checked to avoid occlusal interferences. In this position, one hole is drilled on either side of the microplates and a monocortical microscrew is inserted.

The distractor is removed and the osteotomy line is marked with a small bur or a piezosurgery tip. The osteotomies are completed using a reciprocating microsaw. The segment is now entirely mobilised using fine chisels lingually. The distractor is then refixed in the

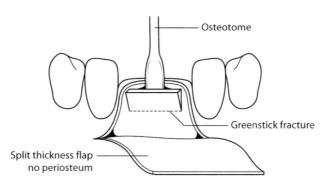

Figure 10.8 Alveolar ridge splitting.

same position and secured with screws. The function of the distractor is finally checked, including possible interference of the distraction rod with the occlusion.

After 5–7 days, the distraction can start at the rate of 1 mm per day. Once the desired bone height is achieved, the consolidation phase sets in, extending over 8–12 weeks. During this period, the distractor is left in place to stabilise the new soft bone. Removal of the distractor is performed with simultaneous implant insertion.

Complications

Specific complications of distraction osteogenesis include relapse, infection, inappropriate distraction vector, asymmetrical distraction, device loosening, device failure and fusion error.

Transalveolar osteotome sinus lift

This procedure is designed to increase the density and height of bone where at least 5 mm of height is available. Compression of the adjacent bone and elevation of the sinus floor is accomplished using osteotomes via a transalveolar approach. The sinus floor may be elevated up to 5 mm without perforation of the sinus membrane.

Procedure

A mid-crestal incision is made without vertical releasing incisions. Small-diameter pilot drills and implant drills are used to prepare the implant site. It is important to underprepare the implant site by 0.5–1 mm smaller than the intended implant width. The implant site should be prepared with careful consideration to avoid perforation of the sinus floor. There should be 2 mm of bone between the most apical extent of site preparation and the maxillary sinus floor (*Figure 10.9*). At this point, a tapered osteotome with a concave cup-ended tip is applied vertically into the implant site and used to create a greenstick fracture of the maxillary sinus and push the sinus floor apically, increasing the length of the implant preparation. The concave and cutting edge of the osteotome tip will both harvest bone from the adjacent walls and compress the bone in an apical direction. The mallet force should be carefully controlled to prevent membrane perforation. A second tapered osteotome with a larger diameter than the first is used to increase both the width and vertical height of the osteotomy. Round-tipped osteotomes may be used as depth guides between osteotomies to confirm the preparation height. The last osteotome used should be 0.5 mm less than the implant width. To optimise, preserve and condense bone, the use of commercially available magnetic mallet kits should be considered. After instrumentation of the membrane superiorly, additional space is created to house particulate bone graft. Many surgeons will not perform further internal sinus membrane manipulation once the desired height of implant is achieved by intrusion alone. Implant placement may then be performed with or without additional grafting material.

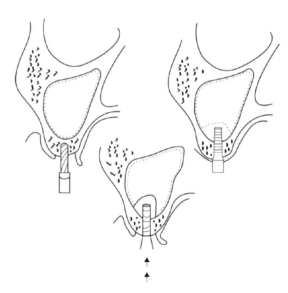

Figure 10.9 Transalvoelar osteotome sinus lift.

TOP TIPS AND HAZARDS

- Autogenous bone is considered the gold standard due to its osteoblastic, osteoinductive and osteoconductive properties.
- Cancellous grafts vascularise more rapidly than cortico-cancellous grafts.
- The mandibular symphysis provides blocks of cortico-cancellous bone measuring up to 1.5–2 cm in length, 1 cm in height and 4–7 mm thickness.
- The mandibular ramus provides cortico-cancellous blocks of bone measuring up to 3 cm in length, 1 cm in height and 4 mm thickness.
- Implants may be placed simultaneously with open sinus floor augmentation with 1 mm or more of native bone height if there is adequate width of 8 mm.
- Implant length may be heightened with the use of the transalveolar osteotome sinus lift. Preparation for implantation should be approximately 2 mm from the sinus floor prior to intrusion.

Bailey & Love's Essential Operations Bailey & Love's Essential Operations
Bailey & Love's Essential Operations Bailey & Love's Essential Operations
Bailey & Love's Essential Operations Bailey & Love's Essential Operations

PART 2 | Oral surgery and implantology

Chapter 11

Craniofacial Implantology

Greg Boyes-Varley, Dale Howes

INTRODUCTION

There are a variety of surgical techniques which can be used in the craniofacial region to facilitate an implant-supported prosthetic rehabilitation in patients. Modified reconstruction procedures can be applied when the facial skeleton has insufficient bone for conventional implant placement, and bone grafting is advocated to create adequate bone volume for implant placement to restore the severely resorbed or resected jaws. Newly grafted bone should ideally remain load-free to allow consolidation and revascularisation for 4 months, thus staged bone graft techniques increase the overall treatment time. There are, however, options for immediate loading depending on the types of implants used.

ZYGOMATIC IMPLANTS, INCLUDING QUADS AND PTERYGOID IMPLANTS

Continuous bone resorption and maxillary sinus pneumatisation is thought to cause maxillary atrophy, which can be unbearable for denture-wearers. The zygomatic implant provides the clinician with an alternative to bone grafting procedures. Brånemark designed the technique for use in 1989, with a reported success rate of 97%.

The implant body traverses the posterior maxillary alveolus, lateral sinus wall into the body of the zygoma, with sub-crestal angular correction of the coronal aspect of the implant allowing for appropriate tooth position. The use of a 55° restorative head (Southern Implants, Irene, South Africa) is preferable to reduce

the buccal cantilever by 20%, with implant placement close to the crest of the edentulous ridge, allowing restorative clinicians to achieve ideal tooth position in the posterior maxilla.

Diagnostic radiology

Radiological assessment of the maxilla can be used to detect maxillary sinus pathology, and evaluate alveolar bone volume and zygomatic body size. Recommended radiological views are panoramic and occipitomental (OM) views, to detect bone height and sinus pathology, and radiological digital imaging data (DICOM) from medical computed tomography (CT) scans, which facilitate stereolithographic model manufacture for surgical planning and prosthodontic rehabilitation. Cone beam CT (CBCT) technology is somewhat superior in tooth-loss cases.

Surgical technique

The position of the incisura of the zygoma is fixed and provides a superior pivot point for the zygoma implant. The apical exit point of the implant in the inferolateral orbital margin should avoid orbital perforation. Using the implant apex as a pivot point and moving the head distally in the maxilla uprights the restorative head into the first molar site, instead of the second premolar site (*Figure 11.1*).

Depending on the patient's anatomy, the lateral sinus wall is engaged by the implant for optimal position; occasionally the body of the implant may be outside the bony envelope (*Figure 11.2*). The head of the implant in the maxillary alveolus is placed as close as possible to the mid-alveolar position of the ridge.

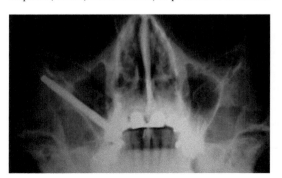

Figure 11.1 Occipitomental radiograph

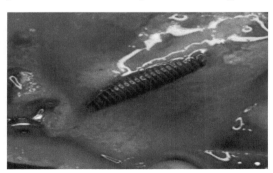

Figure 11.2 Lateral maxillary wall.

Zygomatic implant placement is usually performed under general anaesthesia. However, it is possible to undertake this procedure under sedation and local anaesthesia. *Figures 11.3–11.7* illustrate the process of implant placement.

Crestal mucosal incision extends from maxillary tuberosity to tuberosity (for bilateral implant insertion), periosteal elevation exposes the maxilla, piriform aperture, infraorbital nerves and the inferior aspect of the body of the zygoma. A lateral window in the superolateral aspect of the maxillary antrum is created, with sinus mucosa reflection. The proposed point of entry of the fixture into the zygomatic bone is demarcated through the sinus window (*Figures 11.3* and *11.4*).

Site preparation follows with graded twist drills. Care is taken not to perforate into the orbit or infratemporal fossa (*Figure 11.5*).

The zygomatic implant (55° head angulation, Southern Implants) is placed and a guide pin positioned for appropriate fixture rotation ensuring optimal position (*Figures 11.6* and *11.7*).

Balshi describes the use of quadratic zygomatic implants for maxillary rehabilitation using only two zygomatic fixtures per quadrant with rehabilitation of the atrophic maxilla with a fixed prosthesis of 10/12 teeth, avoiding extensive bone grafting (*Figures 11.8–11.15*).

Quad zygomatic implant placement uses the premolar site and canine or lateral incisor positions. Care should be taken to avoid perforation into the inferolateral aspect of the orbit. Postoperative radiology is mandatory to establish the implant position.

Immediate loading of the implants with a fixed temporary polymethyl methacrylate (PMMA) prosthesis is possible, which remains in place for 3–4 months and is then replaced with a permanent zirconia prosthesis.

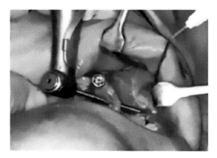

Figure 11.5 Trans-maxillary drill into the zygoma.

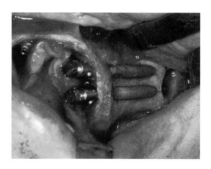

Figure 11.6 Implant placed.

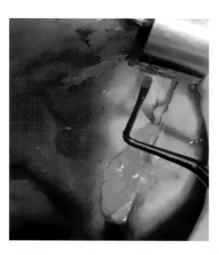

Figure 11.3 Osteotomy in supero-lateral sinus wall.

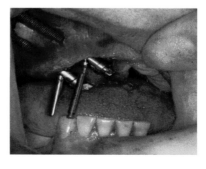

Figure 11.7 Guide pin.

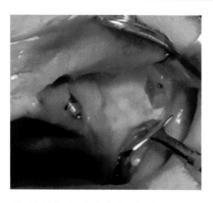

Figure 11.4 Initial pilot hole in body of zygoma.

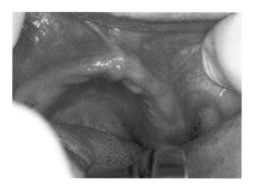

Figure 11.8 Edentulous ridge.

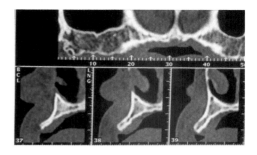

Figure 11.9 Cone beam computed tomography of maxilla.

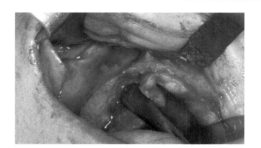

Figure 11.10 Exposed ridge.

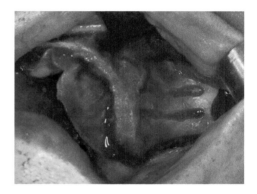

Figure 11.11 Osteotomy sites maxilla.

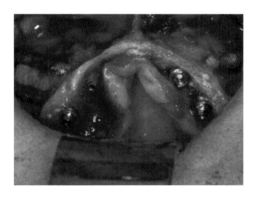

Figure 11.12 Implants *in situ*.

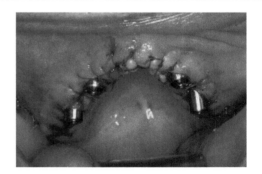

Figure 11.13 Implants exposed.

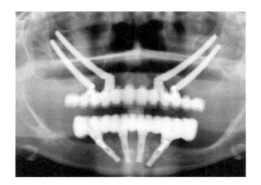

Figure 11.14 Final radiograph.

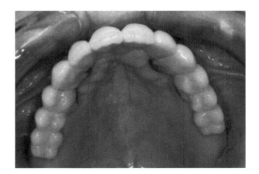

Figure 11.15 Final prosthesis.

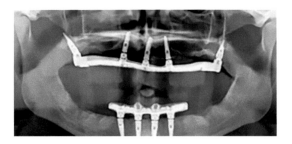

Figure 11.16 Pterygoid implant.

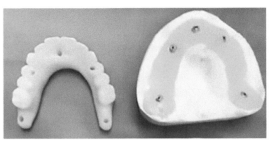

Figure 11.17 Pterygoid prosthesis.

Pterygoid implants

The posterior maxilla is limited due to sinus pneumatisation, and using the tuberosity and pterygoid plate region is an alternative to sinus lifting procedures. Pterygoid implants can be used to provide distal anchorage for a prosthesis if there is insufficient bone in the posterior maxilla. This acts as an alternative or adjunct to sinus grafting procedures and zygomatic implant placement. A root form implant with a narrow apex is best suited. A full-thickness flap is raised to the most distal aspect of the maxillary alveolar crest. Preparation of the site is feeling for cortical bone at the junction between pterygoid plates and the maxilla, on average 15 mm from the crest. The cortical bone in this area provides a predictable site for immediate loading (*Figures 11.16* and *11.17*).

Narrow apex zygomatic implants

The original design of the zygomatic implant body has been modified many times over the past 20 years by various manufacturing companies. The first significant change of the implant body in 2001 was the changed head angulation to 55°, then, in 2003, smooth shafted implant bodies were introduced for oncology and, in 2009, the prosthetic screw channel in the implant head was closed (Southern Implants).

In 2016, narrow apex implants were introduced as many surgeons found it difficult to predictably place two conventional zygomatic implant bodies into small zygomas and the introduction of the Zygan and Zygex (Southern Implants) implant bodies was advocated, in combination with a smooth shafted midsection (*Figure 11.18*).

The narrow apex implant allows for a reduced number of revolutions of the implant body within the alveolus and reduces compression, frictional heat generation and potential fracture of the buccal alveolar bone. The introduction of a purer titanium, with two significant advances in the production of the metal (a vacuum-assisted remelt, VAR and a new rolling mills process, RMP) produced an implant body with a 40% improvement in fatigue strength and the ability to produce a stronger pure titanium implant body.

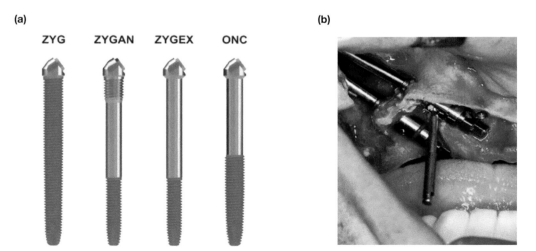

Figure 11.18 (a) Zygomatic implant range. (b) Quad Zygan implants.

ZYGOMATIC IMPLANTS AND GUNSHOT RECONSTRUCTION

Facial trauma from gunshot wounds is common in some parts of the world. Midface gunshot wounds ablate tissue structures in the path of the missile, akin to oncology resection following maxillectomy. Similar treatment protocols are used to rehabilitate these patients. The area of cavitation between the entrance and exit wounds produces hard and soft tissue defects, secondary missile defects of bone, fractured tooth fragments and soft tissue destruction. Initial treatment is resuscitation, debridement, facial bone fracture reduction and soft tissue closure. Further details in the management of ballistic injuries are provided in *Chapter 21*.

Prosthetic rehabilitation usually takes place 3–6 months after the initial repair. 3D Spiral CT and CBCT imaging are useful, and the implant choice is site-specific with a combination of standard and zygomatic implants using immediate loading protocols.

Maxillary defects resulting from ablation/avulsion injury can be functionally and aesthetically rehabilitated with standard implantology and fixed-removable prosthodontic principles.

ZYGOMATIC IMPLANTS AND ONCOLOGY RECONSTRUCTION

Tumours of the craniofacial region can result in facial disfigurement because of the tissue damage due to direct tumour damage and following surgical intervention. Surgery and subsequent radiotherapy can modify the life-supporting functions of mastication and speech due to altered facial soft and bony anatomy. Dental rehabilitation requires functional and aesthetic considerations when planning the proposed reconstruction.

Reconstruction depends on the resultant bony and soft tissue defect, and obturation requires a close working relationship between the surgical and prosthetic teams. Prosthetic designs have evolved and osseointegration has revolutionised facial reconstruction in these cases. A major advantage of initial endosseous implant rehabilitation over vascularised free flaps is the ability of the surgeon to inspect the resection cavity for recurrent disease opposed to periodic radiographic assessment with the CT, magnetic resonance imaging (MRI) and positron emission tomography (PET) scans. The placement of endosseous implants facilitates prosthodontic rehabilitation, which allows for aesthetic and functional replacement of ablated hard and soft tissue, and minimises the use of silicone bulbs, obturators and dentures.

Phase 1: Diagnosis

Incisional biopsy is performed to obtain a definitive histological diagnosis and tumour grading, facilitating optimal surgical and postoperative radio/chemotherapy protocols. Patients undergo standardised preoperative radiological survey, including orthopantomogram, and staging CT/MRI scans. A stereolithographic model is constructed from the CT DICOM data and resection surgery is simulated with optimal implant positions and confirmation of prosthetic design (*Figures 11.19–11.21*). A surgical guide and temporary obturator is made.

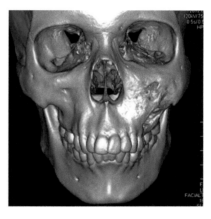

Figure 11.19 Computed tomography scan.

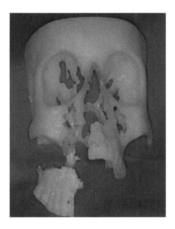

Figure 11.20 Simulated surgery.

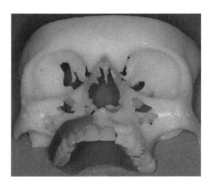

Figure 11.21 Obturator design.

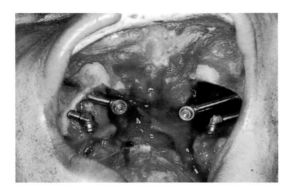

Figure 11.22 Zygomatic implants in the zygomatic stump.

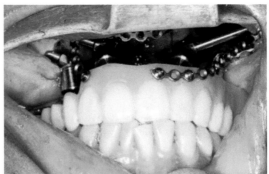

Figure 11.23 Temp obturator in place.

Phase 2: Tumour resection, immediate implant placement and obturation

Surgical access and airway management is decided upon by the surgical team and maxillectomy with adequate resection margins is carried out, together with frozen sections of the resection margins to ensure complete tumour excision.

Implant placement

The objective of implant placement is to 'recreate' the buttresses of the maxilla for appropriate force distribution of the prosthetic rehabilitation. A combination of standard and modified zygomatic 'oncology' implants is used to lower the restorative platform to the level of the palate (Southern Implants) (*Figure 11.22*).

After implant placement, an obturator is modified intraoperatively to restore normal soft tissue facial contour if a soft tissue vascularised flap is not planned at resection surgery. The obturator is secured by transosseous titanium screws, and soft tissue wound edges are closed (*Figure 11.23*).

The fixed dento-alveolar segment is manufactured by the laboratory, as well as a smaller palatal interim obturator.

Postoperative radiographs are taken to confirm the position of the implants within the bone and the prosthesis is firmly secured to the implants intraorally (*Figure 11.24*).

Phase 3: Maintenance

The surgical site is monitored by the oncologist and reconstructive teams for adequate postoperative healing and long-term recurrence. Prosthetic maintenance is ongoing, and extensive soft tissue change occurs in the first year. The obturators require peripheral adjustment and regular oral hygiene instructions.

Occasionally, the patient may request that the removable obturator be replaced with a soft tissue flap to seal the oral from the nasal environment due

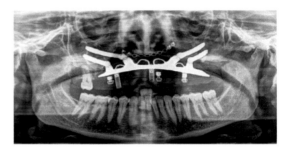

Figure 11.24 Radiograph of implants.

to persistent air, fluid and food escape. In such cases, the patient is investigated for tumour recurrence and if found to be tumour-free, a microvascular free tissue is used to seal the oral from the nasal cavity usually with a radial forearm or anterolateral thigh free flap (*Figure 11.25*).

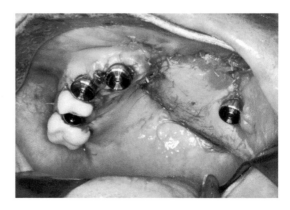

Figure 11.25 Implants *in situ* with facial forearm free flap in defect site.

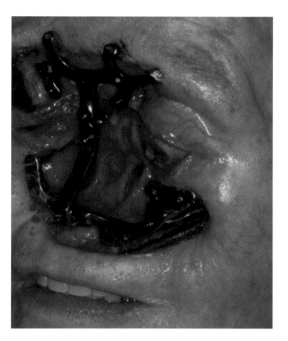

Figure 11.26 Facial dolder bar.

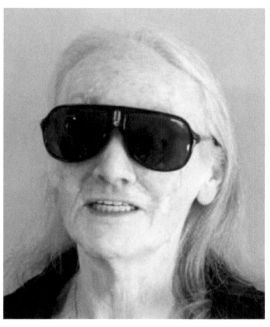

Figure 11.27 Final prosthesis.

NASO-MAXILLARY RECONSTRUCTION AND CRANIAL IMPLANTS

Malignant tumours presenting in the anterior maxilla and nasal area often require complex naso-maxillary resection and rehabilitation using a combined intraoral and extraoral prosthesis (*Figures 11.26* and *11.27*).

Nasal prostheses are generally implant retained with sufficient anchorage using two standard zygomatic fixtures placed horizontally in combination with standard implantology into the anterior maxillary floor.

MICROVASCULAR FREE TISSUE TRANSFERS IN COMBINATION WITH ONCOLOGY ZYGOMATIC IMPLANTS

Permanent palatal defect closure with autogenous free vascularised tissue can be achieved with a zygomatic implant perforated microvascular soft tissue flap (ZIP flap) technique as described by Butterworth and Rogers (2017).

Zygomatic implants placed at primary resection surgery perforate the soft tissue reconstruction flap and support a fixed maxillary dental prosthesis. The technique allows rapid return to function and appearance following low-level maxillary resection, even where radiotherapy is required as an adjuvant treatment postoperatively. The technique is a single-stage improvement on the two-stage technique where maxillary defects are reconstructed with radial forearm free flaps with subsequent zygomatic implant placement used to support the provision of a bar-retained overdenture.

TOP TIPS AND HAZARDS

- Careful planning is the key to a successful prosthetic rehabilitation. The prosthodontist and maxillofacial laboratory team should be involved from the beginning.
- Achieving a satisfactory prosthesis involves multiple adjustments over several weeks, which some patients may find frustrating and cumbersome. Therefore, appropriate counselling is paramount before the treatment starts.
- A tissue transfer reconstructive option may be desired for those who lack the level of manual dexterity required to be able to use a prosthesis.

ACKNOWLEDGEMENTS

The authors wish to acknowledge the contribution made by Southern Implants for technical development of the zygomatic oncology implants and EvoDental (UK) for photogrammetry concepts.

FURTHER READING

Balshi JT, Wolfinger GJ, Petropoulos VC. Quadruple zygomatic implant support for retreatment of resorbed iliac crest bone graft transplant. *Implant Dent* 2003;**12**:47–53.

Boyes-Varley JG, Howes DG, Davidge-Pitts KD, et al. A protocol for maxillary reconstructions following oncology resection using zygomatic implants. *Int J Prosthodont* 2007;**20**:151–61.

Boyes-Varley JG, Howes DG, Lownie JF, et al. Surgical modifications to the Brånemark zygomaticus protocol in the treatment of the severely resorbed maxilla: a clinical report. *Int J Oral Maxillofac Implants* 2003;**18**:232–7.

Butterworth C, Rogers S. The zygomatic implant perforated (ZIP) flap: a new technique for combined surgical reconstruction and rapid fixed dental rehabilitation following low-level maxillectomy. *Int J Implant Dent* 2017;**3**:37

Lekholm U, Wannfors K, Isaksson S, et al. Oral implants in combination with implants. A 3-year retrospective multicenter study using the Brånemark implant system. *Int J Oral Maxillofac Surg* 1999;**28**:181–7.

PART 3 | Trauma
Bailey & Love's Essential Operations Bailey & Love's Essential Operations
Bailey & Love's Essential Operations Bailey & Love's Essential Operations
Bailey & Love's Essential Operations Bailey & Love's Essential Operations

Chapter 12

Facial Trauma Assessment and Emergency Procedures

Rebecca Exley, Ioanna Dimasi

INTRODUCTION

Facial injuries are commonly seen in the hospital setting and are caused by interpersonal violence, road traffic accidents (RTAs), falls, industrial accidents and in sports. It is important to establish a systematic approach to the assessment of the facial skeleton and manage promptly and appropriately all soft and hard tissue injury patterns. Patients can be classified into those who present with isolated facial injuries and those combined with other injuries. The latter are often managed in a major trauma setting.

It is mandatory to manage all trauma patients as per the Advanced Trauma Life Support (ATLS) Protocol. While a brief description of ATLS principles will be discussed in this chapter, the main focus is on the initial emergency and diagnostic management with reference to the role of the Oral and Maxillofacial (OMF) Surgeon.

INITIAL ASSESSMENT: ATLS PRINCIPLES

It is crucial to understand how oral and maxillofacial injuries might impact aspects of the ABCDE assessment. An OMF surgeon can play an essential role in both the primary and secondary surveys. The treating clinician must stabilise and reassess at every step before moving to the next stage.

Airway and C-spine

Identify any bleeding from the oral cavity or dental fragments, which can obstruct the airway. Consider endotracheal intubation if neck wounds or haematomas cause airway obstruction. For this, rapid sequence induction is required while maintaining C-spine immobilisation.

The airway can be obstructed in mandibular fractures that compromise the anterior tongue attachment (e.g. symphyseal fractures or bilateral angle 'bucket handle' fractures). This can lead to posterior displacement of the tongue and loss of the airway.

Head injuries can also impair the level of consciousness and tongue position.

Assessment

The assessment should begin by inspecting the oropharynx for any foreign bodies. A suction can be used to aid assessment, especially if there is bleeding or secretions. It is crucial to account for missing teeth by history, examination and imaging. High-flow oxygen is applied with the aim of saturations of 94–98%.

- Consider the history of the injury
- Inspect
- High-volume suction
- Jaw manoeuvres – jaw thrust. Mandibular fractures may be stabilised with a bridle wire
- Airway adjuncts – oropharyngeal or nasopharyngeal airways
- Consider endotracheal intubation with or without the aid of a bougie
- Surgical procedures (*Figure 12.1*) – cricothyroidotomy

Emergency procedure

Cricothyroidotomy

- Extend neck if possible – consider history and protect the C-spine.
- Establish landmarks:
  ○ Thyroid cartilage notch
  ○ Cricoid cartilage
  ○ Cricothyroid membrane in between.

- Prep the skin.
- Anaesthetise the skin if time permits.
- Make a 2–3-cm vertical incision through the skin followed by a 1–2 cm transverse incision through the cricothyroid membrane with a large blade. Insert the scalpel handle and rotate 90°.
- Insert special tube or a paediatric endotracheal tube (size 5/6).

Note: In the case of devastating neck injury or swelling, laryngeal trauma thyroid or cricoid disruption then formal tracheostomy should be considered.

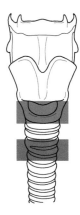

Figure 12.1 The larynx demonstrating points of surgical access. The emergency anterior neck access point is via a cricothyroidotomy (blue box), the semi-elective access is via a tracheostomy (red box).

Breathing

Auscultation of the lungs as well as percussion should be performed in the acute setting. Inhalation of foreign bodies may compromise breathing causing stridor or stertor. Of particular interest are dental injuries, where fragments of the tooth or the whole tooth can be aspirated. It is important to establish whether there is any missing dentition and the location during examination. If the teeth fragments cannot be identified, a chest radiograph should be scrutinised and reported by a radiologist.

Circulation

Injuries to the soft tissues of the face and scalp as well as the oral cavity and the nose can bleed profusely, compromising the circulating volume. A thorough clinical examination is paramount and any active bleeding should be stopped. Intraoral bleeding can be challenging in the acute setting as access is often limited by the endotracheal tube (ETT), or the cervical hard collar. An assistant can maintain C-spine immobilisation to allow for the front of the collar to be temporarily removed. This permits the mouth to be opened and the oral cavity to be inspected. A laryngoscope or bite blocks can be used to aid visualisation.

Shock should be recognised and managed with judicious fluid resuscitation, initially a 1-litre bolus of warmed crystalloid should be given, and the response assessed. Severe shock activates the major haemorrhage protocol, the patient can be given a bolus 1 g tranexamic acid intravenously followed by an 8-hourly IV infusion to help slow the bleeding. Fresh frozen plasma (4 units) and packed red cells (4 units) should be given in a 1:1 ratio and cryoprecipitate 2 pools should be considered.

Emergency procedures

Skin haemorrhage control

- Local measures: apply point pressure on the bleeding area and consider using tranexamic acid or adrenaline-soaked gauze. Local anaesthetic containing adrenaline can be injected (unless contra-indicated).
- Tacking sutures can be used to stop active bleeding in the emergency setting. Use any available type of suture material and take 'big bites'.
- Place a pressure dressing but care must be taken to avoid pressure necrosis.
- In the case of major vessel injury, it may be possible to place a clamp and surgical tie. Good lighting, retraction and suction are essential.

Intraoral haemorrhage control

- Local measures: additionally absorbable haemostatic dressing can be used to pack the area in combination with primary closure using absorbable sutures. If the patient is awake and able to do so they can apply direct pressure or bite on the gauze.
- For intraoral lacerations that bleed excessively and do not stop with pressure, surgical diathermy can be deployed if available.

Disability

The Glasgow Coma Scale (GCS) score should be calculated at this stage. Any head or C-spine injury should be identified as it can have a significant impact on patient management. Severe head injuries will affect the consciousness of the patient. Blood glucose should be measured, and hypoglycaemia corrected in consultation with the anaesthetic team. For blood glucose <4.0 mm/L, give an initial dose of 50 mL 10% glucose per minute until the patient has regained consciousness.

Exposure

The patient should be assessed as a whole, and further injuries identified and managed if applicable.

A secondary survey should be completed after the primary survey, making sure that appropriate management is initiated. This is a head-to-toe examination to identify potential injuries.

An 'AMPLE history' should also be taken:
- **A**llergies.
- **M**edication.
- **P**ast medical history including tetanus status.
- **L**ast meal.
- **E**vents leading to injury.

SYSTEMATIC APPROACH: ASSESSMENT AND MANAGEMENT

For the purpose of assessment and treatment, the facial skeleton can be divided into thirds: upper, middle and lower third. The first part of the examination should involve inspection of the soft tissues. The aim is to appropriately manage active bleeding soft tissue injuries as they can compromise the circulation of the patient. The next step is to palpate all the bony landmarks and assess for any deformities that might indicate an underlying fracture.

Upper third

Related anatomy

Injuries of the upper third of the skull (*Figure 12.2*) may involve the frontal bone as well as the frontal sinuses and the anterior skull base. It is therefore paramount to inspect for any soft tissue injuries and assess their extent.

Steps for assessment

- Assess for any lacerations
  - Note any haematoma or active bleeding from the temporal vessels or scalp
- Nerve deficit

- Sensory, to the supraorbital and supratrochlear nerve distribution
  - Motor, the frontal branch of the facial nerve
- Palpate over the superior orbital rims and assess for any steps
  - Palpate the supraorbital bar and bony orbit
- Assess if there is a potential base of skull fracture
  - Crepitus or surgical emphysema around the frontonasal region
  - Battles' sign, cerebrospinal fluid (CSF) otorrhea or rhinorrhoea

Management

It is important to close and dress any lacerations over the fracture to prevent any infections. Scalp and forehead lacerations should be repaired. Historical and examination features of a head injury, as well as patterns involving the frontal sinus, should be managed in conjunction with a neurosurgeon. Patients with a CSF leak are also managed by a neurosurgeon and are considered separately in this book (see *Chapter 19*).

Middle third

Related anatomy

Midfacial fractures comprise one of the following fractures, which may occur in isolation or in combination: naso-orbital ethmoid (NOE), nasal, nasomaxillary, zygoma, orbital, Le Fort.

Steps for assessment

- Assess any lacerations, note any bruising, abrasion, soft tissue loss
- Visual assessment: visual acuity (Snellen chart), red-light desaturation, ocular motility (by moving the finger in a H-shaped pattern), pupil response, relative afferent pupillary defect (RAPD)

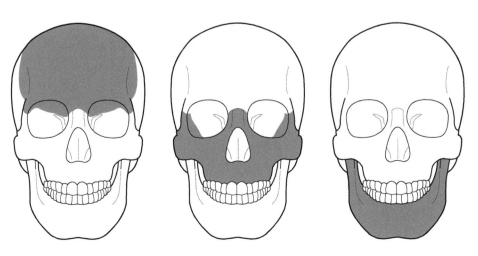

Figure 12.2 For convenience the facial skeleton is divided into thirds. Upper third (left), middle third (middle) and lower third (right).

- Subconjunctival haemorrhage and its posterior limit
- Inspect the patient from above and assess for any obvious enophthalmos or proptosis
- Inspect the patient from the front and assess for any obvious hypoglobus, enophthalmos, chemosis or telecanthus
- Assess medial canthal tendons
  - Palpate over the lateral, inferior orbital rims and assess for any steps, note any asymmetry of the frontozygomatic suture, zygomatic arch, malar prominences, buttress and nasal bones
  - Assess for sensation over the infraorbital and zygomatic nerve distribution
  - Palpate for any maxillary disjunction against the rest of the craniomaxillofacial skeleton
  - Assess the nasal septum for septal haematoma, which necessitates early evacuation
  - Epistaxis should be managed urgently by tamponade packing if non-responsive to 15 minutes of pressure and ice. Topical vasoconstrictors and chemical cautery using silver nitrate can be considered in addition to nasal packing
  - Inspect the hard and soft palate

Orbital emergencies

Retrobulbar haemorrhage may cause orbital compartment syndrome. This is a sight-threatening emergency. Suspect if there is severe pain, difficulty opening the lids, ophthalmoplegia, tense, proptosed globe with loss of vision. Medical management may be initiated but prompt decompression should occur. Early involvement of an ophthalmologist is essential.

Emergency procedures

Orbital compartment syndrome	Rapid loss of vision within the hour. Pain, proptosis, CN III palsy.
Superior orbital fissure syndrome	Possible injury to CNs III, IV, V1 and VI, ophthalmoplegia, ptosis, proptosis, fixed dilated pupil, loss of corneal reflex.
Orbital apex syndrome	As above, (CNs III, IV, V1 and VI) and CN II optic nerve.

- Eyes
  - Lateral canthotomy and cantholysis (*Figure 12.3*). The lateral cantholysis is vision-saving and should be considered routinely in high-energy mechanisms in cases of marked soft tissue swelling, globe proptosis, ophthalmoplegia, significant orbital pain and loss of vision. In the unconscious patient, often with significant orbital fracture, the surgeon should have a low threshold
  - This may not be enough and, subsequently, definitive emergent surgical decompression may be required
- Nose
  - Anterior nasal packing
  - Posterior nasal packing (Foley catheter and bismuth iodoform paraform paste [BIPP])
- Maxilla
  - Repositioning
    - Trans-palatal wire
    - Bite blocks

(a)   (b)

(c)

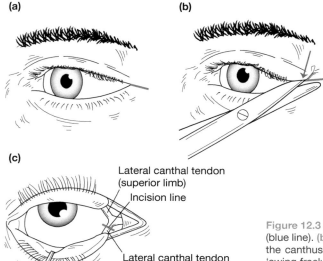

Lateral canthal tendon (superior limb)

Incision line

Lateral canthal tendon (inferior limb)

Figure 12.3 (a) For lateral cantholysis, the incision is marked (blue line). (b) Following administration of local anaesthesia, the canthus is divided with sharp scissors. The lid should 'swing freely' laterally. (c) Cantholysis of the inferior limb of the lateral canthal tendon.

Lateral canthotomy and cantholysis

Relevant anatomy

The medial and lateral canthal ligaments contain the eye within the orbit. The lateral canthal tendon has two branches (superior and inferior); cutting one or both relieves pressure on the globe.

- Supine positioning, stabilise head.
- Antiseptic prep (i.e. aqueous betadine).
- Infiltrate 1–2 mL of 1 or 2% lignocaine with adrenaline lateral canthus with a fine needle.
- Horizontal skin incision lateral to the canthus with a 15 blade.
- Haemostatic forceps to clamp and crush the lateral canthus to the rim of the orbit for a minimum of 20 seconds.
- Canthotomy: use sharp scissors to cut down to the lateral orbital rim 1–2 cm.
- Cantholysis: divide the inferior or both crus of the lateral canthal ligament with scissors. 'Strumming' with scissors identifies any remaining ligament.
- Successful division of this tendon allows the lower lid to swing.

Note: a confused or uncooperative patient may require sedation, children are likely to require general anaesthesia.

Lower third

Related anatomy

Airway compromise can occur due to haemorrhage, oedema and foreign bodies in addition to direct trauma. In the event of airway uncertainty, there should be a low threshold for intubation with provision made for a failed intubation attempt.

Steps for assessment

- Lacerations intra/extraoral
- Inspect for disruption of the mandibular ring
- Sublingual haemorrhage is pathognomonic of mandibular fracture(s)
- Malocclusion, anterior or lateral open bites
- Dental and dentoalveolar injury
- Palpate the mandibular contours, ramus, lateral and inferior borders, symphysis and parasymphysis
  - Any discontinuity should be examined digitally
  - Suspect a second fracture
  - Pain on restriction of opening may localise the fracture site

Medical management of retrobulbar haemorrhage

Oxygen therapy 95% O_2.
Mannitol 20% IV, 1.5–2 g/kg over 30 minutes, first 12.5 g over the first 3 minutes.
Acetazolamide 500 mg IV.
Steroids methylprednisolone 100 mg.
Topical beta-blockers.

White eye blowout 'trapdoor fracture'

Typically occurs in young patients.
- Painful restriction of eye movement.
- Oculogastic and oculocardiac reflexes.
  - Nausea and vomiting, and bradycardia due to raised vagal tone secondary to the entrapment of soft tissue.

- Palpate the glenoid fossa and temporomandibular joint
- Trismus or limited mouth opening
- Nerve deficit
  - Numbness in the distribution of the mental nerve
  - Note function of the marginal mandibular nerve
- Evaluate parotid gland function

Emergency procedures
- Emergency stabilisation
  - Wires: bridle wire
  - Bite block

Dentoalveolar fractures

This is a fracture of the facial bones that involves a segment of the alveolus with or without injury to the associated teeth in that segment.

Steps for assessment
- Inspect for gingival lacerations, vestibular ecchymosis, malocclusion, steps in the occlusion, extrusion, intrusion and luxation injuries
- Palpate for mobility

Management

Closed repositioning and fixation with dental splint (composite, wire, vacuum formed retainer). If associated with more extensive fractures (e.g. Le Fort), open reduction and internal fixation (ORIF) may be required.

Tooth fracture

- Enamel fracture with or without dentine exposure.
- Pulp exposure: the fracture involves the enamel, dentine and exposes the pulp.
- Crown-root fracture: this fracture involves enamel, dentine and cementum with or without pulpal exposure.
- Root fracture: involves dentine, cementum and pulp.

Tooth luxation

- Lateral luxation: lateral displacement of the tooth in its socket often with an associated fracture of the alveolar plate.
- Extrusion: the tooth is axially displaced from the socket.
- Intrusion: the tooth is axially displaced into the socket.
- Avulsion: the tooth is luxated completely from the socket.

Segmental alveolar fracture

- Fracture of the alveolar process, which may or may not involve the socket of the teeth.

TOP TIPS AND HAZARDS

- The technique of needle cricothyroidotomy is a lifesaving procedure with which all trainees must be familiar.
- Direct digital pressure to stop haemorrhage will not only help to stop further loss of blood but also help to organise equipment and materials required for definitive management.
- If there is suspicion of retrobulbar haemorrhage, one must not seek confirmation on imaging. Surgical and medical management must be instigated at once.

FURTHER READING

Perry M. Advanced Trauma Life Support (ATLS) and facial trauma: can one size fit all? Part 1: Dilemmas in the management of the multiply injured patient with coexisting facial injuries. *Int J Oral Maxillofac Surg* 2008;**37**:209–14.

Perry M. Acute proptosis in trauma: retrobulbar hemorrhage or orbital compartment syndrome—does it really matter? *J Oral Maxillofac Surg* 2008;**66**:1913–20.

Perry M, Holmes S. *Useful "First Aid" Measures and Basic Techniques. Atlas of Operative Maxillofacial Trauma Surgery.* Springer; 2014, pp. 89–112.

Perry M, Holmes S. *Manual of Operative Maxillofacial Trauma Surgery.* Springer; 2014.

Perry M, Dancey A, Mireskandari K, Oakley P, Davies S, Cameron M. Emergency care in facial trauma—a maxillofacial and ophthalmic perspective. *Injury* 2005;**36**:875–96.

Chapter

13

Management of Facial Soft Tissue Injuries

Martin Duplantier, Siavash Siv Eftekhari, Baber Khatib, R. Bryan Bell

INTRODUCTION

The management of facial soft tissue injuries is a critical component of trauma care. There is a great variability in complexity, ranging from superficial injuries that require simple approximation to injuries that involve vital structures and extensive reconstruction.

A basic understanding of the wound healing process is necessary when repairing facial soft tissue injuries. Wound healing can be divided into three phases: inflammation, proliferation and maturation. It is important to note that wounds only gain 3–7% of normal tensile strength by 2 weeks, thus initial healing relies heavily on the sutures. Therefore, the suture material and suturing technique used are important for treating facial soft tissue injuries.

CLASSIFICATIONS OF SOFT TISSUE WOUNDS

Lacerations: Usually have sharp edges. Washout with water and debridement, primary closure of layers should be performed. Lacerations can be broken down into several categories:

- Simple lacerations: tension-free closure
- Stellate lacerations: special attention to the flap tip to preserve blood supply. Half-buried mattress suture can be utilised
- Flap-like lacerations: avulsion injuries without the loss of tissue

Contusions: Refers to the bruise caused by oedema and haematoma in subcutaneous tissues resulting from blunt compressive injuries. Usually require observation and no surgical intervention unless infection declares itself.

Abrasions: Superficial damage to the skin no deeper than epidermis. Keeping the wound clean and moist is usually all that is required for treatment.

Avulsions: Involves a level of tissue loss. Minimal tissue loss usually is of little consequence as undermining the surrounding tissue still allows for tension-free primary closure. Larger areas of tissue loss may require skin graft, local tissue flaps or free tissue transfer.

Facial wounds can be categorised as clean or contaminated. Fresh clean wounds are usually in no need of prophylactic antibiotics. The rate of infection increases and is directly related to the length of time that has elapsed since the initial injury. Skin wounds are usually contaminated with *Streptococcus* and *Staphylococcus*. Wounds that involve mucosal lining of the oral cavity are contaminated by oral flora. Through-and-through lacerations between oral cavity and facial/neck skin are considered contaminated. The number of bacteria present in the wound is more important than the type of bacteria in causing infections. Simple lacerations and abrasions have low bacterial content and therefore do not require prophylactic antibiotics.

Contaminated and complex wounds (*Figure 13.1*) such as crush injuries, the presence of foreign bodies, oro-cutaneous communications and animal or human bites lead to higher bacterial inoculation and higher

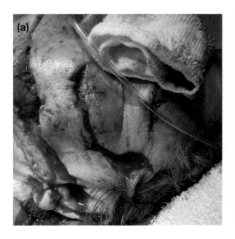
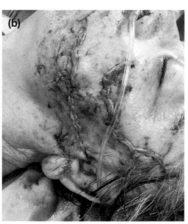

Figure 13.1 Complex lacerations secondary to a motor vehicle collision. Critical structures involve the facial nerve and parotid duct. Careful approximation and tension-free soft tissue eversion after washout completed demonstrates minimal tissue loss.

rates of infection. In these situations, appropriate antibiotic coverage is recommended and absolutely required in animal/human bites. Additionally, prophylactic antibiotics can be considered in the presence of immunosuppression or significant comorbidities such as diabetes, chronic steroid use, malnutrition, etc. It is also paramount to ensure up-to-date tetanus immunisation.

INITIAL EVALUATION

The evaluation of facial soft tissue injury begins in the secondary trauma survey after the patient is in stable condition. The facial wounds are inspected from the scalp to the neck. The depth, length, shape complexity and involvement of specific facial subunits are observed.

The wounds should be pulse irrigated with saline or balanced salt solutions. It is not the type of irrigation solution used that effects wound infection, but the mechanical action of high-pressure irrigation that is important for successful outcomes. A psi of 7 pounds is required to remove adherent bacteria from a wound, which cannot be achieved with bulb irrigation. A helpful tip to achieve this pressure is to use an 18-gauge needle attached to a 35-mL syringe for effective jet stream irrigation. The use of undiluted hydrogen peroxide as an irrigant should be avoided as it inhibits wound healing and may cause tissue necrosis. Scrubbing of the wound with a brush may be undertaken if necessary but should be done sparingly to spare further damage to soft tissues. All devitalised soft tissue should be debrided and excised to create sharp healthy wound margins that will facilitate aesthetic closure.

During clinical examination, it is imperative to assess and document injury to critical structures including the brain, eye, facial nerve, trigeminal nerve, nasolacrimal system, and salivary glands or ducts. Consultation with subspecialists in ophthalmology and/or neurosurgery should be obtained as indicated.

PRINCIPLES OF SOFT TISSUE REPAIR AND WOUND HEALING

Clean wounds may be closed primarily up to 48 hours following the initial injury. A relatively short delay in the definitive repair of soft tissue injuries may be indicated if the underlying facial bones have been fractured and require surgical reduction. Temporary repair of the lacerations will minimise the risk of wound infection and prepare the wound bed for skeletal surgery on a semi-elective basis.

Primary wound closure should be attempted if feasible. Wounds should be closed in layers to place minimum tension on the superficial skin closure and aid in the eversion of skin edges to minimise scar widening. Tension across a wound decreases blood flow, which leads to necrosis of wound edges and increased connective tissue growth in the proliferation phase and to widening of scars in the remodelling phase. Skin flaps should be appropriately undermined so wound edges can be everted, which will minimise scar depression. Achieving good haemostasis is critical, as haematoma formation is a major cause of infection and wound breakdown. If adequate haemostasis cannot be achieved, then drain placement should be considered.

Delayed primary wound closure is usually indicated in patients who have extensive high-energy tissue loss and/or devitalised tissue, such as those caused by high-velocity gunshot wounds (*Figure 13.2*). These wounds generally require serial washouts and debridement before primary closure can be attempted. Delayed repair of contaminated injuries and bite wounds to the face is not recommended, as early primary closure results in less scarring. In the case of significant tissue avulsion, local flaps, regional flaps or free tissue transfer may be needed to adequately restore tissue to previous form and function.

The following general guidelines summarise the management of soft tissue injuries:

1 Perform adequate washout and debridement prior to definitive repair
2 Handle tissue gently to minimise trauma
3 Achieve complete haemostasis
4 When suturing, perform layered closure and ensure that skin margins are relaxed without tension and everted
5 Use fine sutures such as 5-0 or 6-0 sizes for skin closure. Use 3-0 or 4-0 absorbable sutures for deep layers
6 Properly align key landmarks, such as eyebrows and the vermilion border of the lips
7 Delay scar revision for a minimum of 6 months

INJURIES TO FACIAL STRUCTURES REQUIRING SPECIAL TREATMENT

The lip

Lip injuries can cause aesthetic and/or functional problems. Accurate re-approximation of the vermilion border of the lip is critical to achieve an aesthetically acceptable result. An irregular vermilion border or mismatch of more than 1 mm becomes clinically noticeable. Deeper wounds to the lip should be closed in layers to re-approximate the orbicularis oris muscle as this muscle is important for oral function and lip competence.

Avulsive injuries to the lip can still be repaired primarily with minimal to no functional or aesthetic defects if no more than about 25% of the upper or lower lip is lost. For more extensive avulsive tissue loss, local flaps such as the Abbe–Estlander flap can be used to rotate tissue into the avulsed area. The Abbe flap is well suited for both upper and lower lip reconstructions and is generally indicated for repair of vertical defects of both vermilion and cutaneous lip tissue that do not

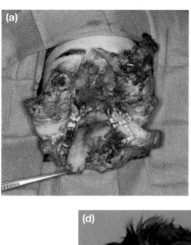
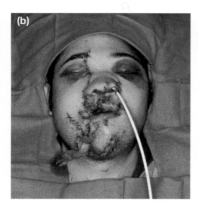
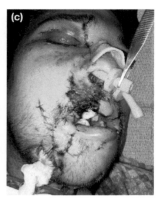
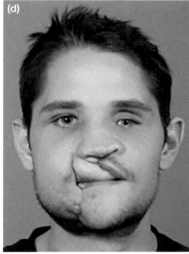
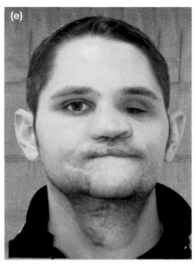

Figure 13.2 (a) Initial washout and minimal selective debridement of a self-inflicted gunshot wound. (b) Initial repair with particular attention to key anatomic landmarks. Note early venous congestion of upper lip. (c) Soft tissue necrosis of right upper lip, philtrum. (d) Delayed repair, osteocutaneus fibula free flaps for maxilla and mandible. (e) Soft tissue revision, delayed Abbe flap and fibula flap debulking.

involve the commissure. Injuries that involve the oral commissure can be reconstructed with a Karapandzic flap, which is designed to re-establish the circumoral sphincter by rotating and advancing the remaining innervated orbicularis oris muscle. A case of extensive lip laceration repair is shown in *Figure 13.3*.

The ear

Initial evaluation of injuries to the ear should include examination of external and internal structures such as the tympanic membrane and a gross hearing exam to rule out sensorineural hearing loss. The auricle is the portion of the external ear most commonly involved in trauma, and consists of a thin central area of relatively avascular cartilage. Importantly, it receives most of

its blood supply from the thin overlying layer of skin. Meticulous approximation of both skin and cartilage is necessary to assure favourable wound healing and prevent chondritis or tissue necrosis. The cartilage should be covered by skin and a bolster dressing is generally recommended to minimise the risk of haematoma formation, which can cause ear deformities such as 'cauliflower ear' (*Figure 13.4*).

Simple ear lacerations are usually easily treated under local anaesthesia. The general principles of wound repair are the same for the ear as they are elsewhere on the face, with 5-0 or 6-0 monofilament sutures recommended. In simple lacerations, there is usually no need for sutures in the cartilage of the auricle.

In partial ear avulsion, the type of reconstruction depends on the size of the defect and the region of

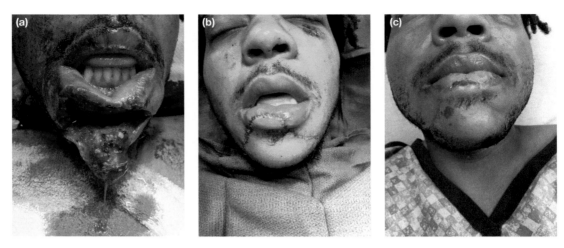

Figure 13.3 (a) Full-thickness knife laceration to lower lip/mentum. (b) Layered closure including intraoral mucosa, orbicularis oris/mentalis muscle and skin/mucosa. Careful approximation of vermilion–cutaneous junction. (c) 1 week postoperative visit showing no tissue loss and recreation of normal anatomy.

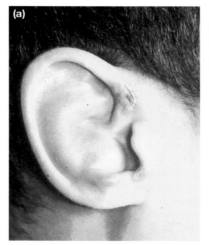
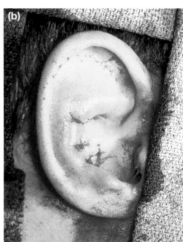

Figure 13.4 (a) Ear haematoma. (b) Haematoma drained and mattress sutures placed to reduce risk of 'cauliflower ear'.

the helix affected. In general, acquired defects of the superior auricle no larger than 2 cm can be repaired primarily by advancing the helix in both directions by making releasing incisions. Middle auricle defects 2 cm or smaller can again be closed primarily with the help of Burow triangles to allow approximation of tissue without tension. Larger avulsive segments may require microvascular anastomosis, although it is very rare to find good vessels for anastomosis, particularly in the avulsed segment. Depending on the amount of cartilage lost, a variety of techniques involving local skin flaps, contralateral conchal cartilage graft and rib cartilage graft can be used.

The treatment of avulsive ear injuries depends on the amount of tissue loss. For total avulsions, the severed ear should be evaluated for the possibility of

microsurgical reattachment or post-auricular pocket techniques. Prosthetic rehabilitation of the external ear can also be considered in cases of significant tissue loss.

Eyelid and nasolacrimal apparatus

The eyelids function to protect the globe from injury, maintain moisture and aid in channelling tears through the canalicular system. The anatomic layers of the eyelid include the skin, alveolar tissue, orbicularis oculi muscle, tarsus, septum orbitale, tarsal (meibomian) glands and conjunctiva. The grey line is defined by the junction of skin and mucosal membrane of the eyelid. Tarsal plate is important for eyelid support. The muscular layer overlying the tarsus is anchored to the lateral and medial canthal ligaments. The orbital septum is

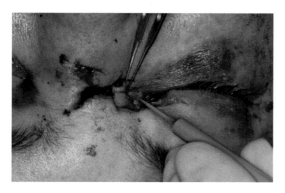

Figure 13.5 Canulation of inferior punctum of nasolacrimal duct system.

attached to the periosteum circumferentially in support of the retro-orbital contents. A thorough examination of the globe, lacrimal drainage system and visual acuity are needed whenever eyelid injuries are present.

Lacerations to the eyelid can be classified into those that involve the lid margin and those that do not. Simple lacerations that do not involve the lid margin can be repaired primarily with small sutures, ideally 6-0 in size. Deep sutures are not recommended in the lower eyelid as inadvertent suturing of the orbital septum can lead to ectropion. If the attachment of the levator muscle to the superior portion of the tarsus is involved, care should be taken to repair this to prevent ptosis. In injuries where the lid margin is involved, accurate re-approximation of this structure is most important. The most important structures of the lid margin that must be realigned are the meibomian glands orifices, lash line and grey line. Avulsive injuries to this region can be treated with

full-thickness skin grafts from the post-auricular region which offers the best colour match. The eyelid avulsions can usually be closed primarily if less than 25% of the length of eyelid is lost. If more is lost, then options such as a lid switch flap can be used

A laceration near the nasolacrimal duct system requires prompt exploration and possible repair (*Figure 13.5*). If injury occurs to the upper or lower cuniculus, placement of silicone tubes through the severed ducts can help preserve drainage and prevent epiphora. The stents will remain in place for 8–12 weeks. The inferior canaliculus drains roughly 70% of tears, but often only one intact canaliculus can provide adequate drainage (*Figure 13.6*). If chronic epiphora exists, dacryocystorhinostomy can be performed.

The nose

Detailed examination of the nose requires use of a nasal speculum with good lighting and suction. Epistaxis should be controlled and nasal bone fractures, septal haematoma and gross deviation of nasal septum must be ruled out before repair of soft tissue injuries. Nasal septal haematomas require evacuation to prevent possible septal necrosis and nasal collapse/saddling.

Soft tissue repair of the nose is based on which subunit has been injured or deformed. Repair of nasal mucosa should be attempted with thin absorbable sutures. Exposed septal cartilage does not pose any difficulty as long as the mucosa is intact on the other side of the septum. In situations of mucosal injury or need for further nasal/septal support after repair, a Doyle open lumen splint can be placed in the naris to optimise healing. Full-thickness lacerations of the nose should be repaired in a layered fashion, re-approximating the mucosa, cartilage and skin. Avulsive wounds of the nose

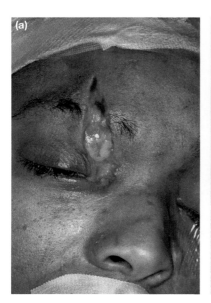
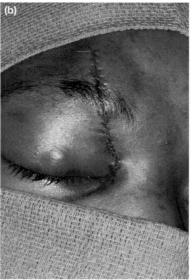

Figure 13.6 (a) Complex medial orbit laceration including eye, lid, puncta. (b) Repair of medial laceration with cannulation (silicone monocanalicular stent).

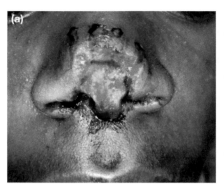 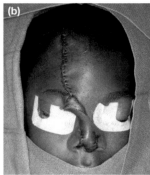 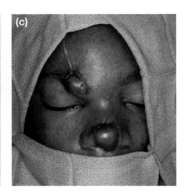

Figure 13.7 (a) Dog bite injury to nasal tip, cartilage intact. (b) Paramedian forehead flap reconstruction. (c) Flap takedown and defatting 3 weeks later.

may be repaired with full-thickness skin grafts, ideally from the post-auricular location. With larger more involved defects, local flaps such as a nasolabial flap or paramedian forehead flap may be used (*Figure 13.7*).

The scalp

Anatomic layers are well described by the convenient acronym 'SCALP': Skin, Subcutaneous Connective tissue, Galea Aponeurosis, Loose areolar tissue and Pericranium. The first superficial three layers are united as one and are difficult to separate. The scalp is highly vascularised and can be a major source of blood loss, haemostasis is critical.

Defects less than 3 cm can typically be closed in a simple, layered fashion. Approximation of the galea is important as it helps offset tension, decreasing the risk of alopecia while also eliminating dead space. If indicated, galea releasing incisions can be performed. In large contaminated avulsive injuries, the use of drains, secondary intention healing or vacuum-assisted closure (VAC) should be considered. In significant avulsive injuries, local rotation/advancement flaps, skin graft or vascularised tissue transfer can be used.

Facial bite wounds

About 15% of animal bite wounds involve the facial structures. The majority inflicted by dogs involve children. Bites are complex injuries contaminated with a unique polymicrobial inoculum. Puncture wounds can have higher infection rates as they involve deep inoculation of pathogens. Crush injuries can cause infections with lower bacterial counts in the wound due to resultant tissue ischaemia. Ear and nose human bite injuries have the highest infection rates due to the inevitable cartilage exposure. Despite these complexities, facial bite wounds generally display low infection rates due to the rich blood supply of the area. Antibiotic prophylaxis is required to cover the broad mixture of aerobic and anaerobic organisms with the most common being:

- Dogs and cats: *Pasteurella* spp.
- Humans: *Eikenella corroends*
- All bites: *Viridans streptococci* and *Streptococcus anginosus*

Furthermore, post-exposure prophylaxis for rabies must be considered if the suspicion is high. Following the principles of tissue repair in combination with infectious prophylaxis can yield a favourable outcome. A close follow-up of these patients is needed.

TOP TIPS AND HAZARDS

- Initial evaluation of the extent of facial soft-tissue injury includes thorough cleansing and removal of wound contaminants (e.g. dirt, glass).
- Lacerations can be repaired with up to 24 hours' delay, with excellent results.
- A low threshold should be maintained for taking a patient to the operating room for evaluation and repair of soft tissue injuries.
- Photographic documentation of injuries and repair is imperative.
- Radiographic evaluation should be performed to rule out fracture or presence of foreign bodies.
- Avoid shaving the eyebrow to facilitate injury evaluation.
- All patients with periorbital injuries should be evaluated for ocular injuries.
- Avulsed or amputated tissue can often be restored successfully.
- Amoxicillin/clavulanate is the antibiotic of choice for animal bites. Clindamycin ± fluoroquinolone or trimethoprim/sulfamethoxazole are recommended for patients with penicillin allergies.
- Re-approximation of the vermilion border should be performed prior to injection of vasoconstrictive local anaesthetic agent for repair of lip lacerations.

ACKNOWLEDGEMENTS

We thank Suhail K. Mithani and Eduardo D. Rodriguez for allowing us to use 'TOP TIPS' from the second edition of *Operative Oral and Maxillofacial Surgery*.

FURTHER READING

Markiewicz MR, Callahan N, Miloro M. Management of traumatic trigeminal and facial nerve injuries. *Oral Maxillofac Surg Clin North Am* 2021;**33**:381–405.

Niamtu III J. Local anesthetic blocks of the head and neck. In: *Simplified Facial Rejuvenation*. Berlin, Heidelberg; Springer; 2008. pp. 29–44.

Powers MP, Beck BW, Fonseca RJ. Management of soft tissue injuries In: *Oral and Maxillofacial Trauma*. Philadelphia: WB Saunders; 1991. pp. 618–48.

Rieck KL, Fillmore WJ, Ettinger KS. Late revision or correction of facial trauma-related soft-tissue deformities. *Oral Maxillofac Surg Clin North Am* 2013;**25**:697–713.

Shupak RP, Williams FC, Kim RY. Management of salivary gland injury. *Oral Maxillofac Surg Clin North Am* 2021;**33**:343–50.

Bailey & Love's Essential Operations Bailey & Love's Essential Operations
Bailey & Love's Essential Operations Bailey & Love's Essential Operations
Bailey & Love's Essential Operations Bailey & Love's Essential Operations

PART 3 | Trauma

Chapter 14

Contemporary Maxillofacial Fixation Techniques

David Powers, Darin Johnston

INTRODUCTION

Maxillomandibular fixation (MMF) is critical to successful reconstruction and rehabilitation in craniomaxillofacial trauma and pathology. Early methods included a single wire spanning a fracture and wrapped around adjacent teeth, known simply as a 'bridle wire'; a Barton bandage consisting of gauze wrapped around the skull, chin and neck; and Gunning splints that combined retrofitted patient dentures with circumferential wires around the mandible, piriform and/or zygoma. These largely historical procedures are still occasionally indicated, depending on the austerity of the location, resources and access to care.

Current methodology usually incorporates some form of metallic framework overlying the dental arch, which is either secured to the teeth using individual wires or anchored to the adjacent bone using mono-cortical screws. This framework may have integrated surgical lugs or hooks to allow for varying degrees of fixation between the maxillary and mandibular arches with elastics or stainless steel surgical wires. The goals of MMF are to:

- Identify, establish and maintain correct occlusion
- Support anatomic reduction of fractures
- Minimize trauma to the periodontium
- Prevent loosening of the framework

Application of the correct principles of anatomy, dental occlusion, metallurgy and bone healing physiology should allow the surgeon to maximize the effects of intermaxillary fixation.

PREOPERATIVE CONSIDERATIONS

Indications for MMF include reduction of facial fractures in conjunction with internal fixation. It may be indicated for definitive primary treatment of maxillofacial fractures in cases of significant comminution, minimally displaced mandibular fractures with favorable muscle vectors if a patient wishes to avoid an open procedure, significant comorbidities which preclude extensive open treatment, intracapsular condyle fractures and fractures isolated to the dental alveolus.

Furthermore, MMF to immobilize the mandible can facilitate bone graft stability following reconstruction of

large mandibular defects. Lastly, it is indicated to establish and/or maintain intraoperative occlusion during orthognathic surgery, total joint replacement and mandibular resection.

Preoperative investigations and contraindications

A thorough history and physical exam should be conducted to identify comorbidities such as seizure disorders, alcoholism, nutritional concerns, developmental delays, homelessness, etc. These are contraindications to postoperative MMF. However, the benefits of MMF can still be harnessed intraoperatively. Confirming pre-existing malocclusions and midline discrepancies can prevent frustration and confusion when attempting to set and secure intraoperative MMF.

TECHNIQUE

Step 1: Preparation

Local or regional anesthesia combined with intravenous sedation may allow for safe and effective treatment. If general anesthesia is used, the airway is typically secured with a nasal endotracheal tube (ETT). Some surgeons may elect to use an armored/reinforced oral ETT, particularly in cases of partially dentate or mixed dentition patients. Trauma and pathology that involves the upper and midface may require submental intubation or tracheotomy.

Step 2: Determine method of MMF

If MMF is indicated postoperatively, then some form of framework or 'arch bar' is secured to the dental arch. These frameworks include an Erich arch bar, Risdon cable, or bone anchored arch bar. If MMF is only needed intraoperatively, then interdental wiring without a framework may be sufficient. Interdental wiring techniques include embrasure wires, Ivy loops, and Gilmer wires. Lastly, intermaxillary fixation (IMF) screws can be used for both intraoperative and postoperative MMF. The specific steps for each technique are described below.

Step 3: Apply framework or interdental wiring

Erich arch bars

- An Erich arch bar (*Figure 14.1*) is measured and trimmed such that it terminates at the posterior aspect of the first molars
- A 24-gauge or 26-gauge wire is passed atraumatically through both embrasures of a posterior tooth. It is easiest to pass the circumdental wire from lingual/palatal to labial/buccal
- The wire is pulled apically with constant gentle force and twisted down to secure the arch bar to the tooth. Care is taken to ensure the wire is apical to the height of contour, preventing wire displacement secondary to transmission of jaw opening forces and loosening of the framework
- The twisted wire is then trimmed, and the end is twisted clockwise and folded to prevent injury (*Figure 14.2*)
- This is repeated for each tooth around the arch. As the Erich arch bar itself elongates during placement, it is recommended to complete placement of the entirety of the arch bar placement from one direction only to prevent 'bunching' of the arch bar, generally seen in the midline/anterior portion of the arch. Excess arch bar material should be trimmed at the posterior edge of the terminal lugs

> **TOP TIPS**
> - To prevent wire deformation and subsequent loosening of the framework during the postoperative period, the wire should be stretched prior to being passed and twisted down.
> - The trimmed and folded wire ends are positioned between lugs to preserve space for elastics and wire loops.
> - It is beneficial to maintain the patient in occlusion when tightening the circumdental wire in areas where the arch bar spans a fracture.
> - Placement of arch wires around each tooth to stabilize the arch bar, especially in the anterior segment, is critically important as when the patient attempts to open their mouth the anterior segments are the first to undergo forces of deformation which result in loosening of the arch bar and loss of MMF.

- The patient is then held in occlusion and MMF obtained with elastics and/or 26-gauge wire loops
- Erich arch bars are preferentially recommended for comminuted fractures of the dentoalveolar table

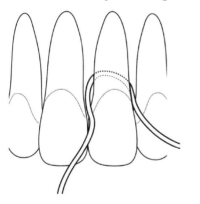
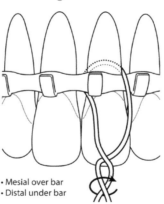
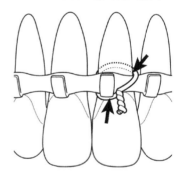

- Mesial over bar
- Distal under bar

Clockwise twist

Figure 14.1 Application of Erich arch bar.

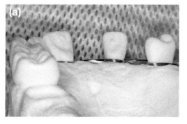
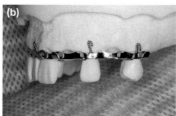
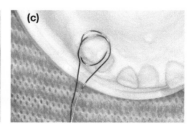

Figure 14.2 A circumdental wire secured below the height of contour (a). Finished ends turned clockwise and folded (b). A wire lasso may be helpful in partially dentate segments (c).

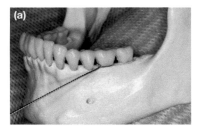 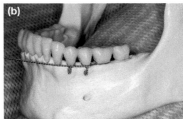 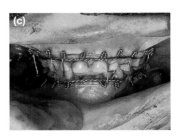

Figure 14.3 Twisted Risdon cable trimmed to reach the contralateral posterior tooth (a). Secured with circumdental wires (b). Clinical application in pediatric patient with bilateral mandibular body fractures (c).

Risdon cable

- A long 24-gauge wire is twisted and secured to the most posterior stable tooth. The wire is then twisted on itself to form an ad hoc arch bar (*Figure 14.3*)
- It is secured with circumdental wires similar to an Erich arch bar as described above
- These wires are trimmed, twisted and folded to create lugs for elastics or wire loops
- The patient is then held in occlusion and MMF obtained with elastics and/or 26-gauge wire loops

TOP TIPS

- The low-profile Risdon cable is useful for primary and mixed dentition.

Bone anchored/'hybrid' arch bar

- The arch bar is measured and trimmed similar to an Erich arch bar
- A locking bone screw is passed through the center eyelet and secured trans-mucosally to the alveolar bone (*Figure 14.4*). Once the screw obtains a bony purchase, the eyelet is lifted off the mucosa
- The screw is then driven into the bone until the threads lock the screw head into the eyelet. This maneuver allows for the arch bar to be anchored to the bone without compressing the underlying mucosa, but places the arch bar at risk for deformation should continued force be applied to the screw once it engages with the locking threads
- The remaining eyelets are repositioned to avoid vital structures or fracture lines, and secured in an anterior to posterior direction (*Figure 14.5*)
- Removal of unused eyelets is recommended to prevent mucosal overgrowth through the eyelet, resulting in a condition which is uncomfortable for outpatient clinical removal without appropriate regional or intravenous anesthesia

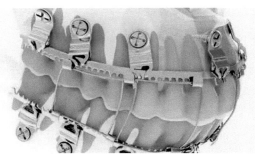

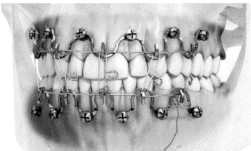

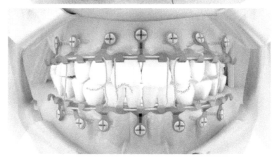

Figure 14.4 Commercially available systems.

TOP TIPS

- Each commercially available system has a unique design to minimize gingival overgrowth and prevent iatrogenic damage to tooth roots.
- Significant cost-savings can be realized due to shortened operative time.

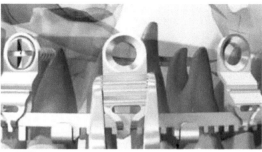
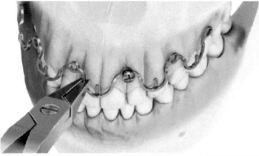
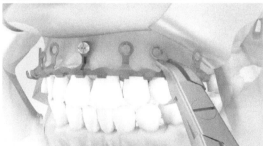

Figure 14.5 Screw eyelets adjusted by sliding (top), stretching (middle) and bending (bottom).

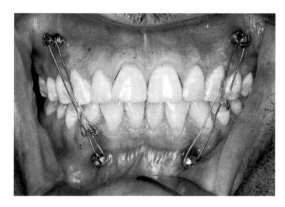

Figure 14.6 Intermaxillary fixation screws positioned adjacent to canine teeth.

- One of the drawbacks of IMF screws is that when properly placed the mechanics of the appliance may result in the slight development of a posterior open bite as all forces for immobilization are directed anteriorly

TOP TIPS

- IMF screws can be maintained postoperatively for MMF and guiding elastics.
- Placement distal to the mental foramen on the mandible places the inferior alveolar nerve at risk, while positioning in regions other than the piriform rim and buttress on the maxilla may result in instability due to the thin maxillary bone.

IMF screws

- The screw is secured trans-mucosally into alveolar bone. Firm pressure is often required; however, care should be taken to avoid penetrating tooth roots. Typically, four screws are placed adjacent to the maxillary and mandibular canines (*Figure 14.6*)
- The screw head has eyelets for passing wire and forming loops to obtain MMF. Some screw heads also accommodate elastics

Embrasure wires

- A 24-gauge or 26-gauge wire is passed between embrasures of opposing teeth. The wire is left untwisted until all planned wires have been passed. Typically, four wires are used at the molar–premolar embrasure and premolar–canine embrasure (*Figure 14.7*)
- The patient is then held in occlusion and the wires are twisted down, trimmed and folded
- Acceptable dentition and periodontal health are necessary for this treatment modality

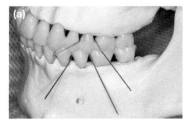
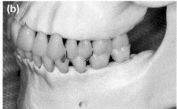
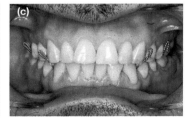

Figure 14.7 Embrasure wires (a–c).

- Commercially available plastic 'zip ties' can be used for embrasure wires

Gilmer wire/Ernst ligature

- A 24-gauge or 26-gauge wire is passed around a single tooth (Gilmer) or woven around two adjacent teeth (Ernst) and twisted down to ligate the tooth/teeth. The twisted wire tail is trimmed long
- The same is repeated on additional teeth in the maxilla and mandible
- The patient is held in occlusion and the long tails of opposing teeth are twisted together to obtain MMF (*Figure 14.8*)
- Once clinically appropriate, the twisted tails can be released and folded to create lugs for guiding elastics (*Figure 14.9*)

Step 4: Apply MMF

The teeth are then brought into a stable and repeatable occlusion. Clues such as mamelons and wear facets will aid in reestablishing the premorbid occlusion. If the arches do not passively align and occlude appropriately, and a premorbid malocclusion has been ruled out, then the adjacent alveolus and facial bones should be inspected. Causes include occult or incompletely reduced Le Fort, palatal or alveolar fractures; subluxated teeth; and incorrect spacing at a site with an avulsed tooth adjacent to a fracture. Once the correct occlusion is passively repeatable the maxillary and mandibular arches can be linked together with elastics, stainless steel wire loops or both. There are many elastic sizes and forces available, the most common forces being medium (4 oz.), heavy (6 oz.) and extra heavy (8 oz.) Generally, the correct elastic is one that maintains a secure occlusion with the minimal required force. Stainless steel wire loops are usually 26–28 gauge.

POSTOPERATIVE CARE AND POSSIBLE COMPLICATIONS

Emesis is a primary concern for patients and healthcare providers, particularly in the immediate postoperative period. When a patient is in MMF, aspiration of gastric contents can be life-threatening. For this reason, all patients in MMF should be provided with the means and education to quickly release the wire or elastic fixation. This unfortunate scenario can be avoided with proactive coordination between the surgeon and anesthesia providers. Perioperative administration of anti-emetics, avoidance of pro-emetic anesthetic agents and gastric suctioning at the conclusion of the surgery should all be employed.

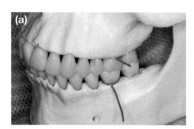 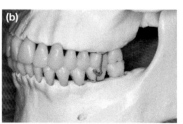 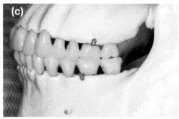

Figure 14.8 Gilmer wires secured to opposing teeth (a), twisted together for MMF (b), trimmed and folded for guiding elastics (c).

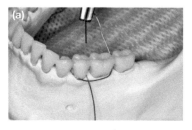 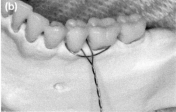 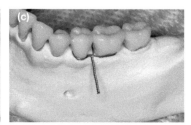

Figure 14.9 Ernst ligature (a–c).

Adequate nutritional intake while in MMF should be optimized perioperatively. Hospital dieticians and case managers, if available, can help identify and provide good sources of liquid nutrition. Nursing staff can educate patients to use simple and atraumatic methods of administering nutrition.

Orthodontic wax can be provided to cover MMF hardware to minimize mucosal trauma. Topical anesthetic rinses can also be used, as needed, for palliation. Standard oral hygiene practices should be encouraged to minimize inflammation of the periodontium.

Loosening of the arch bar framework and wire loops can compromise postoperative MMF, and adjustments in the clinic may not be well tolerated by patients. Therefore, prevention is paramount and best accomplished with consistent application of correct technique.

FURTHER READING

Carlson AR, Shammas RL, Allori AC, et al. A technique for reduction of edentulous fractures using dentures and SMARTLock hybrid fixation system. *Plast Reconstr Surg Glob Open* 2017;**5**:e1473.

Engelstad ME, Kelly P. Embrasure wires for intraoperative maxillomandibular fixation are rapid and effective. *J Oral Maxillofac Surg* 2011;**69**:120–4.

Khelemsky R, Powers D, Greenberg S, et al. The hybrid arch bar is a cost-beneficial alternative in the open treatment of mandibular fractures. *Craniomaxillofac Trauma Reconstr* 2019;**12**:128–33.

Madsen M, Tiwana PS, Alpert B. The use of risdon cables in pediatric maxillofacial trauma: a technique revisited. *Craniomaxillofac Trauma Reconstr* 2012;**5**:107–10.

Bailey & Love's Essential Operations Bailey & Love's Essential Operations
Bailey & Love's Essential Operations Bailey & Love's Essential Operations
Bailey & Love's Essential Operations Bailey & Love's Essential Operations

PART 3 | Trauma

Chapter 15

Mandibular Fractures

Christopher Vinall, Michael Perry

ESSENTIAL SURGICAL ANATOMY

Morphologically, the mandible is a U-shaped bone, and can be divided anatomically into:

- Symphysis
- Parasymphysis
- Body
- Angle
- Ramus, coronoid and condyle

Of particular note are:

- The many muscle insertions (which can either support or displace fractures (*Figure 15.1*)
- The teeth (which together with the periodontal ligament can act as a source of infection)
- The periosteum (which can assist fracture stability)
- The inferior alveolar nerve (which together with the mental nerve, can be injured at the time of fracture, or during their repair)

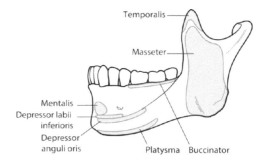

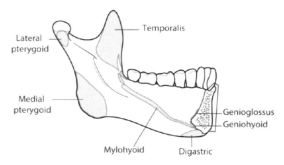

Figure 15.1 Outer and inner view of the mandible showing muscle attachments.

The muscles of mastication and the suprahyoid muscles are the principal movers of the mandible. Considerable forces can be generated; hence certain fractures can significantly displace and remain painfully mobile. Conversely, the masseter and medial pterygoid muscles attach to much of the ramus and therefore splint fractures, and maintain blood supply. Ramus fractures (as distinct from the condyle) rarely need operative repair.

The genioglossus and geniohyoid are attached to the midline genial tubercles – mobile fractures in this region may lead to loss of tongue support and airway compromise.

The canine teeth have long roots and the mandibular third molar teeth are often partially erupted and weaken bone locally, accounting for the frequency of fractures in these regions. In young patients, the periosteum may resist fracture displacement at the time of impact and in minimally displaced fractures may facilitate non-operative management. If divided by injury or surgical exposure, displacement can more readily occur.

PREOPERATIVE CONSIDERATIONS

Assessment

Assessment of mandibular (and other) injuries commonly occurs in one of two scenarios:

- High-velocity injuries with synchronous surgical comorbidity, ATLS principles apply. The importance of inclusion of the head and neck in the primary and secondary survey cannot be under-represented
- The 'walking wounded' – isolated facial injuries only

Clinically the following signs may be elicited to varying degrees:

- Pain, especially on talking and swallowing
- Drooling
- Swelling
- Altered bite
- Numbness of the lower lip
- Trismus and difficulty in moving the jaw
- Loosened teeth
- Mobility of fractured segment
- Bleeding from the periodontium
- Sublingual haematoma

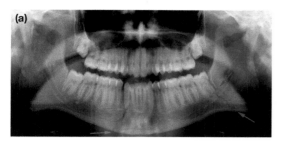

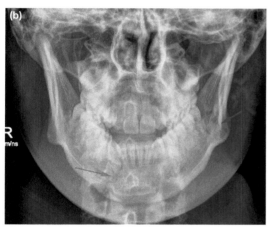

Figure 15.2 Angle + parasymphysis fracture. (a) Preoperative orthopantomogram. (b) Preoperative PA mandible view.

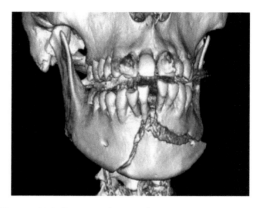

Figure 15.3 Preoperative 3D-CT reconstruction mandible.

Imaging

Deciding on the most appropriate imaging to evaluate the fracture/fractures depends on whether the patient presents with a suspected isolated injury or has suffered multiple trauma. If a low-energy isolated fracture is suspected, an orthopantomogram and a posteroanterior (PA) view will be adequate, which afford excellent interpretation of the teeth and supporting structures (*Figure 15.2*).

It should be noted that fractures of the condylar head are often difficult to see on a plain film view. The symphysis is difficult to evaluate because of the overlap from the cervical spine. A lower occlusal view is useful for evaluating fractures in this region in particular, the anterior lingual plate or consideration of computed tomography (CT) (*Figure 15.3*).

CT imaging would be the preferred choice in the following circumstances:

- High-energy injuries or in patients unable to undergo routine radiography (due to the presence of torso, cervical spine or brain injuries)
- Complex fractures with segmentation
- Suspected pathological fracture
- Associated condylar neck or head fractures

First aid measures

Pain relief may be achieved by infiltration of local anaesthesia around the fracture, or if possible, by an inferior alveolar nerve block.

Bridle wires to splint mobile fracture segments together should be considered when delays in repair (i.e. surgery the next day) are anticipated. This will serve to stabilise the fracture segments, and provide a significant amount of pain relief for the patient (*Figure 15.4*).

A soft cervical collar can be used to support the mandible.

Timing of surgery

In view of patient comfort, mandibular fractures should be treated at the first available opportunity. There is usually no need to explore on admission if outside daylight hours unless there is active bleeding, or instability of the airway. Although simple fractures may be treated under local anaesthesia, most cases are managed under endotracheal anaesthesia. It is essential to discuss choice of intubation with the anaesthetist to ensure that the tube is placed away from the dental occlusion. This is commonly achieved via nasotracheal intubation, occasionally submentally, or if associated with other significant injuries, by tracheostomy.

OPEN OR CLOSED TREATMENT

Treatment can be considered as either 'closed' or 'open'.

Closed treatment

This comprises analgesia, a soft diet until a firm callus forms (usually around 4–6 weeks) and, if required, intermaxillary fixation (IMF).

Indications for closed treatment

This is appropriate in cases of no or minimal displacement, no or minimal fracture mobility and no infection, where there is the possibility of obtaining pre-injury

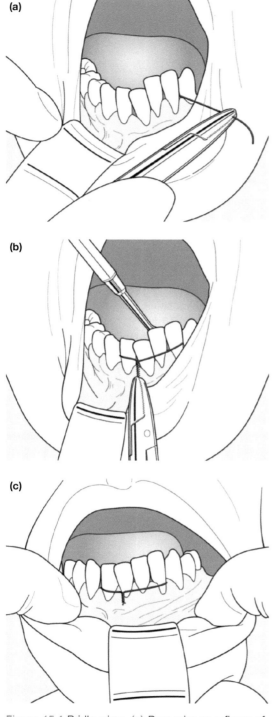

(a)

(b)

(c)

Figure 15.4 Bridle wires. (a) Pass wire as a figure-of-eight around one or preferably two teeth, either side of the fracture (must be firm). (b) Reduce fracture and tighten wire ends. Ensure wire is below maximum bulbosity of the teeth (in the cervical margin). (c) Wire tightened.

occlusion, and there is good patient cooperation and follow-up.

Open treatment

This is indicated when closed treatment is inappropriate or has failed. With open reduction and internal fixation, surgical exposure of the fracture site and anatomical reduction is carried out. There are two options for fixation with open treatment:

Load bearing fixation: This requires an external approach to place rigid plates that can bear all the forces during function at the fracture site. Rigid fixation is achieved. It is required in cases of bone fragment instability such as comminuted, pathological or continuity defect (*Figures 15.5* and *15.6*).

Load sharing fixation: Studies have shown that 'micro movement' following 'semi rigid' fixation encourages callus formation and healing. Instead of large rigid plates, smaller ones are placed along well-defined 'zones of tension' arising at the fracture site according to Champy principles (*Figure 15.7*), effectively converting them into 'zones of compression'. For this fixation to work there needs to be good abutment and interdigitation of the fracture ends. Fixation can be placed transorally and secured with monocortical screws. The technique relies on satisfactory interdigitation of fracture ends, and is contraindicated if this is missing.

STEPWISE OPERATIVE TECHNIQUE

Intraoral approach

Angle fractures

These can be partly splinted by the medial pterygoid and masseter muscles but are often displaced and mobile. Fractures at this site have been classified as vertically and horizontally favourable, or unfavourable, depending on the orientation of the fracture and tendency for it to displace by the pull of these muscles (*Figure 15.8*). This can occur when the periosteum has been ruptured or stripped from the bone allowing displacement to occur.

Access can be made through a variety of incisions, sited along or lateral to the external oblique ridge down to bone. As a general principle, surgical wounds should not lay over any metalwork.

The fracture is then manipulated, while re-establishing the occlusion (with intermaxillary fixation) until it is anatomically reduced.

A four-hole miniplate is placed along the buccal surface of the reduced fracture and fixed with 6-mm screws via a transbuccal approach, whereby a trochar is passed through the cheek. The transoral propeller twist plate is no longer standard of care.

Following fixation of the miniplate, the IMF is removed. The wound is irrigated and checked for haemostasis. Wound closure is achieved with a simple interrupted resorbable suture.

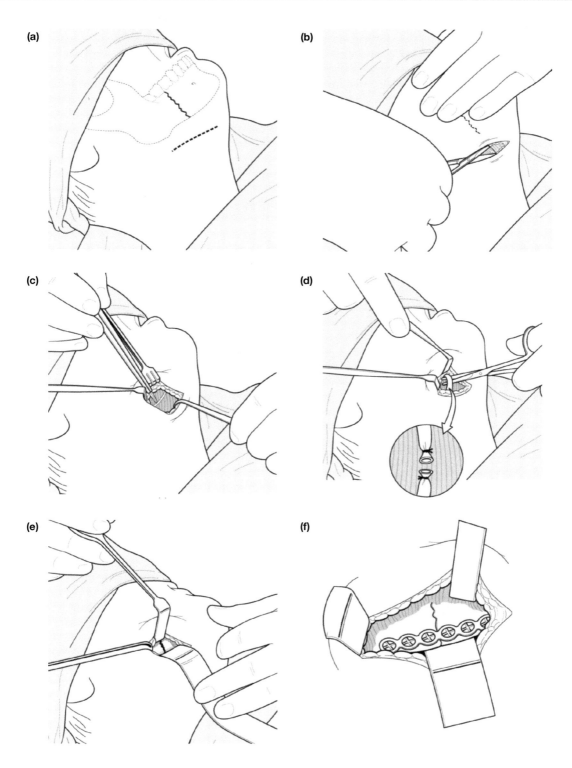

Figure 15.5 External approach to lower mandibular border. (a) Place skin incision in suitable crease (remember nerve anatomy). (b) Following incision, carefully deepen wound through platysma. (c) Watch out for the mandibular branch of VII (bipolar is showing nerve, not frying it!). (d) The facial vessels may need division and ligation. (e) Incise and lift periosteum to expose fracture. (f) Fracture repaired (this is not compression plating).

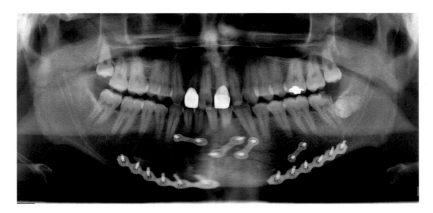

Figure 15.6 Postoperative mandibular reconstruction.

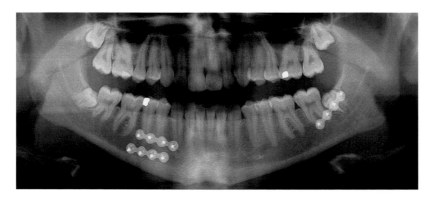

Figure 15.7 A well-reduced fracture according to Champy principles. Note two plates placed at the right parasymphysis and one at the left angle – this has been placed by the transbuccal technique, which is the evidence-based approach to this fracture, the propeller twist plate is no longer standard of care.

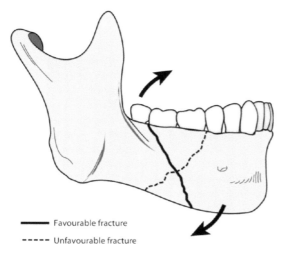

── Favourable fracture

---- Unfavourable fracture

Figure 15.8 Favourable and unfavourable angle fractures (note: tendency to displace).

Symphyseal and parasymphyseal fractures

There are several approaches to the anterior mandible. A two-layer stepped incision placed in the sulcus is the preferred access. Very often the branches of the mental nerve can be seen through the mucosa and protected.

Two miniplates are required to resist torsional forces following muscle pull.

Place the lower miniplate along the lower border. Care is required with drilling the upper miniplate (dental roots). Many surgeons place the holes 5 mm or more below the apices, to avoid damage.

Ramus fractures

These rarely need repair. The attached muscles of mastication effectively splint any fractures. If the occlusion is significantly disrupted, elastic IMF may be applied.

Extraoral approach to lower mandibular border

Referring back to *Figure 15.5*:

- Place skin incision in suitable crease (remember nerve anatomy)
- Following incision, carefully deepen wound through platysma
- Watch out for the marginal mandibular branch of cranial nerve VII
- The facial vessels may need division and ligation
- Incise and lift periosteum to expose fracture
- Fracture repaired

The use of preoperative antibiotics is common practice to reduce postoperative complications following repair of mandibular fractures. There is currently no universal acceptance of duration, and 3 days for most cases would seem to be appropriate.

Steroids (dexamethasone) are given in the perioperative phase to reduce facial swelling.

POSTOPERATIVE CARE

This comprises antibiotics and analgesia. Postoperative radiographs may be taken to confirm adequate repair.

If applicable, patients should be advised to quit smoking, and also given advice on soft diet and appropriate nutrition for 6 weeks. Good oral hygiene is very important.

Regular follow-up for 6 weeks is recommended.

SPECIAL CONSIDERATIONS

Tooth in the fracture site

The indications for tooth extraction are as follows:

- The tooth interferes with fracture reduction
- The tooth is fractured. Devitalised roots act as a nidus for infection
- Tooth with advanced dental caries
- Tooth with established periodontal disease
- The presence of associated pathologies such as cysts or pericoronitis

If the tooth is elevated, precise reduction and immobilisation of the fracture can be difficult particularly if bone has been removed in the process. For this reason, if the tooth has to be removed, it is easier to plate the fracture first, then remove the plate before elevating the tooth.

Fractures in children

Mandibular fractures in young children are uncommon as the facial skeleton is less prominent, and bone elastic. In addition, children do not tend to get as involved in risk-taking activity as their elders. The condyle is the most common fracture site. As a general rule, condylar

fractures without significant malocclusion can be managed with a soft diet and early initiation of jaw movement. Occasionally a period of temporary intermaxillary fixation (no more than 7–10 days) may be appropriate to stabilise the fracture fragments, optimise patient comfort and allow for bony healing.

Management of displaced fractures at other locations of the mandible is often dictated by the stage of dental development (*Figure 15.9*). If open reduction and internal fixation is planned to repair the fracture, then careful placement of the load sharing fixation is important to avoid damage to the developing dentition.

Miniplates and screws applied to the growing mandible will become internalised (*Figure 15.10*). As the mandible grows, new bone formation occurs on the lateral surface with resorption on the lingual surface. If plate removal is required, it should be performed less than 3 months following placement of the fixation. Leaving a miniplate *in situ* and allowing it to become internalised will not interfere with growth of the mandible.

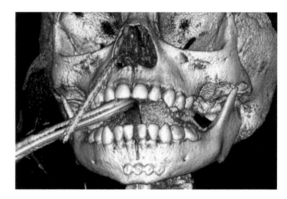

Figure 15.9 The diagnosis of a fractured symphysis was made on the history and examination. Note the position of the miniplate is low, and this has corrected the vertical anomaly, but there is spacing between the teeth – this would be expected to resolve with growth.

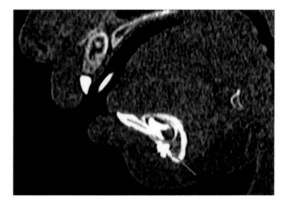

Figure 15.10 In this sagittal view, note the screw is short (4 mm) and is away from the follicle (red arrow).

Infected mandibular fractures

Infection of fractured mandibles is common and management depends on the type of infection, fixation used and state of the overlying tissues. Infection may complicate up to 20% of intraoral access incisions. The postoperative radiograph is crucial in assessment of fracture healing, and while there is a trend to not take them, subsequent management may be compromised.

Superficial wound infection with mild wound dehiscence can be managed by regular oral saline mouth rinse, smoking cessation and antibiotic treatment and weekly review until healed. Significant dehiscence requires consideration of IMF with Leonard buttons, arch bars, or orthodontic brackets, and weekly review. Imaging, in particular a CT, is useful to demonstrate bone pathology and also loss of fixation, and to evaluate spread of infection to other tissue spaces.

If loss of fixation, or significant space infection is identified, then management depends on the degree of swelling of the soft tissues. If the overlying skin is intact and not too swollen, then the preferred treatment is a lower border approach, removal of osteosynthesis material and biofilm. The fracture site requires copious saline irrigation. Any granulation tissue, and bone sequestra at the fracture site needs to be removed.

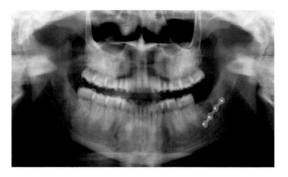

Figure 15.11 This left angle fracture was reduced well. There were no adverse operative findings. The patient was a smoker.

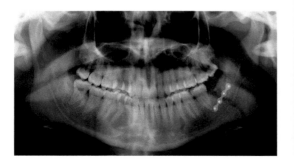

Figure 15.12 At 6 weeks, the patient presented with pain and swelling, and an orthopantomogram showed radiological evidence of osteolysis at the fracture site.

Bleeding at the margins of the fracture site following wound debridement is important to ensure the bone is vital. When the surgical site is clean and the fracture reduced, a load bearing osteosynthesis plate is placed (*Figures 15.11–15.13*). Surgical postoperative drains are maintained for 48 hours.

If the soft tissue envelope is compromised by a space infection, gross oedema, or skin breakdown, then external fixation is used following surgical drainage to stabilise the major fragments to support resolution of infection (*Figure 15.14*).

Following resolution of infection, then a load bearing osteosynthesis can be used.

Continuity defects following removal of necrotic bone have traditionally been bone grafted at a second operation, but may be considered more acutely if rigid fixation and a clean operative bed are obtained, and there is no oral communication. The iliac crest normally provides a suitable donor site.

Edentulous mandible fractures

Fractures associated with the atrophic edentulous mandible often have a poor outcome especially when the height of the mandible is 10 mm or less. Outcome is compromised by poor blood supply and slow healing, especially in patients with multiple medical comorbidities and osteoporotic bones (*Figure 15.15*). IMF is not possible (no teeth) and any periosteal stripping jeopardises the blood supply. A direct relationship between the height of the bone in the fractured area and the complication rate is classified according to Luhr (*Table 15.1* and *Figure 15.16*).

The treatment options for the fractured edentulous mandible are as follows:

- Soft diet and regular review to allow union. This is an appropriate option in frail patients with undisplaced fractures. Close observation is required as these patterns frequently become displaced

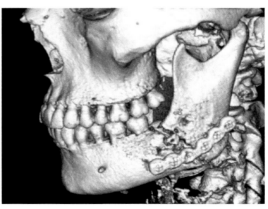

Figure 15.13 The fixation must demonstrate three bicortical screws in sound bone on each side of the fracture.

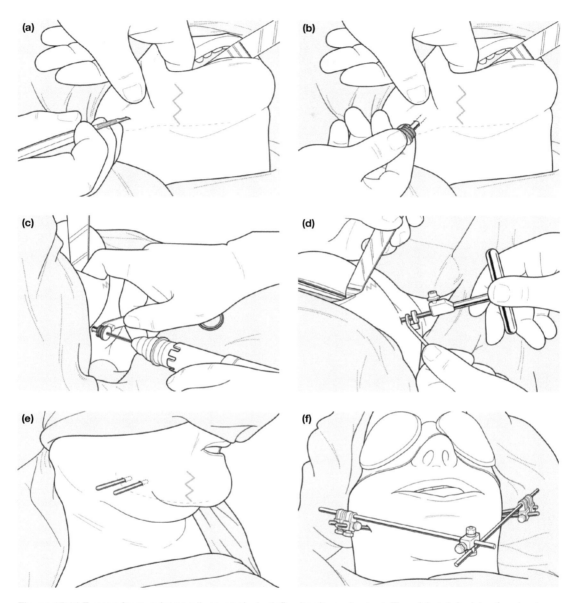

Figure 15.14 Expose fracture intraorally to precisely define its site and extent. Then (a) stab incision for pin placement, (b) pass pointed trochar down to bone, (c) replace inner pointed trochar with drill guide and drill bicortical hole, (d) remove drill guide and place pin (depth gauge may be used), (e) repeat so that there are two pins either side of fracture, (f) completed arrangement.

Luhr class	Criterion: Height mandible (mm)
I	16–20
II	11–15
III	<10

TABLE 15.1 Luhr class and height of the mandible

- Closed reduction using the patient's dentures or customised 'gunning splints', to the maxilla and mandible to allow IMF. This is largely a historical treatment and required fixation of the denture to the mandible by circummandibular wires, and to the maxilla using circum-zygomatic, peralveolar or piriform fossa wires
- Internal fixation using miniplates. Usually effective in simple fractures providing the height of the mandible is significantly above 20 mm

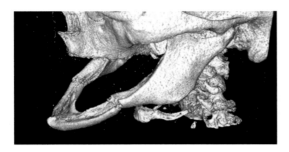

Figure 15.15 The bilateral fracture of the body is known as a bucket handle fracture and is inherently unstable due to the muscle pull.

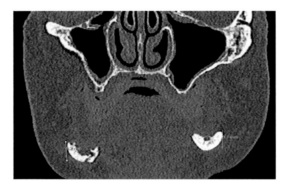

Figure 15.16 This coronal view with bilateral measurements <1 cm indicates a Luhr III.

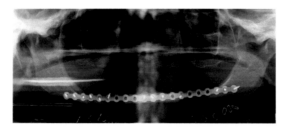

Figure 15.17 Well-reduced fracture but subsequent prosthodontic rehabilitation is complex.

- Internal fixation using heavier reconstruction plates (*Figure 15.17*). Appropriate for comminuted fractures particularly if the height of the mandible is less than 20 mm

TOP TIPS AND HAZARDS

- Fractures of the mandible in restrained supine patients is not a good mix. Never leave such patients unattended.
- Comminution implies high energy and the risk of significant airway swelling.
- Check the hyoid and larynx for associated injuries.
- Beware patients who repeatedly ask to sit up – this may indicate airway difficulties.
- Vomiting is best managed by tilting the trolley head down, rather than attempting to log roll the patient.
- Missing teeth must be accounted for. Both a chest x-ray and soft tissue view of the neck may be required.
- A sublingual haematoma is pathognomonic of a mandible fracture and may also compromise the airway.
- The mandible commonly fractures in two places – if you see one fracture look for another.
- If removing an associated tooth, plate the fracture first, take the plate off and remove the tooth. This can help in unstable fractures.

FURTHER READING

Benson PD, *et al.* Reconstruction of clinically infected mandibular fractures: bone grafts in the presence of pus. *J Oral Maxillofac Surg* 2006;**64**:122–6.

Franciosi E, *et al.* Treatment of edentulous mandibular fractures with rigid internal fixation: case series and literature review. *Craniomaxillofac Trauma Reconstr* 2014;**7**:35–42.

Perry M, Holmes S. Mandibular fractures. In: *Atlas of Operative Maxillofacial Trauma Surgery*, M. Perry, S. Holmes (eds). London: Springer-Verlag; 2014.

Wolfswinkel E, *et al.* Management of pediatric mandible fractures. *Otolaryngol Clin North Am* 2013;**46**:791–806.

Bailey & Love's Essential Operations Bailey & Love's Essential Operations
Bailey & Love's Essential Operations Bailey & Love's Essential Operations
Bailey & Love's Essential Operations Bailey & Love's Essential Operations

PART 3 | Trauma

Chapter 16

Condylar Fractures

Roger Currie, David Laraway

INTRODUCTION

Condylar fractures are an important subgroup of mandibular fractures both in presentation and management. Fractures may present in isolation or in conjunction with other mandibular fractures, or as a component of a panfacial injury. The fracture pattern, level of dentition, prognosis of remaining dentition and age of the patient are all important factors in its management.

Incidence and classification

The literature has various figures for the incidence of condylar fractures, from 30 to 50% of all mandibular fractures. The commonest cause of presentation in the UK is a result of interpersonal violence. Over 80% of fractures are unilateral, with the highest incidence in the age range of 20–39 with at least a 2:1 sex ratio (male:female).

Classification of condylar injuries has been difficult. This is in part due to the number and types of classification in use. These may relate to anatomical position, that is, condylar neck or may relate to displacement of the condylar fragment. Previously, classifications have included Speissl and Schroll, MacLennan and Lindahl. In 2005, as part of the SORG study, Loukota et al. published a subclassification of condylar fractures which is both pragmatic and clinically useful as it aids visualisation and consideration of treatment options when combined with degree of overlap (in mm) and angle of displacement.

The presence of multiple classification systems, some of which have great detail (with accompanying complexity of use as noted in the review by Powers) has made it challenging to compare treatment strategies and outcomes, especially between units. The review by Powers is helpful in supporting the classification noted below, but also in clarifying the definition of displacement, meaning bony contact still within the fossa and dislocation, being outside the fossa.

Minimal displacement

Displacement <10° or overlap of bone edges by <2 mm, or both.

Moderate displacement

Displacement between 10° and 45° or bone overlap >2 mm, or both.

Severe displacement

Displacement >45° or loss of bone overlap, or both.

Although surgeons may disagree on which classification is the most useful, few would disagree on the need for robust reproducible data to compare outcomes of the various operative approaches.

Definitions

- Dicapitular (through the head of the condyle) fracture: the fracture starts in the articular surface and may extend outside the capsule (*Figure 16.1*).
- Fracture of the condylar neck: the fracture line starts above line A, and in more than half (the fracture distance) runs *above* line A – High condylar fracture.

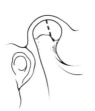 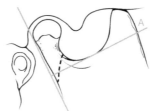 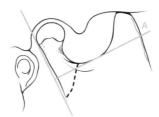

| Dicapitular fracture | Fracture of condylar neck | Fracture of condylar base |

Figure 16.1 Classification of condylar fractures. (Modified from Loukota RA, et al. *Br J Oral Maxillofac Surg* 2005;43:72–3.)

- Fracture of the condylar base: the fracture line runs behind the mandibular foramen and in more than half the distance *below* line A – Low condylar fracture.
- Line A: a perpendicular line through the sigmoid notch tangential to the ascending ramus.

IMAGING

Imaging in two planes is the normal investigation, usually an orthopantomogram (OPT) and postero-anterior (PA) mandible. With the advent of spiral computed tomography (CT) scanning, some surgeons may have a CT as an initial investigation. A CT may well be helpful with bilateral fractures, gross medial displacement and impacted fractures where a contra-lateral open bite is present due to the 'crushing' of the condylar head. Cone beam CT (CBCT) is a new addition to the available imaging options and may be useful in both diagnosis and follow-up.

CT of the condyle is mandatory prior to under-taking open operative management to ensure commi-nution and fracture location, as well as head position, is fully appreciated prior to surgery. Medical CT or CBCT are appropriate for this.

TREATMENT OPTIONS AND OUTCOMES

- No treatment
- Closed reduction (management)
- Open reduction
- Endoscopically assisted
- Free plating and grafting

Debate over operative surgical management has been intense over the last decade with two consensus conferences and a recent prospective randomised multi-centre study. There is a definite trend towards more surgeons adopting open reduction as standard of care according to increasingly accepted criteria.

Patient-specific variables also impact on treatment decisions: age, ability to cooperate; other facial frac-tures and comorbidity all influence the management decision.

Surgical variables include experience, fracture location (and imaging) and available instruments, for example, endoscopic and intracapsular fracture man-agement.

It is important to note several things at this point. Surgical (open) management of the condyle can be safely deferred for several days and is feasible beyond 1–2 weeks. As such it is entirely appropriate to defer a case until there is suitable assistance available, and all imaging is complete in most cases. This means that most open condyle cases are carried out during week-day semi-elective operating.

It is also appropriate in borderline cases to con-sider a 'trial of elastic IMF'. This can be utilised for 1–2 weeks to attempt to correct very minor occlusal dis-crepancies, and if the trial fails, the patient can proceed to open surgery.

A suggested treatment protocol is outlined in *Figure 16.2*, and the ideal outcomes of treatment are listed in *Table 16.1*.

TABLE 16.1 Ideal outcomes of condylar fracture treatment
Pain-free mouth opening >40 mm
Pain-free lateral excursions >6 mm
Stable and pain-free occlusion
Normal facial and jaw symmetry

No treatment

This is appropriate when no occlusal discrepancy or functional impairment exists.

Closed reduction (management)

This is a blanket term, which implies no 'open' inter-vention (*Table 16.2*). In common practice, it would involve the placement of Arch Bars, Splints, IMF screws or Rapid IMF™. All of these allow the placement of elastic intermaxillary traction/fixation.

The precise postoperative course can vary from 2 weeks to 3 months using guiding elastics, with most surgeons using elastics for 2–4 weeks. It is now well accepted that there is no place for wire IMF.

Closed management was the previous treatment of choice for both displaced and non-displaced frac-tures. Many surgeons had concerns about damage to the facial nerve with open reduction and it was not clear that reduced fractures gave better results. Com-plications of closed management can include painful or limited opening, deviation on opening, malocclusion and loss of posterior facial height. Outcome studies per-formed by Ellis confirm malocclusion, occlusal canting and loss of posterior facial height in patients treated with closed management compared with open reduc-tion. The facial asymmetry was notable at 6 weeks.

TABLE 16.2 Indications for closed management
Condylar neck fractures in children <15 years
Very high condylar neck fractures without dislocation
Intracapsular fractures

Open reduction

Open reduction is not a new concept, having been proposed in certain defined circumstances by Zide and Kent in 1983. The impact of technology (*Table 16.3*) and increased understanding of both the biomechanical

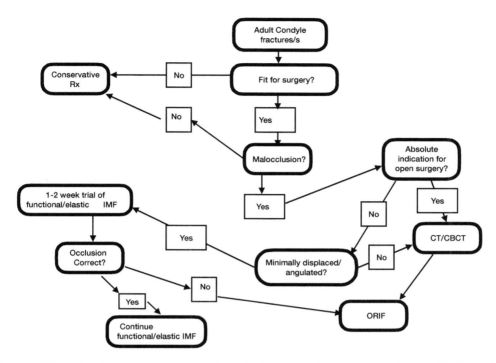

Figure 16.2 Flow chart for open management of mandibular condyle fractures. *Abbreviations:* CBCT, cone beam CT; CT, computed tomography; IMF, intermaxillary fixation; ORIF, open reduction and internal fixation; Rx, prescription.

TABLE 16.3 Impact of technology	
Plates	Including new three-dimensional designs
Imaging	Computed tomography and cone beam computed tomography
Instruments	Endoscope 90° screwdriver and drill

TABLE 16.4 Indications for open reduction
Adult cases with:
Failure of conservative management
Malocclusion with good prognosis for occluding teeth
Panfacial injuries, to establish posterior face height
Contraindications for closed treatment (poorly controlled seizures, alcohol/drug addiction, eating disorders/poorly controlled mental health problems)
Lateral dislocation
Intracranial displacement of the condylar head
Relative indication: 10° angulation/2-mm overlap

and functional advantages of plating, supported by good randomised studies, have encouraged surgeons to re-evaluate open reduction, and for others to explore endoscopically assisted reduction.

The principles of open management are similar for all fractures and include accurate reduction, stable internal fixation, preservation of blood supply and early active mobilisation. With open reduction of condylar fractures, the main specific concerns are facial nerve weakness/paralysis and scarring.

Much work has been carried out on evaluating open reduction (*Table 16.4*), and various surgical approaches have been described including submandibular, retromandibular with transparotid access, pre-auricular, coronal and rhytidectomy. If midfacial access is required, then a coronal approach may well be helpful; however, for the majority of cases a retromandibular incision parallel to the posterior border of the mandible with transparotid dissection will allow

safe exposure of the fracture. No trial evidence exists comparing the various access approaches; these can be broadly considered as either deep or transversing to the course of the facial nerve.

Pragmatism should be applied to the shortening and angulation figures when considering open reduction. It is common for surgeons to accept shortening up to 5 mm and angulations of greater than 10° with reported acceptable outcomes – consider the whole patient and not simply the imaging.

The commonest method of fixation is 2.0-mm titanium semi-rigid plates, with two plates, or specifically

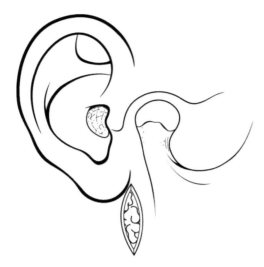

Figure 16.3 Retromandibular (transparotid) incision.

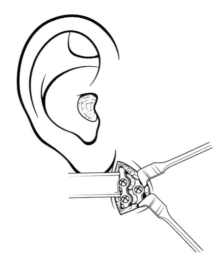

Figure 16.4 Fracture exposed and reduced.

designed three-dimensional plates with 8- or 6-mm screws.

A 70% success rate has been reported by Davis with free grafting alone or in conjunction with a ramus osteotomy in cases when adequate reduction and fixation could not be obtained.

Management of isolated unilateral condylar fracture

Although there are an array of possible approaches to the ramus/condyle, here we will focus on the retromandibular approach, due to its versatility, simplicity and good outcomes. For complex and very high fractures, any of the utility approaches to the temporomandibular joint (TMJ) can be utilised as needed.

Informed consent must be obtained, including discussion of likely complications such as scarring and facial nerve damage, although there is good evidence that permanent damage is rare.

Under endotracheal general anaesthesia the patient is prepped and draped, allowing access to the oral cavity for downward distraction of the ipsilateral angle to aid reduction. An intravenous dose of antibiotic is given at induction. Ideally, two assistants are required for retraction and mandibular manipulation. A small plug is placed in the external auditory meatus. The retromandibular incision is marked 1 cm distal to the posterior border of the ramus, approximately 2 cm in length (*Figure 16.3*).

Wide dissection in the superficial layer above the parotid fascia is carried out to facilitate retraction. The parotid fascia is divided sharply and with blunt dissection under direct vision. If encountered, the facial nerve branches are retracted out of the operative field. Once the masseter muscle is exposed, the surgeon uses a finger to palpate the underlying fracture and a vertical

incision is made down to bone. Subperiosteal stripping exposes the fracture, although the condylar fracture can be 'trapped' in the muscle and require careful dissection.

With retraction in a superior/inferior direction and use of a thin-bladed retractor behind the posterior border, the mandible can be displaced downwards and backwards with occlusal pressure, which increases the space and aids fracture reduction. Once fracture reduction has been achieved, adequate fixation is required. Some surgeons use intraoperative IMF, others will handhold the occlusion while it is fixed.

Options for plate fixation include one 2-mm plate of greater plate rigidity or two 2-mm plates placed as far apart as possible. Newer 3D plates may offer some ease of application. It is important to insert at least two screws (6–8 mm) in the distal aspect of the proximal fracture; placing the superior screw without the mandible in occlusion then re-reducing the fracture and placing the second screw, prior to fixation of the distal fragment, can facilitate this. A fracture gap can open at this point and a two-hole spaced plate with the space over the fracture is useful to close this gap by placing the superior screw and then securing manual reduction of occlusion with inferior traction on the distal screw holes of both plates to close the fracture gap prior to placing the final three screws (*Figure 16.4*).

The wound is closed in layers with attention to closing the masseter muscle and the parotid fascia/superficial musculoaponeurotic system (SMAS) prior to skin closure with non-resorbable sutures (*Figures 16.5–16.7*).

Endoscopically assisted reduction of condylar fractures

While open reduction has become more accepted, groups of surgeons have looked at using newer

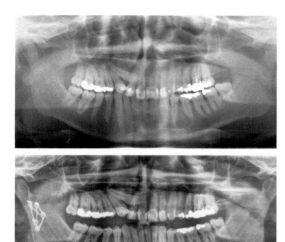

Figure 16.5 Combined pre- and postoperative OPTs.

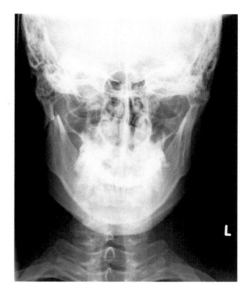

Figure 16.6 Preoperative PA mandible radiograph.

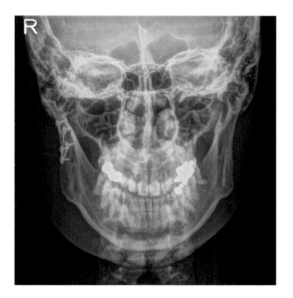

Figure 16.7 Postoperative PA mandible radiograph

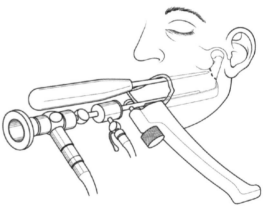

Figure 16.8 Endoscopic principle.

technology and applying this within maxillofacial surgery. Endoscopically assisted reduction is a good example, as it reduces the risk to the facial nerve and minimises scarring. Work done on the development of this technique confirms that there is a long and steep learning curve and that laterally displaced fractures are much easier than medially displaced fractures, and like all endoscopic procedures the surgeon must be able to convert to an open procedure to complete the surgery if needed.

With this development, the plating companies have designed and produced special instruments to facilitate endoscopically assisted reduction; however, most institutions have the basic light sources, monitor banks and camera attachments. The endoscopic approach uses an intraoral or submandibular approach along with a transbuccal access for some fixation (*Figure 16.8*).

Using the intraoral approach, a ramus incision similar to that for a mandibular osteotomy is made and the masseter muscle stripped to create the optical cavity. A 4-mm 30° endoscope with an adapted retractor provides direct vision and this is aided by a Freer elevator with built-in suction. Under vision and with special instruments, the fracture is manipulated and reduced. This may require extensive dissection at the posterior border or the sigmoid notch, and occasionally downward traction may be needed, which can be digital occlusal pressure or a wire at the angle.

The transoral approach can be used to place screws using an adaptable plate holder or a 90° screwdriver, although this can be difficult in a tight soft tissue envelope. Occasionally, a second transbuccal stab may be needed to use a threaded fracture manipulator, 'the screw on a stick', which can be used to place the initial screw in the proximal fragment.

Further refinement of all techniques will be required as challenges exist with difficulty reducing medially displaced fractures, a limited surgical cavity compared with other endoscopic procedures, the need for special training and instruments, and the reducing morbidity and treatment time of direct surgical access. It is fair to say that the initial enthusiasm for the endoscopic approach has waned somewhat, partly in response to comparable facial nerve outcomes via open approaches, added to the complexity of the instrumentation and the technical challenges of endoscopic surgery.

Dicapitular fractures

Dicapitular fractures, which include intracapsular fractures, represent a surgical challenge (*Figure 16.9*). Various surgical approaches have been described, centred on placement of screw fixation into the head to reduce and stabilise the fracture (*Figure 16.10*). The pre-auricular incision affords good access and avoids the transection of the cartilaginous auditory canal. Fixation is technically challenging and may be accomplished by lag screw osteosynthesis or the use of sonic weld.

These are extremely difficult cases to manage surgically, and are frequently managed in a closed manner. The outcomes in closed reduction are generally compromised with reduced mouth opening and compromise of envelope of jaw movement, but open reduction also has potential complications including facial nerve damage, as well as failure of fixation, and late resorption. Currently, management of these fracture patterns remains under debate.

Paediatric fractures

Children with condylar fractures are a very different group. Children exhibit a regenerative capacity that adults do not and will regenerate condylar form and function while adults compensate at an occlusal level with loss of posterior facial height.

The question is when do children become adults with respect to the need of ORIF. This is probably around the age of 13 and due consideration should be given to manage these in an open manner if indicated. Younger patients managed by closed reduction often require long-term follow-up as they can in rare circumstances present in later years with developmental abnormalities including asymmetry, hypoplasia or ankylosis.

Non-surgical management should be the rule for the paediatric population, with open reduction internal fixation for specific unusual cases only, especially older children.

Panfacial fractures

One of the clear indications for open reduction of condylar fractures is an associated midfacial fracture. The correction of vertical height aids the correction of the midfacial deformity and should be carried out when the mandibular fractures are reduced, perhaps before definitive midface correction.

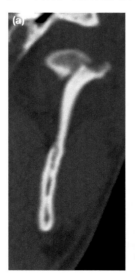
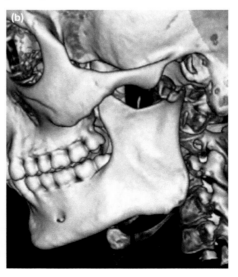

Figure 16.9 Intracapsular fracture with shortening, associated malocclusion. (a) Preoperative coronal image. (b) Preoperative three-dimensional image.

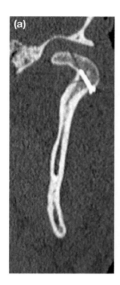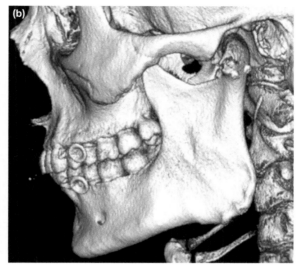

Figure 16.10 Postoperative views show good fixation and restoration of joint occlusal surface and posterior bone height. The patient had restoration of full temporomandibular joint function. (a) Postoperative coronal image. (b) Postoperative three-dimensional image.

Bilateral fractures

When associated with a symphyseal fracture this can lead to mandibular widening and great care must be taken to ensure accurate reduction at the symphysis or a postoperative malocclusion will be evident, in spite of anatomical condylar fracture reductions.

If two fractures are present it is ideal to fix both; however, at least one needs to be fixed to regain height.

POSTOPERATIVE MANAGEMENT

Good postoperative care with elastic traction for closed management and jaw exercises and clear postoperative instructions for open or endoscopic treated fractures are needed.

TOP TIPS AND HAZARDS

- Treat the patient, and the occlusion, not the radiograph.
- Ensure you have adequate assistance.
- Start with easier low laterally displaced fractures when starting open reductions.
- Do not attempt a high medially placed fracture as your first.
- Give clear postoperative instructions.
- Consider endoscopic approaches only when you master open surgery.
- Use new technology to aid treatment, e.g. three-dimensional plates.

Complications

These include malocclusion, condylar necrosis (with associated open bite), wound infection (rare <1%), hypertrophic scarring, facial nerve weakness (transient or permanent), sialocele and fixation failure.

FURTHER READING

Adbel-Galik, Loukota RA. Fractures of the mandibular condyle: evidence base and current concepts of management. *Br J Oral Maxillofac Surg* 2009;**48**:520–6.

Downie JJ, Devlin MF, Carton ATM, Hislop WS. Prospective study of morbidity associated with open reduction and internal fixation of the fractured condyle by the transparotid approach. *Br J Oral Maxillofac Surg* 2009;**47**:370–3.

Ellis E, Simon P, Throckmorton GS. Occlusal results after open or closed treatment of fractures of the mandibular condylar process. *J Oral Maxillofac Surg* 2004;**58**:260–4.

Loukota RA, Eckelt U, De Bont L, Rasse M. Subclassification of fractures of the condylar process of the mandible. *Br J Oral Maxillofac Surg* 2005;**43**:72–3.

Powers DB. Classification of mandibular condylar fractures. *Atlas Oral Maxillofac Surg Clin North Am* 2017;**25**:1–10.

Bailey & Love's Essential Operations Bailey & Love's Essential Operations
Bailey & Love's Essential Operations Bailey & Love's Essential Operations
Bailey & Love's Essential Operations Bailey & Love's Essential Operations

PART 3 | Trauma

Chapter 17

Zygomatic Fractures

Christopher Vinall, Michael Perry

INTRODUCTION

Fractures of the zygomaticomaxillary complex are one of the most common injuries encountered by the maxillofacial team. A thorough understanding of this aesthetic and functional area of the facial skeleton is important to provide the best possible outcome for the patient. Terminology can be confusing: 'zygoma', 'zygomaticomaxillary', 'malar', 'tripod' and 'tetrapod' are all terms used to describe essentially the same injury – a fracture of the zygomaticomaxillary orbital complex (*Figure 17.1*). Apart from isolated zygomatic arch fractures, all other fractures involve part of the orbital floor and lateral orbital wall to some extent. These are termed impure orbital fractures. Therefore, assessment of the orbit (and eye) is an integral part of management.

ESSENTIAL SURGICAL ANATOMY

The cheek is supported by the zygomatic bone. This articulates with the frontal bone at the frontozygomatic (FZ) suture, with the maxilla medially and with the temporal bone posteriorly and within the orbit. The body of the zygoma provides the aesthetic projection of the cheek and together with the supraorbital ridge affords some protection to the eye. Inferiorly, the body of the zygoma forms approximately the lateral two-thirds of the infraorbital rim, which is important for lower eyelid support.

Consequently, any displacement in this area can affect eyelid function. Vertical displacement of the entire zygoma can lower the lateral canthus and lateral attachment of the globe with it (Whitnall's tubercle). This can result in diplopia, hypoglobus and an anti-mongoloid slant to the eye (*Figure 17.2*).

The facial skeleton is not a solid structure, but contains several 'cavities', notably the sinuses, orbits and nasal cavity. Around these, the bones condense to form a series of vertical struts known as 'buttresses'. The zygoma forms part of the lateral buttress. Horizontally buttresses also exist but are much thinner. Consequently, the facial skeleton is very good at resisting vertically directed forces (biting, chewing), but is relatively weak at resisting horizontal forces (i.e. during most injuries). These buttresses are a key element to facial repair and the support for any fixation.

The temporalis muscle passes beneath the zygomatic arch to insert into the coronoid process of the mandible. Displaced fractures of the zygomatic arch can therefore impede mouth opening by interfering with this. The muscle is invested in the temporal fascia, which arises from the skull and passes down to insert into the zygomatic arch. This is important surgical anatomy and forms the rationale for the Gillies approach. The masseter muscle passes up from the mandible and attaches to the body of the zygoma and its arch. This may have a role in the postoperative displacement of fractures that have not been adequately fixed.

(a)   (b)

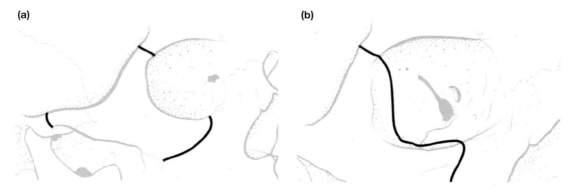

Figure 17.1 Fracture configuration.

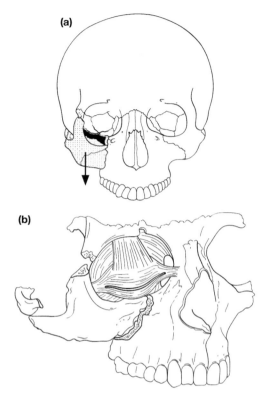

(a)

(b)

Figure 17.2 Downward displacement results in vertical ocular dystopia and an anti-mongoloid slant.

The zygoma and maxilla support many of the periorbital and perinasal muscles attached to the periosteum. In extensive repairs, degloving of much of these bones may be required. Resuspension of the soft tissues is important during wound closure to prevent soft tissue ptosis or sagging postoperatively. The infraorbital nerve supplies sensation to most of the cheek and the ipsilateral half of the nose and upper lip. This passes along the floor of the orbit and exits the infraorbital foramen approximately 1 cm below the infraorbital rim, approximately midway along its length. The infraorbital canal and foramen form a plane of weakness and are often implicated in these fracture patterns. The nerve is at risk during fracture propagation and subsequent repair.

PREOPERATIVE CONSIDERATIONS

Assessment

Several classifications exist. A practical one would be to consider fractures as follows:

- Isolated
  - Zygomatic arch
  - Infraorbital rim
- Minimally displaced

- Displaced fractured
- Comminuted fractures
- Associated with midface or complex orbital fractures

With the exception of isolated arch fractures, all zygomatic fractures extend into the orbit. Following the assessment of the head and neck (remember the ABCs [airway, breathing, circulation]), the eye therefore takes priority over any fractures. Check the following:

- Visual acuity
- Evidence of globe injury – involve Ophthalmology colleagues
- Diplopia
- Any signs of entrapment require a comprehensive orthoptic assessment

Clinical features of a fracture may include the following:

- Pain
- Periorbital bruising and swelling
- Limitation of eye movements with diplopia
- Altered sensation of cheek/upper lip
- Restricted jaw movements
- Subconjunctival haemorrhage and chemosis
- Surgical emphysema
- Flattening of the malar prominence (often masked by swelling immediately after injury)
- Palpable infraorbital step
- Anti-mongoloid slant
- Unilateral epistaxis (due to bleeding into the maxillary sinus)
- Enophthalmos
- Exophthalmos
- Hypoglobus (vertical ocular dystopia)
- Dysocclusion (premature contact on ipsilateral molar teeth, due to flexing of the upper dental arch)

Imaging

This has been an evolving subject as computed tomography (CT) scanning has gained acceptance and adoption. Plain radiology is technically challenging to achieve predictable diagnostic material and in addition demands cooperation of the patient, who may be intoxicated. As a result, accident and emergency images are frequently poorly centred, non-symmetrical, poorly penetrated and not diagnostic. Occipitomental (OM), lateral face and submental vertex (SMV) are often taken. They are assessed using McGrigor lines. On occasion step deformities can be seen; however, a fluid level is common. The orbit is simply not visualised or interpreted reliably.

CT allows for visualisation in axial, coronal and sagittal dimensions, and interrogation for soft tissue involvement (*Figure 17.3*). In contemporary facial trauma surgery, high-energy mechanisms are common, orbital floor and medial wall components need diagnosing and planning for surgery. In addition, the

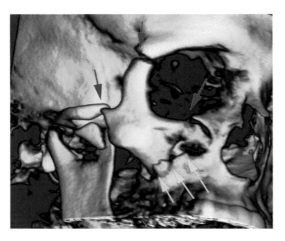

Figure 17.3 This reformatted scan demonstrates the complexity of the case. Note the segmentation of the articulations (blue arrows), and the buttress (yellow arrows) is surgically best approached following elevation of the bone, which will reposition the fragments by 'ligamentotaxis'.

three-dimensional position of all the individual fragments allows for decisions on surgical access, methods of reduction and sites of osteosynthesis.

Immediate advice

These fractures rarely require urgent intervention and can be assessed as an outpatient. In the interim, patients should be advised not to blow their nose to avoid surgical emphysema. The concern here is not the air, but the associated contamination (mucus, etc.), which can pass into the orbit and the soft tissues of the cheek through the fracture. This can result in orbital cellulitis, both a sight- and potentially life-threatening condition if untreated. Patients may also be advised not to fly, although there is no good evidence base for this.

In high-energy trauma, massive medialisation of the zygoma may contribute to an orbital compartment syndrome and may be managed according to a standard orbital protocol including cantholysis (see *Chapter 12*). Occasionally, an urgent decompression by zygomatic elevation may be required.

Indications for reduction and timing of surgery

When there is clinical and radiological evidence of a displaced zygomatic fracture, indications include the following:

- Facial deformity
- Loss of lower eyelid support
- Ocular dystopia
- Limitation of mandibular opening
- Sensory nerve deficit thought to be due to nerve compression

Timing of treatment depends on the degree of swelling and the general condition of the patient (notably any head or ocular injuries). Surgery does not need to be carried out on an immediate basis but planned according to service opportunities (i.e. within a few days). However, significant swelling may interfere with accurate preoperative clinical assessment, as well as compromising the surgical conduit reducing the predictability of an ideal aesthetic result. In addition, the assessment of the reduction on the operating table would also be technically challenging. It is a truism that the most difficult fracture to assess clinically is the total closed reduction. In practice, the surgical window is between 5 and 15 days. If delayed, then the reduction is more difficult and accurate placement of the fragments less predictable as the callus interferes with the reduction. Acceptable results can still be obtained up to 5 weeks after injury, but this may require mobilisation by osteotomising the articulations and an increase in the number of access incisions and plating.

STEPWISE OPERATIVE TECHNIQUE

There has been a general move towards open reduction and internal fixation, placing at least one plate, typically either a 'buttress' plate or one across the FZ suture. This is based on the concerns regarding masseteric and other forces acting on unsupported reduction over the ensuing weeks. A buttress plate can be placed transorally and an FZ plate via a small upper blepharoplasty incision. In both cases scarring is virtually invisible. It must be appreciated that the choice of operative fixation site and number of them is based on the phenotype of the fracture and surgeon preference.

The orbital incision, described in the orbital chapter (*Chapter 18*) is required if there is associated ocular malposition or functional problems. The technical challenge of managing a comminuted infraorbital margin should not be underestimated and may be facilitated by removal of fragments and plating *ex vivo*.

Approach and reduction techniques include the following:

- Temporal approach (Gillies) (*Figure 17.4*)
- Percutaneous or 'malar' hook (*Figure 17.5*)
- Eyebrow approach – via upper blepharoplasty incision (*Figure 17.6*)
- Keen approach (intraoral) (*Figure 17.7*)
- Coronal access for telescoped zygomatic arch and significant comminution (see *Chapters 19* and *24*)

Sequencing is stereotypical and may be achieved:

1. Address the FZ suture first, if it is significantly displaced. The purpose of the fixation is to re-establish the vertical height of the fracture and hopefully the correct height of the lateral canthal/Whitnall's attachments.
2. The zygomatic arch if telescoped or a discontinuity pattern to establish the anterior projection of the

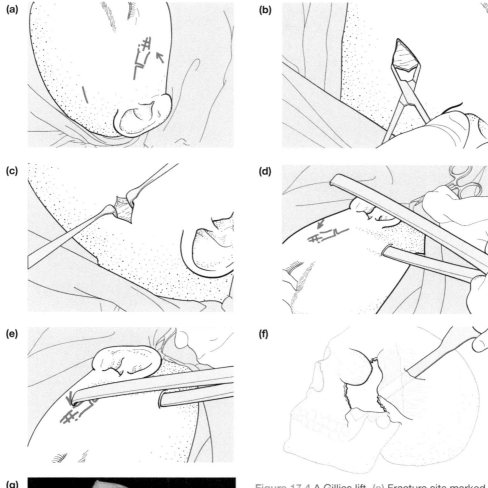

(a)

(b)

(c)

(d)

(e)

(f)

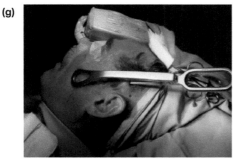

(g)

Figure 17.4 A Gillies lift. (a) Fracture site marked. 2-cm skin incision in the temple. (b) Following skin incision blunt dissect down to temporalis fascia (TF). Watch out for superficial temporal artery. (c) TF is incised and lifted off the temporalis muscle. A curved clip is good for this. (d) The elevator is passed deep to the TF towards the zygoma. Try passing a Howarth periosteal elevator before – it helps open up the correct plane. (e) Make sure the elevator is under the bone before lifting (do not use the skull as a fulcrum). Schematic/operative view immediately prior to lift. (f) Surgical anatomy of lift. (g) Rowe elevator inserted to reduce the fracture.

zygomatic prominence. The arch is also frequently bowed, and this is extremely difficult to diagnose in a closed reduction.

3   Reduce and repair the lateral buttress. This is undertaken via an intraoral approach. In many cases, this may be the only procedure required if (1) and (2) are not significantly displaced. This plate provides mechanical stability. This will NOT obviate the need of an FZ plate if there is any displacement at this site.

4   Assess the infraorbital rim/orbital floor (force duction test) and expose if necessary.
5   Consider the need for bone grafting the buttress. This is rare and more likely in high-energy injuries.
6   Careful resuspension of the cheek prior to closure.

Antibiotics and steroids

Antibiotics are not generally prescribed at initial presentation. A common protocol would be intravenous

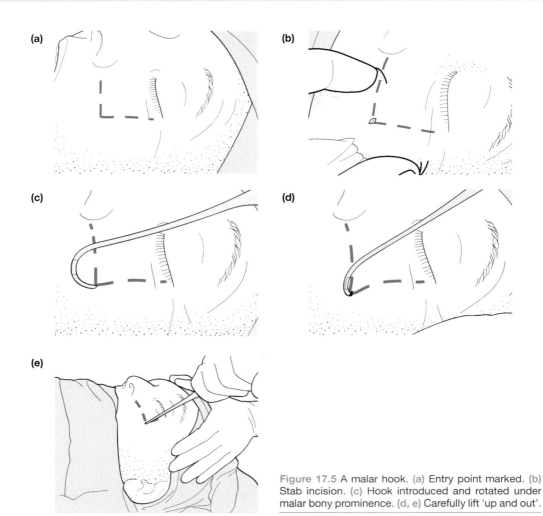

(a)

(b)

(c)

(d)

(e)

Figure 17.5 A malar hook. (a) Entry point marked. (b) Stab incision. (c) Hook introduced and rotated under malar bony prominence. (d, e) Carefully lift 'up and out'.

antibiotics and steroids (dexamethasone) at induction of general anaesthesia. Postoperatively, one dose of dexamethasone and two doses of intravenous antibiotics are probably all that is required. This topic is open to considerable controversy.

Isolated arch fractures

These can often be reduced via a Gillies approach or transorally. They are usually stable, but occasionally can fall back down. If so, they may need support. Alternatives include the following:

- Accept this and deal with any problems secondarily
- Suturing an external splint along the arch (suturing is passed deep to the arch and tied over the splint) – the Zimmer orthopaedic finger splint is ideal
- Open reduction and internal fixation (ORIF) via a pre-auricular or coronal incision

POSTOPERATIVE CARE

The main concerns here are to ensure that the fracture stays in the correct position, and that serious complications such as loss of sight and severe infections do not develop. As patients wake up, they may be initially agitated, and the repaired site must be protected from inadvertent injury. Various ways of achieving this are possible, but having the site clearly marked and an alert recovery/ward nurse go a long way to achieving this. Swelling and bleeding behind the globe can occur, which unrecognised can result in loss of vision. Careful observation of the eye is therefore important in the immediate postoperative period. Patients should be advised not to blow their nose.

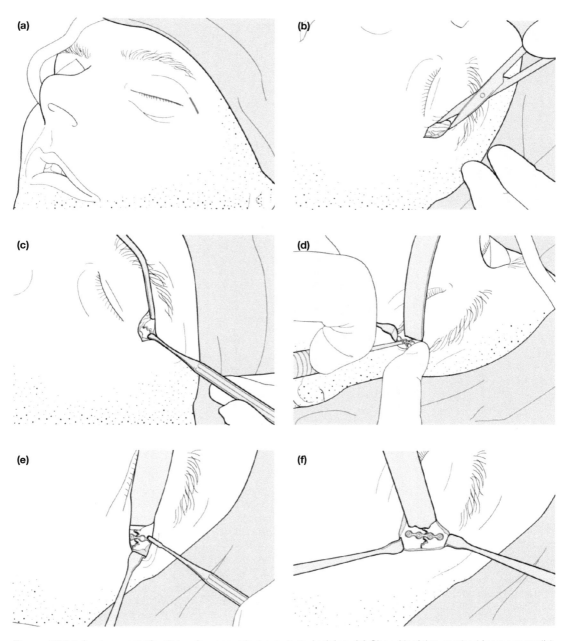

Figure 17.6 A frontozygomatic plate, via upper blepharoplasty incision. (a) Site of incision marked in upper eyelid. (b) Following skin incision, dissect down to periosteum. (c) Incise periosteum and elevate to expose fracture. (d) Some fractures are easily elevated and plated. If very displaced, screw plate to lower half of fracture first. (e) Use a small-hooked instrument or wire to lift and reduce the fracture by applying force through an unused upper hole (do not damage the plate). Drill and screw the other hole. (f) Place second screw. If correctly reduced, this will accurately restore the vertical height.

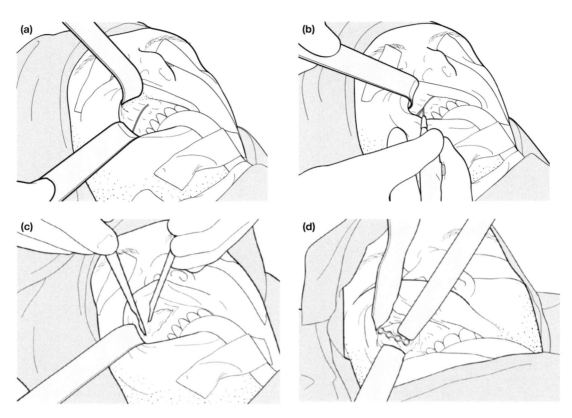

Figure 17.7 A buttress plate. (a) Mucosa marked allowing cuff to close. (b) Incision with knife or cutting diathermy (care with metal retractors). (c) Subperiosteal dissection to expose fractures. (d) Following fracture reduction (Gillies, hook or via incision) open reduction and internal fixation (ORIF) with four-hole plate (usually).

POSSIBLE COMPLICATIONS AND HOW TO DEAL WITH THEM

Retrobulbar haemorrhage/orbital compartment syndrome

Proptosis following injury or repair needs to be evaluated quickly and carefully. The concern here is loss of sight following retinal/optic ischaemia. For this reason, the eye is put under careful observation, usually until the next day. Progressive pain, deteriorating vision, proptosis and ophthalmoplegia are the main signs to check. Once the orbit/zygoma has been reduced, the orbit becomes a closed space and swelling is contained, resulting in an orbital compartment syndrome (OCS). For this reason, steroids are variably prescribed postoperatively. The key to urgency of treatment is the visual acuity; if the vision is normal, decompression is not required. Rarely do such cases need to return to theatre, but if they do it should be remembered that an OCS may not release blood. If the proptosis is severe, decompression will be required. Intravenous acetazolamide, mannitol, steroids and a lateral canthotomy buy time while theatre preparations are being made (see *Chapter 12*). If in doubt, globe tension should be measured by a 'Tono-Pen' or another suitable device.

TOP TIPS AND HAZARDS

- If the eyelids are swollen, gently pressing on them (not the globe) for a few minutes reduces this significantly to assess visual acuity.
- Numbness of the cheek and upper lip is an important sign that should generate a high index of suspicion for orbital or cheek bone fracture.
- Remember the nasolacrimal duct during infraorbital/eyelid access.
- Isolated arch or simple fractures which are incomplete at the FZ suture are the most suitable for closed reduction.
- Arch fractures with associated coronoid fractures are at risk of ankylosis.
- Correct alignment of the sphenozygomatic suture (lateral orbital wall) is a good on-the-table indication that the fracture is correctly reduced.
- A force duction test should be performed at the end of any reduction. As the fractures realign, orbital soft tissues may become trapped.
- Beware of late enophthalmos – follow patients closely.
- Place sticky tape over the repaired site. Do not draw on the patient – they may try and rub it off.
- Not all vision-threatening proptosis is due to retrobulbar haemorrhage (RBH).

FURTHER READING

Brucoli M, Boffano P, Broccardo E, et al. The "European zygomatic fracture" research project: The epidemiological results from a multicenter European collaboration. *J Craniomaxillofac Surg* 2019;**47**:616–21.

Buchanan EP, Hopper RA, Suver DW, Hayes AG, Gruss JS, Birgfeld CB. Zygomaticomaxillary complex fractures and their association with naso-orbito-ethmoid fractures: a 5-year review. *Plast Reconstr Surg* 2012;**130**:1296–304.

Cornelius CP, Audige L, Kunz C, Buitrago-Tellez CH, Rudderman R, Prein J. The Comprehensive AOCMF Classification System: Midface Fractures – Level 3 Tutorial. *Craniomaxillofac Trauma Reconstr* 2014;**7(Suppl 1)**:S068-91.

Lu W, Zhou H, Xiao C, Shen Q, Lin M, Fan X. Late correction of orbital-zygomatic-maxillary fractures combined with orbital wall fractures. *J Craniofac Surg* 2012;**23**:1672–6.

Perry M, Holmes S. Fractures of the cheek: zygomatico-maxillary complex. In: *Atlas of Operative Maxillofacial Trauma Surgery*, Perry M, Holmes S (Eds). London: Springer-Verlag; 2014.

Chapter 18

Orbital Trauma

James Padgett, Duaa Al-Sayed, Michael Williams

INTRODUCTION

The orbit is involved in a high proportion of blunt force facial injuries – approximately 40%. Most commonly these are in conjunction with more extensive midfacial injuries often associated with fractures of the zygomatic, maxillary or nasoethmoidal complexes. A second group of 'pure' orbital fractures exist and these occur in isolation from the outer frame. These are often referred to as blowout fractures, or more accurately isolated wall or floor fractures. The primary aim of treatment is to restore form and function to the orbit, recreating the suspension and support of the globe, relieving entrapment, enabling free movement of the eye.

ANATOMY

The orbit comprises an outer frame within which the walls are described as floor, medial wall, roof and lateral wall (*Figure 18.1*). The outer frame is strong and forms part of the midfacial buttressing system. However, the walls, particularly the floor and medial wall, are extremely thin (lamina papyracea – paper thin), accounting for the frequency of fractures in these areas. The floor has a Lazy S shape in sagittal plane, it is concave upwards in the anterior third but then becomes convex upwards in the posterior two-thirds (post-bulbar bulge blending into the key area medially).

Anteriorly there are four walls at the orbital rim. Deeper in the orbit, the medial wall and floor blend, and at this point the orbit becomes a three-walled pyramidal structure. This forms an important postero-medial

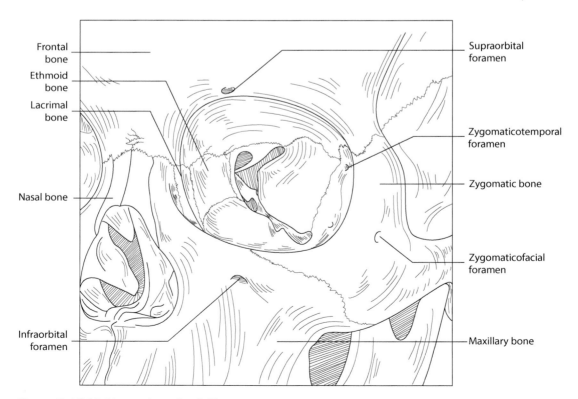

Figure 18.1 Orbital bones, front view (left).

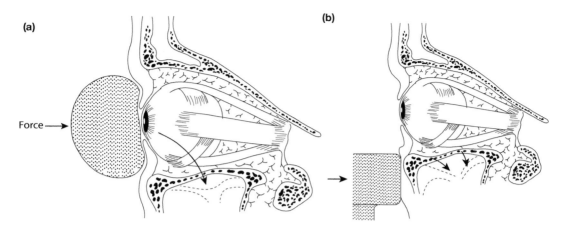

Figure 18.2 Proposed mechanisms involved in blowout fractures. (a) Conductive theory. (b) Hydraulic theory.

bulge which has also been coined the 'key area' of Hammer. The anterior and posterior ethmoidal arteries pass cranial to the ethmoid and a potential source of bleeding. Passing through the floor is the inferior orbital fissure, which often represents the lateral limit of floor fracture as the bone becomes denser in this region.

At the orbital apex, the medially located optic canal passes through dense bone of the sphenoid transmitting the optic nerve together with the central artery of the retina. More laterally, the superior orbital fissure transmits branches of the ophthalmic division of trigeminal nerve together with the superior and inferior branches of the oculomotor nerve, the trochlear and abducens nerves. Anterior to the globe, the upper and lower tarsal plates are attached to the medial and lateral walls by the medial and lateral canthal ligaments. This tense fascial sheath constitutes a 'fifth wall' of the orbit, thereby forming a closed box.

MECHANISM OF INJURY

Two theories have been proposed to explain the mechanism of isolated orbital fractures. In the Hydraulic theory, it is proposed that a force applied to the outer orbital rim leads to a transient increase in intraorbital pressure, leading to a 'blowout fracture'. The Conductive theory proposes a transient deformation of the rim which remains intact but the transmitted force leads to a fracture at a weaker area within the orbit (*Figure 18.2*) as orbital injuries rarely lead to significant ocular injury. Both mechanisms probably coexist.

INITIAL ASSESSMENT

Visual acuity must be assessed at an early stage and enquiries made regarding the presence of diplopia and periorbital paraesthesia.

Traumatic optic neuropathy (TON) is uncommon and presents secondary to either direct or indirect trauma to the optic nerve. Management is controversial and historically has included mega dose steroids and surgical exploration and decompression. Examination should include assessment of the periorbital soft tissues – the presence of a subconjunctival haematoma without posterior limit indicates a likely breach in the orbital periosteum. Red colour desaturation is an important early sign, which when combined with a positive swinging light test may indicate reduced optic nerve function, a relative afferent pupillary defect (RAPD). In the unconscious patient, pupillary reactions take on further importance. If the eye of the injured side is closed, then optic nerve function can be assessed with a bright light while assessing for consensual reflex.

Examination proceeds with palpation of the outer frame, following which eye movements are carefully assessed in the nine cardinal positions of gaze carefully documenting any presence of restriction or diplopia.

INVESTIGATIONS
Orthoptic assessment

This is mandatory and includes formal assessment of acuity, and testing of eye movements in cardinal positions of gaze, pupil movements and cover testing. This may be supplemented by Hess charts and fields of binocular single vision (*Figure 18.3*).

Radiology

The imaging modality of choice for orbital trauma is computed tomography (CT), ideally with sagittal, coronal and 3D reformats. With improvement in image quality and tissue differentiation, an alternative to CT is cone beam CT (CBCT). This has repeatedly been

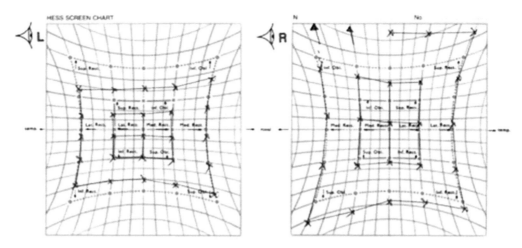

Figure 18.3 Hess charts indicating left orbital floor fracture. Note restricted movements in left chart but overcompensation in uninjured right eye.

shown to be adequate and reliable in the preoperative diagnosis of orbital floor and wall fractures. It has the added benefit of significantly reduced doses of radiation.

Intraoperative imaging

Intraoperative CT or CBCT can be used to assess on table the position of the implant, enabling immediate revision/repositioning as necessary. An intraoperative revision of 22.7% has been reported by one such unit using intraoperative imaging, potentially obviating the need for repeat surgery in that cohort.

Guidance systems offer an alternative to intraoperative imaging, using preoperative CT data integrated with navigational equipment to allow real-time intraoperative imaging of dissection depth and instrument positioning in a multiplanar format. Furthermore, by highlighting the posterior limit and margins of the plate, implant positioning can be estimated. However, many experienced surgeons would suggest deep orbital dissection is safe by following sound anatomical principles.

Postoperative imaging

The decision to obtain postoperative imaging has to be based on sound clinical assessment weighing up the risk of radiation exposure. As with preoperative imaging, CBCT is becoming a more common modality. However, it has been suggested that if clinical restriction is evident postoperatively, conventional multislice CT is preferable to adequately demonstrate the extraocular muscles and tissue.

PAEDIATRIC INJURIES

Paediatric orbital fractures are less common, the walls of the orbit being much thicker as a consequence of the undeveloped paranasal sinuses. When they do occur, they can lead to a true trap door (green stick) fracture, often incarcerating orbital tissue. These are commonly missed injuries due to the absence of other signs. As there is minimal periosteal disruption, there can be an absence of subconjunctival haemorrhage, therefore often being referred to as the 'white eye' fracture. It is imperative to operate and release the entrapped tissues as soon as possible, many emphasising within 5 days.

TREATMENT

Ocular function is the single most important consideration in the management of these injuries. This takes on even greater importance should poor or absent vision exist in the uninjured eye, this can be a contraindication for surgical repair, even accepting a minimal degree of enophthalmos in certain cases.

For 'complex' injuries, it is essential that the outer frame is treated first, restoring the antero-posterior and lateral dimensions of the orbit. This means the wall fractures are then repaired in exactly the same way as for an isolated injury.

Small, isolated injuries with no evidence of enophthalmos or diplopia can be safely observed and, in many cases, no operative intervention will be required. However, larger defects are likely to lead to a significant enophthalmos which can be difficult to correct later, therefore most would favour early operative repair. Other indications for operative intervention include significant entrapment and diplopia.

OPERATIVE PROCEDURE

- The patient is supine with a slight degree of head up under hypotensive anaesthesia
- Both eyes should be exposed and protected with eye shields

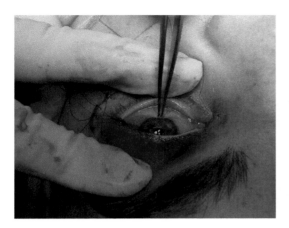
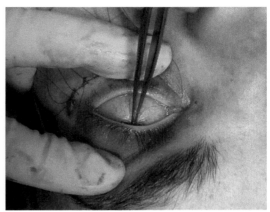

Figure 18.4 Forced duction test which should be performed preoperatively and on completion of repair to exclude entrapment.

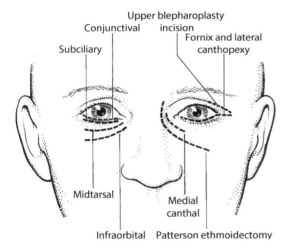

Figure 18.5 Diagram showing various surgical approaches to the orbit.

- Forced duction test performed to assess any restriction in ocular motility (*Figure 18.4*)
- The floor can be approached by either a lower eyelid incision (anterior lamellar) or a transconjunctival incision (posterior lamellar) with or without a transcaruncular or lateral canthotomy extension
- There are three lower eyelid incisions (*Figure 18.5*). The midtarsal incision is regarded as the most predictable
- Incision through skin followed by careful sharp dissection through orbicularis oculi to reach the tarsal plate. Meticulous haemostasis with bipolar forceps is essential
- Using careful retraction with a Desmarres retractor, a clear plane is revealed between orbicularis oculi and tarsal plate and the orbital septum more inferiorly

- Finally, sharp dissection onto the anterior surface of the infraorbital rim (*Figure 18.6*)

The transconjunctival approach gives excellent exposure of the orbit and is probably the approach of choice for larger defects. Dissection can be pre- or post-septal. The pre-septal approach is more complicated with significant advantages with respect to containment of the orbital fat and septum preservation. The post-septal approach is often preferred as it is technically easier.

- Retract the lower lid anteriorly with a Desmarres retractor, a malleable retractor can be placed directly behind the orbital rim, thus placing the tissues under tension (*Figure 18.7*)
- The conjunctival incision is then made, preferably made with a needle point monopolar at a low setting (e.g. 8)
- Retractors are then repositioned inside the wound allowing further dissection, directly to the anterior surface of the orbital rim

Whichever approach is used, the periosteum on the anterior aspect of the orbital rim is now incised, thus minimising herniation of periorbital fat.

- The periosteum is easily elevated over the rim and dissection proceeds in a downward direction before passing posteriorly until the anterior margin of the floor defect is identified
- At this point 'out flank' the defect identifying the margins. The lateral wall of the orbit is robust and easy to establish a subperiosteal plane
- The inferior orbital fissure is then identified and can be safely coagulated and divided to give much improved access

For greater exposure, the approach can be combined with a lateral canthotomy. For this procedure, a small skin incision passes through the fornix between

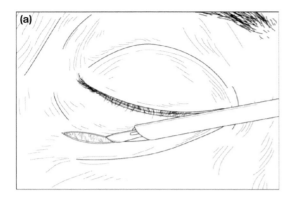

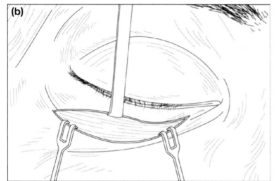

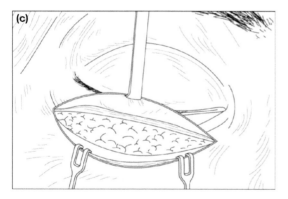

Figure 18.6 (a) Midtarsal skin incision. (b) Retraction of wound edge revealing plane between orbicularis occuli and the tarsal plate. (c) Incision on anterior wall of orbital rim to give access to orbital floor.

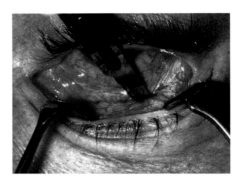

Figure 18.7 Transconjunctival incision. Retraction of lower eyelid with Desmarres retractor combined with tension applied with blunt malleable retractor inside orbital rim to place tissues under tension prior to division with needle point diathermy.

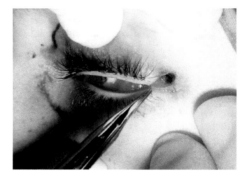

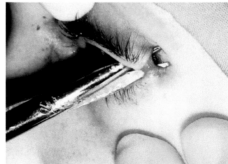

Figure 18.8 Lateral canthotomy, following skin incision the lower canthal band is identified and divided.

the upper and lower eyelids following which the lower limb of the lateral canthus can be divided (*Figure 18.8*).

Involvement of the medial wall is common in high-energy mechanisms, and while historically a coronal flap was used, establishing a common plane between the orbital and coronal incisions is technically challenging. The transcaruncular extension to the transconjunctival approach has revolutionised surgery to this region and is usually used in isolation.

Technique

- Traction sutures are placed at the medial portion of the lower and upper lids at the level of the tarsus
- The carancul is fixated with forceps and then the pica is grasped. A retro-carancular incision is made through the conjunctiva using dissecting scissors
- This incision is made in the direction of the posterior lacrimal crest

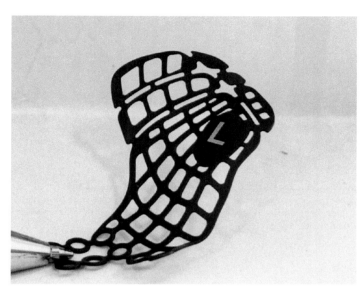

Figure 18.9 Synthes matrix preformed orbital plate.

- Stevens scissors are then used to bluntly dissect to the medial orbital wall, posterior to the posterior lacrimal crest, along the semilunar folds and medial to Horner's muscle
- After vertical incision of the periorbita, posterior of the insertion of Horner's muscle, the medial orbital wall is exposed

Combining the transcaruncular approach with the lateral canthotomy approach already described can give 270° of exposure, enabling dissection around the medial, inferior, lateral walls of orbit, and zygomatico-frontal (ZF) suture.

The posterior limit of dissection should be to the posterior margin of the defect but in deep orbital trauma there is clearly a limit to how far dissection can proceed without endangering the optic nerve. It has been suggested that subperiosteal dissection should not proceed beyond 35 mm from the orbital rim but this guideline should not be used in the presence of an unreduced orbital rim fracture.

Reconstruction

Simple single wall defects can be restored with a single sheet of PDS (polydioxanone sulphate) or medpor sheet. The established preferred material of choice for large orbital reconstructions is titanium, which may be achieved by either stock plates, preformed contoured plates or individualised CAD CAM constructions. CAD CAM reconstructions are expensive but probably provide the safest constructs in complex patterns.

Anatomically preformed orbital plates come in small and large sizes and are size appropriate (*Figure 18.9*).

The plates have a segmented design allowing adaptation of both the medial extension and floor length together with fixation screw holes to accurately locate the plate onto the orbital rim. These recognise the importance of the 'key area', having a 'rigid zone' in the posterior orbit to allow a consistent form in this region. They are probably the material of choice in the moderate orbital defect or for impure fractures that require orbital rim reconstruction prior to orbital repair.

- Following selection and insertion of the implant, assess pupillary level and enophthalmos
- The forced duction test is repeated (see *Figure 18.4*)
- Once the surgeon is happy with the reconstruction, the implant is secured ideally with titanium screws, prior to closure
- It is essential to re-suture the periosteum to suspend the malar fat pad
- The muscle is not closed
- Skin is gently apposed with interrupted 6:0 nylon sutures or continuous subcuticular closure with 5/0 nylon
- Many surgeons choose not to close the conjunctiva, reducing the risk of entropion in transconjunctival approaches
- Postoperative orbital observations including visual acuity, pupil reactions, ocular movements and most importantly increasing pain. A clear protocol should be established
- The patient should be nursed at 45° to reduce periorbital swelling. They should be encouraged to mobilise their eyes and avoid nose blowing

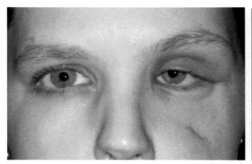 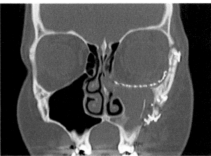

Figure 18.10 Enophthalmos clinical sequelae and imaging. There is a malunion of the left zygomatic bone and the orbital implant is malpositioned, being too low on the medial wall (note the natural upward and medial slope of the uninjured right floor which has not been replicated). This has led to an expansion of orbital volume and enophthalmos as a consequence.

COMPLICATIONS

Blindness

This is the most important complication of orbital surgery, but the incidence is extremely low.

Diplopia

Diplopia is often worse after surgery due to oedema or haematoma but is likely to improve over the following few weeks. Regular orthoptic follow-up is required to ensure improvement, indicate reoperation or referral to a strabismus surgeon.

Enophthalmos

Enophthalmos is largely due to inaccurate restoration of orbital volume, often requiring secondary correction (*Figure 18.10*).

Retrobulbar haematoma

A retrobulbar haematoma follows bleeding within the orbit and can either be intraconal or extraconal. As bleeding continues pressure increases within the orbit leading to an orbital compartment syndrome and pressure on the optic nerve with signs of reducing visual acuity, ophthalmoplegia and pain leading to a fixed dilated pupil. This can occur either following the initial injury or following surgical intervention. Emergency medical measures include the use of steroids, mannitol and acetazolamide, combined with surgical intervention, a lateral canthotomy and inferior cantholysis to give temporary control prior to urgent formal surgical exploration and drainage (*Chapter 12*).

TOP TIPS AND HAZARDS

- Remember sight comes first, visual acuity and full ophthalmic examination for all.
- Close working relationship with ophthalmic surgeons.
- Maintain high index of suspicion of orbital injury in all mid-third trauma.
- Assess integrity of orbital frame.
- Accurate recording of size and location of defect using high-resolution axial scanning with coronal and sagittal reformatting.
- Children require urgent treatment.
- Plan access incisions with regard to size and location of defect, coexisting fractures and choice of repair material.
- Close observation in the postoperative period.

FURTHER READING

De Riu G, Meloni SM, Gobbi R, Soma D, Baj A, Tullio A. Subciliary versus swinging eyelid approach to the orbital floor. *J Craniomaxillofac Surg* 2008;**36**:439–42.

Ellis E, 3rd, Tan Y. Assessment of internal orbital reconstruction for pure blow out fractures: cranial bone grafts versus titanium mesh. *J Oral Maxillofac Surg* 2003;**61**:442.

Evans BT, Webb AA. Post traumatic orbital reconstruction anatomical landmarks and the concept of the deep orbit. *Br J Oral Maxillofacial Surg* 2007;**45**:183.

Kontio R, Suuronen R, Salonen O, Paukku P, Konttinen YT, Lindqvist C. Effectiveness of operative treatment of internal orbital wall fractures with polydioxanone implant. *Int J Oral Maxillofac Surg* 2001;**30**:278.

Kwon JH, Moon JH, Kwon MS, Cho JH. The differences of blowout fracture of the inferior orbital wall between children and adults. *Arch Otolaryngol Head Neck Surg* 2005;**131**:723.

Bailey & Love's Essential Operations Bailey & Love's Essential Operations
Bailey & Love's Essential Operations Bailey & Love's Essential Operations
Bailey & Love's Essential Operations Bailey & Love's Essential Operations

PART 3 | Trauma

Chapter 19

Craniofacial Trauma

Robert P. Bentley

BACKGROUND

Craniofacial injury patterns almost universally result from high-energy transfer and are optimally managed in dedicated trauma centres with a multidisciplinary team including OMFS, Neurosurgery and Ophthalmology. Suboptimal outcomes may have implications with respect to mortality and morbidity requiring multiple revisions.

CLASSIFICATION

A useful working classification of fractures involving the frontobasilar region was suggested by Bernstein et al. who divided the injuries into central, lateral and complex groups. The central group includes fractures involving the central anterior skull base and cribriform region adjacent to the frontal, ethmoidal and sphenoidal sinuses (*Figure 19.1*). The lateral group include frontal bone fractures associated with the orbital roof, but lateral to the frontal sinus (*Figure 19.2*) and finally the complex group involving all areas often bilaterally (*Figure 19.3*).

This classification anatomically describes the fracture pattern, defines surgery and predicts possible functional sequelae. Central injuries are far more likely to involve sinus-related problems, whereas lateral injuries are more often associated with orbital and globe issues.

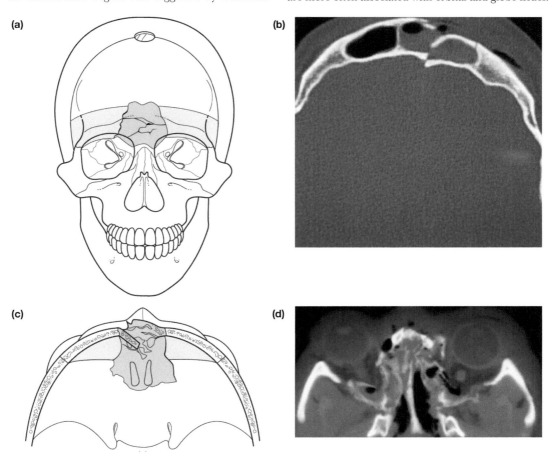

(a)   (b)   (c)   (d)

Figure 19.1 Central injuries.

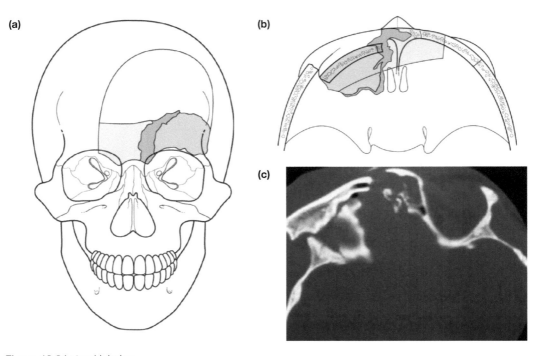

Figure 19.2 Lateral injuries.

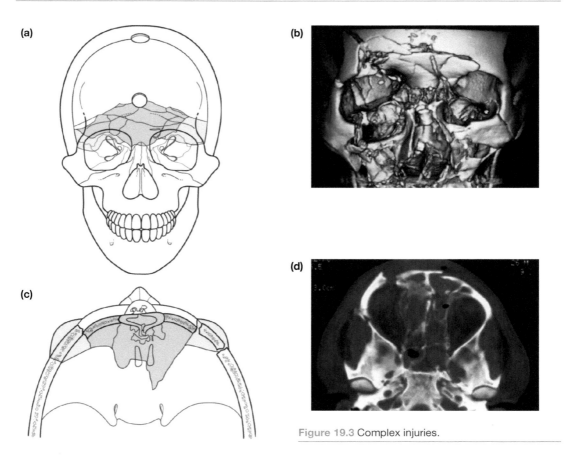

Figure 19.3 Complex injuries.

CLINICAL ASSESSMENT

Predictably, 30% of this patient cohort will have another major life-threatening injury and 20% will have associated cervical spine injury. Advanced Trauma Life Support (ATLS) assessment is mandatory. Comprehensive assessment including neurosurgical and ophthalmological consultation in addition to full facial assessment should be considered.

Any nasal or middle ear discharges should be tested for beta-2 transferrin to detect the presence of cerebrospinal fluid (CSF).

RADIOLOGICAL ASSESSMENT

Computed tomography (CT) assessment permits accurate visualisation of the fracture patterns in all three planes with three-dimensional reconstructions, aiding the surgeon to develop an operative plan.

INDICATIONS FOR COMBINED CRANIOFACIAL REPAIR

Surgical goals of a combined repair are to prevent the late sequelae of infection, prevent cosmetic deformity and minimise functional deficits.

- Central injuries, involving significant displacement of the anterior fossa floor and posterior wall of the frontal sinus
- Lateral injuries, involving the roof of the orbit leading to contour deformity, globe displacement or ocular motility disturbance
- Compound injuries with penetrating injuries or bone loss
- Growing fractures with dural lacerations, involving the orbit

Principles underlying prevention of late infective sequelae

The principles underlying prevention of late infective sequelae include:

- Accurate dural repair
- Achieving a functionally safe frontal sinus
- Repair of a deficient anterior skull base
- The use of vascularised pericranial flaps to help seal off the dura from the nasal cavity

Dural tears in communication with the nasal cavity and paranasal sinuses are common and place the patient at an increased risk of developing meningitis. There is no doubt that risk of infection is significantly increased by the presence of a CSF fistula, and early cessation should not be reassuring. Repair should be undertaken if the CSF leak has not stopped after 14 days.

Principles underlying prevention of post-traumatic cranio-orbital deformity

The key to craniofacial repair is accurate anatomic reconstruction of the frontal bandeau thus defining a platform for facial height, width and projection, as well as allowing for accurate restoration of the convexity of the orbital roof.

TIMING OF SURGERY

While acute neurosurgical intervention may be required, craniofacial intervention typically is planned at 10–14 days, following initial neurological recovery and resolution of periorbital swelling. Precise timing may be influenced by intracranial pressure monitoring.

SEQUENCING OF SURGICAL PROCEDURE

Anaesthesia

The choice of intubation depends on the injury pattern, and ventilation requirements. Nasotracheal intubation allowing restoration of occlusion may need to be converted to an oral tube for nasal manipulation. Tracheostomy is an option, especially if a prolonged period of postoperative ventilation is predicted.

Position of the patient

The patient is placed supine in a head ring ensuring enough support to prevent excess head mobility but allowing good access to the vertex and posterior scalp. Neurosurgeons often prefer that a Mayfield clamp is used but it must be ensured that the neck is not flexed.

Adequate exposure

True anatomical reduction can only be facilitated if there is full exposure of the fracture pattern in a subperiosteal plane, sensitive to local anatomical structures (facial nerve, globe, trigeminal nerve). Adequate skeletal fixation of bone fragments, and accurate soft tissue redrape minimises the risk of resorption.

Coronal scalp access is modified depending on the fracture pattern to allow for various forms of pericranial graft, and also may be extended to access the mid-facial region.

Incision design must take into account the hairline and is best placed along the vertex of the scalp in a wave form with the first curvature directed posteriorly from the tragus with an amplitude of 3 cm, keeping all aspects within the hairline.

Total head shaving is not necessary, but a 3-cm width shave along the incision line is helpful. The hair may be treated liberally with chlorhexidine gel which allows the hair to be gathered into clumps and secured with elastic bands.

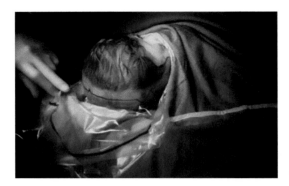

Figure 19.4 Patient preparation, positioning and draping.

The whole site can be prepared with aqueous iodine after simple eye ointment has been applied to each eye. Surgical drapes are secured to the posterior aspect of the proposed incision line with staples and the patient is positioned slightly head up. Be aware that unexpected air emboli may infrequently complicate any cranial procedure with head-up tilt (*Figure 19.4*).

Incision

The incision is marked and the scalp infused in the subgaleal space. Distension of this space has the added benefit of reducing haemorrhage and defining the plane for subsequent dissection.

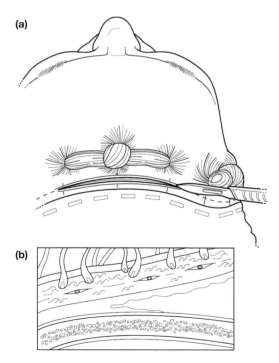

Figure 19.5 Initial incision.

The initial incision is performed with a No. 10 scalpel blade to the level of the hair follicles in the mid part of the outlined flap for a distance of 5 cm (*Figure 19.5*). The incision is deepened using a needle-point diathermy (Colorado MicroDissection Needle®), through the galea to enter the subgaleal space. This procedure may be aided with gentle traction upwards and outwards with cat's paws inserted into the wound margins. Having located the subgaleal layer, further dissection is achieved by placing McIndoe scissors with their tips up beneath the galea and opening the points widely creating a pocket which protects the underlying pericranium. This allows safe extension of the skin incision with the cutting diathermy. As dissection progresses and the scalp flaps become more mobile, haemostasis is obtained with the use of bipolar forceps rather than the use of Raney clips. This reduces blood loss, improves the surgical field and makes final scalp closure easier. Dissection progresses to the pre-auricular region below the superior temporal line on the temporal fascia. Note the dissection is beneath the level of the temporoparietal fascia, which is a continuation of the galea and is important as the temporal branch of the facial nerve runs either on its deep surface or within it. Damage to this branch of the facial nerve results in weakness of the forehead and partial ptosis due to loss of innervation to the frontalis, corrugator, procerus and occasionally a portion of the orbicularis oculi.

Anterior flap elevation proceeds easily in the hydro-dissected subgaleal layer by maintaining tension on the flap with Langenbeck or Cairns retractors. Dissection proceeds using the sweeping action of a No. 10 scalpel blade or use of a ceramic monopolar diathermy blade; blood loss is minimal if the correct plane is not violated. As the dissection proceeds, tension laterally is dealt with by incising the superficial layer of the superficial temporal fascia (*Figure 19.6*). As the flap is dissected inferiorly and anteriorly, an incision is made in the superficial temporal fascia at an angulation of 45° from a point 2.5 cm above the superior aspect of the lateral orbital margin, to a point at the base of the zygomatic arch. This is Pitanguy's line. This incision is best performed

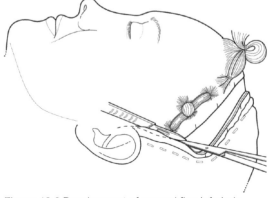

Figure 19.6 Development of coronal flap inferiorly.

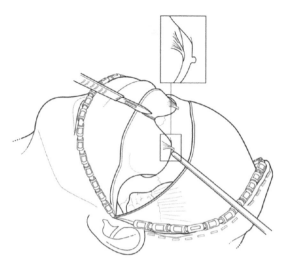

Figure 19.7 Release of supraorbital neurovascular bundle.

with a No. 15 scalpel blade. The yellow colour of the superficial temporal fat pad seen separating the superficial and deep layers of the temporal fascia is a constant landmark. The incision is now extended superiorly to the temporal line and inferiorly to the zygomatic arch with dissecting scissors.

The choice of pericranial flap depends on the fracture configuration and likely integrity of the neurovascular axis. If an anteriorly based flap is required, then the pericranium may be incised posteriorly using cutting diathermy to above the superior temporal line anteriorly. This extension is usually ideal to cover any base of skull defect without tension. Alternatively, if the viability of the anterior pedicle is at risk, then laterally based flaps may be raised with lateral pedicles. In either case, sharp subperiosteal dissection allows reflection of the flap inferiorly to the superior and lateral orbital margins.

Final anterior extension exposes the surpraorbital neurovascular bundles. These are often in a notch, in which case they may easily be freed. In a proportion of cases, there is a true foramen, which may be freed by inserting the tip of a 5-mm fine osteotome into the foramen and tapped inferomedially and then inferolaterally (*Figure 19.7*).

Further subperiosteal dissection along the nasofrontal articulation may be encouraged by a vertical incision of the periosteum on the undersurface of the flap along the medial orbital rim to the level of the medial canthal tendon, which should not be violated.

Laterally, having now incised through the superficial temporal fascia and joined this superiorly with the reflected pericranium, subperiosteal dissection on the zygomatico-frontal junction may continue to the body of the zygoma, facilitated by incising the periosteum on the zygoma. It is important to keep the superficial

temporal fat pad intact. The temporal branch of the facial nerve is safe in the flap beneath the reflected superficial temporal fascia.

In extensive fracture patterns, the lateral flap may be mobilised still further by extension in the pre-auricular skin crease facilitating full subperiosteal exposure of the zygomatic arch to the lateral canthal tendon.

Small soft tissue lacerations are repaired meticulously during the initial presentation. Occasionally, very large facial lacerations may have to be incorporated into the line of the incision so as not to risk the vascularity of the flap. Caution should be exercised as these usually offer poor access and may restrict the size of craniotomy required. Unless exceptionally large, extension of lacerations is to be avoided.

Craniotomy

The primary indication is to effect definitive intracranial inspection and dural repair if indicated. This will depend on the site of injury and suggested craniotomies are shown for central, lateral and complex injuries. Burr holes should be placed to minimise subsequent aesthetic problems and to allow a low frontal craniotomy to manage the frontal sinus with minimal brain retraction to inspect and facilitate dural repair and explore the orbital roof and anterior fossa. For this reason, burr holes may be placed laterally in the region of the pterion after reflection of the temporalis muscle in this region. This allows low access to the horizontal cut of the craniotomy and may be covered with temporalis at the end of the procedure. Parietal burr holes may be repaired by specific cover plates. The craniotomy is raised using a craniotome with a cut out clutch to perforate the skull without damaging the dura. Accessory burr holes are placed according to the size of the bone flap and joined with a side cutting and end guarded craniotome, to avoid damage to the dura. The last cut is made across the midline posteriorly to allow instant access to the sagittal sinus if torn. Finally, the bone flap is raised using blunt dissection from the underlying dura. Exposure should now permit easy tension-free retraction of the frontal lobes and allow inspection of the anterior and posterior walls of the frontal sinus, orbital roof and cribriform regions.

If there are sub-basal dural lacerations, retraction may already have been facilitated by loss of CSF; alternatively, an osteotomy of the frontal bandeau may further aid access (*Figure 19.8*). A planned dural incision allows basal dural lacerations to be approached with minimal brain retraction, especially of the basal region, without damage to the olfactory tracts.

The frontal bandeau has strategic importance to restore frontal projection, width and height. It also provides articulation with the zygomatic and naso-orbito-ethmoid structures thus defining central and lateral midfacial position. The zygomatic arch also defines facial projection and is easily reconstructed, thus predictable reduction of these fractures provides the basis

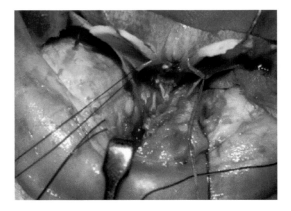

Figure 19.8 Temporary osteotomy of frontal bandeau.

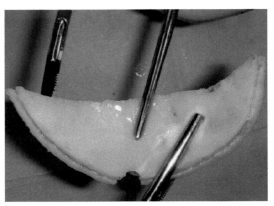

Figure 19.9 Craniotomy splitting with fine saw.

for the accurate reposition of the entire pan-facial sequence and in addition demonstrates the size of defects of the orbital roof and anterior skull base to be reconstructed.

Inner frontal table bone grafts may be harvested at this point. The cortices may be split initially using a fissure burr to define the plane between them, and the split is completed using a reciprocating saw, flexible osteotomes or piezo saw (*Figure 19.9*).

Outer cortical grafts may be obtained from the temporoparietal region overlying the non-dominant hemisphere. The graft is outlined with a fissure burr and cut through the outer cortex. The bone immediately outside the segment may be reduced in height using an acrylic burr, and a slim osteotome can then be introduced into the diploic space and the graft harvested. Bleeding is arrested with resorbable haemostatic agents, giving some bulk to the haematoma, which can then be redraped with the periosteum to help minimise the subsequent depression.

Osteosynthesis is by titanium plates with low-profile screws 1–1.3 mm in diameter used to ensure stability. The orbital roof must be reconstructed accurately to avoid orbital dystopia and exophthalmos. Bone grafting or titanium reconstruction partitions the brain from the orbital contents avoiding pulsatile exophthalmos from a traumatic encephalocele. Following reconstruction of the anterior cranial fossa and removal of the sinus mucosa and posterior wall of the frontal sinus (cranialisation), any dural repair by suturing and dural substitute is facilitated. Following this, vascularised pericranial grafts can be introduced. These may be fed anteriorly beneath the frontal lobes and secured by compression supplemented with fibrin glue to obtain a watertight seal and close off the nasopharynx from the anterior fossa. With respect to laterally based flaps, these may be introduced from the region of the lateral craniotomy cut. Finally, the craniotomy segment may be repositioned without compressing pericranial graft and adjusted to give the most cosmetically acceptable result.

Closure

Regimented soft tissue resuspension will achieve the best aesthetic immediate result and prevent long-term ptosis of the craniofacial soft tissue elements.

- Temporalis must be repositioned correctly following plugging of any burr hole with bone dust
- The inferior aspect of the incised superficial temporal fascia is attached to the temporal fascia at a slightly higher level, to help further support the soft tissue drape of the face
- The lateral canthus is repositioned to a drill hole placed accurately to restore the anatomical position
- The periosteum at the inferior orbital margin (if orbital access utilised) must be repaired – the superficial muscular aponeurotic system (SMAS) invests the orbicularis oculi and so indirect support can be achieved

A surgical drain is placed beneath the flap with the inferior aspect reaching into the side having undergone the most extensive dissection to avoid collection in this region. Haematoma will compromise the frontal bone flap. This is not placed on suction to avoid provoking a CSF leak. If CSF leakage is a real concern, then placement of a lumbar drain for a period of 5–7 days is favoured by some to allow time for the dural repair to establish itself. The scalp is closed with 2/0 resorbable suture, with care taken to use only the galea which allows for good soft tissue support and apposition of the wound margin. It is important to accurately align the scalp flap both laterally and vertically, a step deformity is considerably irritating to the comb.

A well-fitting head bandage is placed, making sure to cover the wound in the first instance with a non-adherent dressing and then absorbent swabs and cotton wool across the forehead and behind the ears before fitting a well-placed crepe bandage under slight tension. This avoids pressure necrosis overlying the drain and forehead regions. The dressing and drain are maintained for 24 hours, and when the drain is removed the tract of the drain is pressed firmly for several minutes to avoid bleeding along the tract.

POSTOPERATIVE CARE

The patient will be managed postoperatively in the neurosurgical high-dependency unit. The decision to extubate is dependent on intraoperative considerations such as frontal lobe manipulation, CSF leakage and positioning of a spinal drain, blood loss and temperature control, and the medical and surgical comorbidities of the patient. A short period of maintained intubation is common and may be advisable. A tracheostomy has the advantage in this cohort of patients to allow the intensivists flexibility. Antibiotics are usually continued for at least three postoperative doses and depending on the anterior fossa and dural repairs, as well as CSF leakage, may be extended for several days.

Management of the frontal sinus

The treatment of the frontal sinus is controversial and written about extensively in the literature, with low levels of evidence. This is further complicated by the long-term nature of major complications with heterogeneity of treatment and presentation to other centres without access to notes or surgeon's memories. There has been a consensus about what one is hoping to

achieve, namely a 'safe sinus' with the least intervention necessary. The frontal sinus is of variable size and is lined by respiratory epithelium that communicates via the frontonasal duct with the middle meatus of the nose. The duct is again in a variable structure, being well defined in some instances, but in more than 60% of cases achieves its drainage via communication with the ethmoidal air cells (*Figure 19.10*).

Frontal sinus fractures occur in approximately 2–15% of facial fractures and are associated with anterior skull base involvement but may occur in isolation involving either the anterior wall, posterior wall or floor with associated duct injuries (*Figure 19.11*). They cause cosmetic deformity and functional problems including chronic sinusitis (up to 60%), meningitis (6%), mucopyocele, osteomyelitis and cerebral abscess formation indicating surgical management.

Cosmetically obvious defects are surgically managed by open reduction with a limited coronal flap and miniplate or titanium mesh fixation. Reduction can be assisted by placing 2-mm screws into the main fragments and elevated using forceps prior to fixation (*Figure 19.12*).

In more fragmented patterns, the fragments are removed, and laid out on a moist swab in anatomical position, with necrotic or damaged mucosa removed leaving all viable mucosa. The remaining mucosa will help seed subsequent re-epithelialisation of the repaired sinus. Defects can be repaired by titanium mesh or outer table bone graft.

Fractures of the frontal sinus floor may result in damage to the frontonasal duct, which may subsequently lead to obstruction with mucocele formation. While stenting of the ducts may lead to uncertain outcome, the sinus exenteration is more predictable. This involves temporary removal of the anterior sinus wall and all the mucosal lining is removed meticulously by curetting and acrylic burr. The mucosa of the nasofrontal duct is mobilised and inverted through the infundibulum. The ducts are sealed by free or pedicled pericranium, temporal fascia or even oxidised cellulose, and a cancellous particulate bone graft placed to obliterate the sinus. The anterior wall is then reconstructed.

Isolated posterior wall fractures with more than 5 mm displacement are associated with dural tears – often with a CSF leak – and should undergo cranialisation. Following low craniotomy and posterior wall removal, allowing all the sinus mucosa to be excised, the duct mucosa is inverted and covered as previously described. In addition, cortical bone is placed over the duct orifice, and bone dust and milled bone obtained from the posterior wall is packed above it (*Figure 19.13*). Following dural repair, the vascularised pericranial flap is then placed across the infundibulum and bone graft or even introduced into the tear (*Figure 19.13*), so as to be supported beneath the frontal lobes with its vascularised surface against the bone graft. The flap is secured with fibrin glue to achieve a watertight seal.

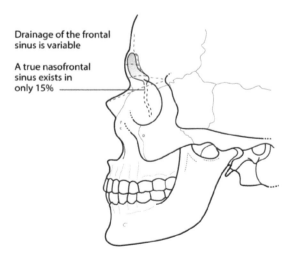

Drainage of the frontal sinus is variable

A true nasofrontal sinus exists in only 15%

Figure 19.10 Anatomy of the frontal sinus and nasofrontal duct. The frontal sinus is a pyramidal, air-filled cavity lying within the lamina of the frontal bone creating an anterior and posterior wall to the sinus. Drainage of the frontal sinus is variable. A true nasofrontal duct exists in only 15%.

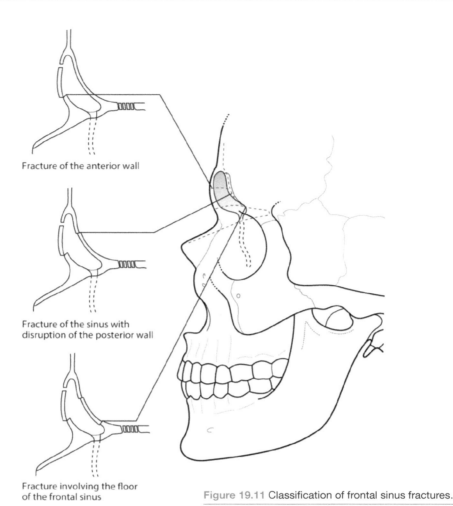

Fracture of the anterior wall

Fracture of the sinus with disruption of the posterior wall

Fracture involving the floor of the frontal sinus

Figure 19.11 Classification of frontal sinus fractures.

COMPLICATIONS

Infection

This may be immediate in the form of meningitis, brain abscess or subdural empyema, often related to failure to debride and gain adequate closure, or reduce dead space. Treatment involves antibiotic treatment with broad spectrum cephalosporins and metronidazole, together with reoperation and removal of infected bone prior to interval secondary reconstruction.

Late infection may be associated with the presence of a mucocele due to an obstructed frontal sinus or CSF fistula that will need to be addressed. Mucocele formation may complicate 10% of unoperated cases and require removal of the frontal sinus and formal cranialisation (*Figure 19.14*).

Cerebrospinal fluid fistulas

Fistulas are relatively rare in closed injuries affecting only 2%, which rises to 9% in open or penetrating head injuries. Suggested investigations involve fine cut coronal CT or T2-weighted magnetic resonance imaging (MRI) with contrast. Alternatively cisternograms are more invasive and the use of fluorescein intrathecally combined with nasal endoscopy has been shown to be of benefit in defects that are difficult to identify. Repair may be achieved endoscopically, particularly if the fracture pattern extends to the sphenoid, or requires revision surgery.

NASOETHMOIDAL FRACTURES

Background

Nasoethmoidal (NOE) fractures are complex and unforgiving related to anatomical and aesthetic reconstruction and also due to the consequences of the close proximity to the skull base and frontal sinus, the orbital contents, and walls and lacrimal apparatus. These patterns follow high energy transfer during anterior compression and subsequent failure of the pneumatised

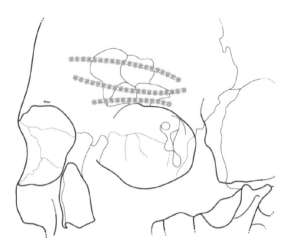

Undisplaced fractures of the anterior wall require no sugical intervention

Displaced fractures of the anterior wall should be reduced and fixed in the anatomical position to restore normal forehead contour

Figure 19.12 Reduction of anterior wall fracture of the frontal sinus.

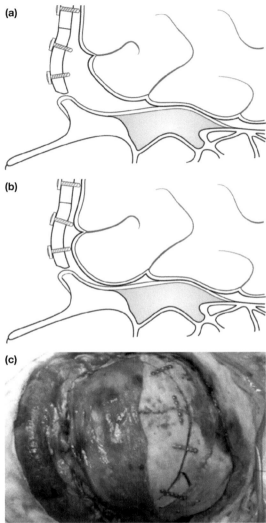

(a)

(b)

(c)

Figure 19.13 Frontal sinus cranialisation.

ethmoidal air cells and weak medial walls of the orbit result in extremely comminuted high value anatomical structures, with poor surgical access. Predictable management requires understanding of the medial canthal tendon and attachments to the central fragment of the nasomaxillary complex. The medial canthal tendon attaches to the medial orbit by superficial and deep limbs attached to the anterior and posterior lacrimal crests, respectively. The punctae of the upper and lower canaliculi within the lid margins continue to canaliculi extending behind the medial canthal tendon into the lacrimal sac. The anterior horizontal tendon is attached firmly to the anterior lacrimal crest and is stronger than the posterior limb attached to the posterior lacrimal crest, which serves to hold the eyelids against the globe in a posterior fashion. It is this medial and posterior relationship that has to be reconfigured in injuries involving the medial canthal tendon if the palpebral shape is to remain unaltered and the tarsal plates are to be supported in close apposition to the surface of the globe.

NOE fractures come as a spectrum, ranging from localised dislocation to those which are segmented and extend into the orbit and skull base. A classification of these injuries has been described by Markowitz, depending on the relative displacement of the medial canthal tendon, as types 1–3 (*Figure 19.15*).

Sequencing of nasoethmoidal fractures

Sequencing follows the following pattern:

- Exposure
- Reduction and stabilisation of the frontal bandeau and anterior fossa floor
- Restoration of the frontonasal angle
- Reconstruction of the outer orbital frame
- Repair of the medial orbital wall
- Reduction and fixation of midfacial buttresses
- Restoration of the medial canthal tendon
- Repair of the lacrimal system
- Closure
- Nasal plaster and septal splints

(a)

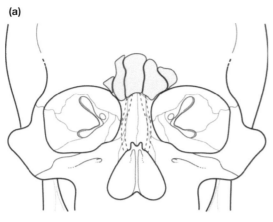

(b)

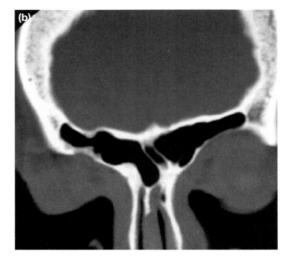

(c)

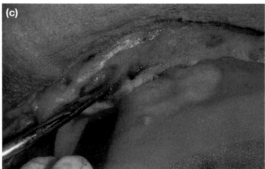

Figure 19.14 Aetiology of mucocele formation. The risk of infection is linked to communication between the nasal cavity and dural tears via the frontal sinus. The aetiology of a mucocele appears to be related to obstruction of the nasofrontal duct in a diseased or injured frontal sinus.

(a)

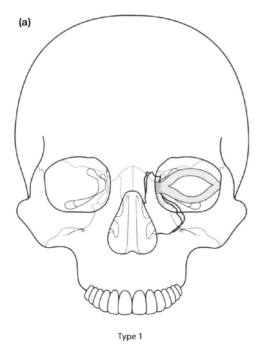

Type 1

(b)

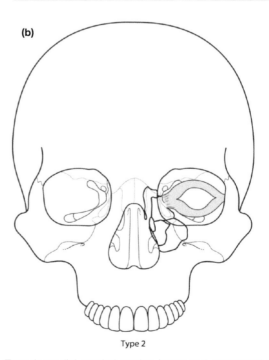

Type 2

Figure 19.15 Classification of nasoethmoidal fractures. Type 1: medial canthal tendon intact and connected to a single large fracture fragment. Type 2: comminuted fracture, medial canthal tendon attached to a single bone fragment. (*Continued*)

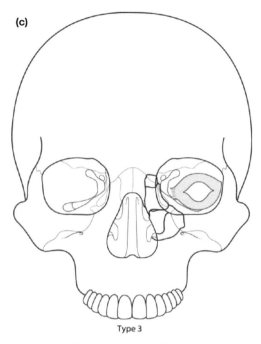

Type 3

Figure 19.15 (*Continued*) Classification of nasoethmoidal fractures. Type 3: comminution extends to the medial canthal tendon insertion site at the level of the lacrimal fossa with avulsion of the tendon.

Exposure

The approach of choice is the coronal flap modified to reach the nasal bridge by incising the periosteum over the nasal bridge. Orbital and transoral approaches may also be required depending on the type and degree of comminution.

The frontal nasal angle must be restored by reduction of the fracture and fixation with low-profile plates. Primary bone grafting using split calvarium may be required if grossly comminuted. It is important to ensure that the central fragment is reduced correctly as it is frequently impacted. A slim osteotome can be introduced and used to lever the impacted fracture element inferiorly.

Care should be taken not to avulse any remaining medial canthal tendon attachment. Orbital dissection of the medial wall is complex and it is potentially difficult to triangulate the position.

NOE fractures are commonly part of a wider panfacial pattern and strategic reduction of all of these individual elements facilitates ultimate reduction (*Figure 19.16*).

The medial orbital wall defects may be repaired with adaptive titanium plates, which can be placed from the orbital aspect.

The medial canthal ligament in type 1 injuries already will have been stabilised by reduction of the

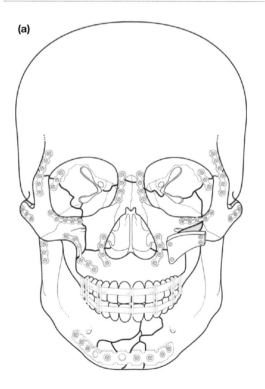

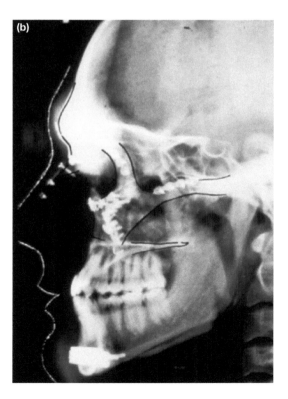

Figure 19.16 Reduction and alignment of midfacial buttresses.

fractures. In type 2 and 3 injuries, however, there is usually the need to identify the ligament with the aid of a canthopexy wire. Specialised wires are available (DePuy Synthes). A stainless-steel needle is passed externally through the medial caruncular region emerging interiorly through the inner surface of the down-turned coronal flap through the identified medial canthal tendon confirmed by grasping the area behind the lacrimal apparatus with toothed forceps and sequentially observing the effects on the medial canthal tendon. The wire is placed through the final hole of a cantilevered plate attached anteriorly to the frontal bone (*Figure 19.17*).

The lacrimal sac and duct must be considered at risk in these injuries. Accurate fixation of the fractures will help, but damage to the system is common particularly if associated with lid lacerations medial to the punctum. Obvious duct disruption can be managed by the use of mini-monoka stents depending on the

experience of the surgeon, appreciating that injudicious attempts at passing catheters may cause damage to the remaining canaliculus. Further dacryocystorhinostomy may be necessary, even in those cases where the duct has been repaired.

Complications

Aesthetic blunting and vertical discrepancies of the medial canthal tendon are best dealt with through a combination of osteotomy and reattachment of the tendon if necessary; this latter point depends on the angle of the medial canthus. In general terms, trying to shorten the tendon without addressing the widening of the bone will not correct the defect.

Epiphora should be investigated by an ophthalmic surgeon, usually with a dacryocystogram and either the duct repaired or, more likely, a dacryocystorhinostomy. Cerebral sinus thrombosis, fistulas, infection and mucocele formation associated with frontal duct injuries and anterior fossa floor injuries may need to be dealt with. A final complication involves orbital volume changes to the associated medial wall defects.

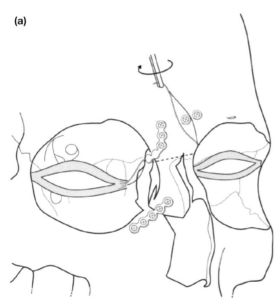

(a)

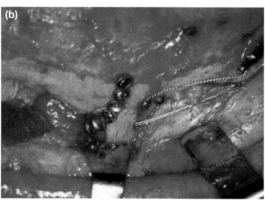

(b)

Figure 19.17 Alignment of medial canthal tendon using tendon wire and medial orbital plate.

TOP TIPS AND HAZARDS

- Treat these injuries as part of a multidisciplinary team in specialised centres.
- Identify and treat appropriately associated life-threatening injuries.
- Outline a clear team plan for operation and sequencing on operation board.
- Avoid facial nerve injury by division of superficial temporalis fascia.
- Mobilise supraorbital bundle with osteotomes.
- Preserve pericranial flaps.
- Ensure accurate soft tissue resuspension following coronal flap.
- Use orbital plate to help give support for insertion of medial canthal tendon.

FURTHER READING

Bell RB, Dierks EJ, Brar P et al. A protocol for the management of frontal sinus fractures emphasizing sinus preservation. *J Oral Maxillofac Surg* 2007;**65**:825–39.

Donald PJ. Management of frontal sinus fractures. *J Trauma* 2007;**62(Suppl)**:S91.

Ellis E 3rd. Sequencing treatment for naso-orbito-ethmoid fractures. *J Oral Maxillofac Surg* 1993;**51**:543–58.

Markowitz BL, Manson PN, Sargent L et al. Management of the medial canthal tendon in nasoethmoid orbital fractures: The importance of the central fragment in classification and treatment. *Plast Reconstr Surg* 1991;**87**:843–53.

Shumrick KA. Endoscopic management of frontal sinus fractures. *Otolaryngol Clin North Am* 2007;**40**:329–36.

Bailey & Love's Essential Operations Bailey & Love's Essential Operations
Bailey & Love's Essential Operations Bailey & Love's Essential Operations
Bailey & Love's Essential Operations Bailey & Love's Essential Operations

PART 3 | Trauma

Chapter 20

Middle Third Fractures

Simon Holmes

INTRODUCTION

The middle third of the facial skeleton is a collective of structures situated between the skull base and the occlusal plane. At a superficial level, these fractures are considered eponymously with respect to René Le Fort's classification but in reality there is considerable overlap with fractures of the zygomatic complex and nasoethmoidal regions. The fracture patterns are frequently not pure and often complicated, and subject to considerable individual variation. While the classification system pervades, each level of maxillary fracture has its own structural, aesthetic and functional challenges, and each has a distinct surgical strategy to manage these. In contrast to isolated mandibular and zygomatic fractures, these patterns are frequently associated with high levels of energy transfer and can also be implicated in vision threatening and extension into the anterior skull base.

APPLIED ANATOMY

The bulk of the central middle third of the facial skeleton is composed of the paired maxillary bones which separate the oral cavity from the nose, support the teeth, form the lateral aspect and floor of the nose together with forming the orbital floor and medial aspect of the orbital rim. The bone thickness of the maxilla varies according to specific regions which have surgical significance. This was first articulated by Gruss and Mackinnon in the 1980s. The thick areas form in response to occlusal forces and form thick vertical buttresses (*Figure 20.1*); these are utilised in the piriform region of the lateral nose and the zygomatic buttress by the trauma and orthognathic surgeon for fixation, the posterior pterygoid buttress is not available for fixation. The vertical strength of the maxilla is in stark contrast to that of horizontal strength which is comparatively poor and results in structural frailty to anterior–posterior compressive forces. The bone between the buttresses is comparatively thin and weak and segments readily.

Subsequently, horizontal facial buttresses have been added to the concept (*Figure 20.1*): superiorly, the frontal bar of the upper facial subunit; inferiorly, the maxillary alveolus and palatal processes, with a contribution from the horizontal process of the palatine bone. The middle horizontal buttress is composed of the zygomatic arches, body of the zygomatic bones

and the infraorbital rim. These transversely orientated supportive elements link the zygomaticomaxillary processes and nasomaxillary processes.

The other osseous components that articulate with the maxillae are also involved in middle third injuries and include the paired zygomatic bones which both fracture and remain attached to the maxillae, or segment separately which leads to both significant variation in fracture pattern together with difficulty in description and classification. The ethmoid is also vulnerable to compression forces and will segment in a variety of patterns and potentially involve the cribriform plate and, as such, high-level Le Fort injuries (2 and 3) should be considered as potentially extending into the intracranial compartment and cerebrospinal fluid leak should always be suspected in these injury patterns.

The midface articulates with the skull base at roughly 45° downwards and backwards, the robust

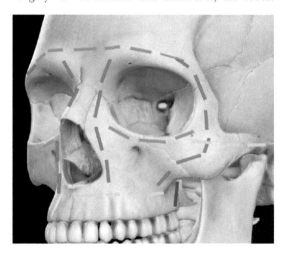

Figure 20.1 The buttresses illustrated. The red lines are thickened in response to the occlusal forces and therefore are used for surgical fixation. The green transverse buttresses define the width of the face, and are commonly used to cross-reference the other surgical fixation points. The yellow lines denote the zygomatic arch and occlusal arch, defining the anterior projection of the zygomatic prominence and the position of the upper maxilla accordingly. The pterygoid buttress represented by the blue line is hidden and therefore not utilised surgically, but will provide strength post healing if aligned.

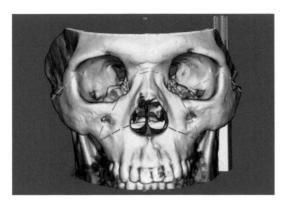

Figure 20.2 The Le Fort classification lines: Le Fort I – blue, Le Fort II – red, Le Fort III – green.

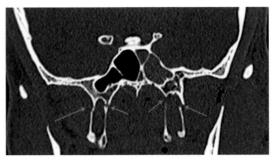

Figure 20.3 Coronal computed tomography scan at the level of the pterygoid plates. Fractures are indicated by red arrows. This radiological finding should always be sought in suspected maxillary fractures.

nature of the osteology of the skull base influences the signs of fractures with an apparent lengthening of the midface with anterior open bite as the complex is positioned posteriorly.

The blood supply of the middle third is significant and intellectually represents an anastomosis between internal and external carotid artery systems. In addition, the named branches are often passing through bone canals which tend to hold the vessels open and frustrate compression to arrest bleeding.

CLASSIFICATION

In view of the inherent complexity and variability of the fracture patterns, a precise classification is almost impossible. Although numerous authors have tried to devise classification systems, there has not been acceptance nor adoption. The classification system of Le Fort has endured and still has some relevance (*Figure 20.2*). It must be appreciated that Le Fort based his system on cadaveric studies where he inflicted considerable violence on his subjects and then dissected and described what he had achieved. There is a ceiling on how much damage an apparently slight Frenchman can inflict, which explains how his patterns of fracture were categorised simply, and why fractures of the palate were excluded.

Le Fort I: This is a low-level fracture (blue line) and is easily conceptualised to the oral and maxillofacial surgeon as the fracture pattern is replicated in a Le Fort I osteotomy. The fracture lies horizontally, passing from the piriform aperture to the zygomatic buttress. The fracture also involves separation of the lateral nose and the nasal septum.

Le Fort II: This fracture pattern (red line) passes from the zygomatic buttress to the orbital margin. It then passes medially across the orbital floor and medial walls (ethmoid) to the frontal process of the maxilla.

Le Fort III: This fracture passes (green line) from the lateral aspect of the orbit and in doing so sections the zygomatic arch and lateral orbital wall, and then

across the orbital floor and frontal process of the maxilla. As such, this separates the facial skeleton from the cranial base and is sometimes termed craniofacial disjunction.

Points to note

- Fractures of the maxilla all involve the pterygoid plates (*Figure 20.3*)
- All fractures are bilateral and can be any combination and multiple. It is therefore common to see mixed patterns of 1 and 2 and 3 bilaterally
- The only exception to the above two rules is if there is a palatal split which 'completes the fracture' (*Figure 20.4*)

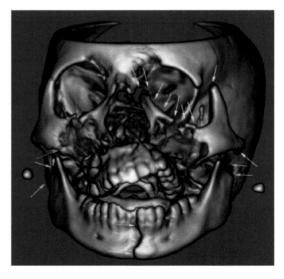

Figure 20.4 A panfacial fracture: Le Fort I (blue arrows), Le Fort II (red arrows), Le Fort III (yellow arrows), palatal fracture (purple arrows). The mandibular component includes a midline symphysis and bilateral condylar fractures in green.

PREOPERATIVE CONSIDERATIONS

These injury patterns are associated with high energy transfer and so the surgeon must consider potential intracranial extension, as well as potentially sight-threatening ocular complications. In addition, the injury must include assessment according to Advanced Trauma Life Support (ATLS) principles, in particular to cervical injuries. Midfacial bleeding can be declared with significant epistaxis or concealed within the soft tissue swelling or by postnasal bleeding (*Figure 20.5*).

The physical examination should be thorough and simply reading the computed tomography scan will not inform the detailed treatment plan required.

- Fracture characteristics
  - Abnormal maxillary mobility
  - Malocclusion (*Figure 20.6*)
  - Midfacial lengthening
  - Split palate
  - Dentoalveolar involvement
- Ophthalmic
  - Visual acuity
  - Globe injury
  - Pupillary reaction
  - Diplopia
  - Abnormal globe position
- Neurosurgical
  - Glasgow Coma Score
  - CSF rhinorrhoea

Physical examination involves a detailed extra- and intraoral examination of all of the potential fracture articulations. The forehead should be stabilised, and the maxilla grasped and moved. Abnormal mobility of the teeth-bearing region signifies a Le Fort I, that of the teeth and nasal bridge a Le Fort II, and that of the infra-orbital margins a Le Fort III. Intraoral examination allows dentoalveolar assessment and determination of the presence of a split palate. An impacted, immobile maxillary fracture may exhibit a dull note when tapping the teeth ('cracked cup sign').

Nasoethmoidal extension

Nasoethmoidal (NOE) injuries are central midface fractures forming an integral part of the higher-level injuries: Le Fort II and III fractures. NOE fracture management may be particularly complex and is dealt with in *Chapter 19*. On occasion NOE fractures may present with concomitant maxillary fractures – in which case the NOE could be thought of as a segmented Le Fort II or III pattern (*Figure 20.7*).

Extremes of age

Older patients often have very thin and brittle bones, particularly when edentulous. This may have particular relevance when determining what kind of fixation to use and whether simpler 'closed' methods should be contemplated. Young patients may not have fully formed sinuses and exhibit unusual patterns of injury.

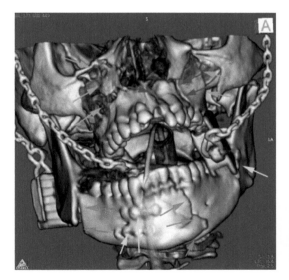

Figure 20.5 Le Fort II (green arrows), segmented maxilla and palate (blue arrows). Right angle of mandible and left parasymphysis (red arrows) – previous fractures (yellow arrows). This patient had bleeding and an attempt to arrest this was made using bite blocks. These are not well located due to the inherent instability of the fracture pattern. Subsequently, bridle wires placed including a transpalatal wire were used to improve the stability and the bleeding arrested.

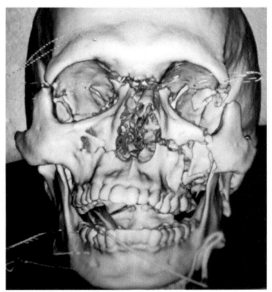

Figure 20.6 Fracture at left Le Fort I and III levels on the patient's left side, and Le Fort III on the right. Note the significant three-dimensional distortion and resulting malocclusion.

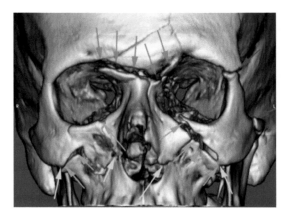

Figure 20.7 A complex pattern. There are Le Fort I (yellow arrows), II (green arrows) and III (blue arrows). Common to the Le Fort II and III is the nasoethmoidal involvement (red arrows). Note that the Le Fort III component could also be described as a zygomatic fracture, but is in effect a segmented Le Fort II.

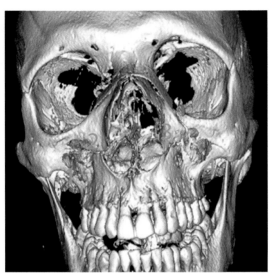

Figure 20.8 In minor displacements with no occlusal disturbance then a conservative plan with either observation or the use of intermaxillary fixation could be considered. This may be an important option should the patient not be considered fit for surgery. Note consideration should be of each buttress 1–4 in turn.

The child's maxilla will be full of developing teeth, again posing potential problems for the use of internal fixation.

PLANNING TREATMENT

Conservative management

A conservative option is possible if there is no disturbance in the dental occlusion, no functional ocular compromise, no significant aesthetic disturbance and no abnormal mobility (*Figure 20.8*). Often Le Fort fractures are 'radiological fractures' and simply require a period of observation. As with all conservatively managed facial injuries involving the dental occlusion, advice on a soft diet for a period of 3–4 weeks is prudent, and if the maxillary antrum is involved in the fracture pattern, then a period of 2 weeks to discourage nose blowing and to sneeze with an open mouth will minimise the risk of surgical emphysema.

In elderly patients with significant medical or surgical comorbidities who are edentulous, conventional management has been championed. This is because the occlusion can be corrected by provision of a new denture. While the author has heard stated from very senior colleagues that "I have never seen a non-union in a maxilla", he certainly has seen this. It should be considered that these are often osteopenic individuals and if the pillars do not align satisfactorily then it is unrealistic to expect poor bone to form a large callus. Edentulous maxillary fractures should therefore be treated on their merits.

Surgical management

Surgical management of the middle third injury must work in concert with management of other injuries which commonly coexist in high energy transfer cases. In addition, it is important to allow some resolution of swelling to allow for exploitation of surgical access planes and also to assess facial bone position intraoperatively.

Airway

Consultation with the anaesthetist is essential. As these are fracture patterns that result in malocclusion, then the airway must be separated from the oral cavity. This may be achieved by an anatomical approach – nasotracheal intubation, or non-anatomical in the form of a tracheostomy. Often a patient with middle third injury will have thoracic injuries, or neurosurgical considerations that make a strong case for tracheostomy.

A nasotracheal tube may require a tube change to an oral tube or laryngeal mask to facilitate management of complex nasal fractures.

Midfacial fractures can bleed spectacularly on mobilisation and due consideration should be made to facilitate transfusion, particularly if bleeding on admission was noted, or in grossly segmented fracture patterns.

Intermaxillary fixation

In all cases of maxillary fracture, malocclusion and subsequent management may be facilitated by the use of intermaxillary fixation (IMF). Choice of method is a matter of personal preference. The author prefers Leonard buttons, as they are quick to apply and allow for both wire and elastic IMF. Their use is contraindicated in physiological spacing, and if there are missing teeth. Although the trend is for a move away from the use of IMF toward anatomical fixation, there are still clinical situations where its use is of benefit:

- When there are two fracture patterns that can cause an anterior open bite, for example, bilateral condylar and Le Fort fractures
- Presence of intra-arch dentoalveolar fractures – in these cases the loose teeth of one arch can be splinted by the opposing teeth
- Presence of degloving soft tissue injuries of the maxilla
- Missing condylar head

Surgical access

This is planned to aid reduction and expose the fracture elements that require fixation. There are often several treatment options to manage some elements by closed reduction to avoid extended exposure, but the treatment plan must be decided prior to the patient being anaesthetised. There is never the option to 'cut as you go' in these fracture types.

In essence, there are three levels of surgical access:

- *Transoral access:* this is a mucosal incision running from first molar to first molar across the labial fraenum. This is conducted using a cutting diathermy leaving a small free gingival cuff. Following mucosal incision, the diathermy is angled 45° down to cut to bone thus avoiding the buccal fat pad. The anterior maxilla and piriform aperture require subperiosteal degloving and the floor of the nose exposing as with a Le Fort I osteotomy
- *Orbital access:* this may be accessed by a number of approaches, by an anterior lamellar (blepharoplasty or first lid crease incision) or posterior (transconjunctival) lamellar incision. In the author's view, the transconjunctival preseptal approach with a McCord lid swing represents a major leap forward in terms of profound surgical access with excellent aesthetics. This has been practised for many years at the author's institution with large numbers of cases with long-term follow-up and a minimal complication rate. The extent of the dissection will depend on the size and position of the orbital defect but the rim must be exposed to sound margins. Should a McCord cantholysis be required, then it is important to perform this prior to a coronal incision, and repair it after closure of the scalp
- *Coronal access:* this is required in cases of displacement of the zygomatic arch in Le Fort III patterns, or if displacement affects the nasofrontal junction. It is also required should there be anterior skull base involvement in conjunction with neurosurgical liaison. The importance of the zygomatic arch in predicting zygomatic projection was a seminal observation by Joe Gruss and not much has

changed since 1985 when he described it. If the arch is 'off ended' then predictability can greatly be improved by putting the arch out to length. Exposure of the arch is a highly technical procedure and must be designed to include the temporal fascia over temporalis to avoid damage to the facial nerve as per Al-Kayat and Bramley. The versatility of this approach is demonstrated by the opportunity to expose the posterolateral orbit by reflecting temporalis in the temporal fossa, and also by the ability to perfect soft tissue suspension (see below)

Reduction

This is achieved via a number of techniques depending on the fracture pattern. In grossly comminuted cases, the reduction of the maxilla can usually be achieved by digital pressure. If the fracture is impacted, then use of Rowe disimpaction forceps is required. These are placed under the dissected nasal mucosa and the palatal mucosa. The oral component is usually padded with a silicone tube. It is crucial to check that this remains on the instrument post reduction. This manipulation may restart or worsen the leakage of cerebrospinal fluid. This should be anticipated prior to surgery and discussed with neurosurgery.

Sequencing

The principle of maxillary reduction involves placing the maxilla in the correct occlusal position and then reconstructing the previously described pillars. As these maxillary patterns are typically involved in high energy transfer particularly AP compressions, then concomitant fracture patterns involving the mandible are seen. This mandibular AP compression pattern may involve condylar neck and midline symphysis, which makes for a complex three-dimensional challenge.

The order of reduction is termed sequencing (*Figures 20.9–20.11*) and follows established order in broad terms according to the work of Manson (inside out) and Gruss (outside in), and most surgeons do a combination of both (*Figure 20.12*). The difference is academic if the bones ultimately are in the correct place, but the weighting of the NOE by Manson reflects the complexity of management of this fracture element. In addition, if a fracture element is perfectly reduced then there is considerable wisdom in fixing that articulation earlier thus simplifying the pattern.

- Outer circle: this involves the mandible from condyle to condyle. Caution is needed with symphyseal fractures – it is always easy to 'open the fracture' thus introducing a deformity. The sagittal fracture of the maxilla is also addressed now with miniplates across the fracture. The frontal bandeau is reconstructed next which defines the articulation with the NOE and frontozygomatic (FZ) regions (*Figure 20.13*). Fixation of the zygomatic arch establishes facial projection, FZ plating is an

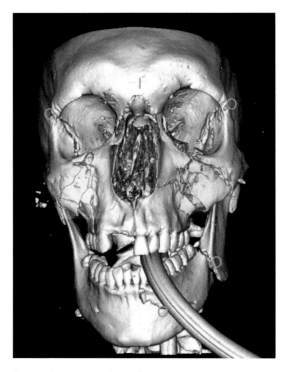

Figure 20.9 Three-dimensional computed tomography scan with a complex panfacial pattern. There are elements of Le Fort I and II in the maxilla (shaded areas). The sequencing can be conceptualised in terms of reducing and fixing of the outer ring (O) and inner ring (I) using intermaxillary fixation to localise the maxilla, and then connecting and ratifying (C).

anatomically important articulation which defines the position of the zygoma in three dimensions
- Establish occlusion: this puts the maxilla in the correct position, to reconstruct the pillars, and emphasises the importance of correct reconstruction of the mandible. IMF is important in this application and acts 'as another pair of hands'
- Reconstruction of the pillars: this both aligns and stabilises the pillars and reduces the central midface to allow final alignment of the orbital margins and NOE segments
- Orbital floor management

Fixation

The majority of midface injuries are fixed internally using low-profile titanium plates and screws (typically, 1.5 and 1.3 mm). The fundamental principle is to plate at least three out of four vertical buttresses and put all other articulations 'out to length'. Should a buttress not have enough residual bone, then consideration should be given to bone graft.

Soft tissue resuspension

This is an area of increasing importance. The evolution in trauma surgery to achieve anatomical fixation comes with extended soft tissue degloving, and therefore separates the facial suspension ligaments. This may be seen as an advantage in coronal access to lift the soft tissues and resuspend. In addition, deep closure of the orbital incision exploits the anatomical property of investiture of the superficial musculoaponeurotic system (SMAS) of orbicularis oculi.

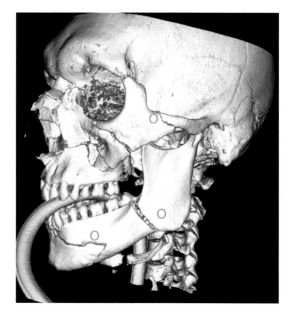

Figure 20.10 Left lateral view showing the outer ring (O).

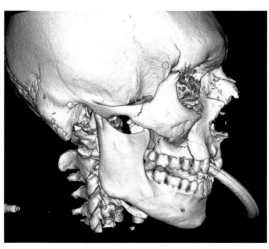

Figure 20.11 Right lateral view showing the outer ring (O).

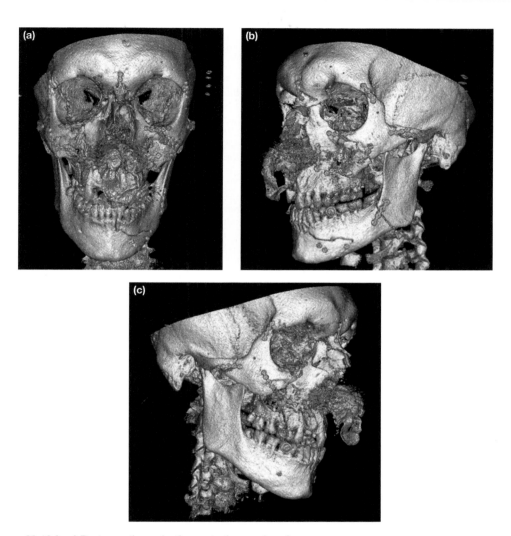

Figures 20.12 (a-c) Postoperative reduction, note the nasal pack.

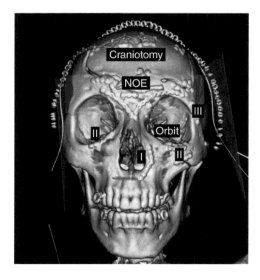

Figure 20.13 The importance of the frontal bandeau. There are components of Le Fort I, II, III. The craniotomy was required for front sinus exenteration and cranialisation, but the complex shape of the bandeau requires anatomical reconstruction to site the 'footplate' of the nasoethmoidal (NOE) and frontozygomatic regions.

POSTOPERATIVE CARE AND RECOVERY

With anatomical reduction, major postoperative sequelae are unusual. On occasion malocclusion can require ongoing management, either in the short term with elastic IMF, or later with an orthognathic approach.

Medium-term complications with respect to the scalp with poor scars and rarely with temporal hollowing are revised and fat grafted. Complications of the orbital approaches can be seen but are usually easily managed in conjunction with an ophthalmologist. We have observed <10 entropion in 20 years with over 250 transconjunctival incisions per annum; these were managed with posterior lamellar augmentations with oral mucosa, and we manage lateral canthal malposition at an incidence of <1%.

TOP TIPS AND HAZARDS

- Midface fractures may be difficult to detect as they may be hidden beneath soft tissue swelling. All components, including the orbital, nasal and dental aspects are frequently underestimated.
- CT scanning is the imaging of choice and should be considered early to fully appreciate the extent of fractures.
- Surgical intervention is often delayed until associated head injury and facial swelling have resolved. This time should be utilised to develop a comprehensive surgical treatment plan, and the surgery undertaken within 2 weeks if possible.
- Secondary correction is never as easy as primary anatomic repositioning of the basic midface structure. The planned intervention should be performed without further compromise to the damaged brain and should not need to wait for full recovery from brain injury.

FURTHER READING

Gruss JS, Mackinnon SE. Complex maxillary fractures; role of buttress reconstruction and immediate bone grafts. *Plast Reconstr Surg* 1986;**78**:9–22.

Manson PM, Clark N, Robertson B *et al.* Subunit principles in midfacial fractures: The importance of sagittal buttresses, soft tissue reductions, and sequencing treatment of segmental fractures. *Plast Reconstr Surg* 1999;**103**:1287–306.

Moss CJ, Mendelson BC, Taylor GI. Surgical anatomy of the ligamentous adhesions in the temple and periorbital regions. *Plast Reconstr Surg* 2000;**105**:1475–90.

Perry M, Holmes S. Fractures of the middle third of the facial skeleton. In *Atlas of Operative Maxillofacial Trauma Surgery: Primary Repair of Facial Injuries.* Springer; 2015, pp. 245–75.

Hanratty J, Perry M. Panfacial fractures. In *Atlas of Operative Maxillofacial Trauma Surgery: Primary Repair of Facial Injuries.* Springer; 2015, pp. 529–63.

Bailey & Love's Essential Operations Bailey & Love's Essential Operations
Bailey & Love's Essential Operations Bailey & Love's Essential Operations
Bailey & Love's Essential Operations Bailey & Love's Essential Operations

PART 3 | Trauma

Chapter 21

Ballistic Maxillofacial Trauma

Mohammed A. Al-Muharraqi

INTRODUCTION

"Those who wish to be a surgeon should go to war"

Hippocrates (460–370 BC)

Since the conception of maxillofacial surgery during the two World Wars, many lessons have been learned regarding management of maxillofacial trauma. Experience gained from the treatment of injuries during conflict has contributed to development of treatment protocols based on sound scientific principles with the aim of helping the patients regain quality of life both functionally and aesthetically. Although every generation of maxillofacial surgeons has lived through a major global conflict since World War 1, very few have personally experienced the management and fewer have been deployed into war zones.

Tissue disruption associated with ballistic injury can be daunting. Identification of the physiological anatomical planes can be extremely challenging as a result of catastrophic haemorrhage, and destroyed soft and hard tissues. The head, face and neck are three distinctly separate regions that respond differently after ballistic trauma.

- The neck: projectiles passing through it which miss the vertebrae produce a narrow linear permanent wound tract (PWT) with mortality and morbidity related to involvement of the neurovascular and aerodigestive components
- The face: projectiles passing through it ricochet off the bony skeleton, significantly increasing energy deposition, and it can be very difficult to ascertain the PWT (*Figure 21.1*) even with three-dimensionally reconstructed imaging. The blast wave of explosive weapons can also cause expansion of air-containing bones without superficial penetration of the overlying skin
- The head: the effect of a projectile penetrating the skull is the most devastating of the three body areas because of the closed vault. Penetrating head injuries continue to be associated with poor outcomes

Pathways of care for ballistic maxillofacial injury may vary, but level 1 trauma maxillofacial surgeons are mobilised in most circumstances, although local first-line providers are often alone for the first 24 hours of injury. The wounding capacity of firearms is an important issue, which affects surgeons with little knowledge of weapons. Hence, understanding basic definitions and characteristic clinical findings of ballistic and blast wounds is an important tool in the armamentarium of any practicing maxillofacial surgeon. Treatment protocols remain poorly defined where reconstructive principles proven in the civilian sector are modified and applied in ballistic maxillofacial trauma. Recent experience from Iraq and Afghanistan has done much to clarify these.

UNDERSTANDING THE PATHOPHYSIOLOGY OF BALLISTIC MAXILLOFACIAL TRAUMA

Understanding how ballistic weapons interact with soft and hard tissue is fundamental to management. Ballistic maxillofacial trauma includes injuries that are sustained either directly by, or secondary to, firearms and explosive devices in both military and civilian settings, which differ in cause and pattern:

- Low-velocity devices (handguns and shotguns)
- Energised fragments (improvised explosive devices)
- High-velocity devices (rifles) (*Figure 21.2*)

Maxillofacial ballistic trauma in urban settings is usually due to low-velocity weapons, in contrast to most injuries sustained during recent conflicts that resulted from energised fragments and a minority from high-velocity rifles.

The wounding power of weapons causes energy transfer and cavitation (temporary and permanent) of tissue from both high- and low-velocity projectiles. It is wrongly assumed that low-velocity projectiles cause less maxillofacial injury. Surgeons will understand wounding power and the consequences of ballistic injury to the head and neck by appreciating the basic mechanical properties of the projectile expelled toward the target, the correlation between the projectile (velocity, profile, shape, stability, fragmentation, expansion and secondary impact) and subsequent energy transfer, and the anatomic properties of the head and neck (*Figure 21.3*).

Terminal ballistics attempts to describe the complex interaction of a projectile (*Figure 21.4*), target tissue and any protective elements preventing or modifying penetration.

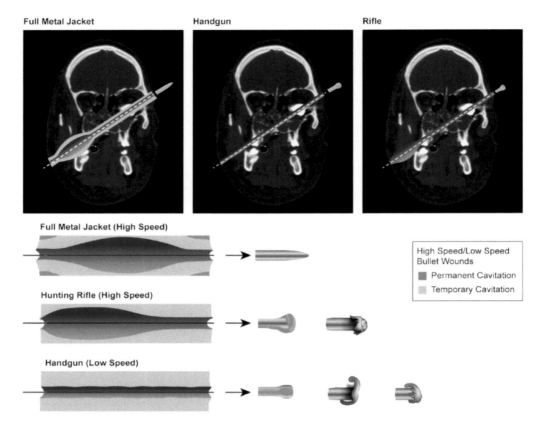

Figure 21.1 The projectile's mass and velocity determine its energy, which transfers into living tissue, and results in cavitation. The highest energy bullets can form the largest cavities and have the greatest potential for tissue injury and damage. The cavity formed is either temporary or permanent [permanent wound tract (PWT)]. Temporary cavitation reverses following the passage of the bullet, but the stretch effects may result in longer lasting tissue injury. The figure also illustrates the spectrum of bullet integrity ranging from an intact non-deformed bullet (in jacketed bullets) to a mushrooming deformation of the tip (in non-jacketed bullets). The military ordinance jacketed projectile causes the most damage without losing form.

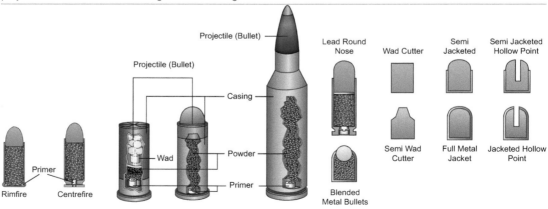

Figure 21.2 A cross-sectional diagram of the composition analysis of a shotgun shell, a handgun cartridge and a rifle cartridge, as well as an illustration of the features of various common bullet types. Each cartridge consists of a projectile, casing, propellant (gunpowder or cordite) and a primer. The different cartridge designs are made to change the projectile's mechanical property when used, hence increasing or decreasing the wounding capacity. A common example is the Jacketed Hollow Point (JHP) designed to expand rapidly when hitting the target, which increases the wounding potential of the bullet and decreases the chances of overpenetration.

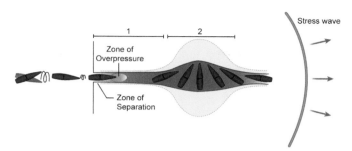

Figure 21.3 Idealised ballistic performance of a military rifle bullet in air and through tissue penetrating from left to right (bullet tumbling, shown here within a short distance for illustrative purposes, normally requires a certain penetration depth, and the declining precession of the bullet in air, which intensifies upon entering tissue). The wound track displays an initial narrow channel or neck (1), but subsequently widens owing to bullet yawing and tumbling (2). A bullet's initial passage through tissue creates a crush cavity, characterised by the shape of its nose and its depth of penetration. At the point of impact, a stress wave is formed, which rapidly spreads ahead without actual tissue movement; secondarily, separation at the projectile–tissue interface results in temporary cavity formation behind the bullet. A larger permanent wound cavity (red) indicates the true extent of tissue death and is composed of injury from tumbling of the bullet, bullet fragmentation and cavitation injury. The temporary cavity causes radial expansion of the wound track in a spindle-shape fashion (yellow), outlined at its maximum by the dashed line. The stretch cavity is temporary and cannot be seen by imaging.

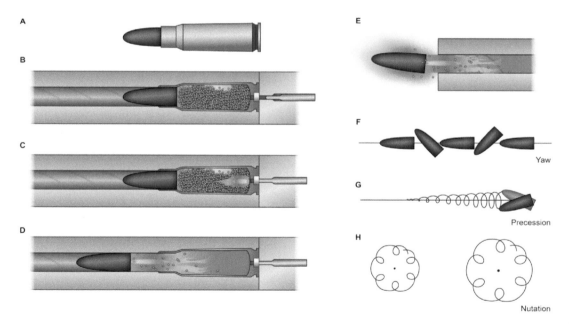

Figure 21.4 An artistic drawing of a rifle cartridge, (a) intact, (b) in the rifle chamber before firing with the cartridge case cut across demonstrating the centrefire primer and powder propellant. (c) The irreversible firing process activates the firing pin which strikes the primer, producing an explosion. (d) This ignites the powder generating propellant gases, which accelerate the bullet down the barrel, while attaining rotation (spin) as it encounters the rifled bore. (e) While exiting the muzzle, slight deviation of the bullet body from its axis of flight occurs. (f) Yaw: movement along the longitudinal access of the projectile. (g) Precession: rotation of the projectile around the centre of mass. (h) Nutation: small circular movement along the projectile tip. Yaw and precession decrease as the distance of the bullet from the barrel increases, and along with nutation, are terms associated with shooting from a distance. A low degree of yaw affords tight control of the projectile in flight, allowing one to hit with better precession. If the yaw is excessive, the projectile would be uncontrollable because of tumbling along the path of fire. Projectiles tumble within the target, causing increased damage after striking hard tissue, or with deformation of the projectile.

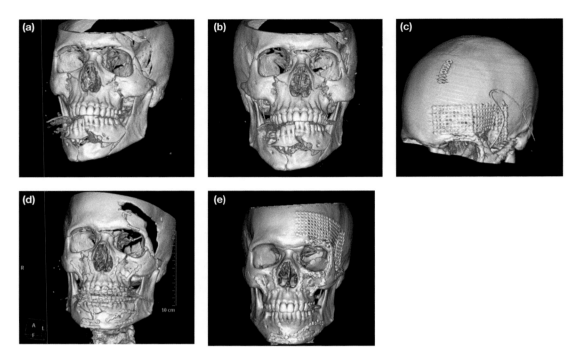

Figure 21.5 A 3D computed tomography (CT) scan of a patient (a, b) who sustained panfacial fractures following a 'jet-ski' petrol tank explosion. The upward force of the blast is demonstrated in the form of primary blast injuries (sudden increase in air pressure after the explosion affecting bones that contain air); and tertiary injuries (being thrown by the explosion and colliding face first with the sea surface); and quaternary blast injuries (having soft tissue thermal second and third degree burn damage to the face). To avoid surgical fatigue, the maxillofacial team carried out the surgeries in two stages, starting with the lower and midface (c, d), followed by the orbits and cranial vault when he was cleared neurologically. The final image (e) is a 3D CT scan of the same patient 4 years post open reduction and internal fixation and multiple surgeries with wound debridement and grafting.

High-velocity bullets generally deposit more energy than explosively propelled fragments, which is increased if tumbling occurs. Contemporary thinking in the pathophysiology of terminal ballistics is important as the interaction between a projectile and the tissues that it penetrates results in production of a PWT. This is the area of irreversibly damaged tissue that requires exploration and debridement in most body regions until healthy adjacent tissue is found.

Maxillofacial damage caused by blast injuries is defined as primary, secondary, tertiary or quaternary.

- Primary blast injuries are caused by the sudden increase in air pressure after an explosion, and they affect bones that contain air, this is the defining feature of a high-energy explosive
- Secondary injuries are caused by energised fragments propelled by the blast
- Tertiary injuries occur when the casualty is thrown by the explosion and collides with nearby objects (*Figure 21.5*)
- Quaternary blast injury is defined as all explosion-related injuries, illnesses or diseases not due to the cause of primary, secondary or tertiary injuries.

This will include burns as well as exacerbation of other disease processes, for example, asthma from breathing toxic fumes

COMPONENTS OF BALLISTIC MISSILES

Table 21.1 presents commonly used terms associated with ballistics and related injuries. As a projectile deforms on striking a target due to its metallurgic composition or as a direct consequence of striking underlying bone, energy transfer to the target and potential injury to associated tissues are increased.

Calibre specifications based on nomenclature used globally can be difficult for the healthcare team to understand. Misperceptions regarding calibre exist because the North Atlantic Treaty Organization and United States (US) military projectiles are described using the metric system, whereas US civilian firearm munitions are generally referred to in measurements relating to inches. Calibre has minimal practical impact on patient care, as the surgical management of a wound caused by a 0.357-inch projectile is no different from

TABLE 21.1 Commonly used terms associated with ballistics

Components of ammunition

Cartridge/round	A unit of firearm ammunition
Propellant	The accelerant that allows for expulsion of the projectile – the more propellant in a cartridge, the greater the velocity of the projectile
Wadding (wads)	A plastic framework with a paper/felt insert that holds the various projectiles together in relation to the propellant, allowing for release of a shotgun cartridge
Primer	The only portion of the projectile with an explosive charge. As the primer is struck by the firing pin (rimfire or centrefire) of the weapon, the explosive charge is activated, igniting the propellant, and sending the projectile on its flight
Casing	The container packaging the round
Primary projectile	The component of the round that is expelled toward the target, sometimes referred to as the 'bullet'
Secondary projectile	Formed due to fragmentation of the primary projectile and/or bone, which can result in producing additional wounding potential, enlarging the size of the permanent cavity
Magnum	A cartridge loaded with either a greater volume or more powerful propellant than the original cartridge design, imparting greater velocity to the projectile

Components of a weapon

Rifling	Helical grooves in the barrel of a weapon that impart spin along the long axis of the projectile
Calibre	The internal diameter of the barrel of a weapon, usually measured in millimetres or fractions of an inch
Gauge/bore	The total number of round lead balls that would fill the diameter of the barrel and weigh 1 pound

Other associated terms

Yaw	Movement along the longitudinal access of the projectile (the degree of yaw is generally <1–2°)
Tumbling	Excessive (exaggerated) yaw
Kinetic energy	The energy an object has owing to its motion – kinetic energy (KE) is equal to one-half the mass (M) of the projectile times velocity (V) squared (KE = $\frac{1}{2}$ MV^2)
Precession	Rotation of the projectile around the centre of mass
Nutation	Small circular movement along the projectile tip
Magnus effect	Lateral crosswind effect of a spinning projectile in flight
Coriolis effect	Spherical shape and rotational properties of the Earth and its orbit, as it applies to the projectile
Permanent wound	The site of initial permanent tissue destruction

that of a wound caused by a 9-mm round and should be directed to the specific anatomic anomaly created by the projectile, not the weapon used.

Handgun injuries tend to 'push away' or stretch soft tissues as opposed to causing avulsion. The characteristic low-velocity wound has a small, rounded entrance wound, causing fragmentation of teeth and bony comminution, often exhibiting no exit wound (*Figures 21.2* and *21.6*). At a distance, *rifle* wounds create a low-energy transfer like those seen with handguns but at close range; the wounding characteristics are different because of the velocity and high-energy transfer. The presence of an exit wound is usually found, which may be stellate and larger than the entry wound. The existence of avulsion soft/hard tissue wounds and fragmentation of the bone can be characteristic findings of rifle wounds.

A shotgun is a long gun that may fire a single pellet (*Figure 21.2*), or numerous pellets, at a low velocity. The gauge of the shotgun is classified as the number of

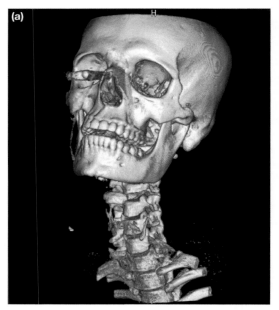

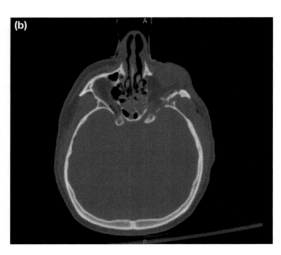

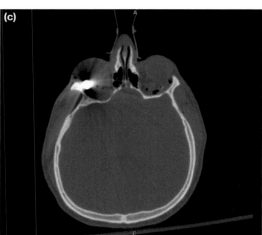

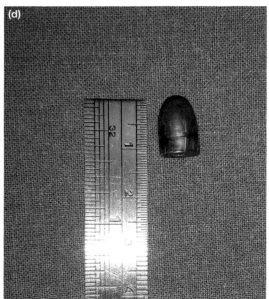

Figure 21.6 A 3D computed tomography (CT) scan (a) of 'low-velocity' handgun, shot at long distance towards the head of the target exhibiting the typical small entry wound, bone fragmentation and no exit wound. The axial CT scans (b, c) demonstrate the small entry wound in the left temporal fossa, transecting the left orbital cavity, then crossing the midline diagonally upward (medial wall of left orbit, ethmoid process and lateral wall of the right orbit), then coming to rest in the medial wall of the opposite right orbit. The patient was brought to hospital intubated where he was taken to emergency theatre and had both eyes undergo prophylactic canthotomy until a CT scan was taken to assess the state of the optic nerves, rule out retrobulbar haemorrhage and triangulate the exact resting place of the bullet. The intact non-deformed bullet/projectile (d) (a 7.62 mm × 25 mm Tokarev projectile without the casing) was only retrieved surgically following full ophthalmological assessment where it was removed via a transconjunctival approach. Much of the bullet's kinetic energy was spent as a result of an apparently distant shot, which explains the absence of significant bone injury and bullet deformation.

lead balls/pellets placed together, equalling the interior diameter of the barrel. In close-range injuries, the effect of the gas that is discharged under pressure into the wound also needs to be considered. Shotgun pellet injuries depend on the distance between the weapon and the target at the time of discharge or the size of the pellet scatter. The closer the shotgun is to the patient, the more dramatic the injury is to the hard and soft tissues, as some of the ballistic material will exhibit high-energy properties.

TREATMENT PROTOCOL

Timings for the treatment of military and civilian maxillofacial injuries vary depending on the mechanism of injury and the environment within which they are sustained. In either case, 'damage-control' surgery should commence within an hour, as definitive treatment of maxillofacial wounds is often delayed, especially during conflict as the facial region itself is rarely associated with appreciable mortality.

Stabilise the patient: Immediate care (0–120 minutes)

This stage is based on the principles of Advanced Trauma Life Support (ATLS), but military personnel are taught a modified version of this, where control of catastrophic haemorrhage precedes securing the airway because exsanguination is more likely to threaten life. Securing the airway by whatever means necessary with a low threshold for a surgical airway is adopted because of the risk of delayed swelling and the need for additional future procedures. This includes a planned tracheostomy (if time allows), a cricothyroidotomy, or intubation directly or through a defect.

Facial haemorrhage is rarely the sole contributor to hypovolaemic shock, a hallmark of penetrating neck injuries (PNIs), and is often controlled by packing the wound with haemostatic dressings and compressing the site of injury. Ligation of one or both external carotid arteries may be required, but this should be performed only under direct visualisation and after careful identification of the bleeding vessel. Blood volume expansion is also performed at this stage although advanced anaesthetic management allowing permissive hypotension may be employed.

Potentially fatal situations should be identified and prevented (pneumothorax, cardiac tamponade, intraperitoneal haemorrhage or intracranial haemorrhage). Fracture of the cervical spine must always be suspected in those exposed to blast injury.

Penetrating neck injuries

PNIs have been increasingly seen in war zones and urban low-level conflicts, presenting in 11% of all battle injuries with a high mortality. These injuries are associated with the highest mortality in the first 30 minutes post-injury. Death is caused by vascular haemorrhage, spinal cord trauma or a compromised airway. The most commonly affected vessels are the carotids followed by the internal jugulars, resulting in death due to exsanguination within 2 minutes if not treated.

Immediate and deep exploration of PNIs to the platysma reduces mortality dramatically, but this is only recommended following repeated physical examination with validated hard signs indicating underlying injury (*Table 21.2*), which is assisted by computed tomography angiography (CTA) (*Figure 21.7*). PNIs in civilians are primarily due to low-velocity wounds, which is in direct contrast to PNIs in military personnel, which are due to explosive fragmentation.

Surgical management is proposed upon an arbitrary categorisation of the neck into three arteriography zones after Zoon and Christensen: zone I, below the sternal notch (thoracic inlet); zone II, between the sternal notch and the angle of the mandible; and zone III, above the angle of the mandible. Nevertheless, designing a management protocol based on these zones can be misleading as an external wound does not necessarily indicate the trajectory of the projectile.

Haemorrhage in the unstable patient often necessitates ligation of the external carotid and internal

TABLE 21.2 Proposed management algorithm modified from John Breeze and Neil Mackenzie for penetrating neck injuries based on the neck zones

Zone	Significance	Treatment without 'hard signs'*	Treatment with 'hard signs'*
1	Mortality is highest because of the size of vessels and their proximity to the skin surface Vessels are difficult to access	Serial physical examination following CTA Formal arteriography as required	Median sternotomy or left anterior thoracotomy to control haemorrhage by appropriately trained surgeons
2	Management in a military hospital setting continues to be debated	As above However, there is a low threshold for surgical exploration if there are multiple penetrating wounds even in the absence of hard signs	Incision parallel to the sternocleidomastoid or horizontal neck dissection incision if access to the mandible is required
3	High mortality rate and access to vessels is difficult because of the skull base, styloid process and mandible	Serial physical examination following CTA Formal arteriography as required	Temporary division of the mandible or even craniotomy to control a high-carotid injury

* Hard signs: expanding haematoma, active bleeding and neurological deficit. *Abbreviation*: CTA, computed tomography angiography.

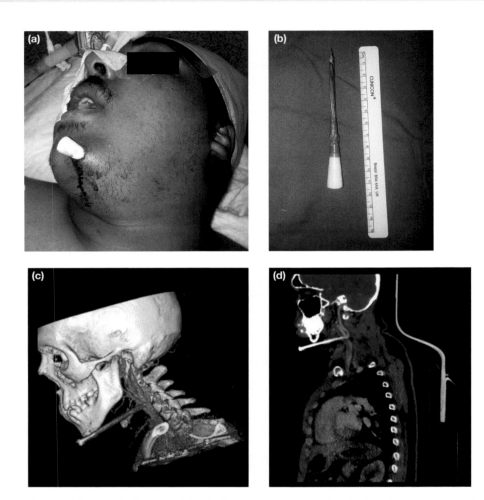

Figure 21.7 A penetrating neck injury in Zone II in a civilian setting (a). This 'home-made' projectile is a sharpened construction nail (10 cm long) fastened to a stabilising plastic 'tale' to assist in flight. It is shot with a fire extinguisher utilised as a propellant towards the target (b). On arrival of the above patient to our trauma unit, he had an emergency computed tomography angiogram (CTA) done (c, d), then was taken to the operating theatre immediately. The CTA demonstrated the proximity of the tip of the projectile to the major neck vessels. The patient did not have any hard signs, but his cervical spine was secured, Advanced Trauma Life Support protocols were followed and he was closely monitored while having his CTA done.

jugular vessels (*Figure 21.8*), which is generally well tolerated unless performed bilaterally. However, repair should be attempted first by lateral arteriorrhaphy or end-to-end anastomosis.

Damage-control maxillofacial surgery (<120 minutes)

This describes when surgical procedures are shortened to the minimum to prioritise short-term physiological recovery over anatomical reconstruction in the seriously injured patient.

Identification of injuries

After initial stabilisation, assessment of such wounds is usually rapid, as injured patients are often taken straight to the operating theatre as part of the overall continuum of damage-control resuscitation. Detailed documentation of all injuries is necessary to coordinate the sequence of treatment with all respective surgical services. It is often in the operating theatre that facial injuries are first assessed, and such an examination must also ensure that lacerations of the scalp, nasal fractures, missing teeth and deep damage caused by small penetrating fragments are not missed.

Obtaining radiographs and stereolithographic models

In most cases, rapid computed tomography (CT) is conducted to assist in intraoperative decisions. Modern CT scanners allow rapid assimilation of data and

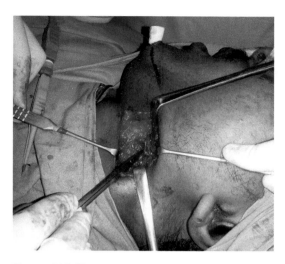

Figure 21.8 The wound was debrided and formally explored following a 5-cm submandibular incision to identify the bifurcation of the carotid artery and to locate the tip of the projectile. The projectile was not pulled out until all major neck vessels were identified, and local bleeding controlled. This is prophylactically done in case immediate ligation was required due to unforeseen trauma in the track of entry/withdrawal of the projectile.

manipulation of conventional cuts to three-dimensional images, which assists visualisation of the skeleton, helps identify foreign bodies and evaluates displaced fracture segments and associated aerodigestive soft tissue extension. CT findings should be the minimum information obtained before surgery (*Figure 21.9*).

Complex trauma is facilitated by fabrication of stereolithographic (SL) models to plan treatment adequately and determine the sequencing of fracture repair. The use of SL models allows preadaptation of surgical plates to obtain proper soft tissue projection and support that otherwise would not be possible to the degree of accuracy obtained by this technique. SL models also allow for wax replacement of avulsed structures or the generation of mirror-image structures, pre-bending of plates, fabrication of templates for contouring of bone grafts, fabrication of custom implants or use of stock alloplasts (*Figure 21.10*).

Serial debridement

The role of serial debridement is important for patients injured during conflict. The injury patterns seen differ in several ways from those seen in a civilian trauma setting: the devastating destruction of soft and hard tissues caused by high-velocity, fragmentation-type injury patterns lead to compromised tissue beyond the visibly damaged tissue; the battlefield environment is grossly contaminated; wound care on the field and

during transport is not ideal; and evacuation off the battlefield is not always swift, leading to increased wound contamination.

Early and aggressive debridement (scrubbing brushes and pulsatile lavage, with copious irrigation and antibiotic solution, e.g. clindamycin), together with surgical dermabrasion of ballistic facial wounds, is required to prevent infection and wound tattooing.

- After the first irrigation, superficial wet-to-dry dressing changes are performed three times per day
- After 48–72 hours, the procedure is repeated
- Next, the surgeon is faced with the decision of when to perform the primary closure. Most facial wounds can be closed within 36 hours of injury, and delayed closure (as advocated for the rest of the body) is rarely necessary
  - If tissue vitality is questionable or if it is not possible to debride the tissue adequately, delayed primary closure is advocated, and the wound is dressed in iodine-soaked gauze
  - If the wound is contused or ragged, 1–2 mm should be sharply trimmed off the edge of the skin to achieve non-contaminated, non-bevelled edges

Experience has shown that removal of all embedded energised fragments can be futile and of no clinical benefit, for example, shotgun pellets (*Figures 21.11* and *21.12*). If severed branches of the facial nerve or a damaged parotid duct are encountered, they should be tagged with a non-absorbable suture for later repair, and the wound should be closed.

Stabilisation of the hard tissue base to support the soft tissue envelope and prevent scar contracture

Owing to the high risk of infection and extensive soft tissue injury, definitive reconstruction is delayed to a secondary stage. A lack of bony support, fibrous tissue and scar contracture dictate the eventual functional and aesthetic result of any reconstruction. Generally, the hard tissue base is stabilised at the time of primary wound closure.

At this stage, temporary reduction and fixation of any facial fracture should be attempted to reduce bleeding and pain and to provide support to the facial pillars. This maintains a tissue plane, which provides easier dissection upon secondary reconstruction with either autogenous or alloplastic materials.

Patterns of facial fractures sustained from ballistic trauma differ considerably from those seen after blunt impact (*Figure 21.13*). These fractures are often comminuted and open to the cutaneous and mucosal surfaces. Explosions can cause blowout fractures of the orbit and facial burns, both of which put the patient at greater risk of orbital compartment syndrome; if this is suspected, lateral canthotomy and inferior cantholysis are necessary (*Chapter 12*).

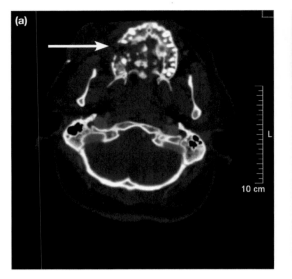

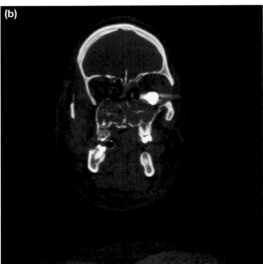

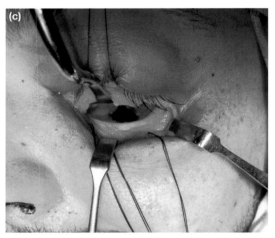

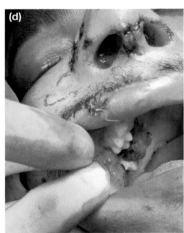

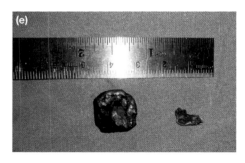

Figure 21.9 A ball-bearing projectile from a low energy blast being identified with a rapid computed tomography scan (a, b). The scan identified the final resting position of the projectile (b) in the left medial orbital wall and assisted in identifying the entry point (white arrow), which was intraoral in the opposite maxillary wall (a, d). From these two data points, the projectile's trajectory could be drawn. The projectile and its fragments were surgically retrieved via a transconjunctival approach to the orbit (c, e).

The use of an external fixator, sometimes with arch bars/wires, can provide anatomical reduction of the mandible and stabilise fragments. Unlike the generic Hoffman the mandible-specific devices are anatomically contoured, which enable the main bar to stand up to 1 cm from the skin surface making it less cumbersome. External fixator pins should not be inserted through infected bone or skin, and they are usually wrapped with antibacterial dressings such as iodine-impregnated ribbon gauze. These pins do not compromise the airway, and no special precautions are required for the release of fixation while the patient is being moved.

Any soft tissue or bony defects may continue to be debrided with the fixation device *in situ*. As the mouth can be opened while the fracture is healing, oral hygiene

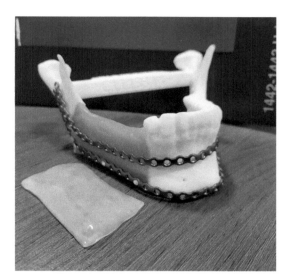

Figure 21.10 Stereolithographic model demonstrates an avulsive defect of the right mandible region with 2.5-mm titanium plates pre-bent to a wax template replacing the avulsed tissue. The adjacent white material moulded in the shape of the wax is a custom porous polyethylene implant spacer to be inserted temporarily in the defect. We use antibiotic impregnated implants to prevent bone-on-bone contact and soft tissue contraction. Refobacin® Revision: antibiotic-loaded bone cement containing both gentamicin and clindamycin.

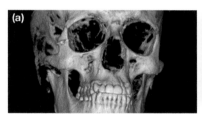
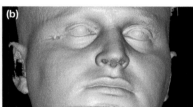
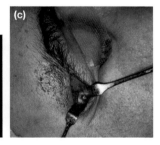

Figure 21.11 An officer who felt 'something hit him' when he discharged his shotgun and the pellets ricocheted off his surroundings. A cone beam computed tomography scan (a, b) demonstrates the embedded metallic bullet fragment in the frontal-process buttress of the right zygomatic bone with the small soft tissue entry point. Patients with these pellets usually become obsessively incessant to have them removed although not clinically necessary. Via a cosmetic lateral eyelid incision (c), the impacted and deformed bullet is identified embedded in the skull.

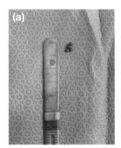
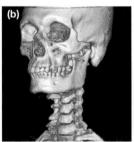
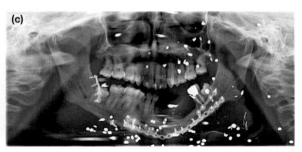

Figure 21.12 One of the reasons for not attempting to remove shotgun pellets is the difficulty in locating them, especially when close to major structures. Even with 3D computed tomography scans and triangulating their location, the procedure can be mutilating. In (a) and (b), the patient was adamant about having these pellets removed which were embedded in his left cheek. They were very close to his parotid gland and facial nerve – both had to be identified before locating the pellets. Note a direct shot to the face is more extensive and a characteristic facial appearance of a patient sustaining a shotgun wound from a distance is the presence of multiple punctate entry wounds, with no significant disruption of the facial features. Close range shots show extreme avulsion. In (c), a panoramic radiograph of a shotgun injury to the lower lateral face, with minor bone injury due to the distance of the shooting is demonstrated. From the main entrance wound corresponding to the circular pellet concentration in the premolar area, ricochet phenomenon and probably the so-called 'billiard ball' effect resulted in some pellets being distributed further posteriorly along the external oblique line.

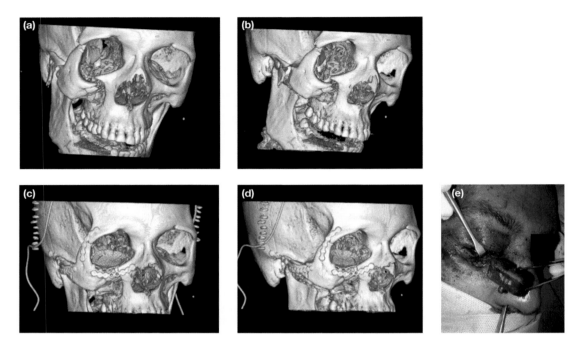

Figure 21.13 Preoperative and postoperative 3D computed tomography scans (a–d) demonstrating a badly displaced right zygomaticomaxillary complex (ZMC) fracture with a blowout of the orbit following being shot at from a distance with a rubber bullet. These are known as 'less-lethal' weapons but are shot from blended shotgun shell that can cause considerable damage especially in the facial region. This rubber bullet (a Soft-Gomm Caliber 8.8 × 10 SAPL®) (e), although shot from a considerable distance, caused the above fracture, and was embedded in the maxillary sinus under the orbits protruding from the skin.

and the patient's nutrition are improved along with trismus because fibrosis and scarring are reduced.

If external fixation of the midface is required, use of a Levant frame (maxilla or zygoma attached to supraorbital ridges) is ideal, as it interferes less than other options, for example, a box frame, when the patient is lying on their side while sleeping.

It may be necessary to combine techniques to produce fewer and larger bony units, which can then be stabilised by an external fixator. Even if the plates are exposed, infection can generally be stabilised with serial debridement and antibiotics until bony stability is achieved by the external fixator, resulting in minimal cosmetic defect.

Early care (120 minutes to 28 days)

The extent of necrosis of soft tissue wounds is more evident at this stage, and it is relatively safe to close wounds primarily if tension-free closure is possible. Deep spaces are debrided further and closed with absorbable sutures to prevent the formation of haematomas, pockets and subsequent infection. Surgical drains with suction bulbs can also be considered.

Replace missing soft tissue component

If primary closure is not possible because of tissue loss and avulsion, it is critical to replace the missing soft tissue before the development of scar contractures or bacteria colonisation (secondary infection). Once scar contractures develop, it is difficult to create a normal soft tissue appearance and almost impossible to rectify this later. The consensus is the use of vascularised tissue where it is the most resistant to secondary infection and scar contracture in these injuries.

Local rotation or advancement flaps may be considered as they provide excellent similarity to healthy skin in tissue coloration, consistency and appearance. Care must be taken not to damage any vessels needed for future anastomoses when local flaps are used. These vessels may already be damaged and require ligation, but, if possible, they should be identified and preserved for future use. Skin grafts are best avoided for the first 5–7 days as the risk of infection remains, and they are more prone to contracture.

The choice of using a local rotational flap versus a free flap is determined based on whether a satisfactory result can be obtained in one surgical procedure or several revision procedures. If a single surgery is planned, rotation of a local flap may be indicated, but if the need for future surgical intervention is necessary, consideration should be given to using free tissue transfer initially and finalising treatment during the secondary and tertiary surgeries with the local flap. Waiting 8–12 weeks after placement of a graft is recommended to allow for maturation before the next surgical procedure at that site.

It is noteworthy that high-energy transfer may result in temporary damage to the microcirculation of the soft tissue at a distance from the permanent wound, which must be considered when planning microvascular anastomoses. Thromboses in the facial vessels up to 3 cm from the macroscopic wound edges are attributed to the effect of the temporary cavities. These vessels begin to repair themselves between 7 and 10 days later. It is recommended that all anastomoses should be made at least 2 weeks after injury if this mechanism is suspected, and if required preceded by angiography. Anastomotic considerations are compounded by the fact that associated injuries to limbs are common and may be catastrophic, which has an impact on the availability of donor sites.

Infectious disease

Infection rates after war-related maxillofacial injuries have been poorly characterised, with rates ranging from 7% to 19%. All wounds due to bullets and fragmentation are inherently contaminated, and contrary to popular belief, the explosive process of firing a bullet does not sterilise it. These projectiles carry contaminants from clothing and skin flora into the wound.

Any soil or debris that is covering explosively propelled devices has the potential to be driven into the wound and cause gross contamination with bacteria. Patients' wounds from modern war zones were colonised by *Acinetobacter baumannii*. The decision to use antibiotics is based on the area of injury and degree of wound contamination. Empirical broad-spectrum antibiotics should be used to provide coverage against staphylococci, enterococci, *Klebsiella*, *Clostridium perfringens* and *Clostridium tetani*. These are given for 10–14 days, with cultures and sensitivities obtained as early as possible to direct treatment.

Patients may present with a confusing clinical picture because of infection of various other wounds or a progression to sepsis; therefore, maintaining vigilant monitoring and early consultation with infectious disease specialists are crucial.

Primary reconstruction and fracture management

Open fractures should be debrided, irrigated and closed temporarily to prevent infection. Except for fractures that compromise the airway or impair haemostasis, repair may be delayed for up to 2 weeks after injury, particularly if a high-energy transfer mechanism is suspected and when all infection has been cleared. Longer delays increase the chance of fibrosis and collapse of the soft tissue envelope. The goal is to obtain the best functional and cosmetic results possible by accurately reproducing the patient's pre-injury skeletal contour and maximising the potential for an accurate facial width and good soft tissue projection after healing. Preoperative planning is of paramount importance, prioritising support of the soft tissue envelope with missing bone replacement.

If the recipient site is contaminated or infected, allogeneic bone has a high tendency for resorption and chronic foreign body reaction. Autogenic bone, particularly bone transferred with periosteal coverage, is less likely to develop late infection and maintains the soft tissue projection obtained.

In cases of significant panfacial trauma that involves the maxilla and mandible, sequencing the treatment is recommended. After securing the airway, the surgeon should reconstruct the mandible in the first stage, ideally within 3–5 days. One of the more common errors associated with panfacial trauma reconstruction is inadequate reduction of the mandibular arch form (gonial width), which results in excessive facial width secondary to splaying. To avoid the potential of surgical team fatigue, lengthy reconstruction of the midface and orbital fractures should be delayed. Taking a break after the mandibular procedures also allows for the creation of dental impressions and splint fabrication.

Contemporary management techniques of mandibular fractures largely depend on miniplate osteosynthesis. However, in the case of serious comminution, periosteal damage and the 'through-and-through' nature of the injury, conventional direct fixation with miniplates is often not appropriate.

After proper fixation of the mandible, attention is directed to the zygomaticomaxillary complex and arch projection. Accurate positioning of the malar prominence and zygomatic arch is best accomplished by direct visualisation of the zygomaticomaxillary and zygomaticotemporal junctions using a coronal flap.

Long-term rehabilitation (1–3 months)

Secondary reconstruction

The objectives of secondary reconstruction are to increase functional activity, correct obvious errors and bony relapses from the primary procedures, improve the patient's cosmetic appearance, and provide enough bone to enable placement of dental implants. These objectives are in a manner analogous to those of oncological reconstruction.

Bone loss may be replaced by either free or vascularised bone grafts, with the latter generally taken from the iliac crest-deep circumflex iliac artery flap, scapular flap (for better bone height) or fibular flap (for better bone length). Great care must be taken with vascularised flaps because of the risk of microscopic vascular damage from the temporary cavity that could place the anastomosis at risk.

Block grafts may mean that it can be difficult to reproduce the vestibular anatomy, with subsequent difficulty in chewing and cleaning. This can be facilitated by a vestibuloplasty incorporating a palatal mucosal graft or a split skin graft taken from the thigh or the arm if other pre-prosthetic surgery wholly for dental indications is planned.

Distraction osteogenesis can provide additional bone, with no donor site morbidity, enabling the overlying soft tissues to adapt to the new bony shape. Although autogenous reconstruction is ideal, alloplastic methods using prostheses have a role in those tissues that are challenging to reconstruct aesthetically.

Facial scarring secondary to ballistic injuries is a significant cosmetic concern where preventive measures outweigh the benefits of secondary management. Early scar excision and revision along with early dermabrasion and use of laser technology to remove tattooing of soft tissue provides the most favourable outcome.

Physiotherapy

Physiotherapy addresses the movement of the temporomandibular joint and electrical stimulation of facial musculature that have been affected by facial nerve injury. This prevents muscle atrophy and encourages facial nerve regrowth in the area of deficit.

Pain management

Post-surgical patients manage their pain with large amounts of opiate analgesics. Centrally mediated pain syndrome has been identified in patients whose pain was not addressed adequately. These patients should be supported while withdrawing from opiate analgesics to an appropriate level of pain medication.

Psychiatric evaluation and support

Facial appearance is an important variable in how patients are perceived by others. Trauma patients must develop additional coping skills throughout their treatment to improve their self-esteem and ability to continue with reconstructive surgery.

Nutrition and speech therapy

Providing nutrition to a recovering surgical patient is of primary concern in healing and maintenance of the immune system. Ballistic injuries remove vital structures for phonation, mastication and deglutition, and even if salvaged or reconstructed, cranial nerve injury results in difficulties in performing these functions. Early placement of percutaneous endoscopic gastrostomy feeding tubes and central catheters may be beneficial.

TOP TIPS AND HAZARDS

- Appreciating the consequence(s) and compositional makeup of the ballistic missile is more important than its velocity or calibre in OMFS ballistics.
- In ballistic wounding, there are two zones of tissue damage: (a) the permanent cavity created by the passage of the projectile, and (b) the potential area of contused tissue surrounding it which is produced by temporary cavitation (manifestation of high-energy transfer to tissue).
- Treatment protocols for OMFS ballistic injuries highlight the importance of serial debridement for effective wound control while favouring early definitive reconstruction.
- Staged treatment and virtual surgical planning are helpful for surgical planning and allow for more predictability. This also determines treatment sequence and decreases operative time.
- Soft tissue injuries in ballistic trauma can exhibit avulsive loss, progressive necrosis and compromised vascularity (wound sepsis), contradicting/delaying potential microvascular soft tissue reconstruction.
- With hard tissue injuries in ballistic trauma, anatomic reduction is the objective; in complex fractures, maintaining large segments of bone as much as possible with soft tissue coverage is the goal.

FURTHER READING

Breeze J, Tong D, Gibbons A. Contemporary management of maxillofacial ballistic trauma. *Br J Oral Maxillofac Surg* 2017;**55**:661–5.

Powers DB, Delo RI. Characteristics of ballistic and blast injuries. *Atlas Oral Maxillofac Surg Clin North Am* 2013;**21**:15–24.

Powers DB, Will MJ, Bourgeois SL, Jr, et al. Maxillofacial trauma treatment protocol. *Oral Maxillofac Surg Clin North Am* 2005;**17**:341–55.

Stefanopoulos PK, Filippakis F, Soupiou OT et al. Wound ballistics of firearm-related injuries--part 1: missile characteristics and mechanisms of soft tissue wounding. *Int J Oral Maxillofac Surg* 2014;**43**:1445–58.

Tong DC, Breeze J. Damage control surgery and combat-related maxillofacial and cervical injuries: a systematic review. *Br J Oral Maxillofac Surg* 2016;**54**:8–12.

<table>
Chapter
22
</table>

Management of Potentially Malignant Oral Mucosal Disorders

Peter Thomson

INTRODUCTION

Potentially malignant disorders (PMD) are recognisable oral mucosal lesions, primarily leukoplakia, but also including erythroplakia, erythroleukoplakia and proliferative verrucous leukoplakia (PVL), which display variable tissue disorganisation and dysmaturation features histopathologically classified as epithelial dysplasia, and precede, in an unpredictable manner, invasive squamous cell carcinoma (SCC) development. There is an overall 12% cancer risk over a mean transformation time of around 4 years, with severe or 'high-grade' dysplasia most at risk. The ensuing morbidity and high mortality consequent upon SCC development remains significant in contemporary practice and, while the objectives of treating PMD have been poorly defined in the past, most authorities agree that preventing malignancy is the priority. This may be complicated, however, by the widespread, often multifocal presentation of disease throughout the upper aerodigestive tract. Current management goals for treatment intervention are summarised in *Table 22.1*, while *Table 22.2* lists the available treatment options.

CLINICAL OBSERVATION

Clinical observation, comprising oral lesion recognition and provisional diagnosis by incision biopsy, photography, routine inspection and patient monitoring, together comprise the traditional PMD management protocol. Unfortunately, this has led in many cases to 'passive observation' of SCC development in a previously identified 'at-risk' patient, which is self-defeating and inappropriate for modern patient care. A period of clinical observation may be appropriate for patients with low-grade dysplasia who stop smoking, who are prepared to address additional risk factor behaviours and attend for regular clinical review. While it is recognised that PMD lesions may improve and/or regress following smoking cessation, it is important that this is carefully monitored. Failure of existing mucosal disease to resolve may indicate that the patient has not stopped smoking or, more significantly, highlight progressive PMD disease exhibiting significant and

TABLE 22.1 Management goals in treating potentially malignant disorders

Diagnostic accuracy

Prediction of clinical behaviour

Early recognition of malignancy

Removal of dysplastic mucosa

Prevention of further disease

Prevent malignant transformation

Patient acceptability and minimal morbidity

Cost-effective

TABLE 22.2 Treatment options for potentially malignant disorders

Clinical observation

Medical treatment

Surgical intervention

irreversible dysplastic change; it is unwise to rely on observation alone for such cases.

MEDICAL TREATMENT

Numerous medical treatments have been proposed over many years to facilitate PMD management, including both local and systemic chemopreventive agents. Therapeutic agents are summarised in *Table 22.3*; their postulated mode of action includes antioxidant and anti-angiogenesis properties, together with targeted epithelial homeostasis and tissue repair mechanisms. Systematic reviews have proved unhelpful in determining their efficacy, however, and few relevant randomised, controlled trials exist in the literature. Documented clinical benefit has rarely followed medical treatment: no evidence of effective long-term resolution of mucosal abnormality, no significant prevention of malignant transformation and no reduction in PMD incidence or recurrence compared with observation

TABLE 22.3 Medical treatments proposed for management of potentially malignant disorders

Vitamins A, C and E

Retinoids

Beta carotene

Lycopene

Ketorolac

COX-2 inhibitors

Bleomycin

Green tea

Antivirals/antifungals

EGF receptor blockade

Curcumin

TABLE 22.4 Surgical approaches for management of potentially malignant disorders

Scalpel excision

Cryotherapy

Interventional laser surgery

Photodynamic therapy

or placebo. Many trials have enrolled small numbers of patients over short study durations, with cases followed for months rather than years post-treatment, which is mandatory for accurate determination of malignant transformation risk. If clinical improvement was observed during a trial, lesions often worsened on cessation of therapy and, because treatment goals were poorly defined, the precise relevance of treatment remained unclear. In addition, side effects in many patients, including dermatitis, skin discoloration, headaches, muscular pain, cardiovascular thrombosis and teratogenicity, may interfere with compliance and prompt treatment withdrawal.

SURGICAL TREATMENT

A fundamental flaw in both observational and medical approaches to treatment is the realisation that incision biopsy sampling provides only a provisional diagnosis. Whole lesion examination is necessary for definitive histopathological classification; it is self-evident that only surgical intervention can effectively remove localised areas of abnormal mucosa. A therapeutic approach that intervenes to diagnose SCC at either a 'potentially malignant' or early invasive phase, and thereby institutes curative treatment, should thus be encouraged. PMD are mucosal conditions only and do not require the extensive treatment modalities necessary for removal and/or destruction of invasive SCC. Critics of surgery correctly observe that no randomised controlled trials of surgical intervention have ever been carried out, particularly a direct comparison of surgery with non-intervention. Nonetheless, surgery is the first choice of many clinicians when PMD lesions exhibit high-grade dysplasia or a significant risk of early SCC development. *Table 22.4* lists the surgical treatment approaches.

Scalpel excision

Surgical intervention by conventional scalpel excision and primary closure of small defects, or by mucosal or skin grafting techniques for large oral defects, has rarely proved popular with clinicians or patients, primarily due to localised post-surgical scarring, contracture and deformity and the frequent failure of skin grafts to take reliably within the unforgiving oral environment. Although very small, isolated mucosal lesions may be excised, this is rarely the way in which PMD presents in practice. Attempts to manage widespread or multifocal PMD disease with such an approach are doomed to repeated failure and are not recommended.

Cryotherapy

Cryotherapy is a technique based on the localised destruction of diseased tissue by application of extreme cold, usually via liquid nitrogen. Although popular in the past for treating soft tissue oral lesions, it is now less commonly used and is not a recommended technique for either PMD or SCC treatment. Significant post-operative pain and swelling result from tissue damage following cryoprobe application, PMD are rarely if ever successfully destroyed and, of course, no excision biopsy is undertaken to establish a definitive diagnosis. This potentially leaves partially treated dysplastic tissue, or even occult SCC, *in situ* to be 'stimulated' by the tissue damage response that can lead to more aggressive lesion behaviour. Both high recurrence and increased malignant transformation rates are reported following cryotherapy use.

Interventional laser surgery

Interventional therapies based on laser surgery have evolved following the demonstrable failure of observational or medical therapies, and the limitations of conventional surgery in treating oral cavity PMD. Laser, the acronym for 'light amplification by stimulated emission of radiation', delivers monochromatic, coherent waves of light energy to target tissue via fibreoptic systems or alternatively a series of articulated arms and mirrors. A photothermal reaction occurs when laser light interacts with tissue; between 60 and 100°C coagulation produces tissue necrosis and/or facilitates localised haemostasis, while at 100°C and above

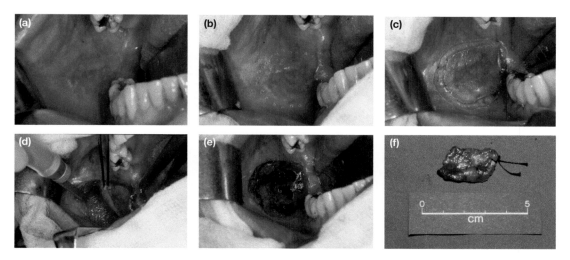

Figure 22.1 Laser excision of (a) buccal erythroleukoplakia which exhibited severe dysplasia on incision biopsy. (b) Excision margin marked 5 mm outside visible mucosal disease. (c) Excision margin established. (d) Dysplastic lesion resected at constant submucosal level. (e) Post-excision laser vaporisation of lesion margins and base to eliminate residual disease and facilitate haemostasis. (f) Excision specimen for histopathological assessment.

vaporisation allows the surgeon to incise tissue, and to either resect or ablate lesions. The carbon dioxide (CO_2) laser is a preferred modality to treat oral mucosal disease, because CO_2-generated laser light is within the mid-infrared range (10 600 nm), close to the spectroscopic absorption peak for water, rendering successful interaction of all oral soft tissues with the laser beam.

The operative technique is illustrated in *Figure 22.1*, which shows excision of a buccal PMD lesion. With a power setting of around 12 W, a handheld delivery device with a laser spot size of 1 mm diameter is used for intraoral use. As CO_2 laser light is invisible, a helium–neon aiming beam facilitates operator guidance to the target and an evacuation system removes smoke and debris from the surgical site. Single-pulse laser mode is used to outline resection margins, which are situated 5 mm outside the apparent clinical margins of the target lesion. Although excision margin placement is based on subjective judgement by the operating surgeon, adjunctive visual examination techniques such as VELscope® have not proved helpful in influencing the intraoperative siting of resection margins or to significantly improve the achievement of disease-free resection margins. Pulse marks are connected using the laser in a continuous mode, deepening the incision to approximately 5 mm in the submucosal plane. Depth of excision is ultimately influenced by the anatomical site, less when involving thin floor of mouth tissue or resections overlying alveolar bone, and by the extent of known dysplasia; severe dysplastic lesions are resected where possible at a deeper level due to the risk of foci of microinvasive or early invasive SCC coexisting. The whole specimen is then excised by undercutting at a constant depth. Following excision, the surgical bed and

all peripheral margins are vaporised using a defocused laser beam to eliminate residual disease, facilitate haemostasis and to effectively extend the treatment field beyond the surgical excision zone. The excision specimen is sutured at one or two points, to aid later tissue orientation, and is then placed in formal saline solution prior to forwarding to the pathology laboratory for histopathological analysis.

Clinically, there is little in the way of immediate postoperative pain, swelling or discomfort and patients may take clear fluids straight away, followed 2 hours later by a gradually increasing soft diet. Excised areas heal well by secondary intention, with a fibrinous cream-coloured coagulum forming over the wound within the first few days followed by re-epithelialisation from surrounding wound edges usually complete within 4–6 weeks. Due to the specific effects of laser vaporisation, a lack of mechanical trauma during surgery and the absence of wound suturing, scarring is usually minimal and excellent aesthetic and functional results ensue. *Figure 22.2* illustrates post-laser surgery healing after excision of a lateral tongue PMD.

Although excision techniques are preferred, there is a limited role for ablation therapy in which surface mucosa only is destroyed, to a varying depth selected by the surgeon and dependent on the pathological lesion treated, using a defocused laser beam. Although tissue is not excised for histopathological examination and abnormal basal epithelium may be left *in situ*, ablation may be used to treat non-dysplastic or mildly dysplastic lesions on tightly bound down alveolar or gingival tissue, where excision can result in slow or non-healing mucosa with painful areas of denuded and ultimately de-vitalised alveolar bone. *Figure 22.3* illustrates laser

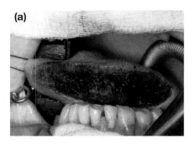
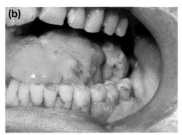
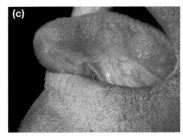

Figure 22.2 Healing post-laser surgery (a) immediately following excision of dysplastic lateral tongue lesion, and (b) 2 weeks post-surgery with creamy fibrinous exudate and pink, healthy granulation tissue. (c) Healing at 2 months with minimal scarring, good appearance and excellent functional mobility.

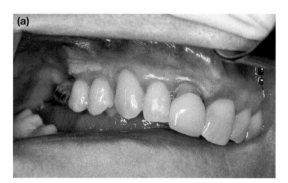
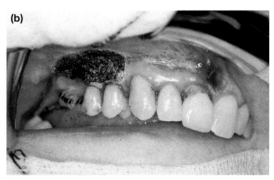

Figure 22.3 Laser surgery ablation (gingiva) showing (a) the pre- and (b) post-ablation appearance of posterior maxillary gingiva, following superficial destruction of a patch of mildly dysplastic proliferative verrucous leukoplakia (PVL).

ablation destruction of a small patch of mildly dysplastic PVL arising on posterior maxillary gingiva.

The CO_2 laser offers precise mucosal lesion excision, full histopathological assessment of tissue specimens and minimal postoperative morbidity; long-term postoperative complications are rare, although patients may experience initial lingual nerve dysesthesia following lateral tongue treatment or intermittent submandibular duct obstruction post-floor of mouth surgery. Specific technical advantages of laser include a relatively bloodless surgical field, improved intraoperative accuracy, reduced postoperative pain and swelling, rapid mucosal re-epithelialisation, limited scarring, reduction in damage to adjacent tissues and the ability to repeat treatment where necessary.

The intrinsic requirement for post-treatment follow-up also helps to facilitate a coordinated and structured patient surveillance strategy. Regular patient review and repeated, detailed clinical examination remain mandatory for all PMD patients following their intervention, although limited data are available to determine the precise length of follow-up or the optimal time intervals between clinic appointments to monitor patients safely post-surgery.

Other lasers in use for oral surgery practice include the neodymium:yttrium-aluminium-garnet (Nd:YAG) or the potassium-titanyl-phosphate (KTP) and a number of various argon and diode variants. There is little evidence to suggest that any one of these is more or less effective than another, and all have their advocates. The CO_2 laser, however, is probably the most utilised and studied in oral surgical practice.

Photodynamic therapy

This is a specialised form of intervention, which relies on cellular destruction by a cold photochemical reaction following activation of a photosensitising drug, such as aminolevulinic acid or temoporfin, by low-power visible light. This technique has been advocated as a non-invasive PMD treatment, although remains primarily a tool for palliative treatment of advanced head and neck SCC. A number of observational studies have reported variable success rates using photodynamic therapy to treat oral leukoplakia, but with inconsistent reporting regarding recurrent disease and to date very limited, often only between 3 and 6 months, or in some cases no follow-up data.

CONCLUSIONS

Early diagnosis of oral SCC and PMD management are areas of contemporary clinical practice in which variability in decision-making and lack of high-quality evidence has confounded treatment initiatives. Combining a defined surgical intervention with detailed patient profiling and active clinical surveillance provides a well-coordinated and methodical clinical management protocol with the potential to stall or even halt the ongoing process of oral carcinogenesis. Clinical outcomes for patients will only improve by earlier detection of SCC and effective management of 'precursor lesions' with malignant potential. As the consequences for an individual patient progressing to SCC can be devastating, there seems little to gain from observational or medical strategies. Interventional laser surgery provides readily available, effective, low morbidity treatment, which is successful in excising PMD mucosal lesions, facilitates early diagnosis of occult SCC and helps reduce the overall risk of SCC development. In the future, PMD patients will benefit from more accurate stratification into 'high-risk' and 'low-risk' categories, with individually tailored treatment protocols based on biomolecular and genetic profiling of cancer risk. While awaiting such refinements, and in the absence of meaningful multicentre, prospective randomised trials, the contemporary approach to interventional laser surgery management is recommended.

TOP TIPS AND HAZARDS

- PMDs are clinically recognisable mucosal precursor lesions that precede, in an unpredictable manner, SCC development.
- Overall malignant transformation rate is 12%.
- Stratification of individual patient risk guides interventional treatment planning.
- Incision biopsies provide provisional histopathological diagnoses only.
- Complete PMD excision provides definitive histopathological diagnosis and reduces same-site malignant transformation risk.
- Complete PMD excision identifies 'occult' early SCC in 12% of cases.
- Active surveillance is mandatory post-PMD excision to identify new-site SCC development.

FURTHER READING

Thomson PJ. *Oral Precancer – Diagnosis and Management of Potentially Malignant Disorders.* Wiley-Blackwell; 2012.

Thomson PJ. Potentially malignant disorders – the case for intervention. *J Oral Pathol Med* 2017;**46**:883–7.

Thomson PJ. *Oral Cancer: From Prevention to Intervention.* Cambridge Scholars Publishing; 2019.

Thomson PJ, Goodson ML, Cocks K, Turner JE. Interventional laser surgery for oral potentially malignant disorders – a longitudinal patient cohort study. *Int J Oral Maxillofac Surg* 2017;**46**:337–42.

Thomson PJ, Goodson ML, Smith DR. Profiling cancer risk in oral potentially malignant disorders – a patient cohort study. *J Oral Pathol Med* 2017;**46**:888–95.

Bailey & Love's Essential Operations Bailey & Love's Essential Operations
Bailey & Love's Essential Operations Bailey & Love's Essential Operations
Bailey & Love's Essential Operations Bailey & Love's Essential Operations

PART 4 | Oncology

Chapter 23

Neck Dissection

Peter A. Brennan, Mark Singh

INTRODUCTION

Many of the surgical principles described in this chapter have not changed significantly since 1906 when Crile published his classic paper describing 132 neck dissections (36 radical and 96 more selective procedures). Only 2 years later, Sir Henry Butlin described a procedure that is essentially the same as a current supra-omohyoid neck dissection (SOHND). Despite this publication of a 'selective' neck dissection, most elective treatment of even the clinically negative (N0) neck during the first half of the 20th century consisted mainly of radical neck dissection (RND). Over the last 20 years, there has been an increasing trend towards selective neck dissection (SND) for the initial management of patients with no clinical evidence of neck metastasis, and in carefully selected patients with nodal metastasis (although its use in the latter remains controversial).

Although SND preserves many vital structures (such as the accessory nerve), the functional results after these procedures are not as good as expected. Shoulder function and pain scores are worse in patients who undergo posterior triangle dissection, which may not recover despite preservation of the accessory nerve. A study found that the variables that contribute most to quality of life scores relating to the neck were age and weight, radiotherapy to the neck and type of neck dissection.

NECK DISSECTION CLASSIFICATION

Neck dissection nomenclature can be confusing; however, it can be simplified as follows:

- Radical neck dissection refers to removal of lymph nodes in levels I–V en bloc with sternocleidomastoid muscle (SCM), internal jugular vein (IJV) and spinal accessory nerve. This operation is both cosmetically and functionally mutilating and is used in gross metastatic disease, involving multiple levels of the neck and when preservation of the above structures would compromise surgical clearance. Although this operation has been regarded as the 'gold standard' for the surgical treatment of metastatic neck disease, it has largely been replaced by more selective surgery.

- Modified radical neck dissection (MRND) refers to dissection of levels I–V but with the preservation of one or more of the following structures: IJV, spinal accessory nerve and sternomastoid. The nomenclature refers to the number of structures preserved (so MRND type I is preservation of one of these structures, MRND type II is preservation of two structures and so on). Both RND and MRND are used when the neck has evidence of nodal metastasis (N+), although there is growing evidence to suggest that SND (see below) has a role to play not only in staging but also in the management of the N+ neck.

- Selective neck dissection: in 1991, the Committee for Head and Neck Surgery and Oncology of the American Academy of Otolaryngology and Head and Neck Surgery indicated that "in all SND, the IJV, spinal accessory nerve and SCM are routinely preserved. If removal of one or more of these structures is necessary, the structure should be listed after the appropriate term for the neck dissection". As a result, SND can easily be confused with MRND and indeed some surgeons use the terms interchangeably. However, SND should refer to the dissection of one or more levels of the neck (with careful preservation of the anatomical structures listed above, as well as other nerves such as the marginal mandibular branch of the facial nerve) rather than all five levels. Examples include the SOHND (levels I–III), lateral compartment neck dissection (levels II–IV) and levels I–IV neck dissection.

TERMINOLOGY OF NECK LEVELS

The most significant change to the well-known Robbins classification was the publication of an updated system in 2002. In addition to the five standard levels, nodal levels were subdivided into levels IA and B, IIA and B (below and above the accessory nerve) and VA and B (above and below the accessory nerve in the posterior triangle) (*Figure 23.1*). The concept of sublevels is clinically relevant as metastasis to level IIB from anterior oral cavity tumours is uncommon and metastases to level VA is rarer still, with studies advocating that the dissection of these levels is not usually necessary.

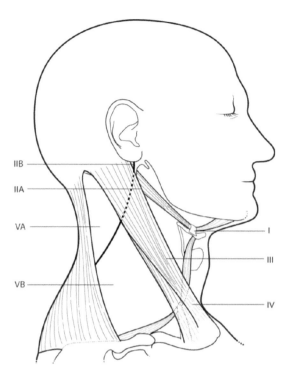

Figure 23.1 Levels of the neck. Level is divided into IA (submental) and IB (submandibular triangles).

PRINCIPLES OF SURGERY

The rationale for neck dissection is based on predictable patterns of lymphatic spread from the primary tumour site, and the relative risk of nodal metastatic disease. Over 30 years ago, Lindberg's clinical study found that the jugulo-digastric and mid-cervical nodes (levels II and III) were the most frequently involved in metastatic disease from the oral cavity. Tumours of the lip, anterior two-thirds of the tongue, floor of mouth and buccal mucosa also metastasise to the level I nodes (submental and submandibular triangles), often bilaterally. Lindberg described the possibility of skip metastasis, avoiding the first echelon nodes and spreading directly to the level III area. More recent studies have found that when levels I–IV are negative, level V is never node positive, supporting the use of the SND for the N0 neck. Despite many published studies, there is still controversy about neck dissection surgery and the reader should refer to specialist textbooks for a full discussion.

When taking trainees through a neck dissection, the authors make the analogy of walking through a jungle. Some structures in the neck (such as the digastric and omohyoid muscles) will help to delineate the path – these are your trusted guides. However, you will also come across many dangers, which if not treated with respect could take you by surprise, sometimes when you least expect it! These include structures such as the phrenic, hypoglossal and marginal mandibular nerves.

TECHNIQUE
Patient position

For all neck dissections, the fully anaesthetised (but unparalysed) patient should be placed supine on the operating table with the head turned away from the side being operated. A sandbag can be used if required to elevate the shoulder. It is sensible to expose the neck from the sternum and lateral clavicle to the ear and lips. Following skin preparation, the drapes need to be secured in place using adhesive strips, sutures or skin clips. It is useful to keep the lower lip exposed (to check for marginal mandibular nerve function).

Choice of incision

This depends on the type of neck dissection being undertaken. Ideally, skin incisions should be placed in natural skin creases, following Langer's lines. The lower border of the mandible, sternomastoid and clavicle can be marked to assist placement of the incision. For a SND, an incision running from the mastoid to submental area 3 cm below the mandible is usually adequate. When levels IV and V are being dissected, it may be necessary to place this incision lower down. The authors routinely use a Schobinger-type incision for MRND (*Figure 23.2*), except in the previously irradiated neck,

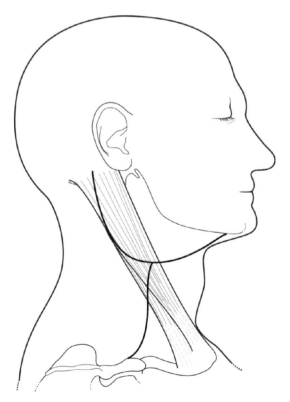

Figure 23.2 Schobinger incision for modified radical neck dissection (MRND).

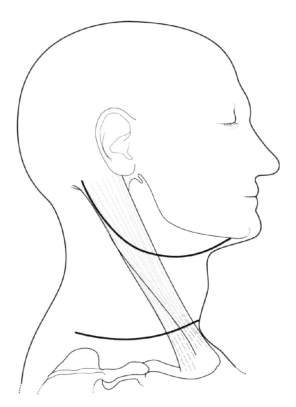

Figure 23.3 MacFee incision. Distance between incisions should be at least 4 cm.

where a MacFee incision is preferred (to reduce the risk of wound dehiscence). When a Schobinger incision is used, it is important not to place the tri-radiate part of the incision over the great vessels, especially if the sternomastoid is removed (risk of wound infection and vascular compromise!). If a MacFee incision is used – this is the correct spelling of the author who described it in 1960 – some spell it McFee! – an adequate bridge of skin between the incisions (of at least 4 cm) is essential to minimise the risk of skin necrosis (*Figure 23.3*). It is important to mark either side of the incisions (using needle and Bonney's blue, or superficially scoring the skin with the back of a scalpel blade) to facilitate subsequent skin closure.

Development of skin flaps

It is usual to raise skin flaps in a subplatysmal plane. Local anaesthetic solution may be injected to facilitate this process. The flaps can be raised using monopolar diathermy (Colorado needle), scalpel or scissor dissection. The authors also like using the Harmonic scalpel for some parts of a neck dissection, but not close to important nerves. With all these techniques, but particularly when diathermy is used, care should be taken in the upper skin flap to minimise damage to

the marginal mandibular nerve, which lies just deep to the platysma muscle in the deep cervical fascia. It can be readily identified as it crosses the facial vessels (FVs) and great care should be taken to preserve this nerve. It is sometimes possible to preserve the great auricular nerve as it crosses the SCM, although the roots (C2,3) are often transected later on in the dissection. In both the submental and posterior triangles, the platysma muscle often fades away and care should be taken to ensure that the skin flap does not become too thick or thin in these areas. It is sometimes surprising just how superficial the accessory nerve can be! The external jugular vein is easily damaged when the inferior skin flap is being raised as it lies immediately deep to the platysma muscle and may need to be ligated. The flaps should be developed beyond the boundaries of the neck dissection to be performed. For a MRND, the flap should be extended to the trapezius muscle in the posterior triangle. The muscle can be brought into view by having an assistant pushing it upwards and forwards or finding its origins at the mastoid. In bulky disease, it may be necessary to leave the platysma on the metastatic nodes, or even include skin in the resection if clinically indicated. In these cases, it is important to plan skin incisions to facilitate subsequent closure.

Start of neck dissection proper: I–IV SND

Where should I start the neck dissection? This is a question often asked by newcomers to this procedure. There are many ways to perform the procedure (inferiorly to superiorly, posterior to anterior and so on), and it is often good to try different methods and to vary these on separate occasions to find a way that works for each operator. Even then, one's routine procedure may need to be modified when, for example, a large metastasis is present in level II, in which case it is often wise to start somewhere else. Also, if one particular area is proving difficult, move on to another region and come back to it. The procedure described below is for a level I–IV SND. The RND and MRND variations are discussed subsequently.

Mobilisation of the SCM

The fascia overlying the SCM is incised along the whole posterior margin length of the muscle and lifted anteriorly. It is possible to preserve the external jugular vein and great auricular nerve (GAN) if mobilised and retracted posterior laterally. If the GAN has to be divided, then it is recommended to bury the proximal stump into the SCM to reduce the risk of annoying neuromas. The dissection is continued close to the muscle in a broad front inferiorly and superiorly around its anterior border. Superiorly, the tail of the parotid and the posterior digastric muscle will come into view on its way to the mastoid process. The SCM is then retracted posteriorly until you reach the posterior

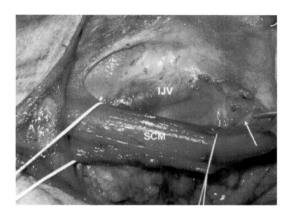

Figure 23.4 Dissection around sternomastoid muscle (SCM) to reveal internal jugular vein (IJV). The accessory nerve is just coming into view (arrow).

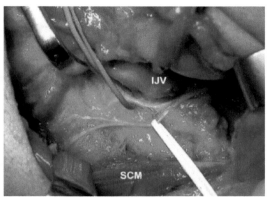

Figure 23.5 Identification of the accessory nerve. In this case, a variant with innervation from a cervical plexus nerve. *Abbreviations*: IJV, internal jugular vein; SCM, sternomastoid muscle.

border of this muscle. The carotid sheath will come into view, initially with the IJV (*Figure 23.4*). This is the lateral limit of the dissection. As one dissects superiorly, the accessory nerve will be found deep to the posterior digastric passing in a medial to lateral direction into the anterior border of the upper third of the SCM. It can often be felt as a cord-like structure. By hugging the anterior border of the SCM in a broad front, this important nerve is easily identified. It is worth noting that this nerve has many anatomical variations (one can be seen in *Figure 23.5*), and it can pass superficial, deep or even through the IJV. By maintaining a broad front, the SCM can be skeletonised away from the underlying deep structures. It can then be retracted with vascular slings. The omohyoid muscle will be seen inferiorly, the tendon of which passes superficial to the IJV. This muscle arbitrarily divides the 'surgical neck' into levels III and IV, although the position of the muscle varies with neck position. For a level IV dissection, the omohyoid is dissected free from the IJV, whereas in a SOHND, the dissection commences superiorly to the upper border of this muscle.

Clearance down to pre-vertebral fascia

The fatty tissue containing nodes posterior to the IJV is carefully incised at the inferior extent of the dissection in a horizontal direction. This is done in stages, so as to not inadvertently go through the thin pre-vertebral fascia. The use of scissor dissection combined with the intermittent use of a wet swab to sweep this tissue off the pre-vertebral fascia enables easy identification of this fascia. The phrenic nerve will be seen under the pre-vertebral fascia passing from lateral to medial on the scalenus anterior muscle (*Figure 23.6*). More laterally at the root of the neck, the upper trunks of the brachial plexus may also be visualised, again under the fascia. The authors routinely extend this dissection laterally to the area over which lies the posterior border

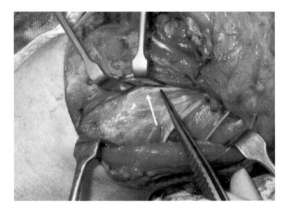

Figure 23.6 Clearance in level IV. The arrow indicates the phrenic nerve under the pre-vertebral fascia.

of the SCM (effectively including the anterior border of level V in the dissection). Once the correct depth has been established, it is quite easy to carry the postero-lateral part of this dissection in a superior direction. This can be facilitated by appropriate retraction and counter-traction. As the dissection proceeds in this way, one will come across cervical nerves that have pierced the pre-vertebral fascia. These can be cut as long as they are superficial to it and the phrenic nerve has been identified. In some cases, it is possible to preserve some of these nerves, thereby maintaining sensation to the skin in the dermatomes supplied by them. As one reaches the accessory nerve superiorly, the sternomastoid is retracted fully, and the level IIB can be cleared down to the muscular floor. The anatomical variations of this nerve should be remembered (it can be anterior [most common] or posterior to the IJV, or even pass through the vein). Level IIB contains the occipital artery, which runs postero-inferior to the posterior digastric muscle.

Once cleared, the fatty tissue can be passed under the accessory nerve in continuity with the neck dissection specimen.

Dissection and clearance around the great vessels

The dissection now proceeds anteriorly onto and around the IJV. The fascia overlying the posterior aspect of the IJV is incised in a broad front (superiorly and inferiorly), and dissection is carried around the IJV itself. The inferior loop of the ansa cervicalis can usually be seen and preserved on the inferior half of the vessel. With a left-sided neck dissection and when approaching the IJV inferiorly in level IV, an attempt should be made to identify the thoracic duct on its posterior surface. It is also vital to identify the vagus nerve (*Figure 23.7*), which usually lies between the IJV and common carotid artery. Superiorly, the hypoglossal nerve will be seen crossing the internal and external carotids. It gives a descending branch (C1) which joins with C2,3 to form the ansa cervicalis. This nerve usually lies antero-lateral to the IJV and should be preserved if possible (if only to show off one's technical expertise!). The sympathetic chain can sometimes be seen on the pre-vertebral fascia deep to the carotid artery, although the dissection itself should not be deeper than IJV.

Anterior dissection

The limits of the anterior dissection are the anterior border of the omohyoid, and the midline of the neck in the submental triangle. The dissection can proceed quite quickly up the omohyoid muscle. Occasionally a large vein is identified (sometimes after it has been cut!) but this is readily ligated. As the dissection reaches the inferior part of the hyoid bone, care should be taken to re-identify the hypoglossal nerve as it passes into the submandibular triangle. The dissection can now continue from the midline along the lower border of the mandible. The mandibular periosteum can be incised

to create a sharp plane of dissection. The submental area is usually quite vascular, due to many branches of the submental vessels. The bleeding is usually controlled with diathermy.

Submandibular triangle

As the dissection passes along the mandible, the mylo-hyoid muscle will come into view. The marginal mandibular branch of the facial nerve should be identified (if this has not already been done) and retracted. The facial vessels can be ligated and retracted superiorly to assist retraction of this nerve (*Figure 23.8*). Having dealt with these structures, it is easy to retract the mylohyoid, exposing the floor of mouth, and enabling easy removal of the submandibular gland (*Figure 23.9*). The lingual (superiorly) and hypoglossal nerves (inferiorly) should be

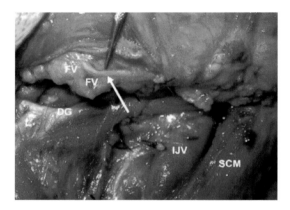

Figure 23.8 Marginal mandibular branch of facial nerve. The facial vessels (FVs) have been ligated. *Abbreviations*: DG, digastric tendon; IJV, internal jugular vein; SCM, sternomastoid muscle.

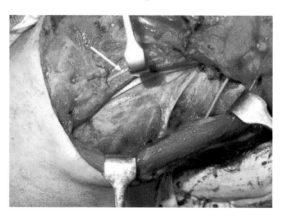

Figure 23.7 Further dissection reveals the vagus nerve and ansa cervicalis (arrow).

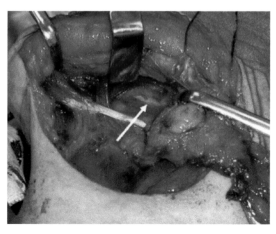

Figure 23.9 Level I clearance. The arrow indicates the lingual nerve.

identified in the floor of mouth and the submandibular ganglion and duct ligated and divided. At the posterior aspect of the gland lies the facial artery, which loops over the posterior digastric and this requires division. If possible, when a microvascular reconstruction is taking place, this artery should be left as long as possible to facilitate subsequent anastomosis. All that remains is to join up the posterior part of the submandibular triangle with the level II dissection. The tail of the parotid can be included here, and the retromandibular vein will need to be ligated. The specimen should be suitably orientated for the pathologist.

Drains and closure

Meticulous haemostasis is paramount for this procedure – the patient should be positioned head down to increase venous pressure to visualise bleeding points. A Valsalva manoeuvre given by the anaesthetist to further increase venous pressure is also often helpful. Two large drains (size 16) should be placed. The authors routinely use 3/0 Maxon to close platysma, with either 5/0 Prolene, skin clips or a running subcuticular suture to close the skin itself.

VARIATIONS: MRND AND RND

In many respects, removal of the SCM makes a neck dissection much easier, although adds morbidity for the patient. With a RND or MRND (when the SCM and IJV are included), the SCM can be cut through superiorly and inferiorly using monopolar diathermy. The IJV itself requires careful ligation both superiorly and inferiorly. The authors place two 2/0 linen ties with a 3/0-silk transfixation suture between them on the IJV being left. On the part of the vein being removed, it is wise to place a transfixation suture as well, as the ties sometimes come off during the dissection giving an unexpected shock. As it is low pressure in the IJV, any bleeding can be temporarily arrested with pressure. If a tie came off superiorly at the skull base, it should still be possible to control bleeding with pressure (even suturing packs in place). Once the SCM and IJV are divided, it is easy to use the cut omohyoid muscle belly to rapidly progress the dissection anteriorly. Ideally, if possible, the accessory nerve should be preserved in a MRND as should the marginal mandibular nerve (*Figure 23.10*).

Level V can be cleared starting initially inferiorly along the clavicle, again down to the level of the pre-vertebral fascia. Large clips (e.g. Roberts) can be used to clamp the fat (and transverse cervical vessels). These are ligated as one proceeds with the dissection. At this point, care should be taken not to inadvertently pull up the subclavian vessels! This can be prevented by initially dissecting straight down through the fat onto the pre-vertebral fascia. It is also possible to damage

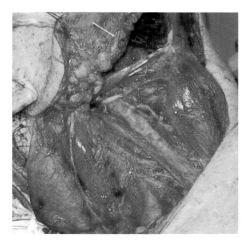

Figure 23.10 Completed modified radical neck dissection type I with preservation of accessory and marginal mandibular nerve (arrow).

the lung apex resulting in a pneumothorax, although this is rare. The accessory nerve can be dissected free and skeletonised from the fat if this nerve is being preserved. The cervical nerves will need to be cut to enable removal of level V but remember that these should only be cut when they are superficial to the pre-vertebral fascia. It may be necessary to cut the inferior belly of the omohyoid.

SUPRA-OMOHYOID NECK DISSECTION

The principles of a more selective procedure are the same as for the levels I–IV neck dissection described above, although it can be technically more challenging. The dissection usually starts inferiorly over the omohyoid muscle and proceeds superiorly as before. As with a levels I–IV neck dissection, it is important to mobilise the SCM muscle and take the dissection posterior to the IJV to sample as many nodes as possible.

EFFECTS OF RADIOTHERAPY

Surgery becomes more difficult in the irradiated neck, and it is often more difficult to preserve structures, particularly nerves such as the accessory nerve. Tissue planes are distorted, fibrosis makes dissection much more difficult and bleeding from small vessels can also be a problem. Furthermore, there is a greater chance of wound breakdown (*Table 23.1*).

TABLE 23.1 Complications of neck dissection

Immediate	
Bleeding	Packing, identify vessel, repair if appropriate (involve vascular surgeons if common or internal carotid [rare])
Pneumothorax	Chest drain
Damage to thoracic duct	Oversew with 3/0 silk. Use sternomastoid or omohyoid Fibrin glue and cyanacrylate can also be used
Inadvertent transaction of nerve	Micro-neural repair
Gross swelling (if both internal jugular veins compromised)	May need tracheostomy
Early	
Chyle leak	Exploration and/or medium chain triglyceride diet (dietician support)
Haematoma	Evacuate depending on size
Infection	Systemic antibiotics/drain if collection
Wound breakdown	Minimise risk with initial choice of incision and two-layer closure re-suturing in theatre
Late	
Shoulder pain/dysfunction	Physiotherapy
Contractures	Physiotherapy

TOP TIPS AND HAZARDS

- Meticulous haemostasis.
- Traction and counter-traction.
- Dissection on a broad front.
- Beware of anatomical variations.
- If you get stuck, start dissecting elsewhere and come back.
- Position patient head down at completion to raise venous pressure and identify bleeding points.

FURTHER READING

Crile GW. Excision of cancer of the head and neck. With special reference to the plan of dissection based on one and hundred and thirty two operations. *JAMA* 1906;**47**:1780–6.

D'Cruz AK, Vaish R, Kapre N et al. Elective versus therapeutic neck dissection in node-negative oral cancer. *N Engl J Med* 2015;**373**:521–9.

de Bree R, Takes RP, Shah JP et al. Elective neck dissection in oral squamous cell carcinoma: past, present and future. *Oral Oncol* 2019;**90**:87–93.

Robbins KT, Clayman G, Levine PA, et al. American Head and Neck Society; American Academy of Otolaryngology – Head and Neck Surgery. Neck dissection classification update: Revisions proposed by the American Head and Neck Society and the American Academy of Otolaryngology – Head and Neck Surgery. *Arch Otolaryngol Head Neck Surg* 2002;**128**:751–8.

Shabtay N. Level IV neck dissection as an elective treatment for oral tongue carcinoma – a systematic review and meta-analysis. *Oral Surg Oral Med Oral Pathol Oral Radiol* 2020;**130**:363–72.

Bailey & Love's Essential Operations Bailey & Love's Essential Operations
Bailey & Love's Essential Operations Bailey & Love's Essential Operations
Bailey & Love's Essential Operations Bailey & Love's Essential Operations

Chapter 24

Access Surgery

Madan G. Ethunandan

INTRODUCTION

Appropriate access to the craniomaxillofacial region is an essential prerequisite to perform any procedure. The complex anatomy and adjacent vital and aesthetically sensitive areas make the design of access procedures important. In this chapter, the relevant anatomy and essential steps in various access procedures are described.

The access procedure should enable identification and protection of critical structures, safe resection of the tumour, not compromise healing and aid reconstruction, allow modification if required and result in acceptable scars. The excellent blood supply in the craniofacial region allows a wide range of soft tissue and bone flaps to be designed, provided one recognises and respects the relevant anatomy.

CORONAL FLAP

The coronal flap provides access to the skull, anterior and middle cranial fossa, upper midface including the nasoethmoid region and orbits, temporal and infratemporal fossa.

The SCALP, an acronym, consists of five layers: **S**kin, sub**C**utaneous connective tissue, galea **A**poneurotica, **L**oose areolar tissue and **P**ericranium (*Figure 24.1a,b*). The first three layers are firmly attached to

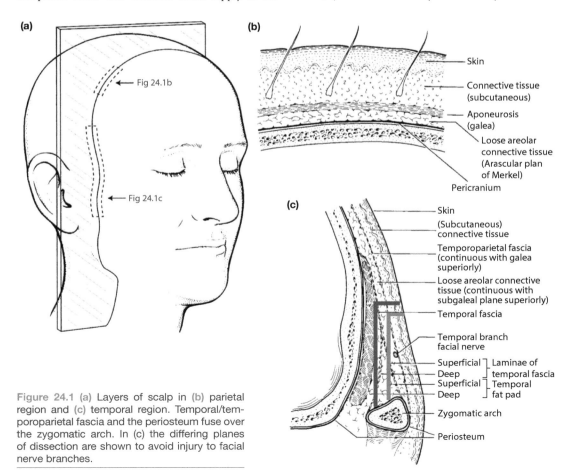

Figure 24.1 (a) Layers of scalp in (b) parietal region and (c) temporal region. Temporal/temporoparietal fascia and the periosteum fuse over the zygomatic arch. In (c) the differing planes of dissection are shown to avoid injury to facial nerve branches.

each other and are raised as a single layer, superficial to the loose areolar tissue. The neurovascular bundle runs within the first three layers. The 'perceived' complexity of the layers in the temporal region can be rationalised, if one were to consider the galea aponeurotica as a single layer which extends to the temporal region as the 'temporoparietal fascia' (synonym – superficial temporal fascia/supra-zygomatic SMAS) and the pericranium extending as the 'temporalis fascia' (synonym – deep temporal fascia) overlying the temporalis muscle. The deep temporal fascia divides about 2–3 cm above the zygomatic arch into superficial and deep layers (*Figure 24.1c*). The temporoparietal fascia, superficial layer of the deep temporal fascia and the periosteum of the zygomatic arch fuse together on the lateral aspect of the zygomatic arch and contain the frontal branch of the facial nerve. The superficial temporal fat pad is present between the superficial and deep layers of the deep temporal fascia, with the deep layer attached to the deep aspect of the zygomatic arch. Dissection deep to the galea and the temporoparietal fascia affords a relatively avascular plane and maintains and preserves the blood supply and avoids damage to the nerves, including the frontal branch of the facial nerve. This 'safe' plane of dissection can be between the temporalis muscle and the 'undivided' deep temporal fascia or (more inferiorly) between the superficial and deep layers of the 'divided' deep temporal fascia (*Figure 24.1c*).

Landmarks of temporal branch(es)

- At least 8 mm in front of the cartilaginous meatus at the zygomatic arch
- At least 1 cm anterior to the upper anterior attachment of the helix

- No higher than 2 cm above the frontozygomatic suture (lateral edge of the eyebrow)

Nerve damage is prevented with dissection deep to the temporal fascia beyond these limits (*Figure 24.2*).

Procedure

The hair along the incision line can be parted or a small strip shaved (*Figure 24.3*). Local anaesthetic containing 1:200 000 adrenaline is infiltrated above the galea for appropriate haemostasis (you know you are in the right plane if increased resistance is felt. If it is easy to inject, you are in the deeper loose areolar tissue plane). The incision is marked from the anterior attachment of the helix and carried over the vault to the opposite side, inside the hairline (*Figure 24.3*). It can stop at the midline, if only unilateral access is required. If repeated access is likely to be required to the cranial skeleton, it would be useful to incorporate a posteriorly directed 'curve', just above the helical attachment to the scalp, to try and avoid injury to the anterior branch of the superficial temporal artery and maintain additional vascularity to the flap. A 'bevelled' incision parallel to the hair follicles is made to minimise alopecia and a 'zig-zag' can be incorporated to avoid parting of the hair along the incision line. In male patients, the likely influence of male pattern baldness should be taken into account.

The incision commences at the vertex between the superior temporal lines and is made with a blade through the galea, up to the loose areolar tissue and the first three layers are raised as a unit. Blunt scissors or a brain retractor can be used to undermine the incision line along this plane, down to the root of the helix

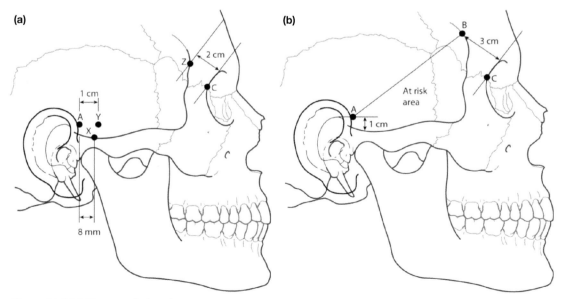

Figure 24.2 (a) The outer limits of the temporal branch(es) of the facial nerve. (b) The temporal branch of the facial nerve is superficial to the temporal fascia anterior to the line A–B.

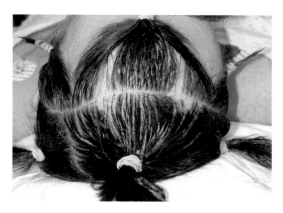

Figure 24.3 With the hair parted the incision is parallel to the hair follicles.

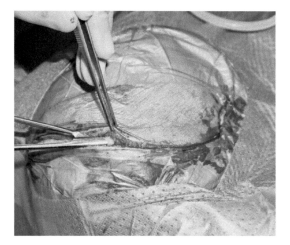

Figure 24.4 The first three layers of the scalp lift as a single unit.

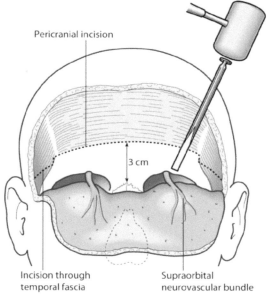

Figure 24.5 Pericranial incision when a pericranial flap is not required. Freeing of the supraorbital neurovascular bundle from canal.

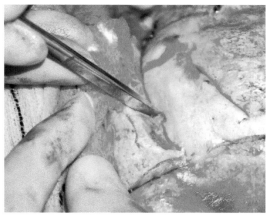

Figure 24.6 Supraorbital neurovascular bundle freed with osteotome.

and with the brain retractor *in situ*, the incision is made down to it (*Figure 24.4*). This allows rapid elevation of the flap, without inadvertent damage to the underlying temporal fascia/temporalis muscle. Dissection is carried forward in the subgaleal plane. Approximately 3 cm above the superior orbital rim the pericranium is incised and the dissection continued subperiosteally (*Figure 24.5*). Resistance is often encountered in the frontozygomatic and frontonasal suture region and around the supraorbital neurovascular bundles. If the supraorbital neurovascular bundle is present within a foramen, rather than a notch, the foramen can be opened with careful use of a fine osteotome (divergent cuts to minimise damage and ease of release) (*Figure 24.6*). The formamina/notch are present on average 32 mm from the midline and the location can often be identified on the scans.

A midline vertical incision in the periosteum aids exposure of the nasal bones and frontal process of the maxilla. Detachment of the medial canthal tendon from the anterior lacrimal crest gives unrestricted exposure of the medial orbit to the optic canal, and the orbital floor to the infraorbital nerve.

The medial canthal tendon must be 'tagged' through the periosteum with a suture for later reattachment to a microplate (*Figure 24.7*). Subperiosteal dissection medially is now possible as far as the floor of the orbit.

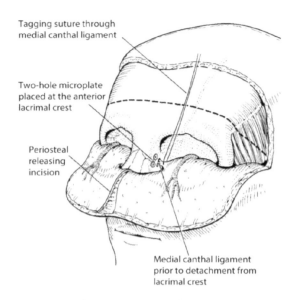

Tagging suture through medial canthal ligament

Two-hole microplate placed at the anterior lacrimal crest

Periosteal releasing incision

Medial canthal ligament prior to detachment from lacrimal crest

Figure 24.7 Midline vertical releasing periosteal incision to aid exposure of nasal bones. Medial canthus 'tagged' with suture for later attachment to microplate.

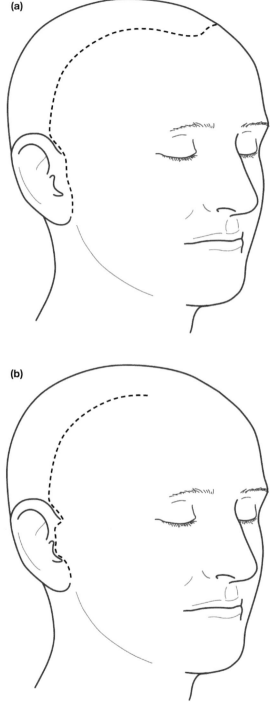

(a)

(b)

Figure 24.8 (a) Incision in skin crease; (b) following the tragus.

To expose the temporomandibular joint, zygoma and lateral orbit, the skin incision is extended inferiorly to just below the cartilaginous meatus, in a naturally occurring skin crease. This could be modified to follow the free edge of the tragus, to make this section less conspicuous (*Figure 24.8a,b*). The dissection is carried forward medially following the cartilaginous meatus. At the upper attachment of the helix the temporalis fascia is incised, about 1 cm above the zygomatic arch, and angled forwards to connect with the supraorbital periosteal incision 3 cm above the superior orbital rim (*Figure 24.9a*). The incision in the temporal fascia is extended vertically to the root of the zygomatic arch, which can be palpated above the cartilaginous meatus. A pocket is created at the root of the zygomatic arch, deep to the periosteum and the soft tissues tented with a periosteal elevator to expose the arch. The soft tissues superior to the arch, on the surface of the temporalis muscle, can be transected down to the periosteal elevator to expose the zygomatic arch and lateral orbit, without damaging the frontal branch (*Figure 24.9a–f*).

Retraction of the temporalis muscle posteriorly provides additional exposure to the temporal fossa and the superior limit of the infratemporal fossa (*Figure 24.9f*).

A pericranial flap could be easily incorporated, by extending the pericranial incision superiorly to the required length, between the superior temporal lines, as an extension of the temporalis fascia incision (*Figure 24.9b–d*). If a pericranial flap is to be utilised, the subgaleal dissection should stop 2 cm above the supraorbital rim, to maintain the vascularity of the pericranial flap.

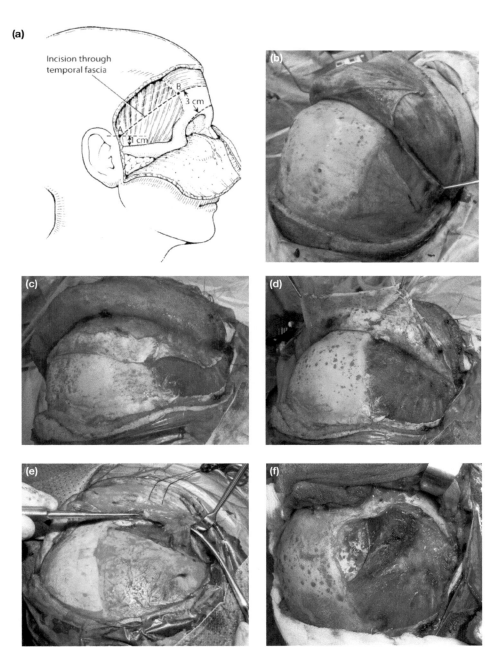

Figure 24.9 (a, b) The incision through the temporal fascia is made along line A–B (see Figure 24.2b) to ensure preservation of the temporal branch of the facial nerve. Complete exposure of the temporomandibular joint (TMJ) and the entire zygoma is possible without damage to the temporal branch of the facial nerve. (c, d) Incorporation of the pericranial flap as an extension of the temporal fascia incision. (e) Creation of subperiosteal tunnels along the zygomatic arch. (f) Exposure of the orbital rim, zygoma, zygomatic arch and temporal fossa.

The periosteum is freed over the lateral and inferior orbital rim, detaching the lateral canthal ligament. Deep circumferential subperiosteal orbital exposure is now easily achieved.

The extent of subperiosteal exposure possible with the coronal scalp flap is demonstrated (*Figure 24.10*).

Closure of the galea and meticulous haemostasis are essential and drains and/or head dressing can be additionally utilised to prevent haematomas.

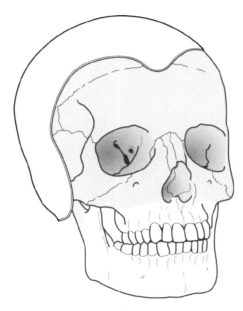

Figure 24.10 Exposure possible with a coronal flap.

TOP TIPS AND HAZARDS

- Inject vasoconstrictor above the galea, make the incision in segments with a blade and use bipolar diathermy to achieve meticulous haemostasis and minimise blood loss.
- Start the incision between the superior temporal line to 'easily' identify the appropriate plane of dissection.
- Stay deep to the galea in the temporal region to avoid injury to the frontal branch of the facial nerve.
- An easier and safer plane of dissection would be between the temporalis muscle and the deep temporal fascia.
- Stop dissection in the subgaleal plane, 2 cm above the supraorbital rims, if a pericranial flap is planned, to preserve vascularity.
- Place deep sutures along the galea for 'tension-free' skin closure, but away from the skin surface to minimise 'stitch' abscesses.
- Alopecia: use a knife for skin incision, meticulous haemostasis with judicious use of bipolar diathermy, tension-free closure.
- Frontal nerve damage: appropriate plane of dissection, care during retraction and judicious use of diathermy in the temporal/pre-auricular region.
- Supraorbital / supra-trochlear nerve damage: Care during dissection in the supraorbital rim region, judicious use of fine/sharp osteotomes when deroofing the supraorbital foramen.

MIDFACE ACCESS

A variety of approaches have been described to access the midface and can be broadly categorised into open and endoscopic approaches. The open approaches can be further subdivided into transfacial, transorbital, transnasal and transoral according to the site of access, and soft tissue and composite flaps based on the components of the mobilised tissue. With the increasing use of endoscopic techniques, the use of complex open approaches continues to reduce, although some still have a very definite role to play. The open and endoscopic approaches are often used in conjunction to improve access and reduce morbidity. This chapter will pertain to the open approaches.

Transfacial approaches

A modified Weber–Fergusson incision provides excellent access to the ipsilateral maxilla and with appropriate extensions, provides additional exposure of the nasal cavity, orbit and ethmoid. The 'nasal' part of the incision can be utilised for a lateral rhinotomy access.

The modified Weber–Fergusson commences with an upper lip-split incision that is made along the philtrum and extended along the alar margins. A 'V' can be incorporated along the nasal floor to improve localisation of the flap during closure. The incision is carried along the alar margin and extended superiorly at the junction between the nasal side wall and dorsal nasal subunit (*Figure 24.11*).

The intraoral incisions are made along the gingival crevice or buccal vestibule and are principally determined by the location of the tumour. A 'V' can be incorporated in the lip mucosa to facilitate accurate approximation at the end of the procedure. The cheek flap is elevated to expose the maxilla. The plane of dissection is principally determined by the extension of the tumour (*Figure 24.12*). A 'tonsil' swab can be placed in the nasal cavity and soft tissues along the piriform rim transected to gain access to the nasal cavity and avoid inadvertent damage to the nasal septum.

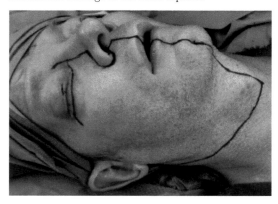

Figure 24.11 Modified Weber–Fergusson incision with Dieffenbach and Lynch extensions.

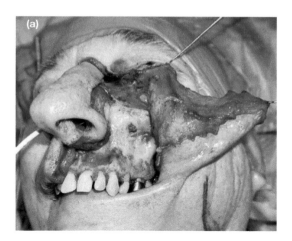
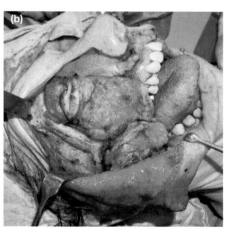

Figure 24.12 Exposure and planes of dissection: (a) subperiosteal, (b) subcutaneous.

Lateral extensions can be incorporated if additional access is required to the orbits and zygoma. This is made along the subciliary/midtarsal skin crease and can be extended laterally along the crow's feet skin crease (*Figures 24.11* and *24.12*). Care is taken to elevate the skin flap 'superficial' to the orbicularis oculi muscle in the eyelid region to preserve function and it is important to avoid 'buttonholes' in the thin skin of the eyelids.

Superior extension (Lynch modification) can be incorporated if additional access is required to the medial orbit and ethmoids (*Figure 24.11*). The nasal sidewall incision is extended superiorly along the medial orbit at least 5 mm medial to the medial canthus, up to the medial end of the eyebrow/medial supraorbital rim. The incision is deepened down to the bone and the frontal process of the maxilla, anterior lacrimal crest and frontonasal suture exposed. The medial canthal tendon is 'formally' identified and detached (*Figure 24.13a*). It is 'tagged' with a 3.0 Prolene suture on a round body needle, for subsequent reattachment (*Figure 24.13b*). The medial orbit can now be exposed with fine periosteal elevators. The fronto-ethmoid suture (FES) in the medial orbit provides an excellent landmark for the position of the anterior and posterior ethmoid (foramen) vessels and optic canal (*Figure 24.14*). These vessels are identified along the suture, skeletonised and ligated/diathermised. The optic canal lies posteriorly in superomedial orbit, in line with the suture. The number of ethmoidal vessels varies frequently (1–3), and over-reliance of the distances between the vessels (24 mm, 12 mm, 6 mm) and the optic canal can be dangerous. The FES can often lie 'above' the cribriform plate and its relationship to the anterior cranial fossa should be 'critically assessed' in the preoperative scans. Osteotomies are best placed below the FES, if 'unintentional' intracranial extension is to be avoided.

The lacrimal sac is identified inferiorly in the lacrimal fossa and can be dissected free for retraction or transection (*Figure 24.13b*).

A medial extension along the glabella skin crease can be incorporated if additional access is required to the nasal bones, roof of the nasal cavity or if a 'nasal' swing is considered (*Figure 24.15*).

The lower eyelid extension can be combined with a similar upper eyelid incision, if a lid-sparing orbital exenteration is planned (*Figure 24.16*).

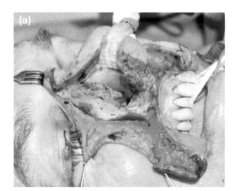
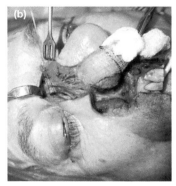

Figure 24.13 (a) Exposed and (b) tagged medial canthus.

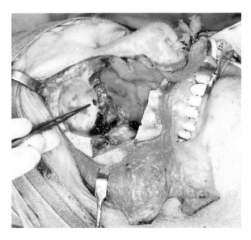

Figure 24.14 Ethmoidal foramen and fronto-ethmoid suture relationship.

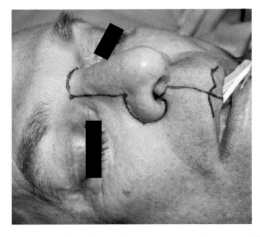

Figure 24.15 Modified Weber–Fergusson incision with glabella extension.

TOP TIPS AND HAZARDS

- Extend the midline skin incision past the vermilion, prior to incorporating the mucosal 'V' to facilitate accurate approximation of the vermilion.
- Tattoo or mark the vermilion if you feel it would help in later approximation
- If a lower eyelid extension is planned, the plane of dissection is ideally above the orbicularis oculi muscle (if eye is preserved).
- Soft tissue 'elevation' is kept to the minimum along the osteotomy sites, if a maxillary swing is planned.
- Formal identification and tagging of the medial canthus is necessary for later reattachment.
- Recognise the 'orientation' value of the fronto-ethmoid suture.
- Beware of using distances between the ethmoidal foramina and optic canal as the 'sole' modality during deep dissection of the medial orbit.
- Unsightly scar: use the modified Weber–Fergusson incision along the philtrum, nasal subunits with 'V' in the nasal floor and lip mucosa. Meticulous layered closure and accurate approximation of the vermilion border.
- Delayed bone healing: minimal soft tissue elevations along the osteotomy sites, pre-plating prior to completion of osteotomy, use fine saw blades and bur, copious irrigation.

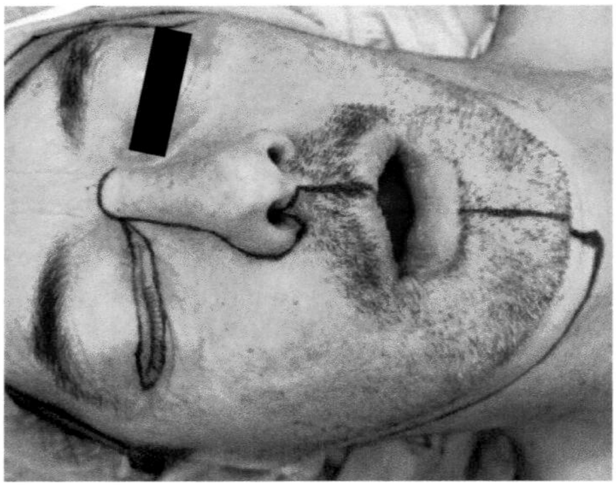

Maxillary swing

Incision

A Weber–Fergusson incision is made with a lateral eyelid extension (nowadays respecting the nasal subunits) (*Figures 24.11* and *24.17a*). A 'V'-shaped

Figure 24.16 Modified Weber–Fergusson incision with marking for eyelid-sparing orbital exenteration and glabella extension.

notch can be incorporated in the mucosal aspect of the upper lip and alar rim, to help accurate localisation of the flap. Subperiosteal stripping is minimised to retain the maximum blood supply to the bone segments.

The incision is taken vertically through the alveolar mucosa and attached gingiva between the upper central incisors. The palatal incision is in the midline extended laterally at the junction of the hard and soft palate behind the maxillary tuberosity (*Figure 24.17b,c*).

The author's preferred approach is to make the incision around the gingival margins of the teeth, extending from the canine tooth on the opposite side to the pterygoid hamulus, deliberately sectioning the greater palatine neurovascular bundle on the side of the osteotomy. The nasopalatine bundle is preserved if the bone cut is between the central and lateral incisor teeth. The palatal soft tissues are elevated to the opposite side (*Figure 24.17d*). This incision avoids the risk of palatal fistulae.

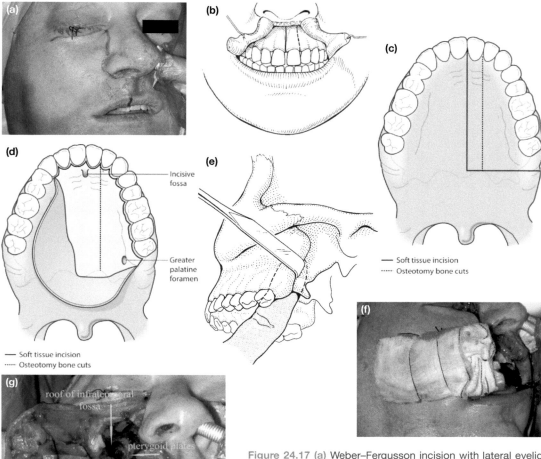

Figure 24.17 (a) Weber–Fergusson incision with lateral eyelid extension. (b, c) Stepped soft tissue and bone cuts avoid later wound dehiscence/fistulae. (d) Alternative (favoured) palatal incision, with the incisive and greater palatine foramina highlighted. (e) Pterygomaxillary dysjunction with osteotome. (f) Mobilised maxilla secured to facial skin with sutures. (g) Maxilla swung laterally to access infratemporal fossa.

Bone cuts

The bone cuts are made with fine saws/a fissure bur/Sonopet® and completed with osteotomes. The mucoperiosteum of the floor/lateral wall of the nose is elevated and the bone cuts made:

- Between the central and lateral incisor teeth, continued paramedially through the length of hard palate into the nasal floor
- Laterally from the piriform fossa, below the inferior turbinate (preserving the nasolacrimal duct) through the anterior maxilla inferior to the infraorbital nerve through the zygomatic buttress back to the pterygoid plates. The infraorbital nerve is sectioned at the infraorbital foramen as it prevents lateral retraction of the maxilla. The nerve ends may be tagged for later anastomosis
- The bone cut posterior to the zygomatic buttress is

angled downwards and may be made either with a fine osteotome or reciprocating saw/Sonopet®, to reduce soft tissue stripping

The maxilla is pre-localised with bone plates:

- Above the incisor teeth anteriorly
- At the frontal process of the maxilla
- On the zygomatic buttress

The maxilla and pterygoid plates are separated with a curved pterygoid chisel placed through a small vertical buccal incision (*Figure 24.17e*).

The maxilla is then out-fractured, pedicled to the soft tissues of the cheek. The maxilla can be secured to the soft tissues with 0/silk sutures over a gauze swab (*Figure 24.17f*). Following nerve division, wide lateral retraction of the maxilla exposes the soft palate, nasopharynx and infratemporal fossa (*Figure 24.17g*).

The buccal pad of fat is within the operative field and immediately available for reconstruction as a pedicled flap. The coronoid process and the attached temporalis tendon may impede access to the infratemporal fossa. A coronoidectomy will improve access and has the added benefit of reducing postoperative trismus.

When closing, an occlusal splint may be used if the bite is not 'positive'. The palatal soft tissues are covered with an acrylic cover plate wired to the standing teeth. Closure of the palatal tissues is completed interdentally. The plates and screws are reapplied.

The maxilla is frequently mobile to a degree at the completion of surgery. The palatal cover plate can be left *in situ* for 6–8 weeks or until maxillary stability is achieved.

Nasal swing

This provides access to the nasal cavity, ethmoids and nasal roof and can be considered for bilateral lesions, when the nasal skin/bones can be preserved. Currently, with the widespread use of endoscopic techniques, its role as a 'sole' access to these lesions is restricted. It is often used for additional access, as part of a wider resection.

A modified Weber–Fergusson incision is made respecting the nasal subunits and allowance is made for a transverse medial extension along the glabella skin crease (*Figure 24.18a*). The soft tissues are retracted laterally and superiorly to expose the nasal bones, frontal process of the maxilla and the piriform rims. The soft tissues overlying the nasal bone are left undisturbed (*Figure 24.18b*). Exposure of the contralateral nasal bones is achieved by undermining in a subperiosteal plane. The underlying nasal mucosa and soft tissue along the piriform rim are released with a diathermy. The soft tissue incisions and the bone cuts are stepped.

The nasal septum restricts complete lateral retraction. The septal cartilage is divided with a cutting diathermy set on 'coagulation' – the damp swab in the opposite nostril prevents accidental trauma to the mucosa of the contralateral lateral nasal wall and the facial skin on the opposite side. The 1-cm strut of nasal cartilage is preserved along the dorsum and columella to prevent collapse (*Figure 24.18c*).

Bone cuts are made with a saw/fine bur/Sonopet® along the frontal process of the maxilla and across the nasal bones (*Figure 24.18d*). The contralateral nasal osteotomy is carried out with fine osteotomes, if necessary, through separate stab incisions. The osteotomy sites are pre-localised with low-profile bone plates, removed and replaced during the final fixation. The nasal bones and the nasal soft tissues are mobilised and retracted to the opposite side (*Figure 24.18e*).

A soft tissue only and soft and hard tissue nasal swing can be combined with a larger midface/craniofacial resection for pathologies involving adjacent structures. The nasal swing links readily with a frontal craniotomy for resection of pathology that also involves the central compartment of the anterior cranial fossa (*Figure 24.18f–i*).

The plates are replaced, and the wound closed in layers (*Figure 24.18j*).

> ### TOP TIPS
>
> - The soft tissue dissection is kept to the minimum, overlying the nasal bones.
> - The osteotomy is planned along the frontal process of the maxilla, which is mobilised along with the nasal bones.
> - Bone cuts are made with a fine saw/bur/ Sonopet®.
> - Create a contralateral subperiosteal pocket and use 'stab' incisions and fine osteotomes to complete the osteotomy.
> - Pre-plate the osteotomies prior to completion.
> - Preserve at least a 1-cm caudal and dorsal strut of septum to prevent nasal collapse.

Per oral

The use of a solely per oral access is determined by the location and size of the lesion, the mouth opening and status of the dentition. An appropriately sized mouth prop/gag with cheek and tongue retractors and traction sutures can be utilised to provide the necessary access to safely carry out the procedure (*Figure 24.19*).

> ### TOP TIPS
>
> - Utilise appropriate retraction to obtain the 'best' access.
> - 'Orthodontic' cheek retractors can be very helpful for additional retraction and protecting the commissures.
> - If teeth extractions are planned, these are best carried out prior to the resection to improve access.

SOFT TISSUE LIP SPLIT

Soft tissue only lip split can provide excellent access to the posterior buccal mucosa and mandible, for lesions that cannot be safely excised through a per oral or cervical approach. The principal disadvantages of the approach are the need for lip-split scar and likely sacrifice of the mental nerve; this must be weighed against improved access. The latter is not a consideration if the inferior alveolar nerve is sacrificed in the subsequent resection. A lip split through the commissure would have to be considered for tumours located close to the commissure to avoid devascularising the segment between the midline lip split and commissure. This would also be a consideration for composite resections involving the adjacent skin.

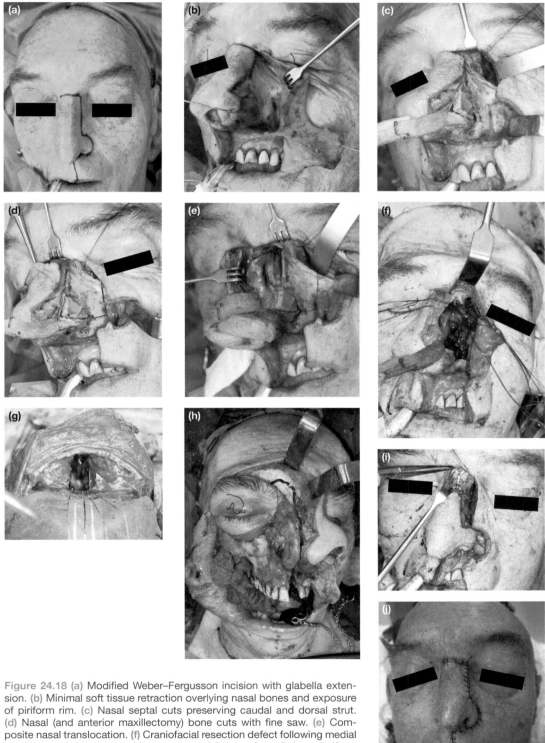

Figure 24.18 (a) Modified Weber–Fergusson incision with glabella extension. (b) Minimal soft tissue retraction overlying nasal bones and exposure of piriform rim. (c) Nasal septal cuts preserving caudal and dorsal strut. (d) Nasal (and anterior maxillectomy) bone cuts with fine saw. (e) Composite nasal translocation. (f) Craniofacial resection defect following medial maxillectomy, frontoethmoidectomy and (g) resection of the cribriform plate. (h) Soft tissue nasal swing as part of craniofacial resection. (i) Nasal osteotomy fixation with pre-localised plates. (j) Wound closure.

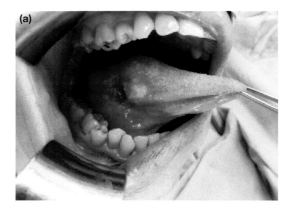

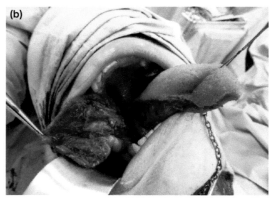

Figure 24.19 Per oral resection with appropriate retraction and mouth opening.

TOP TIPS AND HAZARDS

- Dissection of the anterior mandible is in the subperiosteal plane to minimise damage to the facial and mental nerves.
- Identify the mental nerve and decide if it can be preserved, prior to sacrificing it.
- More posteriorly, the dissection can be superficial or deep to the masseter muscle. If superficial dissection is planned, care must be exercised to prevent damage to the facial nerve branches and parotid duct.
- Avoid midline lip split for tumours adjacent to the commissure and composite resections.
- Mental and marginal mandibular nerve damage: appropriate plane of dissection and identification and protection of the nerves.
- Lip necrosis: avoid 'additional' midline incision for tumours in the commissure region or composite buccal mucosa resections.

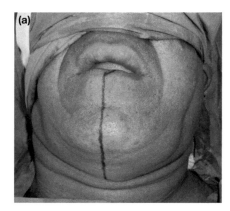

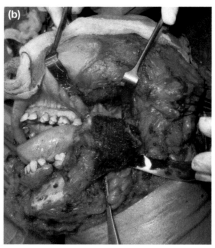

Figure 24.20 (a) Skin markings for soft tissue lip split. (b) Exposure obtained.

A full-thickness vertical incision is made through the midline of the lower lip and extended inferiorly across the midline of the chin/upper neck (*Figure 24.20a*). It continues with an appropriately placed low-neck skin crease incision. A 'V' can be incorporated in the mucosal aspect of the lower lip to facilitate accurate approximation. The cosmetic outcome with a midline chin incision is excellent and reduces the risk of numbness and ischaemia of the ipsilateral chin, associated with a curvilinear incision along the mental fold.

The neck skin flap is raised in the subplatysmal plane up to the lower border of the mandible, taking care to avoid damage to the marginal mandibular branch of the facial nerve. The cheek flap is elevated by detaching the platysma from the lower border of the mandible in the subperiosteal plane. More posteriorly, the dissection can be extended superficial or deep to the masseter muscle (*Figure 24.20b*).

Intraoral soft tissue incisions are placed along the gingival crevice or the lower vestibule and are principally determined by the location of the tumour. The wound is closed in layers, taking care to accurately approximate the vermilion border.

VISOR FLAP

A visor flap can be utilised for lesions in the floor of mouth, tongue and mandible and can be combined with bilateral neck dissections. The incision is marked at an appropriate low-neck skin crease and extends from one mastoid tip to the other (*Figure 24.21a*). The skin flaps are raised in the subplatysmal plane up to the lower border of the mandible, taking care to preserve the marginal mandibular branch of the facial nerve. The periosteum is incised along the lower border of the mandible and a mucoperiosteal flap elevated, taking care to identify the mental nerves (*Figure 24.21b*). Intraoral mucosal incisions are determined by the location of the lesion and the mental nerves might have to be sacrificed to obtain further access or adequate margins. The skin flaps are retracted cephalad with 'penrose' rubber drains (*Figure 24.21c*), which offers excellent exposure of an anterior mandibular/floor of mouth/tongue tumour, allowing en bloc resection and neck dissection (*Figure 24.21d*).

When used as a part of lingual release/pull-through procedure to access a floor of mouth/tongue lesion, the mental nerves and labial/buccal soft tissue can be left undisturbed. The anterior belly of digastric and the mylohyoid muscle are detached from their attachment to the mandible bilaterally, followed by detachment of the geniohyoid and genioglossus from the genial tubercle (*Figure 24.21e,f*). A gingival crevicular incision is made along the lingual aspect of the teeth and the contents of the floor of the mouth and tongue are 'released and pulled through' into the neck (*Figure 24.21g*). Care is taken to preserve the hypoglossal nerve and lingual artery on the ipsilateral side if a portion of the tongue is to be preserved. The pull-through technique and resection of the lesions in the anterior floor of mouth along with the mandible results in loss of attachment of the tongue to the mandible (*Figure 24.21h*). It is essential that the genioglossus and geniohyoid muscles are reattached to the reconstructed mandible to prevent the tongue falling back (*Figure 24.21i*). The wound is closed in layers (*Figure 24.21j*). The advantage of this incision is the avoidance of a lip-split facial scar, which needs to be weighed against the risk of damage to the mental and marginal mandibular branch of the facial nerves bilaterally.

TOP TIPS

- The intraoral labial/buccal vestibular incision is determined by the location of the tumour and can be placed along the vestibule or crevicular margins.
- If the attachment of the tongue and the hyoid apparatus to the anterior mandible is sacrificed, the remnant genioglossus and geniohyoid should be 'formally' suspended to the (reconstructed) mandible with non-resorbable sutures.

TRANSMANDIBULAR APPROACHES

Mandibular swing

Lip-split paramedian mandibulotomy

Although various sites and design of the osteotomy have been described, a straight line paramedian mandibulotomy is currently the most widely used option, as it preserves the attachment of the genioglossus, geniohyoid and anterior belly of digastric muscles and mental nerve. The availability of rigid fixation and fine saws negate the need for step osteotomies and tooth extractions in most cases.

The lip split with a mandibulotomy provides excellent access to the floor of the mouth, mid and posterior third of tongue, tonsillar fossa, soft palate, oropharynx including the posterior pharyngeal wall and supraglottic larynx. Extended posteriorly it provides equally good access to posterior maxillary tumours, infratemporal/pterygopalatine fossa and the parapharyngeal space with vascular control. It can be considered in three discrete stages: division of the lower lip/chin, paramedian mandibulotomy and elevation of the soft tissues of the lingual aspect of the mandible.

A full-thickness vertical incision is made through the midline of the lower lip and extended inferiorly across the midline of the chin/upper neck and continues with an appropriately placed low-neck skin crease incision (*Figure 24.22a*). A 'V' can be incorporated in the mucosal aspect of the lower lip to facilitate accurate approximation.

The neck skin flap is raised in the subplatysmal plane up to the lower border of the mandible, taking care to avoid damage to the marginal mandibular branch of the facial nerve. Intraorally, the incision through the labial mucosa and attached gingiva is stepped, so that it does not lie directly over the planned osteotomy (*Figure 24.22b*). The periosteal elevation and mentalis muscle stripping should be restricted to allow identification and protection of the mental nerve and placement of the plates.

A soft tissue pocket is created by elevating the mucosa off the lingual aspect of the mandible adjacent to the osteotomy. A periosteal elevator is placed in the pocket and an osteotomy carried out between the lower lateral incisor/canine or canine/first premolar region (*Figure 24.22c*). The bone cuts are marked/scored, and the mandible pre-plated prior to completion of the osteotomy (*Figure 24.22c*). The plates are removed and replaced during the final fixation. The mandible is divided with a fine saw taking care to avoid damage to the tooth roots. Occasionally, a tooth has to be removed to facilitate the osteotomy. The osteotomy cuts are in a straight line, as a stepped osteotomy neither aids fixation nor bone union and can increase the risk of damage to the teeth apices and mental nerve.

Following division of the mandible, the mandible is gently retracted laterally, and an incision made along the lingual gingival crevice and the mucoperiosteum

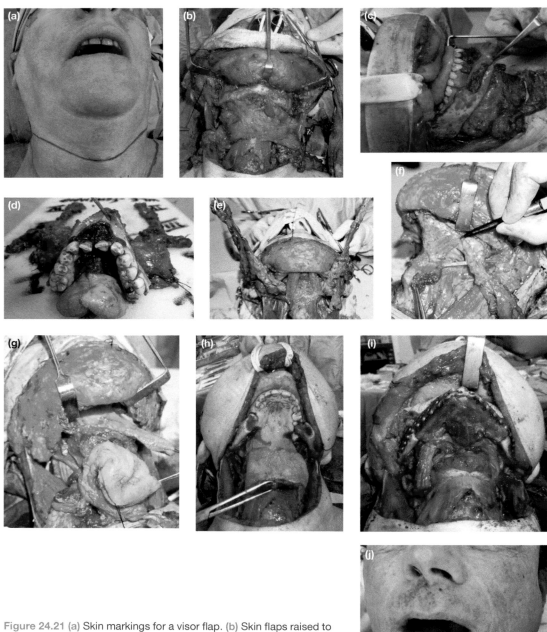

Figure 24.21 (a) Skin markings for a visor flap. (b) Skin flaps raised to lower border of mandible. (c) Exposure obtained. (d) En bloc resection and neck dissection. (e) Exposure of the lower border of mandible and anterior belly of digastric muscles. (f) Anterior bellies of digastric and mylohyoid muscles detached from mandible. (g) Tongue and floor of mouth contents 'pulled through' into the neck with excellent exposure for appropriate resection. (h) Loss of anterior attachment of the tongue. (i) Mandible reconstructed with a composite fibula free flap. Remnants of geniohyoid and genioglossus 'reattached' to neo mandible. (j) Wound closure.

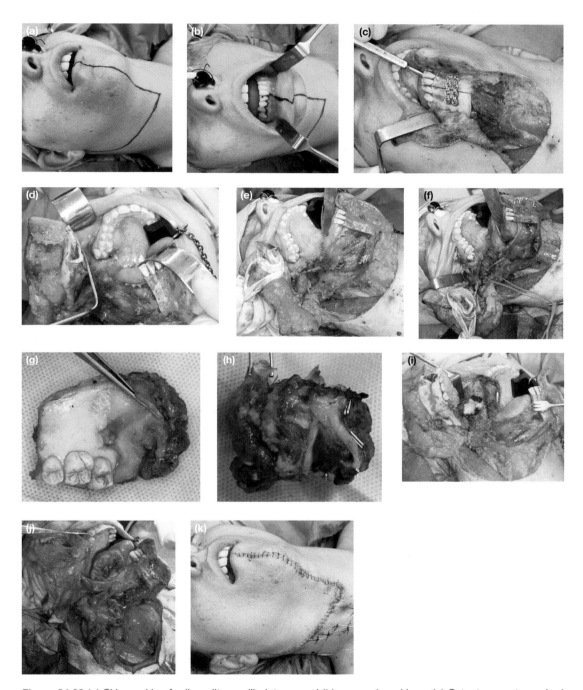

Figure 24.22 (a) Skin marking for lip-split mandibulotomy and (b) mucosal markings. (c) Osteotomy cuts marked with fine saw and the plates pre-localised. (d) Mandible swung laterally – intact lingual periosteum. (e) Detachment of medial pterygoid and stylomandibular ligament for extended mandibular swing. (f) Exposure of lingual and inferior dental nerves for use as roadmaps to the skull base/infratemporal fossa. Early control of the maxillary artery. (g, h) Posterior maxillectomy specimen with contents of infratemporal fossa including mandibular nerve dividing into inferior dental and lingual nerves. (i) Post-resection defect to skull base demonstrating infratemporal, pterygopalatine fossa, foramen ovale and rotundum. (j) Exposure of posterior tongue lesion with in-continuity neck dissection. (k) Wound closure.

elevated off the lingual mandible (*Figure 24.22d*). The mylohyoid muscle is detached along its attachment to the mylohyoid ridge. Further soft tissue dissection is determined by the location of the tumour.

If additional access is required to the infratemporal fossa/parapharyngeal space, it will be necessary to detach the medial pterygoid muscle from the medial aspect of the mandible. In addition, the stylomandibular ligament (at the angle of the mandible) and the sphenomandibular ligament (at the lingula) have to be detached to obtain the best possible access (*Figure 24.22e*). The inferior dental and lingual nerves are identified early and protected and can be utilised as roadmaps to the foramen ovale and skull base. The maxillary artery can also be identified entering the infratemporal fossa, at the neck of the condyle by following the posterior border of the mandible (*Figure 24.22f*). Early identification and ligation can help provide a relatively bloodless field for dissection of the infratemporal fossa (*Figure 24.22g–i*).

The paramedian mandibulotomy also provides excellent access to the posterior oral cavity/oropharyngeal lesions and can be easily combined with in-continuity neck dissection (*Figure 24.22j*).

The lingual gingival crevicular incision facilitates easy closure and avoids placement of the suture line

TOP TIPS AND HAZARDS

- A straight osteotomy in the canine region is ideal and the site is pre-plated prior to completion of the bone cuts.
- The soft tissue and bone cuts are stepped, so that they do not lie on the same plane.
- The lingual soft tissues are retracted following a lingual crevicular incision.
- The medial pterygoid muscle, stylomandibular and sphenomandibular ligaments have to be detached to obtain additional access to the infratemporal fossa.
- The lingual and inferior dental nerves provide excellent landmarks and can be utilised as roadmaps to the skull base and foramen ovale.
- The maxillary artery is identified at the neck of the condyle, as it enters the infratemporal fossa, and ligated early in the procedure to minimise blood loss and improve visibility during infratemporal fossa clearance.
- Delayed bone healing: minimal soft tissue elevations along the osteotomy sites, pre-plating prior to completion of osteotomy, use fine saw blades, burs, osteotomes and copious irrigation. Osteotomy ideally in the canine region.
- Damage to adjacent teeth: design osteotomy where space allows, use fine instruments, consider extraction.

at the depth (sump) of the wound. The mandible is held in occlusion and the plates replaced accurately to obtain the premorbid localisation. The wound is closed in layers (*Figure 24.22k*).

Double mandibular osteotomy

Double mandibular osteotomy provides excellent access to the infratemporal fossa, parapharyngeal space, deep lobe of the parotid and terminal extracranial internal carotid artery adjacent to the skull base, when the oral cavity does not have to be entered.

A low-neck skin crease incision with submental extension is made (*Figure 24.23a*) and the neck skin flap is raised in the subplatysmal plane up to the lower border of the mandible, preserving the marginal mandibular branch of the facial nerve. The lateral aspect of the mandible is exposed in a subperiosteal plane and the mental nerve identified and protected anteriorly. The masseter muscle is detached from the lateral aspect of the ramus of the mandible to expose the sigmoid notch. The anterior bone cuts are fashioned anterior to the mental foramen, between the canine/lateral incisor or canine/first premolar teeth roots. The posterior bone cut is made from the sigmoid notch to the lower border of the mandible, posterior to the lingula and inferior dental canal (similar to a vertical sub-sigmoid osteotomy). The bone cuts are marked/scored, and mandible pre-plated prior to completion of the bone cuts (*Figure 24.23b*). The plates are removed and replaced during the final fixation. Following completion of the osteotomy, the segment of the mandible containing the inferior dental nerve is retracted lateral and superiorly to provide wide access to the parapharyngeal and infratemporal areas (*Figure 24.23c*).

Further soft tissue dissection can be carried out to access specific parts of the medial mandibular area.

The stylomandibular ligament can be detached from the posterior 'condylar' segment to obtain further exposure of the stylomastoid area. The muscular and ligamentous attachments to the styloid process can be

TOP TIPS

- This procedure is considered when intraoral access is 'not' required.
- A lip-split scar is avoided.
- The bone cuts are made anterior to the mental foramen and posterior to the mandibular foramen and inferior dental canal.
- The osteotomy site is pre-plated prior to completion of the bone cuts.
- Styloid process and its attachments can be detached to gain addition access to the post styloid and 'stylomastoid' spaces.

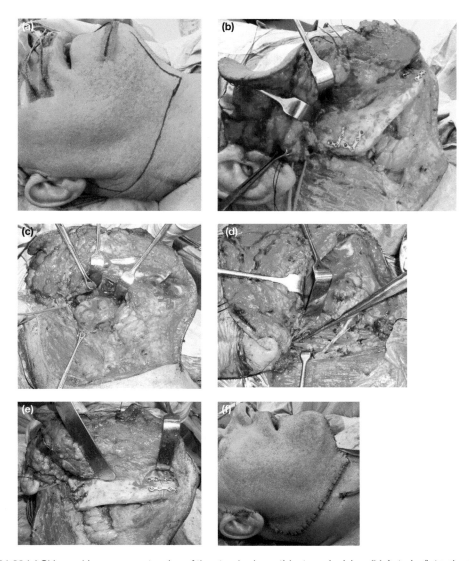

Figure 24.23 (a) Skin markings as an extension of the standard parotidectomy incision. (b) Anterior/lateral mandible exposed and the pre-localised plates across the planned osteotomy. Parotid tumour deep to the facial nerve, just about visible, medial to the mandible along the posterior border. (c) Exposure of the tumour following retraction of the mandible. (d) Exposure obtained to the high internal carotid in the post styloid compartment following resection of the styloid process. (e) Osteotomised segments replaced with pre-localised plates. (f) Wound closure.

detached, and if necessary, the styloid process osteotomised to gain additional access to the 'post styloid' space, terminal extracranial internal carotid and the skull base close to the jugular foramen and lower cranial nerve (*Figure 24.23d*).

The osteotomy sites are re-plated, confirming that the occlusion remains unchanged, and the wound closed in layers (*Figure 24.23e,f*).

This procedure avoids a lip-split scar and helps preserve sensation to the lip, while providing access to the more 'difficult to reach' areas.

Zygomatic osteotomy

Facial translocation techniques allow modular craniofacial disassembly of the facial skeleton to access relatively inaccessible regions of the skull base and nasopharynx. A variety of osteotomies have been described, but with the increased use of endoscopic approaches, the necessity for extensive procedures continues to diminish.

Zygomatic osteotomy, pedicled on the masseter muscle and its subsequent inferior displacement, provides simultaneous exposure of the orbit, temporal and infratemporal fossa. An additional frontotemporal craniotomy links the middle and anterior cranial fossa and the middle cranial fossa with the infratemporal fossa. The extent of the 'zygomatic' osteotomy and the direction of retraction of the temporalis is determined by the site of the pathology. For subcranial lesions (orbit/temporal/infratemporal fossa), the temporalis is reflected superiorly following a coronoidectomy. For combined exposure of the middle/anterior cranial fossa, orbit and/or temporal/infratemporal fossa, the temporalis is reflected inferiorly. The blood supply of the temporalis can potentially be compromised with both superior and inferior reflections.

The zygomatic body, arch and lateral and inferior orbital rims are exposed via a coronal flap (*Figures 24.19* and *24.24a*). Limited subperiosteal dissection is carried out in the lateral orbit to protect the orbital contents. The temporalis is reflected off the lateral orbit in the temporal fossa. The lateral limit of the inferior orbital fissure is identified in the orbit and temporal fossa with a blunt hook. The orbital contents are preserved with a malleable retractor and bone cuts are made with a fine saw/Sonopet®. Superiorly at the frontozygomatic suture, inferolaterally from the lateral infraorbital rim through the body of the zygoma towards the inferior orbital fissure and posteriorly just anterior to the articular eminence (*Figure 24.24b–d*). A sagittal bone cut is then made in the lateral orbital wall from the temporal fossa aspect, extending from the fontozygomatic suture osteotomy to the inferior orbital fissure (*Figure 24.24e*).

> ## TOP TIPS AND HAZARDS
>
> - The lateral aspect of the inferior orbital fissure in the orbit and temporal fossa is an important landmark for orbital and zygomatic osteotomies. It can be identified with a 'blunt hook'.
> - The extent of the osteotomy is determined by the location of the lesion and the need to enter the orbit.
> - The attachment of the masseter muscle to the osteotomised zygomatic complex should be preserved.
> - The osteotomy along the zygomatic arch should be made anterior to the articular eminence, to avoid disturbing the temporomandibular joint.
> - The osteotomy sites are pre-plated, prior to completion of the bone cuts.
> - Trismus is often expected and can be minimised by jaw opening exercises.
> - Damage to orbital contents: meticulous intraorbital subperiosteal dissection and haemostasis, fine malleable retractors for orbital retraction, bone cuts under 'direct' vision.
> - Malposition of lateral canthus: accurate bone re-approximation with pre-plating. Consider tagging lateral canthus prior to detachment and subsequent reattachment.

A more limited zygomatic arch osteotomy can be utilised when orbital access is not required (*Figure 24.24f*). The osteotomy is pre-plated and plates removed and replaced during the final fixation. The cuts are completed and the zygoma mobilised, pedicled inferiorly on the masseter muscle.

Exposure to the infratemporal fossa is limited with a zygomatic osteotomy, which restricts its use to benign pathology, when utilised as a sole means of access. It can, however, be combined, following retraction of the temporalis, with frontotemporal/temporal craniotomy to widely access the anterior and middle cranial fossa, optic canal, superior orbital fissure and for combined middle cranial/infratemporal fossa resections (*Figure 24.24g,h*). Often for more medial middle/anterior cranial fossa pathology and orbital lesions, a lateral/superolateral orbitotomy combined with a craniotomy is sufficient.

Lateral and superior orbitotomies

This approach is useful for lacrimal and lateral/superior/inferior extra- and intra-conal orbital lesions, lesions at the orbital apex and superior orbital fissure, and provides additional access for 'look up' approaches to the anterior and middle cranial fossa and for reconstruction with a temporalis flap following orbital exenteration.

A hemicoronal flap is raised, and the zygomatic complex exposed as described above for the zygomatic osteotomy (*Figure 24.25a*). For isolated lesions, an upper eyelid skin crease with extension into the lateral orbital crow's feet can be utilised (*Figure 24.25b*). The temporalis muscle is retracted posteriorly to expose the temporal aspect of the lateral orbit and the orbital periosteum is elevated from lateral orbital wall (*Figure 24.25c*). The inferior orbital fissure is identified both within the orbit and temporal fossa with a blunt hook. Perforating blood vessels are identified and coagulated prior to division.

The orbital contents are protected with a malleable retractor and the bone cuts are made with a thin saw/Sonopet®. The bone cuts are marked/scored and pre-plated prior to completion of the osteotomy. The plates are replaced during final fixation.

In the case of a lateral orbitotomy; superiorly – just above the frontozygomatic suture; inferiorly – inferior lateral orbital rim along the superior border of the zygomatic arch (the superior border of the zygomatic arch is at the same level as the orbital floor) up to the anterior limit of inferior orbital fissure (*Figure 24.25d*).

The posterior cut is made in the lateral orbital wall with a fine bur/Sonopet® joining the superior bone cut to the anterior limit of the inferior orbital fissure. This is more easily made from the temporal aspect. The bone cuts are pre-plated prior to removal of the osteotomised segment and plates replaced following completion of the procedure.

The lateral orbitotomy can be combined with a superior orbitotomy and is usually performed in conjunction with a frontotemporal craniotomy (*Figure 24.25e*). The craniotomy is best performed initially, and the superior orbital wall delineated from the cranial aspect. The medial extent of the superior orbitotomy can be limited by the extent of the frontal sinus. The supraorbital neurovascular bundle will have to be protected/retracted.

With malleable retractors *in situ*, the superior and lateral orbitotomies can be carried out under direct vision (*Figure 24.25f*). The amount of lateral wall and

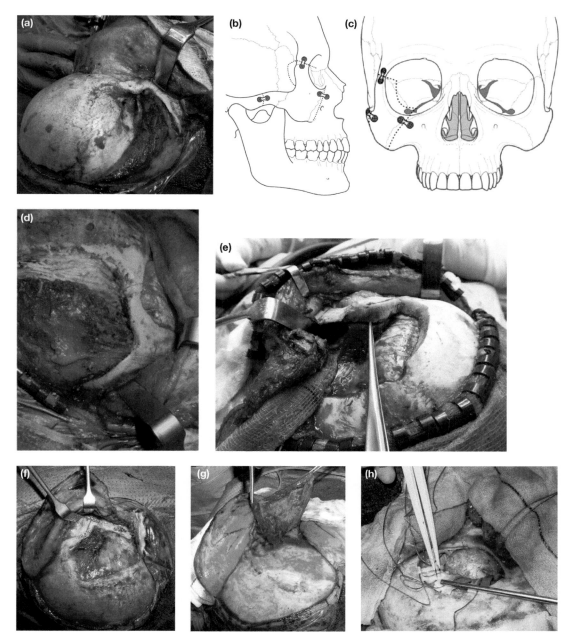

Figure 24.24 (a) Exposure of the zygomatic complex via a coronal flap with additional retraction of the temporalis. (b–d) Bone cuts for zygomatic osteotomy. (e) Sagittal bone cut from the temporal aspect of the lateral orbital wall. (f) Planned zygomatic arch osteotomy with pre-localised plates. (g) Retraction of the temporalis to facilitate a temporal craniotomy. (h) Exposure of the lesion in the middle cranial fossa floor following retraction of the zygomatic arch and temporalis muscle.

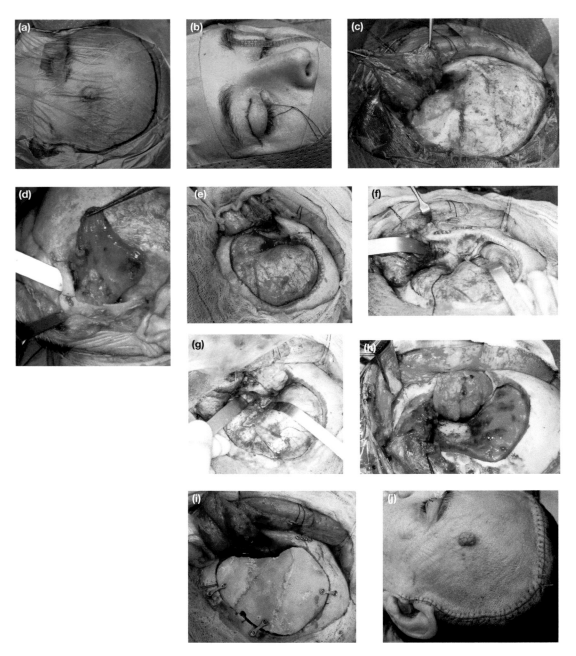

Figure 24.25 (a) Hemicoronal incision with pre-auricular extension. (b) Upper eyelid skin crease incision with lateral crow's feet extension. (c) Exposure following retraction of the temporalis. (d) Lateral orbitotomy bone cuts with pre-localised plates. (e) Exposure following frontotemporal craniotomy. (f) Bone cuts for a superolateral orbitotomy with pre-localised plates *in situ*. (g, h) Exposure following superolateral orbitotomy. (i) Bone flaps replaced with pre-localised plates. (j) Wound closure.

roof included in the orbitotomy can be customised according to need. This provides excellent exposure of the superior orbital contents, superior orbital fissure and optic nerve/canal (*Figure 24.25g,h*). This can also be used for 'look up' approaches to the superior anterior and middle cranial fossa lesions. The bone flaps are replaced (*Figure 24.25i*), and the wounds closed in layers (*Figure 24.25j*).

TOP TIPS

- The lateral aspect of the inferior orbital fissure in the orbit and temporal fossa is an important landmark for orbital and zygomatic osteotomies. It can be identified with a 'blunt hook'.
- The extent of the osteotomy is determined by the location of the lesion.
- The superior surface of the zygomatic arch is in line with the floor of the orbit and is a useful landmark for bone cuts in the lateral orbital rim.
- The osteotomy sites are pre-plated prior to completion of the bone cuts.
- The use of Sonopet®/Piezo blades enables controlled bone cuts and avoids adjacent soft tissue damage.

CONCLUSIONS

Multiple routes are available to the clinician to access the pathology in the craniomaxillofacial region. The technical aspects of the individual procedures are described in detail, along with the potential alternatives and a progressive algorithm. An understanding of the relevant anatomy, a critical analysis of the extent of the lesion, exposure required and potential reconstruction help in determining the most appropriate choice of procedure. There is no substitute to working within well-functioning teams to obtain the relevant clinical experience.

ALGORITHMS

The following algorithms provide a potential sequence that can be considered for progressively increasing access for pathologies in the head and neck region. The algorithms 'exclude' endoscopic approaches that can be used in isolation or in combination with open access for lesions especially in the oral cavity, nose, orbit, anterior skull base and retromaxilla.

1   *Access to buccal mucosa*

Per oral access

↓

Soft tissue lip split (midline/commissure lip split)

↓

Composite resection (skin/mucosa involvement)

↓

Compartment resection (skin/mucosa/bone involvement)

2   *Access to tongue*

Per oral access (anterior/lateral tongue)

↓

Lip-split mandibulotomy (lateral/posterior tongue/extensive floor of mouth involvement)

↓

Visor / lingual release (extensive bilateral tongue/floor of mouth involvement)

3   *Access to mandible*

Per oral access (limited crestal involvement/ marginal mandibulectomy)

↓

Transcervical/submental extension (lateral mandible ± floor of mouth involvement/ segmental mandibulectomy)

↓

Soft tissue lip split (lateral/posterior mandible/ extensive floor of mouth/parapharyngeal involvement/segmental mandibulectomy)

↓

Visor flap (bilateral mandible/floor of mouth involvement)

4 **Access to maxilla***

Per oral access (crestal/infrastructure involvement)

↓

Modified Weber–Fergusson (more extensive maxillary involvement, but no significant orbital/ ethmoid or posterior extension)

↓

Modified Weber–Fergusson with Dieffenbach extension (maxillary with significant orbital involvement)

↓

Modified Weber–Fergusson with Lynch extension (maxillary with significant ethmoid involvement)

↓

Lip-split mandibulotomy ± modified Weber–Fergusson (posterior maxillary, maxillary with significant posterior extension)

↓

Maxillary swing (posterior maxillary/posteromedial extension to nasopharynx)

↓

Facial degloving approach (anterior/bilateral maxillary lesion that cannot be accessed with per oral approach and need to avoid facial scar)

* Consider early coronoidectomy to improve access.

5 **Access to nasal cavity***

Per nasal (small anterior lesion)

↓

Lateral rhinotomy (ipsilateral nasal lesion)

↓

Nasal swing (soft tissue) – bilateral lesion, able to preserve nasal skin

↓

Nasal swing (soft tissue/nasal bone) – bilateral lesion, able to preserve skin and nasal bone)

↓

Facial degloving approach (bilateral/inferior lesions, able to preserve nasal skin)

↓

Le Fort I osteotomy (bilateral/inferior lesions)

* With the widespread use of endoscopic techniques, the need for open approaches as the 'sole' access modality continues to diminish.

6 **Access to orbitotomies**

(a) *Lateral orbitotomy (lateral lesions/temporalis – orbital reconstruction)*

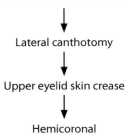

Lateral canthotomy

↓

Upper eyelid skin crease

↓

Hemicoronal

(b) *Lateral/superior orbitotomy (supero-lateral lesions/combined cranio-orbital lesions)*

Hemicoronal/bicoronal flap with frontotemporal craniotomy

(c) *Inferior orbitotomy (inferior lesions)*

Lower eyelid skin crease incision

7 **Access to parapharyngeal space (deep lobe parotid/post styloid compartment pathology)**

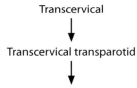

Transcervical

↓

Transcervical transparotid

↓

Double mandibular osteotomy (no oropharyngeal mucosal involvement)

↓

Lip-split mandibulotomy (oropharyngeal mucosal involvement)

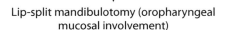

TABLE 24.1 Common access procedures to the various sites*

Access	Procedure
Oral cavity	Per oral
	Soft tissue lip split
	Lip split with access mandibulotomy
	Visor flap
Maxilla	Per oral
	Modified Weber–Fergusson
	Modified Weber–Fergusson with Lynch and eyelid extensions
	Lip-split mandibulotomy
	Facial degloving
	Combinations
Infratemporal fossa	Modified Weber–Fergusson with eyelid extension and early coronoidectomy (with maxillectomy)
	Lip-split mandibulotomy
	Coronal flap with zygomatic osteotomy
	Maxillary swing
	Combinations
Nasal cavity	Per nasal
	Lateral rhinotomy
	Nasal swing
	Le Fort I osteotomy
	Facial degloving
Pterygopalatine fossa/nasopharynx	Maxillary swing
	Transpalatal approaches
	Le Fort I Down fracture ± midline split
Orbit	Various soft tissue incisions
	Lateral orbitotomy
	Superior orbitotomy
	Inferior orbitotomy
	Combinations

* Excludes endoscopic approaches, which can be utilised alone or in combination with the open approaches.

FURTHER READING

Al-Kayat A, Bramley P. A modified pre-auricular approach to the temporomandibular joint and malar arch. *Br J Oral Surg* 1979;**17**:91–103.

Chatni SC, Sharan R, Patel D et al. Transmandibular approach for excision of maxillary sinus tumors extending to the pterygopalatine and infratemporal fossa. *Oral Oncol* 2009;**45**:720–6.

Ethunandan M. Infra-temporal fossa and pterygopalatine fossa. In Brennan PA, Standring S, Wiseman SM, editors. *Gray's Surgical Anatomy*. Elsevier; 2019.

McGregor IA, McDonald DG. Mandibular osteotomy in the surgical approach to the oral cavity. *Head Neck Surg* 1983;**5**:457.

Smith GI, Brennan PA, Webb AA et al. Vertical ramus osteotomy combined with a parasymphyseal mandibulotomy for improved access to the parapharyngeal space. *Head Neck* 2003;**25**:1000–3.

Bailey & Love's Essential Operations Bailey & Love's Essential Operations
Bailey & Love's Essential Operations Bailey & Love's Essential Operations
Bailey & Love's Essential Operations Bailey & Love's Essential Operations

PART 4 | Oncology

Chapter 25

Resection of the Mandible and the Maxilla

Panayiotis A. Kyzas

INTRODUCTION

This chapter outlines the principles of bony resection of cancer involving the mandible or the maxilla. This chapter is firmly based on the doctrine of surgical resection planning using information derived from imaging and clinical examination. In essence, "tumour, anatomy and biology guide the resection plan". Surgeons must think outside the box, moving away from past dogmata, having a clear understanding that each case must be looked at individually; resection must be planned and trialled well before entering the operating theatre. These principles are from knowledge in treating oral cavity squamous cell carcinoma. However, these are transferable to cases where bone resection is needed for malignant salivary gland tumours or in some selected cases of odontogenic tumours. Jaw resection for osteonecrosis is an altogether different concept (not an oncological resection) and thus, it is not discussed in this chapter.

RESECTION OF THE MANDIBLE

Resection principles

Surgical oncology is founded on the doctrine of 'clear resection margin'. The aim and endpoint of any onco-logical resection for oral cancer (including resection of the mandible) is a clear margin.

When planning mandibular resection, one needs to ascertain whether the tumour invades the mandible or not. In most cases without mandibular bone invasion, a marginal mandibulectomy (rim resection) is the approach of choice, if that is dictated by the tumour resection planning. Cases with frank bone invasion and/or marrow involvement require segmental mandibulectomy.

It is now widely accepted that cancer enters the mandible at the point of contact. In the dentate mandible, this is usually the junction of the attached and non-attached gingivae. In the edentulous mandible, this is more likely at the crest of the ridge. The histological pattern of the tumour (cohesive/pushing versus non-cohesive/infiltrating) is linked to the pattern of invasion (shallow/erosive pattern for cohesive tumours versus deeper invasion for infiltrative tumours). However, the pattern of mandibular invasion cannot be reliably predicted based on the histology of the biopsy alone; therefore, mandibular resection planning relies heavily on imaging.

Assessment of mandibular invasion

Searching for the 'holy grail' of the ideal preoperative imaging modality to assess mandibular invasion has led to several conflicting publications. Clinicians now agree that the most reliable way of assessing mandibular invasion (and the extent of it) is via combined imaging modalities (*Table 25.1*). A dual-phase contrast high-resolution computed tomography (CT) scan will highlight mandibular cortical erosion in detail. Its high resolution allows images to be viewed at a slice width of 0.9 mm. This allows accurate patient-specific planning (PSP), utilising specialised computer software and 3D printing. Ultimately, the bone resection is aided by pre-made guides using the CT data (dicom files). A magnetic resonance imaging (MRI) neck is a widely accepted imaging modality for staging the primary tumour and the neck in oral cavity cancer. Despite its low-resolution abilities (images are viewed at a slice width of 3 mm at best), it is superior to CT in assessing bone marrow invasion and perineural spread. Therefore, in an ideal setting, both modalities should be utilised to assess mandibular invasion. An orthopantomogram (OPG) is always taken as part of the work-up for every patient with oral cavity tumour, primarily to allow dental assessment prior to radiotherapy. Although mandibular invasion in large tumours can be seen on the OPG, its value in resection planning is extremely limited. Positron emission tomography–computed tomography (PET–CT) has limited value in the precise anatomical delineation of mandibular tumours.

TABLE 25.1 Imaging modalities for mandibular invasion: current gold standard

Use the imaging modalities below together, to aid maximum resection accuracy

1. High-resolution dual-phase contrast CT neck	a. Use CT dicom files for PSP-3D plan
2. MRI neck	b. OPG is always taken but of limited use
	c. If only one imaging available, choose CT

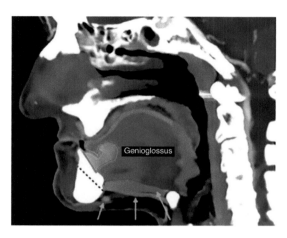

Figure 25.1 Rim resection of the anterior mandible for an anterior floor of mouth tumour. Note the direction of the rim resection vector and the inferior exit cut, below the muscular insertions. (Reproduced from *Br J Oral Maxillofac Surg* 2021;**59**:5–15.)

Methods of mandibular resection

The endpoints of any mandibular resection procedure for malignant disease are first and foremost an R0 resection, followed by trying to reduce morbidity and achieve the best possible functional and cosmetic outcome. The two main approaches for mandibular resection are discussed in detail below.

Marginal mandibulectomy (rim resection)

The definition (and main advantage) of the marginal mandibulectomy/rim resection is that the continuity of the mandible is kept intact. This is achieved in most instances by preserving the lower border of the mandible. On occasions, it is the upper border of the mandible that remains, ensuring continuity of the jaw. These rare cases include, for example, reverse rim resection for submandibular salivary gland tumours abutting the lower mandibular border.

Preserving the continuity of the mandible is associated with a better functional and cosmetic outcome; however, this should never take priority over adequate oncological clearance. Indeed, the functional and cosmetic outcomes of an appropriately planned and executed mandibular reconstruction following segmental mandibulectomy are comparable to those following rim resections.

A rim resection of the mandible is usually performed in the coronal or the sagittal plane. This is guided by the primary tumour. Let us take, for example, the case shown in *Figure 25.1*. This anterior floor of mouth tumour does not invade the mandible, but it abuts the lingual periosteum close to the insertion of the genioglossus/geniohyoid muscles. Without a rim

resection, there is a great risk of a histologically involved inferior/deep margin. A marginal mandibulectomy in the coronal plane, with an oblique vector as shown on the image, ensures an R0 resection.

A posterolateral floor of mouth tumour requires a different thought process (*Figure 25.2*). The posterior mandibular alveolus is medial to the basal mandibular body and corresponds to the origin of mylohyoid muscle at the mylohyoid line. It is crucial to know whether the tumour involves the mylohyoid muscle or not, as if it does not, it will be well separated from the lingual aspect of the mandible inferior to the mylohyoid ridge. In this case, the rim resection is easily done at the sagittal plane, orientating the saw almost vertically, starting behind the alveolus and extending anteriorly as far as needed. However, when the tumour involves or goes through the mylohyoid muscle but does not invade the mandible, the rim resection needs to be almost through-and-through, up to lower border of the mandible (conceptually similar to a sagittal split osteotomy). This is technically more difficult and requires a combined approach through the neck (for the lower border cortical cut) and intraorally (superior bone cut and anterior/posterior lingual cuts). When the tumour extends buccally, or wraps around the mandible without invasion or in cases of markedly atrophic mandible, it may not be possible to preserve mandibular integrity with a rim resection and a mandibular segmental resection and reconstruction is needed. In most cases of posterolateral mandibular rim resection, a coronoidectomy is also performed, to prevent postoperative trismus.

A rim resection can be used for benign odontogenic tumours in which there is sufficient residual bone to safely maintain continuity. A rough guide is that a minimum of 10 mm of residual bone is required, otherwise the risk of pathological fracture is significant and a segmental mandibulectomy and reconstruction is employed as the safest option. This becomes even more

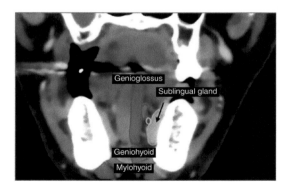

Figure 25.2 Rim resection of the posterolateral mandible for a lateral floor of mouth tumour. Note the importance of mylohyoid muscle invasion in planning the extent of the resection. (Reproduced from *Br J Oral Maxillofac Surg* 2021;**59**:5–15.)

important when the mandible is edentulous. In edentulous mandibles with Class V and VI Cawood–Howell classification, there is insufficient bone height to safely perform a marginal resection for malignant disease.

It is therefore clear that the decision to perform a rim resection of the mandible, and the extent of it, is largely dependent on imaging. Intraoperatively, the extent of rim resection can be aided by periosteal stripping, which assesses the extent of tumour invasion into the mandible from the surrounding soft tissues (e.g. when a tumour abuts the mandible). This, however, should be used with caution, as it is not as reliable in areas at risk of an involved margin, such as the muscle insertion lines described above.

Segmental mandibulectomy

In this procedure, both the upper and lower borders of the mandible are included in the resection, thus creating a breach in the continuity of the mandible. This mandates reconstruction of the mandible, which almost always involves composite free tissue transfer and increases donor site morbidity. Without reconstruction, the functional and aesthetic results are generally poor.

The extent of any segmental mandibulectomy is based on the preoperative planning, which is aided by imaging, as described above. Care must be taken to ensure an adequate margin on the inferior alveolar nerve; previous cases of local relapse in the masticator space in cases with clear bony and soft tissue margins have highlighted the importance of perineural involvement (PNI) in locoregional disease control. As a minimum, a lateral segmental mandibulectomy should commence in front of the mental foramen and finish behind the lingula, to incorporate all the intraosseous course of the inferior dental nerve. A preoperative MRI scan can identify perineural spread beyond the lingula, thus making further resection of the inferior alveolar nerve necessary; this can be up to V3 on the base of skull and/or requiring intraoperative frozen sections.

Careful evaluation of the preoperative imaging is the hallmark of segmental mandibulectomy. The extent of soft tissue resection should not be underestimated, and this is often what guides the choice of the composite free flap that will be used for reconstruction. On some occasions, even facial skin overlying the mandible needs to be excised. The extent of the resected segment usually corresponds to the soft tissue element of the tumour that directly invades the mandible. However, there are occasions when mandibular resections need to be much more aggressive, such as in primary intraosseous carcinomas or osteosarcomas.

The modern era of mandibular resections dictates these to be guided by 3D-printed surgical stents (guides – *Figure 25.3*).

CT dicom files are processed by specialised software, recreating a 3D image of the mandible. The surgeon has a planning session with the reconstructive scientist, where they plan the resection margins based on

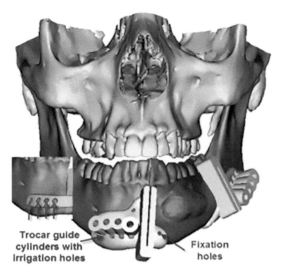

Figure 25.3 An illustrative example of mandibular segmental resection using surgical guides.

the principles discussed above (PNI/soft tissue extent/bone marrow involvement). 3D-printed surgical guides are then created as accurate indicators of the planned resection margins. The same guides provide drill-holes to secure pre-bent or milled mandibular fixation osteosynthesis plate(s), which ensure perfect condylar positioning and dental occlusion postoperatively (*Figure 25.4*). The era of using temporary external fixation and/or intraoperative plate bending/adaptation now belongs to the history books. As one can see from the examples below (*Figure 25.5*), the PSP-3D approach is

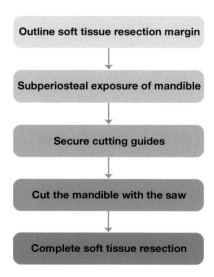

Figure 25.4 A roadmap to segmental mandibulectomy.

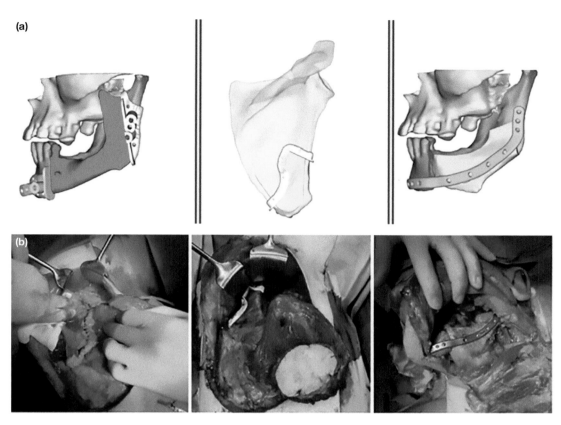

Figure 25.5 (a) Segmental mandibular resection and reconstruction planning with the use of 3D printing. (b) Clinical implementation of the above plan.

now the standard of care for mandibular resections and reconstructions, ensuring adequate surgical margins, reducing intraoperative time, aiding dental rehabilitation and pushing the boundaries in composite free tissue transfer.

In technical terms, a segmental mandibulectomy is an easy procedure. Once the surgeon establishes access to the buccal aspect of the mandible (either via facial skin resection, if required, or via the buccal soft tissue resection margin), the surgical guides are secured in place. The lingual soft tissue margin is marked and the mandibulectomy bone cuts are performed with a saw. Once the bone cuts have been made, the mandible is delivered into the neck; this allows completion of the lingual soft tissue resection.

In benign disease, when a segmental mandibulectomy cannot be avoided, one can occasionally preserve the integrity of the inferior alveolar nerve, by dissecting it free and allowing it to lie in the soft tissues overlying the reconstructed bone. This avoids the morbidity of lip and chin numbness.

There have been many attempts at classifying mandibular segmental resections (Jewer, Brown), but none of the proposed classification systems are used routinely in daily practice. Personalised image-aided resection

planning is much more important than strict adherence to classification systems.

In most cases of segmental mandibulectomy, the condylar process can be preserved. This is important as with appropriate reconstruction, a mandible with both temporomandibular joints (TMJs) can function adequately. However, there are occasions when disease extent dictates condylar disarticulation and resection of the TMJ. These cases are technically challenging due to the proximity of the maxillary artery (which needs to be controlled) and the risk of traction injury to the facial nerve. It used to be almost impossible to obtain accurate reconstruction in these cases, as residing a plate and a bony flap into the glenoid fossa was extremely difficult – it was merely a surgical guess. This issue has now improved with the PSP-3D planning aids, although it is not completely resolved.

RESECTION OF THE MAXILLA

Resection principles

Achieving an R0 resection in maxillary/midfacial tumours is a surgical challenge. Because of that, the most common manifestation of disease relapse in maxillary tumours is local failure, in an anatomically and radiologically predictable pattern. It is fair to say that "tumours know their anatomy" and they will recur in areas not resected/dissected adequately at the time of primary surgery. This is more often the case for posterior/superior maxillary tumours, due to their relative inaccessibility and the proximity of vital structures (base of skull, optical apex, pterygopalatine fossa, infratemporal fossa). The limiting factors in achieving complete excision are poor direct visualisation and inadequate vascular control. In contrast to the above, smaller maxillary/midfacial tumours can be easily resected transorally.

Maxillectomy

Tumours enter the maxilla at the point of contact and spread outside via anatomical routes of minimal resistance. A posterior maxillary tumour will exit posteriorly into the pterygomaxillary fissure and tract upwards, into the pterygopalatine fossa and/or laterally into the infratemporal fossa. From there, tumours can extend upwards towards the skull base and invade foramen ovale (V3) and/or foramen rotundum (V2). Superior tumours can invade the orbit via the inferior orbital fissure (PNI at the course of the infraorbital nerve). Extension into the ethmoids allows access to the tumour to reach central skull base structures (cribriform plate/lamina papyracea) and the medial orbit.

There are two important anatomical considerations when planning a maxillectomy (*Table 25.2*). First, the ablative surgeon needs to determine the relationship of the maxillary artery to the lateral pterygoid muscle to facilitate a controlled and relatively bloodless extended maxillectomy. Understanding the anatomy of this vessel preoperatively allows early proximal vascular control. Careful preoperative evaluation of a high-resolution dual-phase contrast CT allows for mapping the course of the vessel. The second consideration is the point of entry of the ethmoidal arteries into the medial orbit. The emergence point will always be above the level of the cribriform plate; careful evaluation of the preoperative CT scan at the coronal level will allow an accurate assessment of this.

Maxillary resection is guided by the extent of the soft tissue component and by the extension of the tumour into the anatomical spaces and fossae described

TABLE 25.2 Anatomical considerations in maxillectomies

- Course of the maxillary artery
- Aim for early proximal vascular control
- Ethmoidal arteries emergence points

- Identify the relationship of the vessel with the lateral pterygoid muscle on CT scan
- Coronal sections CT scan
- Always above cribriform plate

TABLE 25.3 Brown classification of vertical and horizontal maxillectomy and midface defects

	Vertical classification
I	Maxillectomy not causing an oroantral or oronasal fistula (alveolectomy)
II	Maxillectomy causing oroantral fistula but not extending to the orbit
III	Maxillectomy extending to the orbit (including the orbital floor) but retaining the orbital contents
IV	Maxillectomy with orbital exenteration
V	Orbitomaxillary defect (alveolus preserved)
VI	Nasomaxillary defect (alveolus preserved)
	Horizontal classification
a	Palatal defect only (alveolus preserved)
b	Less than or equal to half unilateral
c	Less than or equal to half bilateral or transverse anterior
d	Greater than hemimaxillectomy

above. The preoperative imaging modality of choice is a high-resolution contrast CT scan. For locally advanced tumours, an MRI scan is useful in ascertaining perineural spread, periorbita involvement and soft tissue extension into the infratemporal/pterygopalatine fossae. A combined imaging modality approach is thus preferred.

Maxillectomy defects are usually quoted using the Brown classification, as illustrated in *Table 25.3*. Although this classification is a useful guide for subsequent reconstruction, one should not deviate from the dogma and endpoint of the maxillectomy procedure, which is complete resection to clear margins (R0).

A Class I maxillectomy (alveolectomy) is a simple transoral resection of low-volume maxillary alveolus disease. It is a very rare procedure and often does not require reconstruction. A Class II (low-level) maxillectomy preserves the floor of the orbit. In this procedure, the superior margin is usually at the level of the infraorbital nerve, and it can be performed transorally. However, depending on the soft tissue extent of the tumour, an access adjunct procedure such as midfacial degloving or Weber–Fergusson approach might be needed. The bone osteotomies for such a maxillectomy need to be done vertically at the alveolus, horizontally at a high Le Fort I level, palatally, as a posterior continuation of the alveolar cut and at the pterygoid plates, where the maxilla is separated from the plates with a pterygoid chisel. PSP and 3D printing is not as widely employed in maxillectomies, compared with mandibular resections; however, our recent experience suggests that it might be of benefit when it comes to the anterior bone margin (superior, lateral and medial) and to plan composite free-flap reconstruction (see *Figure 25.6*).

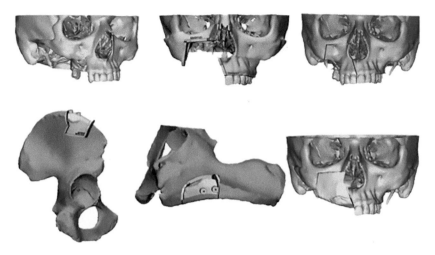

Figure 25.6 3D planning of a class II maxillectomy and subsequent reconstruction. (Reproduced from *Plastic Reconstructive Surgery* 149(2): 359e–361e, February 2022. Wolters Kluwer. Copyright © 2021 American Society of Plastic Surgeons.)

TABLE 25.4 Anterolateral corridor approach

Surgical steps for the anterolateral corridor approach

1	Weber–Fergusson–Dieffenbach skin incision
2	Soft tissue margin anterior face (this may include facial skin)
3	Division of the infraorbital nerve
4	Zygomatic osteotomy – zygoma bone pedicled on masseter muscle
5	Identify the plane between masseter muscle and temporalis tendon
6	Coronoidectomy
7	Enter infratemporal fossa (ITF) by dividing temporalis muscle – ITF dissection
8	Identify infratemporal crest
9	Proximal control of maxillary artery (preop scans)
10	Margin on the pterygoid muscles – direct visualisation of the pterygoid plates
11	Foramen ovale – V3 resection if needed (beware of venous bleeding)
12	Osteotome to the pterygoid plates 0.5 cm from skull base and aiming downwards
13	After pterygoid plates osteotomy, enter and dissect pterygopalatine fossa
14	Complete resection as required (skull base drill-out, orbital exenteration, etc.)

Maxillectomies for more locally advanced tumours are extensive resections requiring a combination of access procedures and careful preoperative planning based on imaging. *Table 25.4* summarises the modified Altemir technique/anterolateral corridor approach for locally advanced posterior/superior maxillary tumours. This technique can be tailored and adjusted depending on the specifics of each individual case.

TOP TIPS AND HAZARDS

Resection of the mandible

- Preoperative imaging with a dual-phase high-resolution CT scan and MRI neck.
- Preoperative surgical planning using PSP-3D.
- Tumours invade the mandible at the point of contact.
- PNI dictates resection behind the lingula and in front of the mental foramen (as a minimum).
- Vector orientation in rim resection is crucial.

Resection of the maxilla

- Preoperative imaging with a dual-phase high-resolution CT scan and MRI neck.
- Proximal vascular control of the maxillary artery and adequate access for direct visualisation of posterior/superior tumours.
- Direct resection of the pterygoid plates via the anterolateral corridor approach ensures a safe resection margin.
- A high maxillectomy is only a part of several ablative procedures required for a locally advanced midface tumour (i.e. orbital exenteration, skull base drill-out, etc.).

FURTHER READING

Brown JS, Shaw R. Reconstruction of the maxilla and midface: introducing a new classification. *Lancet Oncol* 2010;**11**:1001–8.

Kyzas PA. Patient-specific three-dimensional planning for head and neck reconstruction: paradigm shift and refuted myths. *Plast Reconstr Surg* 2022;**149**:359e–361e.

McMahon J, Steele P, Kyzas P, et al. Operative tactics in floor of mouth and tongue cancer resection – the importance of imaging and planning. *Br J Oral Maxillofac Surg* 2021;**59**:5–15.

McMahon JD, Wong LS, Crowther JC, et al. Patterns of local recurrence after primary resection of cancers that arise in the sinonasal region and the maxillary alveolus. *Br J Oral Maxillofac Surg* 2013;**51**:389–93.

Pu JJ, Choi WS, Yu P, et al. Do predetermined surgical margins compromise oncological safety in computer-assisted head and neck reconstruction? *Oral Oncol* 2020;**111**:104914.

Bailey & Love's Essential Operations Bailey & Love's Essential Operations
Bailey & Love's Essential Operations Bailey & Love's Essential Operations
Bailey & Love's Essential Operations Bailey & Love's Essential Operations

PART 4 | Oncology

Chapter 26 | Skull Base and Orbital Tumour Resection

Madan G. Ethunandan, Nijaguna Mathad

SKULL BASE RESECTION

The skull base is an interface between the facial skeleton and the cranial cavity. The floor of the cranial cavity is divided into anterior, middle and posterior cranial fossae. A number of benign and malignant tumours originating from the sinonasal cavity, orbit, ear, skin, parotid gland and temporomandibular joint can invade through the skull base and similarly, intracranial tumours can extend into these structures. Understanding the anatomy of the skull base from above and below is crucial for dealing with pathology in this area.

Management: Key considerations

Options are conservative treatment, surgery, radiotherapy and chemotherapy in combined or sequential order.

All options have advantages and disadvantages, and their effects should be discussed in detail with the patient and their family. The patient's expectations should match the surgical aims to obtain patient satisfaction. In the vast majority of cases, tumour control is a more realistic achievement.

The patient should be discussed in Head and Neck and Skull Base multidisciplinary teams (MDTs), with all the relevant information presented. Scans should be critically evaluated for any extension of the tumour. Once the decision is taken to proceed with surgery, the surgical team must decide whether the intent of such surgery is complete resection, debulking or palliative.

With very extensive tumour, consideration should be given for preoperative radiotherapy or induction chemotherapy to downsize the tumour so that subsequent surgery can be less morbid or to aid organ preservation (e.g. eye).

The majority of patients will need postoperative radiotherapy, and some will have had radiotherapy before surgery. Careful thought should be given to reconstruction of the defects to achieve robust healing. This becomes relevant if endoscopic endonasal resection is considered and the nasal septum is involved in the tumour.

Surgical philosophy has changed over the decades. Preservation of function and patient's quality of life are the overarching principles. Radical excision of the tumour with negative margins is the oncological principle. In finding the balance between these two principles, one must take the patient's wishes into consideration. Careful and thorough preoperative discussion should

take place when preparing a patient for high-risk surgery.

The best outcome for a benign tumour is complete excision. However, if complete excision involves increased morbidity, for example, invasion into the cavernous sinus/orbital apex, then subtotal excision and subsequent radiation treatment for the residuum provide a good compromise to maintain the patient's quality of life. Preserving neurological function, psychological wellbeing and cosmesis are the surgical goals for benign tumours.

Selecting the surgical approach based on the location and its relation to major blood vessels and cranial nerves, and histology will help in maximising the resection and reducing postoperative morbidity.

In parallel with technological advances, several minimally invasive/keyhole transcranial approaches and endoscopic endonasal approaches have been developed in the last two decades and concepts such as skull base 360 and orbit 360 have emerged. Selection of the most appropriate approach is often based on the relationship of the index pathology to the major blood vessels and cranial nerves. Traditionally, skull base and orbital pathologies have been addressed though well-established open procedures such as craniofacial resections.

Skull base 360

A multicorridor 360-degree approach to skull base pathologies may be considered, based on the following aspects:

- The skull base is divided into anatomical compartments corresponding to the cranial fossa and intracranial cisterns. Different corridors are used to reach a specific compartment
- Cranial nerves do not tolerate manipulation. The carotid arteries can be exposed and lateralised to a certain extent, but the cranial nerves should not be manipulated, and therefore provide a major limitation for lateral extension of the anteromedial approaches
- The angles of approach and dissection should be along the same plane. Surgery can only be performed when both the angles are in the same axis, with least manipulation of the critical neurovascular structures

TABLE 26.1 Endoscopic skull base approaches

Sagittal plane

- Transfrontal
- Transcribriform
- Transtuberculum/Transplanum
- Transsellar
- Transclival
  - Superior third
    - Transsellar(intradural)
    - Subsellar (extradural)
  - Middle third
  - Panclival
- Transodontoid and foramen magnum/craniovertebral approach

Coronal plane

- Anterior coronal plane
  - Supraorbital
  - Transorbital
- Middle coronal plane
  - Medial petrous apex
  - Petroclival approaches
  - Inferior cavernous sinus/Quadrangular space
  - Superior cavernous sinus
  - Infratemporal approach
- Posterior coronal plane
  - Infrapetrous
  - Transcondylar
  - Transhypoglossal
  - Parapharyngeal space
    - Medial (jugular foramen)
    - Lateral

- In endonasal approaches, an air compartment is encountered before reaching the bony and cisternal compartments. It is essential that the more superficial compartments are well exposed to adequately expose the deeper compartments
- The ideal corridor is one that enables reaching the lesion with the least morbidity

Approaches

A variety of approaches are available for skull base pathology and are often described in terms of endoscopic (*Table 26.1*) and open transcranial approaches (*Table 26.2* and *Figure 26.1*). Please also refer to *Chapter 24* on access surgery for a more detailed description of individual procedures.

TABLE 26.2 Transcranial skull base approaches

Anteromedial

- Subfrontal
- Interhemispheric
- Transfacial (transmandibular, transmaxillary, lateral rhinotomy)
- Craniofacial/transbasal

Anterolateral

- Subfrontal/supraorbital
- Frontotemporal
- Pterional
- Orbitozygomatic
- Transorbital

Lateral

- Subtemporal
- Preauricular infratemporal

Posterolateral

- Translabyrinthine
- Transpetrous
- Retrosigmoid

Posterior approach

- Midline suboccipital
- Supracerebellar infratentorial

Endoscopic endonasal approaches

Endoscopic endonasal approaches have been organised in modules based on anatomical corridors and described in relationship to the sagittal and coronal planes. Median endonasal approaches are oriented rostrocaudally along the sagittal plane (between the carotid arteries) from the frontal sinus to the second cervical vertebra (*Table 26.1* and *Figure 26.1*). The paramedian approaches (lateral to the carotid arteries) are divided into three different depths: anterior, middle and posterior, corresponding to the anterior, middle and posterior cranial fossa. These approaches are used for a variety of conditions and benign pathologies and increasingly in carefully selected cases, for malignant tumours.

Endoscopic endonasal skull base surgery

Endoscopic tumour resection uses the same principles as surgery through an operating microscope: internal debulking, capsular mobilisation, extracapsular dissection of neurovascular structures, coagulation and removal of the capsule. Depending on the consistency of the tumour, the debulking is carried out with a bimanual suction, ultrasonic aspirator and piecemeal removal.

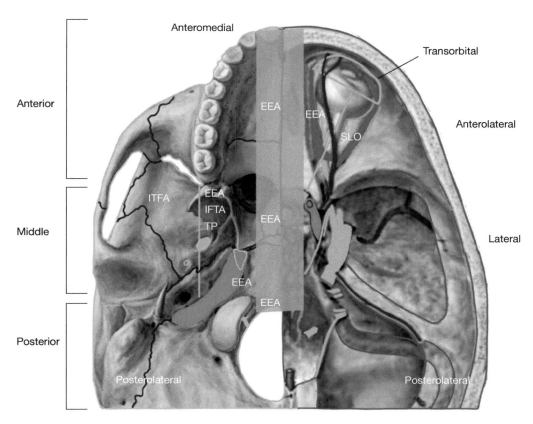

Figure 26.1 Endoscopic and transcranial approaches to the skull base. *Abbreviations*: EEA, endoscopic endonasal approach; SLO, superior lateral orbitotomy; IFTA, infratemporal approach; TP, transpterygoid.

Surgical approach to the ventral skull base from the frontal sinus to the craniocervical junction via the nasal cavity can be performed using an endoscope as the sole visualising tool. Exposure to the paramedian skull base, lateral to the internal carotid artery (ICA), increasingly requires mobilisation of the carotid artery.

Use of neuronavigation, power instruments, intraoperative doppler, neurophysiological monitoring and intraoperative use of indocyanine green fluorescence visualisation of the vessels have made these procedures more effective.

Reconstruction is often multilayered, with the outermost layer being a vascularised flap. The Hadad nasoseptal flap is versatile and is one of the most commonly used flaps. If a nasoseptal flap is unavailable due to involvement by the tumour, then other local flaps such as frontal pericranial and temporoparietal flaps can be used.

The most feared complications are cerebrospinal fluid (CSF) leak and vascular injury; however, widespread use of the nasoseptal flap has significantly reduced the frequency of CSF leaks. Similarly, adequate training and interventional radiological techniques have been most helpful in dealing with vascular injury.

Illustrative cases

Tumours involving the anterior cranial fossa

Case 1: Anteromedial: subcranial resection – medial maxillectomy/ethmoidectomy/subcranial resection frontal sinus/orbital exenteration.

This gentleman presented with recurrent basal cell carcinoma in his medial orbit with extension into the ethmoids and base of frontal sinus (*Figure 26.2a*). Access was gained with a modified Weber–Fergusson incision, respecting the nasal subunits, and the lesion was circumscribed with 1-cm clinical margins and included the medial eyelids (*Figure 26.2b,c*). The main tumour was removed en bloc, but transecting the tumour attached to the base of the frontal sinus (*Figure 26.2d*). The margin of the frontal sinus was delineated with navigation and transillumination (*Figure 26.2e*) and an anterior wall osteotomy performed. The removal of the anterior wall allowed an excellent opportunity to inspect the contents of the frontal sinus and resection of the remanent tumour under direct vision (*Figure 26.2f,g*). The defect was reconstructed with a radial forearm free flap (*Figure 26.2h*).

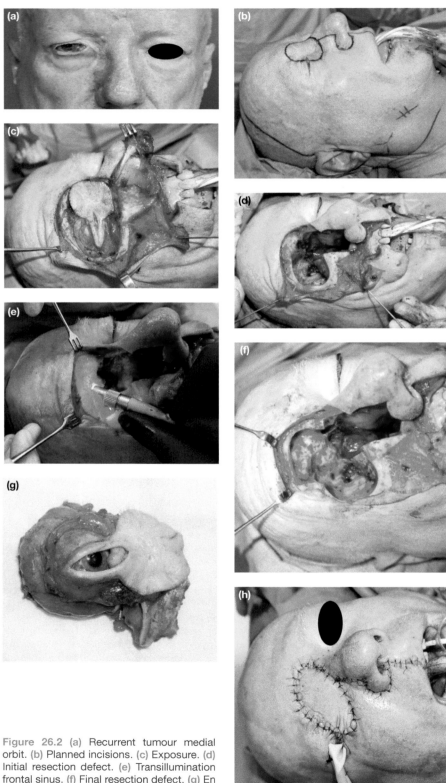

Figure 26.2 (a) Recurrent tumour medial orbit. (b) Planned incisions. (c) Exposure. (d) Initial resection defect. (e) Transillumination frontal sinus. (f) Final resection defect. (g) En bloc resection. (h) Reconstruction.

Tumours involving the middle cranial fossa

Case 2: Lateral: preauricular/infratemporal – resection tumour temporomandibular joint (TMJ), temporalis, parotid, zygomatic arch, temporal bone and dura.

This gentleman presented with an enlarging preauricular lump (*Figure 26.3a*) and the biopsy was reported as a tenosynovial giant cell tumour. Imaging demonstrated involvement of the temporalis muscle, TMJ, zygomatic arch, temporal bone and dura (*Figure 26.3b,c*). A preauricular cervicomastoid incision with hemicoronal extension was utilised (*Figure 26.3d*).

The tumour was circumscribed with adequate margins (*Figure 26.3e*) and then transected in line with the bony defect and excised along with the temporalis muscle, superolateral parotid, zygomatic arch, lateral capsule and articular disc of the TMJ, including the synovium of the glenoid fossa (*Figure 26.3f,g*). The remanent tumour along the bony margins and deep surface was removed down to the middle fossa dura, and the involved dura subsequently excised. The defect was reconstructed with a de-epithelialised anterolateral thigh free flap (*Figure 26.3h*).

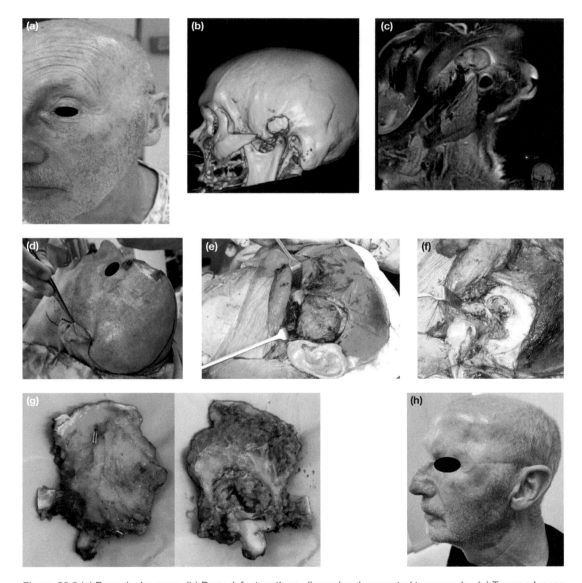

Figure 26.3 (a) Preauricular mass. (b) Bony defect on three-dimensional computed tomography. (c) Temporal mass on magnetic resonance imaging. (d) Planned incisions. (e) Exposure. (f) Initial resection defect – dura intact. (g) En bloc resection. (h) Early postoperative status.

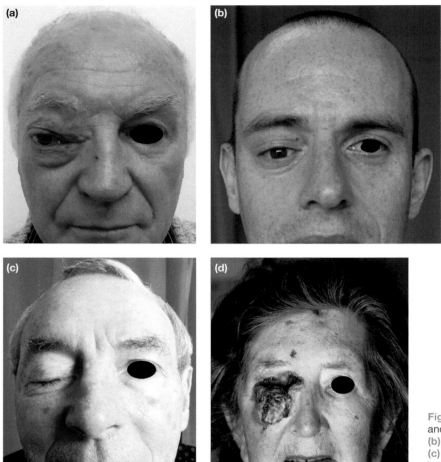

Figure 26.4 (a) Proptosis and ophthalmoplegia. (b) Orbital dystopia. (c) Ptosis. (d) Ulcerated lesion eyelids/orbit.

ORBITAL RESECTIONS

Orbital pathology and clinical presentation

Primary tumours of the orbit can be of epithelial, mesenchymal, vascular, neural, glandular and haematological origin. Tumours can also involve the orbit from the adjacent skin, sinonasal/cranial cavities and metastatic deposits from distant primaries. Pathologies can also be classified as intraconal and extraconal, based on the relationship to the extraocular muscles.

Clinical presentation is often dependant on the location, size and direction of spread of the tumour, in addition to neural and vascular compression/invasion (*Figure 26.4a–d*).

Round-the-clock orbit/orbit 360

The main considerations when excising orbital pathologies are preservation of vision and ocular motility, while undertaking adequate removal. The nature of the

pathology (benign versus malignant) and involvement of the orbital contents and adjacent structures will primarily determine the extent of orbital resection. The best approach to the lesion is determined by the location and extension of the lesion and the need to avoid manipulation of the optic, oculomotor, trochlear and abducent nerves, exiting from the optic canal and superior orbital fissures, if vision and motility are to be preserved.

Using the right orbit for demonstration of the clock model, a medial transconjunctival/transcutaneous approach provides access to the anterior orbit from 1 to 6 o'clock; endoscopic endonasal approaches provide access to the mid and posterior orbits and orbital apex from 1 to 7 o'clock. A lateral orbitotomy provides access from 8 to 10 o'clock. A frontotemporal craniotomy with superolateral orbitotomy extends the access from 9 to 1 o'clock and addition of a zygomatic osteotomy extends this from 6 to 8 o'clock (*Figure 26.5*). These approaches are most suitable for benign and low-grade malignant lesions and are determined by the

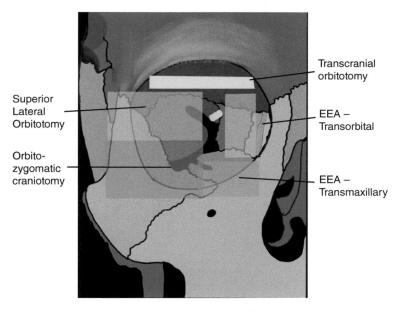

Figure 26.5 Access to intraorbital lesions. *Abbreviation*: EEA, endoscopic endonasal approach.

relationship to the optic nerve and the need to avoid 'crossing' the nerve to access the pathology.

In the case of malignant sinonasal, cranial and skin tumours, secondarily involving the orbit, the extent of orbital resection is determined by extent of orbital involvement.

- Tumours in close proximity to the bony orbit, but not involving it – preserve soft tissue orbital contents ± bony orbit
- Tumours involving the bony orbit, but not involving the orbital soft tissues – resect bone but preserve orbital soft tissue. Consider frozen section of the periorbita
- Tumours involving the periorbita, but not involving the wider orbital soft tissue (fat/muscle) – excise periorbita but consider preserving orbital contents; depends on pathology. Consider frozen section
- Tumours involving the extraocular muscles/intraconal contents – orbital exenteration
- Tumours involving the orbital apex and superior orbital fissure – orbital exenteration
- In cases of focal extraconal soft tissue involvement/focal extraocular muscle involvement – the decision for orbital preservation, partial or complete exenteration will be based primarily on the tumour pathology and prior treatment

Illustrative cases

Orbital preservation

Case 3: Resection tumour superior/lateral orbit/squamous temporal bone: frontotemporal craniectomy/ resection bony superior and lateral orbit/surgical guides/patient-specific implant.

This patient presented with a new metastatic deposit from a thyroid cancer in the left superior/lateral orbit/sphenoid wing/temporal fossa, causing significant pain, proptosis and reducing vision (*Figure 26.6a,b*). A hemicoronal flap with preauricular extension was planned (*Figure 26.6c*) and raised in the subgaleal/subtemporalis fascia plane and the superior/lateral orbital rims/zygomatic arch/frontal and squamous temporal bone was exposed. A preplanned surgical guide was placed, which incorporated the planned resection, including the craniectomy/lateral/superior orbital wall resection (*Figure 26.6d*). The frontotemporal craniectomy was performed initially and the tumour separated from the underlying dura (*Figure 26.6e*). The superior/lateral orbital rim/wall resection was then performed, and the tumour dissected away from the peri orbita, in addition to extradural decompression of the superior orbital fissure and optic canal (*Figure 26.6f*). The defect following the resection was reconstructed using a patient-specific PEEK implant (*Figure 26.6g*). Three weeks following the procedure, the patient presented with excellent position of the globe and retained full range of eye movements and intact vision (*Figure 26.6h*).

Orbital exenteration

When the decision has been made to remove the eye, the extent of resection is primarily dependant on the specific pathology, intraorbital location and the extension (intraorbital/periorbital) of the lesion (*Figure 26.7*).

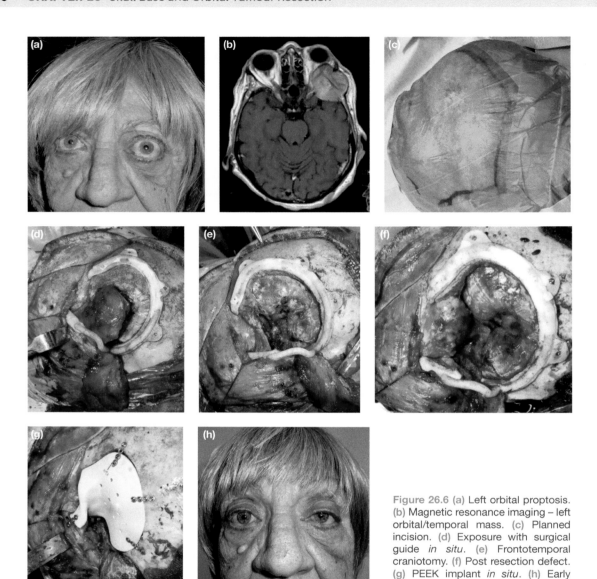

Figure 26.6 (a) Left orbital proptosis. (b) Magnetic resonance imaging – left orbital/temporal mass. (c) Planned incision. (d) Exposure with surgical guide *in situ*. (e) Frontotemporal craniotomy. (f) Post resection defect. (g) PEEK implant *in situ*. (h) Early postoperative status.

- *Evisceration*: surgical removal of the entire 'contents' of the eyeball, leaving intact the scleral shell and the attached extraocular muscles, optic nerve and conjunctiva
- *Enucleation*: surgical removal of the 'entire' eyeball including the sclera and detaching but retaining the extraocular muscles and optic nerve
- *Exenteration*: removal of the entire contents of the orbit – the eyeball, extraocular muscles, lacrimal gland, periorbital fat and optic nerve

Evisceration and enucleation are undertaken for intraocular pathology and predominantly performed by the ophthalmologist. Exenteration is undertaken for more aggressive intraorbital tumours and periorbital

malignant tumours secondarily invading the orbit. The location of the periorbital tumour and the site and extent of orbital involvement will determine the extent of the orbital exenteration.

Sinonasal tumours, especially those arising from the ethmoid and maxillary sinus, intracranial and skin tumours are the most common sites of the primary tumours, which secondarily invade the orbit. In these instances, the contents of the orbit, in addition to the involved bony wall and the primary tumour site, will have to be resected. When an en bloc resection is contemplated, the contents of the orbit are circumferentially dissected free, away from the area of involvement, leaving it attached along the site of orbital invasion, for

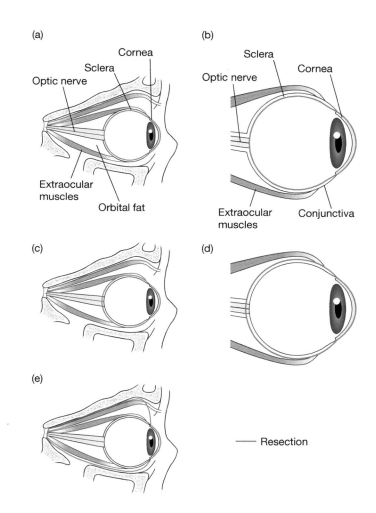

(a)

Cornea
Sclera
Optic nerve

Extraocular
muscles
Orbital fat

(b)

Sclera
Optic nerve
Cornea

Extraocular
muscles   Conjunctiva

(c)

(d)

(e)

——— Resection

Figure 26.7 Extent of orbital resection. (a, b) Evisceration. (c, d) Enucleation. (e) Exenteration.

'en bloc' removal with the primary tumour resection. Decisions will have to be made about preserving the eyelids, eyebrows and uninvolved orbital bony margins to aid reconstruction.

Case 4: Eyelid-sparing orbital exenteration with total maxillectomy/infratemporal fossa clearance.

This gentleman presented with a squamous cell carcinoma of the right maxilla (*Figure 26.8a*) and cross-sectional imaging suggested infiltrative mass lesion in the right maxillary sinus, with extension into the cheek soft tissue, nasal cavity, infratemporal fossa and orbit (*Figure 26.8b*). He was planned for a total maxillectomy, orbital exenteration and infratemporal fossa clearance.

A modified Weber–Fergusson incision, respecting the nasal subunits, was marked with upper and lower eyelid midtarsal extensions for an eyelid-preserving exenteration (*Figure 26.8c*). A glabella and lip-split

mandibulotomy incisions were marked for additional access but were not used. The cheek flap was raised in the subcutaneous plane to retain the soft tissues over the anterior maxilla. The eyelid dissection was carried out in the suborbicularis oculi muscular plane but the soft tissues along the infraorbital rim were left undisturbed. The lateral, superior and medial bony orbital rims were exposed, and subperiosteal dissection carried posteriorly towards the orbital apex (*Figure 26.8d*). Medially, the medial canthus was detached, the lacrimal sac dissected free from the lacrimal fossa and the ethmoidal vessels identified and diathermised (*Figure 26.8e*). The intraoral incisions, maxillary and medial/lateral orbital bone cuts were completed. The maxilla and orbital contents were mobilised inferiorly, which allowed additional access to the orbital apex and the contents transected. The contents of the superior orbital fissure can be diathermised and transected, but additional care should be taken when transecting the

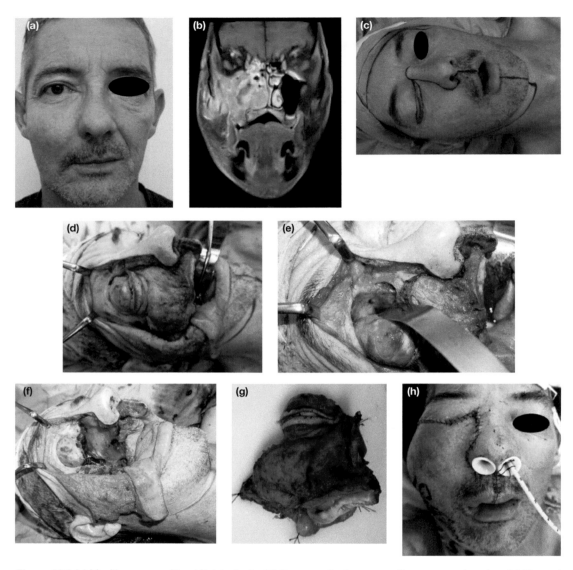

Figure 26.8 (a) Maxillary mass with orbital dystopia. (b) Tumour extent on magnetic resonance imaging. (c) Planned incisions. (d) Exposure. (e) Medial orbital exposure. (f) Resection defect. (g) En bloc resection. (h) Reconstruction.

proximal optic nerve/contents of the optic canal. Haemostasis could be carried out with a curved haemostat and suture ligation, Ligaclip placement with a curved applicator, or judicious use of a diathermy. There is always concern for transmission of diathermy current to the optic chiasm and damage to the contralateral optic nerve and the use of monopolar diathermy should be avoid. The total maxillectomy/infratemporal fossa and orbital exenteration contents were removed en bloc (*Figure 26.8f,g*). The defect following the resection was reconstructed with a musculocutaneous latissimus dorsi-free flap (*Figure 26.8h*).

POSTOPERATIVE CARE/ COMPLICATIONS

Meticulous postoperative care is essential for patients undergoing skull base and orbital surgery. Specific attention should be focussed on level of consciousness (Glasgow Coma Score), visual acuity, pupillary reaction, eye movement, orbital pain and proptosis. Intracranial and intraorbital bleeding, cerebrospinal fluid leak and infections are also of concern and should be identified early and appropriately managed. It is our routine practice for patients undergoing major skull base resection to have a postoperative CT scan, prior to commencement of anticoagulation.

TOP TIPS AND HAZARDS

• Skull base surgery should only be contemplated with appropriate skill mix in a multidisciplinary setting.

• Sound anatomical knowledge (open/ endoscopic) is essential and should also concentrate on linking intracranial and subcranial dissection.

• Many skull base tumours are slow-growing, and clinical and imaging surveillance play a key role in patient management.

• Subtotal tumour resection, particularly for benign and low-grade malignant tumours, will frequently provide adequate tumour control, relief of symptoms and minimise morbidity.

• Key elements in skull base reconstruction are the isolation of intracranial contents from the sinonasal cavities and appropriate support for the frontal/ temporal lobes. Vascularised tissues (local pedicled/free flaps) are most appropriate.

• Functional vision should be preserved where possible when dealing with orbital pathology.

• Brain, cranial nerve and vascular manipulation should be kept to a minimum and will often determine the most appropriate access to the lesion.

• Concepts of skull base 360 and 'round-the-clock' orbit (orbit 360) provide good foundations on which the most appropriate access can be planned.

FURTHER READING

Ethunandan M. Infratemoporal fossa and pterygopalatine fossa. In: Brennan PA, Standring SM, Wiseman SM eds. *Gray's Surgical Anatomy*. Elsevier; 2020. pp. 58–65.

Ganly I, Patel SG, Singh B et al. Craniofacial resection for malignant paranasal sinus tumours: report of an international collaborative study. *Head Neck* 2005;**27**:575–84.

McLaughlin N, Prevedello DM, Kelly DF et al. A multicorridor 360 degree strategy. *Jpn J Neurosurg (Tokyo)* 2011;**20**:190–9.

Paluzzi A, Gardner PA, Fernandez-Miranda JC et al. "Round-the-clock" surgical access to the orbit. *J Neurol Surg B Skull Base* 2015;**76**:12–24.

Wang EW, Gardner PA, Zanation A. A consensus statement on endoscopic skull base surgery: executive summary. *Int Forum Allergy Rhinol* 2019;**9**:S127–S144.

Bailey & Love's Essential Operations Bailey & Love's Essential Operations
Bailey & Love's Essential Operations Bailey & Love's Essential Operations
Bailey & Love's Essential Operations Bailey & Love's Essential Operations

PART 4 | Oncology

Chapter 27
Sentinel Node Biopsy
Moni Abraham Kuriakose, Nirav Pravin Trivedi

BACKGROUND

Lymphatic metastasis generally follows an orderly and predictable pattern of progression beginning with the sentinel lymph node (SLN). It has been demonstrated that the status of the sentinel node predicts the presence of metastasis in the remainder of the nodal basin. Lymphoscintigraphy is now established as a reliable and minimally invasive technique of identifying the sentinel nodes in solid tumours such as breast cancer and melanoma. Since the original description to stage patients with cutaneous melanoma, biopsy of the sentinel lymph node has replaced routine elective lymph node dissection in many anatomical regions. Initial attempts at lymph node mapping using the vital dye and isosulphan blue failed to localise the sentinel nodes in about 20% of cases. The introduction of the handheld gamma probe has improved sensitivity to over 93%. This technique is increasingly being used to evaluate cancer of the breast, colon and vulva, and it is redefining the standard of care for these treatment sites.

Previously untreated head and neck squamous cell carcinomas (HNSCC) are considered to have a predictable pattern of metastasis to cervical lymph nodes. However, clinical experience may not provide fail-safe information with which to direct therapy for individual patients. It has been reported that 16% of patients with SCC of the oral tongue had 'skip metastases', which bypassed what was considered to be the first echelon nodal basin (*Figure 27.1*). This highlights the need for individualised localisation of sentinel lymph nodes.

DETECTION OF SENTINEL NODES

Conventionally, sentinel lymph nodes can be identified by three techniques:

- Isosulphan blue dye
- Static lymphoscintigraphy
- Dynamic lymphoscintigraphy

This is an evolving field and highlights of technical advances are discussed below.

The isosulphan blue-dye technique involves injection of the dye submucously around the tumour. The sentinel lymph nodes are those which are stained blue. As the technique requires visualisation, it is necessary to expose the entire nodal basin, thereby increasing the invasiveness of the procedure. Moreover, the isosulphan blue dye has been proven to have lower reliability than lymphoscintigraphy (*Figure 27.2*).

Dynamic lymphoscintigraphy involves injection of Tc 99-labelled filtered sulphur colloid at the periphery of the tumour. The flow of radiolabelled dye from the primary tumour to the sentinel nodes can be visualised in real time using a gamma camera operating in a continuous mode. The position of the nodes where the radioactivity localises can be marked on the skin using a pen (*Figure 27.3*).

Static lymphoscintigraphy involves identifying the nodes with increased radioactivity using a hand-held gamma probe (*Figure 27.4*). The sentinel node, which is surgically removed, is submitted for various histopathological, immunohistochemistry and molecular

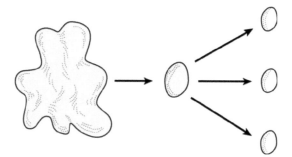

Figure 27.1 The sentinel node is the first echelon node of the nodal basin. Presence of metastasis to the sentinel node defines the status of the rest of the nodes in the nodal basin.

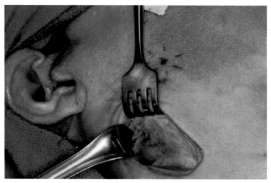

Figure 27.2 Blue-dye technique. (Courtesy of Mark Delacure.)

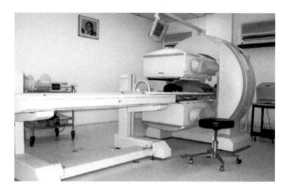

Figure 27.3 Dynamic lymphoscintigraphy under gamma camera.

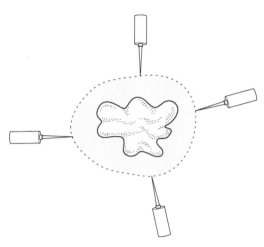

Figure 27.5 Injection of dye into periphery of tumour.

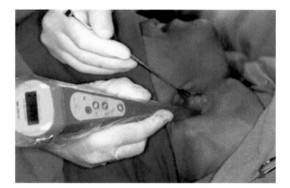

Figure 27.4 Static lymphoscintigraphy with handheld gamma camera.

marker examination for the detection of micrometastasis.

Indication

Sentinel node biopsy is indicated for early stage (T1, T2) SCC of oral cavity with clinically N0 neck.

Contraindications

Sentinel node biopsy is contraindicated in:

- Advanced-stage tumours
- Clinical or radiological evidence of nodal metastasis
- Cases where the neck needs to be exposed for other reasons (exposure of donor vessels for reconstructive surgery)

Lymphoscintigraphy

Injection of the dye

A total of 5 mL of Tc 99-labelled filtered sulphur colloid is loaded into an insulin syringe. Between 1 and 2 mL of the sulphur colloid is injected submucously around the

tumour (*Figure 27.5*). This is performed after isolating the tumour with gauze. Care should be taken to avoid spilling the radioactive material but if this does occur, it should be wiped away with gauze. Allow the patient to rinse the mouth with saline several times to remove any salivary contamination. It is necessary to instruct the patient to avoid swallowing of saliva contaminated with the radioactive material to avoid misleading images in the gamma camera. All the radioactive material and contaminant should be disposed of according to the institutional radioactive material disposal guidelines.

Position of patient under the gamma camera

The patient should be positioned on the gamma camera table similar to that on the operation table, using shoulder bag and head ring. This is important as the position of skin marking can change with neck extension in the operating table.

Dynamic imaging

Beginning immediately after the injections, the patient is positioned with the injection site centred under a large field-of-view dual-head gamma camera. A large field of view, set at 20% window centred on the 140-keV technetium energy peak and fitted with a low-energy, high-resolution parallel hole collimator, is used to follow the disbursement of the radionuclide from the primary site to the cervical lymphatic. Initially, images are captured in an anteroposterior plane to determine the laterality of the sentinel nodes, following which the images are captured in the lateral view (*Figure 27.6*). The images are captured in a continuous mode. The transit time for drainage of the sentinel node in oral cavity cancer is less than 5 minutes. It is a continuous process where tracking of dye into sentinel nodes can be seen on screen. The primary tumour is seen as a large shadow, while a sentinel node is seen as a smaller

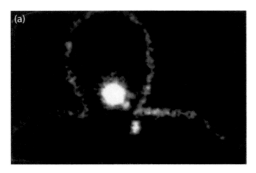

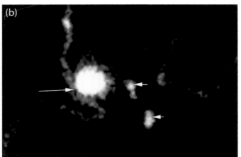

Figure 27.6 Nuclear scan images. Large arrow indicates the primary tumour. Small arrows indicate sentinel nodes.

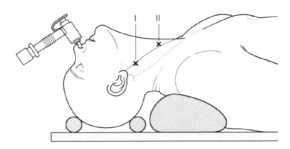

Figure 27.7 Marking of sentinel node externally on neck.

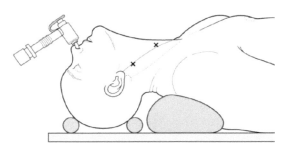

Figure 27.8 Positioning of patient on operation table.

shadow. The number of sentinel lymph nodes can vary from two to three in head and neck cancer.

Marking of sentinel nodes

The position of the sentinel node is marked externally on the neck (*Figure 27.7*). This serves as a landmark for incision in the neck during the surgery. The location of the sentinel node is marked with the guide of a pointer with radioactive tip under gamma camera in a continuous mode. The location where the 'hotspot' of the pen and that of the sentinel node coincide is marked on the skin with an indelible pen.

Anaesthesia

The operation is performed under general anaesthesia. Nasal intubation is preferred to avoid interference in dealing with the primary tumour in the oral cavity.

OPERATION

Position of the patient

The neck must be hyperextended with the shoulders and occiput supported with a head ring. The neck is rotated to the contralateral side. The operating table is tipped with a head-up tilt. The head and neck region is prepared and draped in the standard fashion to expose the neck and oral cavity (*Figure 27.8*).

Surgery of the primary lesion

Emission of radiation from the primary lesion interferes with detection of the sentinel node using the gamma probe, particularly if the node is situated in the region of level I. Excision of the primary lesion in the oral cavity before performing sentinel node biopsy in the neck helps in eliminating this radiation interference.

Neck incision

A transverse neck incision is marked on the neck as in a standard neck dissection. An incision of about 4 cm in length is placed along this marking to access the marked sentinel nodes. Occasionally, it may be necessary to make more than one incision. However, all the incisions should be placed in such a way that these incisions should be later extended to perform neck dissection, should it be necessary (*Figure 27.9*).

Raising flaps

Upper and lower skin flaps are raised in the subplatysmal plane over the region of the marked sentinel nodes (*Figure 27.10*).

Identification of sentinel nodes

Using a handheld gamma camera, the background radiation level is noted in the neck in a position away

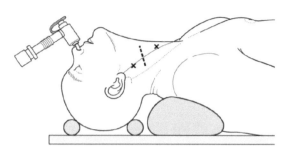

Figure 27.9 Incision in neck.

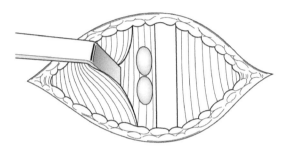

Figure 27.10 Raising of flaps, exposing lymph node groups.

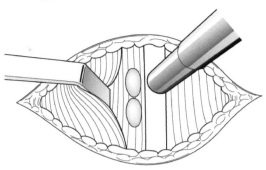

Figure 27.11 Identification of sentinel lymph node with gamma probe.

from the sentinel nodes and primary tumour. Using the skin marking and the handheld gamma probe as guides, the region of the sentinel node is explored (*Figure 27.11*). If there is an increase in count of more than threefold, the background is considered significant. This count is noted as an *in vivo* count. That particular node is removed and the *ex vivo* count is obtained outside the body to confirm it as a sentinel node. Count of node-bed is noted, which should confirm that the identified node is removed. The procedure is repeated to remove all the marked sentinel nodes. The wound is closed in layers. Drains are not usually required.

SENTINEL NODE PATHOLOGIC EVALUATION

The excised sentinel nodes are sent for histopathological evaluation. Further details of histopathological analysis are described in *Chapter 4*. Step-sections of the nodes are obtained along the hilum of the node at 3–4 mm intervals. The tissue is processed by haematoxylin and eosin staining. Immunohistochemistry with pan-cytokeratin antibody or CK-14 polymerase chain reaction may be performed to identify submicroscopic metastasis. The clinical relevance of such lesions is yet to be determined. The feasibility of determining metastatic status by frozen section evaluation also needs to be determined.

POSTOPERATIVE CARE

Sutures are removed on day 7. The final histopathological report is evaluated and if any node shows metastasis, formal neck dissection is carried out.

Follow-up

Regular follow-up should be monthly for the first year, and every 2 months for the second year. Any suspicious neck mass should be thoroughly evaluated with ultrasound scan and fine needle aspiration cytology as deemed necessary.

TECHNICAL ADVANCES FOR IDENTIFICATION OF SLN

In recent decades, new tracer substances have been developed such as ^{99m}Tc-tilmanocept (Lymphoseek) and the combination of ^{99m}Tc-nanocolloid with indocyanine green (ICG). These are beneficial for avoiding 'shine through' effects of tracer, particularly when dealing with floor of mouth lesions. However, additional prospective studies are needed to establish their credibility.

Progress has also been made in intraoperative detection systems, with the emergence of freehand SPECT (FhSPECT) which generates 3D images during the sentinel node biopsy. This new imaging system can provide information about the direction and depth of the sentinel node in relation to the gamma probe, making possible *in situ* biopsy planning. This could contribute to incisions being made at the correct place, thus reducing risk of morbidities.

The high costs of these emerging techniques are the main limit to their clinical use, in particular for FhSPECT and ICG which require setup of an appropriate imaging system in the operative room.

In terms of technical advances in identifying cancer cells in SLN in real time, molecular markers, including CK, PARP and DSG3, are currently under investigation for real-time detection of metastasis.

CONCLUSION

At present, there are no clear guidelines for the management of clinically N0 neck. Lymphoscintigraphy and sentinel node biopsy offer the possibility of minimal invasive management of the N0 neck, avoiding undue morbidity of surgery or radiation, as well as eliminating the risk of regional recurrence. However, efficacy of the procedure and long-term results must be assessed before implementing this in clinical practice.

TOP TIPS AND HAZARDS

- Sentinel node biopsy should be performed in previously untreated patients.
- Care should be taken to avoid spillage of the dye while injecting around the tumour.
- The patient should be instructed not to swallow during injection to prevent ingestion of the dye.
- The position of the patient under the gamma camera should be similar to the position to be adopted in the operating room to increase the accuracy of sentinel node marking.
- If the sentinel node is identified in level I, consider removing the primary tumour first to avoid background radiation.

FURTHER READING

Hamy A, Curtet C, Paineau J et al. Feasibility of radio-immunoguided surgery of colorectal carcinoma using indium 111 CEA specific antibody and simulation with a phantom using 2 step targeting with bispecific antibody. *Tumori* 1995;**81**:103–6.

Liu M, Wang SJ, Yang X, Peng H. Diagnostic efficacy of sentinel lymph node biopsy in early oral squamous cell carcinoma: a meta-analysis of 66 studies. *PLoS One* 2017;**12**:e0170322.

Pijpers R, Collet GJ, Meijer S, Otto SH. The impact of dynamic lymphoscintigraphy and gamma probe guidance on sentinel node biopsy in melanoma. *Eur J Nucl Med* 1995;**22**:1238–41.

Schilling C, Stoeckli SJ, Haerle SK et al. Sentinel European Node Trial (SENT): 3-year results of sentinel node biopsy in oral cancer. *Eur J Cancer* 2015;**51**:2777–84.

Bailey & Love's Essential Operations Bailey & Love's Essential Operations
Bailey & Love's Essential Operations Bailey & Love's Essential Operations
Bailey & Love's Essential Operations Bailey & Love's Essential Operations

PART 4 | Oncology

Chapter 28

Management of Benign and Malignant Skin Lesions

Carrie Newlands, Daniel van Gijn

INTRODUCTION

Facial and head and neck skin lesions are usually obvious to patients and others, and advice is often sought as to their nature, with cosmetic removal of benign lesions regularly requested. Premalignant and malignant skin lesions are increasing in incidence, and this is related to sunshine exposure, an ageing Caucasian population, along with increasing numbers of patients who are immunosuppressed. The head and neck comprise only 12% of the skin surface area of the body but are where most premalignant and malignant skin lesions are seen, with the commonest keratinocyte cancers (KC), basal cell carcinoma (BCC) and cutaneous squamous cell carcinoma (cSCC) cancers affecting this anatomical site in over 80% of cases.

ESSENTIAL SURGICAL ANATOMY

Skin consists of the epidermis and the dermis, and most skin lesions arise from one or more of these layers or from associated appendages. Important surgical anatomical considerations in skin surgery relate to appropriate curative resection margins, specifically where the deep margin may involve or be close to important underlying structures. Areas where there is a known higher risk of histologically close or involved KC margins following attempted curative excision include the medial canthus, the temple and the eyelids.

PREOPERATIVE CONSIDERATIONS

Skin lesion assessment

History specific to skin surgery should include:

- History of the lesion including growth, bleeding, crusting, colour change and previous treatment at the same site
- History of other previous skin lesions
- Family history of skin lesions
- Sunshine exposure including use of sunbeds
- Medical history including antiplatelet and anti-coagulant therapy and immunosuppression

Examination of skin lesions should include:

- Site
- Size
- Shape and symmetry
- Colour(s)

- Border
- Fixity
- Relation to underlying and adjacent structure
- Lymphadenopathy
- Neurology possibly indicative of neural or perineural infiltration
- Dermoscopic features
- Patients with suspected or confirmed skin cancer diagnosis should have a full skin check

Cross-sectional imaging of the primary region is indicated where involvement of deeper structures is suspected and will aid decision making in term of operability.

SURGICAL MANAGEMENT OF COMMON SKIN LESIONS

Benign and malignant skin management is outlined in *Tables 28.1* and *28.2*. Most skin lesions can be diagnosed clinically without the need for a diagnostic non-excisional biopsy. Shave excision (SE) is indicated in specific superficial benign lesions (*Table 28.1*) and usually results in superior cosmesis over formal excisional surgery. SE can be used in indeterminate nodules on the nose, where the diagnosis lies between an intradermal naevus or a BCC, with further surgery and complex repair then indicated for a histological result of BCC. SE should not be carried out if there is a possibility of the lesion being a melanoma, as it is subsequently difficult to determine the tumour thickness, and thus, the pathological T stage and future management.

Low-risk BCC

This includes:

- Superficial and nodular subtypes
- Infraclavicular anatomical sites
- Where the lesion is non-recurrent and the patient immunocompetent
- 1-mm or more histological clearance at all surgical margins

High-risk BCC

This includes:

- Immunosuppression
- Size >20 mm (10 mm on midface)

TABLE 28.1 Benign and malignant skin management

Intervention for the primary lesion	Indications
Five fluorouracil cream	Actinic keratosis including Bowen's disease, superficial BCC
Imiquimod cream	Actinic keratosis, superficial BCC, lentigo maligna
Cryotherapy	Actinic keratosis, low-risk infraclavicular BCC, seborrheic wart, skin tag
Photodynamic therapy	Superficial BCC, actinic keratosis
Curettage and cautery ×3	Low-risk BCC, low-risk cSCC
Shave excision	Seborrhoeic wart, intradermal naevus sebaceous hyperplasia
Punch/incisional biopsy	Unclear diagnosis, particularly where complex reconstruction may be required following excision with curative intent. Biopsy should be dermoscopically directed in possible melanoma (see above)
Excisional biopsy (see margins below)	Epidermal cysts, junctional and compound naevi, suspected dysplastic moles, suspected melanoma
Excision with curative intent with a predetermined surgical margin and immediate repair (see margins below)	Biopsy-proven or clinically diagnosed skin cancers, with well-defined margins in non-critical anatomical sites where complex reconstruction not required
Excision with curative intent with a predetermined surgical margin and delayed repair (see margins below)	Biopsy-proven or clinically diagnosed skin cancers, with one or more of the following factors: poorly defined margins/critical anatomical sites/complex repair required
Mohs micrographic surgery (see *Chapter 29*)	Biopsy-proven or clinically diagnosed KC, with one or more of the following factors: poorly defined margins/critical anatomical sites/complex repair required

Abbreviations: BCC, basal cell carcinoma; KC, keratinocyte cancer; cSCC, cutaneous squamous cell carcinoma.

- Infiltrative/sclerosing/micronodular/basosquamous subtypes
- Presence of perineural infiltration (PNI) or lymphovascular invasion (LVI)
- Recurrent tumour
- One or more close or involved surgical margin

Low-risk cSCC

All the following should be present:

- Patient factors
  - Immune competent
- Tumour factors
  - Not recurrent
  - Diameter <20 mm
  - Not a high-risk site
  - No PNI or LVI
  - Well or moderate differentiation
  - Depth of invasion (DOI) <4 mm
- Margin status
  - 1-mm or greater histological clearance at all surgical margins

High-risk cSCC

- Patient factors
  - Congenital immunosuppressive states
  - Acquired immunocompromise, HIV
  - Steroid, anti-tumour necrosis factor (TNF) methotrexate, azathioprine or hydrochlorothiazide therapy
- Tumour factors
  - Recurrent tumour
  - Diameter 20–40 mm
  - Tumour site ear or vermilion lip or within scar/chronic inflammation
  - PNI involving any nerve <0.1 mm, or dermal nerve only
  - Poor differentiation
  - DOI 4–6 mm
- Margin status
  - One or more close (<1-mm clearance) or involved (tumour cells at cut edge) margin

Very high-risk cSCC

- Patient factors

TABLE 28.2 Benign and non-melanocytic skin lesions – excision margins

Diagnosis (clinical and/or histological)	(Total) peripheral margin of normal tissue suggested to take, in mm	Deep margin should include at least the anatomical layer of: *	Acceptable final any closest histological clearance, in mm
Epidermal cyst	Complete cyst lining plus punctum within a skin ellipse	Complete cyst lining	0
BCC: low risk	4–5	Fat	1
BCC: high risk (consider delayed reconstruction)	5–10	Fat	1
cSCC: low-risk pT1	4	Fat (galea on scalp)	1
cSCC: high risk	6	Fat (galea on scalp)	1
cSCC: very high risk (consider delayed reconstruction)	10	Fat (galea or periosteum on scalp)	1, but consider ART
MCC	10–20	Fat (galea or periosteum on scalp)	1 and then ART
AFX	10	Fat (galea or periosteum on scalp)	2
PDS	10–20	Fat (galea or periosteum on scalp)	5

* Further deeper structures such as muscle or bone or dura may need to be taken to achieve a clear deep histological margin.

Abbreviations: AFX, atypical fibroxanthoma; ART, adjuvant radiotherapy; BCC, basal cell carcinoma; cSCC, cutaneous squamous cell carcinoma; MCC, Merkel cell carcinoma; PDS, pleomorphic dermal sarcoma.

- ● Current or former haematological malignancy, primary immunodeficiency, organ transplant recipient on immunosuppressive treatment
- ● Tumour factors
  - ● Diameter >40 mm
  - ● DOI >6 mm, or beyond subcutaneous fat, or into bone
  - ● High-grade histological subtype
  - ● Significant PNI (defined as tumour cells around a nerve >0.1 mm diameter/or named nerve/ or a nerve beyond the dermis, or tumour cells within any nerve) (UICC 8)
  - ● In-transit metastasis
- ● Margin status
  - ● One or more close (<1-mm clearance) or involved (tumour cells at cut edge) margin with more than one other high or any very high-risk factors

Merkel cell carcinoma (MCC), atypical fibroxanthoma (AFX) and pleomorphic dermal sarcoma (PDS)

If suspected, should undergo incisional biopsy before definitive treatment.

Melanoma

Suspected melanoma should undergo narrow excision biopsy where direct closure is possible. Closure can be by purse string, and any ellipse should be short, to preserve proximal lymphatic channels. Sampling biopsies guided by dermoscopy, or no repair are other options where the primary defect is not suitable for direct closure.

SURGICAL EXCISION AND HISTOLOGICAL MARGINS IN COMMON SKIN LESIONS

Most skin lesion surgery can be carried out under sterile conditions and local anaesthetic, using lidocaine and adrenaline. Levobupivacaine can also be used for postoperative analgesia. Skin preparation should follow NICE prevention of wound infection guidance. Suitable solutions are aqueous povidone-iodine (which can be used around the eyes and ears) and alcoholic chlorhexidine (which should not come into contact with the eyes or tympanic membrane).

This is clean surgery and prophylactic antibiotics are not indicated. In most cases, patients should continue their normal medication including antiplatelet and anticoagulant medication. If extensive surgery is planned, or deeper structures are involved, the risks and benefits of continuing versus stopping required medication should be considered.

Marking the clinical edge of a lesion, using an adjunct such as dermoscopy, loupe magnification and the stretch test, prior to adding a predetermined clinical margin where appropriate, will improve rates of curative surgery. In excisional surgery, the skin should usually be incised at 90° to the skin surface, to aid both resection and reconstruction. In excisional specimens of proven/suspected skin cancer, a marker suture should be placed for orientation. A skin-specific histopathology form aids the pathologist and multidisciplinary team (MDT) discussion.

Close/involved histological margins at the primary site following skin cancer resection

More likely:

- Non-expert/non-MDT attender operator
- At a critical site
- More than one lesion is removed at the same time

Recurrence is more likely with:

- Deep margin or more than one margin involved
- One or more other high-risk/very high-risk factor(s)

Chances of subsequent cure are reduced in:

- Critical anatomical sites such as near the skull bony orifices, for example, the orbit, external auditory meatus or piriform aperture
- Increasing age and comorbidity

Options include:

- Monitoring in low-risk situations for recurrence, particularly in the elderly

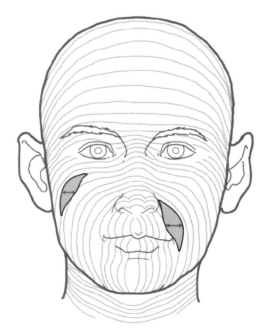

Figure 28.1 Closure of primary defect parallel to inter-pupillary line to reduce anatomical distortion.

- Re-excision of one or more margins with or without delayed repair
- Adjuvant radiotherapy (ART) (KC and MCC)

Reconstruction

None following shave excision, or in specific anatomical sites, for example, upper lateral nose, conchal bowl of pinna.

Direct closure

Consider closure of the primary defect without the darts of an ellipse in thick skin. Design of any wound ellipse should follow relaxed skin tension lines (RSTLs) but should consider possible anatomical distortion. Closure parallel to the interpupillary line will reduce anatomical distortion to mobile structure such as the eyelids and lips (*Figure 28.1*).

Closure of skin should be in layers with deep resorbable sutures to close any dead space and oppose the deep dermis. Skin can be closed with subcuticular, interrupted or continuous sutures or tissue adhesive. Adjuncts to primary closure include achieving a curved scar, and ways to match lengths of an ellipse, not causing distortion by ellipse lengthening of a scar (*Figure 28.2*).

Skin grafts

Full-thickness skin grafting (FTSG) has several advantages over a split skin graft. Graft contraction and donor site morbidity are reduced, and aesthetics are superior. The donor site should be closable primarily. Common FTSG harvest sites to reconstruct head and neck lesions are shown in *Figure 28.3*. Inset of a graft to the primary defect is made with resorbable sutures.

Graft take is likely to be improved by:

- Aseptic surgery
- Careful defatting of the graft
- Gentle tissue handling of the graft and recipient site
- Minimal diathermy to the graft recipient site
- Elimination of air and clot between the graft and recipient bed, by irrigation with saline under the graft post-inset

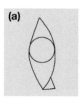 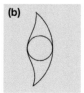 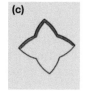

Figure 28.2 Adjuncts to primary closure. (a) Matching line discrepancies by introducing a Burow's triangle; (b) achieving a curved closure and matching line discrepancy; and (c) ellipse shortening of a scar to reduce distortion in an anatomically sensitive area.

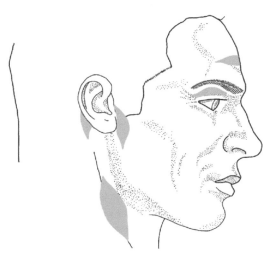

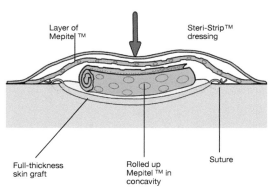

Figure 28.4 Simple dressing alternative to a bolster for full-thickness skin graft.

Figure 28.3 Common full-thickness skin graft donor sites.

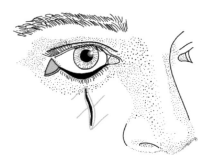

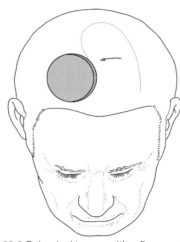

Figure 28.5 Ectropion secondary to contracted scar may be resolved by multiple Z plasties and resection of part of lower eyelid.

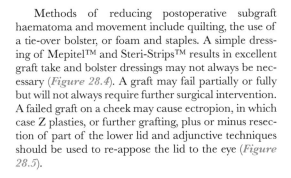

Figure 28.6 Subgaleal transposition flap used to reconstruct full-thickness scalp defect. A full-thickness skin graft is used to reconstruct the secondary defect with periosteum at its base.

Methods of reducing postoperative subgraft haematoma and movement include quilting, the use of a tie-over bolster, or foam and staples. A simple dressing of Mepitel™ and Steri-Strips™ results in excellent graft take and bolster dressings may not always be necessary (*Figure 28.4*). A graft may fail partially or fully but will not always require further surgical intervention. A failed graft on a cheek may cause ectropion, in which case Z plasties, or further grafting, plus or minus resection of part of the lower lid and adjunctive techniques should be used to re-appose the lid to the eye (*Figure 28.5*).

Flap repair

Flap repair is more complex and requires an understanding of tissue laxity and three-dimensional movement. A well-designed flap will have a higher tissue survival success than a skin graft and imports tissue similar to the resected tissue. The most useful sites of laxity for local flap harvest include the skin of the neck, the angle of the jaw, and the preauricular, nasolabial and glabella areas, but will vary with each case.

In most cases, the secondary defect is designed so that maximum laxity is used, with closure in a RSTL if possible, without distortion to mobile structures. Skin flaps in the head and neck are usually raised as a skin and fat flap, but include the galea in the scalp.

On the scalp, a subgaleal flap can be used to close a full-thickness scalp defect and the donor site grafted onto the periosteum (*Figure 28.6*). Scalp flaps should be based caudally and not cross the vascular watershed at the scalp vertex where possible, to maximise flap viability. Interpolated flaps are used to import more distant tissue (*Figures 28.7* and *28.8*).

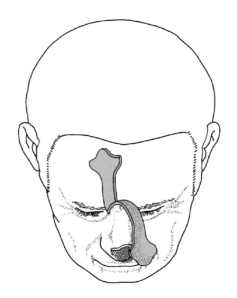

Figure 28.7 Paramedian forehead flap based on the supratrochlear artery.

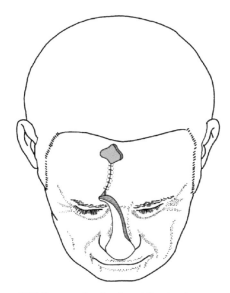

Figure 28.8 Paramedian forehead flap in place.

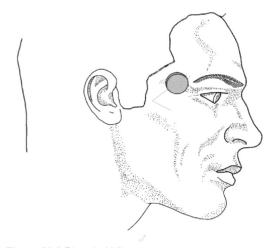

Figure 28.9 Rhomboid flap.

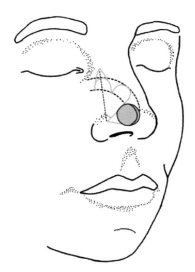

Figure 28.10 Nasal bilobed flap.

Figures 28.9–28.14 illustrate common skin flap examples in specific sites: a rhomboid flap (the 'square peg into a round hole') (*Figure 28.9*), a bilobed flap (*Figure 28.10*), the dorsal sliding nasal flap (*Figure 28.11*), an O to T closure (*Figure 28.12*), a tenzel flap (*Figure 28.13*) and a cervicofacial flap (*Figure 28.14*).

COMMON COMPLICATIONS OF SKIN SURGERY

These include:

- Surgical site infection
- Dehiscence
- Stitch abscess
- Bleeding/haematoma
- Necrosis (significant, partial or minor)
- Nerve injury
- Ectropion or other anatomical distortion
- Delayed wound healing
- Retained resorbable sutures

Patients with skin cancer should be discussed at an MDT as per (inter)national guidance.

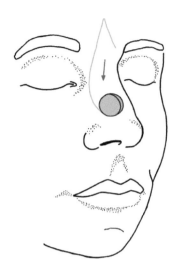

Figure 28.11 Dorsal sliding nasal flap.

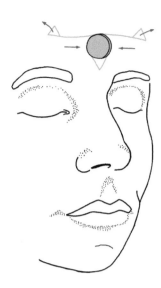

Figure 28.12 O to T closure of forehead defect.

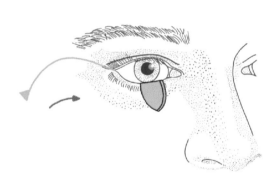

Figure 28.13 Tenzel flap for lower eyelid reconstruction.

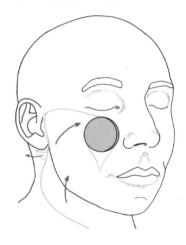

Figure 28.14 Cervicofacial flap to reconstruct anterior cheek defect.

Nodal disease

The management of the N0 and N+ patient in common skin cancers is outlined in *Table 28.3*. Principles include:

- There is no role for elective lymph node dissection (LND) in the N0 case
- Therapeutic LND is indicated in operable N+ cases with macroscopic disease if systemic staging is clear

FUTURE DIRECTION

The role of radiotherapy, and of medical treatment such as targeted treatment and immunotherapy in the management of skin cancer continues to evolve, in the neoadjuvant, therapeutic and adjuvant settings.

TOP TIPS AND HAZARDS

- Beware odd-looking lesions.
- Avoid operating on indolent lesions in the elderly as the risks often outweigh any benefits.
- Beware of over-resecting or disrupting proximal lymphatic pathways when removing a possible melanoma. This can increase false-negative SNB rates and thus deny access to adjuvant systemic therapy (which has a significant survival benefit).
- Have a low threshold for delaying complex reconstruction if further surgery may be needed.

TABLE 28.3 Management and investigation of the N0 patient and suspected nodal disease (cSCC, MCC and melanoma)

Pathology	Clinical or pathological node (N) status	Invx/Imaging	Sentinel node biopsy	Further imaging if SNB/FNA positive	Definitive management of established treatable nodal disease
cSCC	N0	None	May be considered in very high-risk cases	MRI skull base to clavicles CT skull base to diaphragm	TLND
cSCC	N+	USS/FNA CT Chest	N/A		TLND
MCC	N0	CT HN CAP or PET-CT	Offer	N/A	Options of TLND, ART to the primary site, and therapeutic RT to the nodal basin(s), or immunotherapy
MCC	N+	CT HN CAP or PET-CT	N/A	N/A	Options of TLND, ART to the primary site, and therapeutic RT to the nodal basin(s), or immunotherapy
Melanoma pT1a	N0	None	None	None	N/A
Melanoma pT1b	N0	None	Consider	CT HN CAP or PET-CT and MRI brain	Targeted or immunotherapy if SNB +, TLND if FNA +*
Melanoma pT2a–pT3a	N0	None	Offer	CT HN CAP or PET-CT and MRI brain	Targeted or immunotherapy if SNB +, TLND if FNA +*
Melanoma pT3b-pT4a	N0	Consider CT HN CAP or PET-CT and MRI brain	Offer if M0 on scans if done	CT HN CAP or PET-CT and MRI brain	Targeted or immunotherapy if SNB +, TLND if FNA+*
Melanoma pT4b	N0	CT HN CAP or PET-CT and MRI brain	Offer if M0 on scans	N/A	Targeted or immunotherapy if SNB +, TLND if FNA +*
Melanoma any pT stage	N+	CT HN CAP or PET-CT and MRI neck and brain	N/A	N/A	TLND if M0 and adjuvant targeted or immunotherapy*

* Resected Stage III or Stage IV melanoma is followed by targeted or immunotherapy

Abbreviations: ART, adjuvant radiotherapy; CT, computed tomography; CT HN CAP, CT head, neck, chest, abdomen and pelvis; FNA, fine needle aspiration; cSCC, cutaneous squamous cell carcinoma; MCC, Merkel cell carcinoma; MRI, magnetic resonance imaging; N/A, not applicable; PET-CT, positron emission tomography-computed tomography; RT, radiotherapy; SNB, sentinel node biopsy; TLND, therapeutic lymph node dissection; USS, ultrsound scan.

FURTHER READING

Bichakjian CK, Olencki T, Aasi SZ et al. Merkel Cell Carcinoma, Version 1.2018, NCCN Clinical Practice Guidelines in Oncology. *J Natl Compr Canc Netw* 2018;**16**:742–74.

Keohane SG, Botting J, Budny PG et al. British Association of Dermatologists guidelines for the management of people with cutaneous squamous cell carcinoma. *Br J Dermatol* 2020;**184**:401–14.

Nasri I, McGrath EJ, Harwood CA et al. British Association of Dermatologists guidelines for the management of adults with basal cell carcinoma. *Br J Dermatol* 2021;**185**:899–920.

Newlands C, Currie R, Memon A et al. Non-melanoma skin cancer: United Kingdom National Multidisciplinary Guidelines. *J Laryngol Otol* 2016; **130**:S125–S132.

Bailey & Love's Essential Operations Bailey & Love's Essential Operations
Bailey & Love's Essential Operations Bailey & Love's Essential Operations
Bailey & Love's Essential Operations Bailey & Love's Essential Operations

PART 4 | Oncology

Chapter 29

Mohs Micrographic Surgery

Ross O. C. Elledge, Haytham al-Rawi

INTRODUCTION

Mohs micrographic surgery (MMS) was first described in 1941, when Frederick Mohs described a technique involving *in situ* fixation of skin cancers followed by excision. The excised specimen was subjected to horizontal sections from the undersurface to yield a more comprehensive examination of the surgical margin when compared with conventional surgery. In standard excision specimen processing ('bread loafing'), which examines only 0.01% of the entire soft tissue margin, the verdict of a 'complete excision' may well be incorrect, particularly in more aggressive histological subtypes.

In Mohs' original method (termed 'chemosurgery'), each 'stage' of excision lasted a day, as repeated overnight applications of zinc chloride were required in between stages. It was not until 1953 that Mohs began applying the principles to fresh tissue specimens taken under local anaesthesia, significantly shortening the duration of surgery. This technique is the one used by the majority of Mohs surgeons exclusively today. Modern Mohs surgeons are typically dermatologists by background, with expectations regarding training and maintaining competency clearly set out in the *Service Guidance and Standards for Mohs Micrographic Surgery (MMS)* document produced by the British Society for Dermatological Surgery (BSDS).

MMS has the dual advantages of enabling the smallest possible ablative defect while at the same time returning a more comprehensive histological examination (100% of the margin being examined) thereby minimising recurrence rates. The 5-year cure rate is typically in excess of 99% for primary BCC (92.2 – 96% for recurrent BCC) and while it appears more labour and resource intensive, multiple studies have attested to its cost effectiveness when applied to carefully selected cases with clear indications.

PREOPERATIVE CONSIDERATIONS

Indications

MMS may be used for a diverse range of tumour types including basal cell carcinoma (BCC), cutaneous squamous cell carcinoma (cSCC), follicular tumours, melanoma, melanoma *in situ*, dermatofibrosarcoma protruberans (DFSP), microcystic adnexal carcinoma (MAC), sebaceous carcinoma, Merkel cell carcinoma, atypical fibroxanthoma (AFX), extra mammary Paget's disease and others. This list is far from exhaustive, but by far the commonest application of MMS is for the treatment of BCCs and cSCCs meeting the indications outlined below.

Within the practice of the authors, all proposed MMS patients are discussed at the skin cancer multidisciplinary team (LSMDT or SSMDT, i.e. local or specialist) meeting with reference to clinical photographs and with clear reasons given for consideration. Reasons to consider MMS may include:

- Aggressive histological patterns (e.g. morphoeic, infiltrative or micronodular subtypes of BCC)
- Clinically poorly defined borders
- Critical anatomical location (e.g. central face, periorbital, etc.)
- Recurrent lesions or arising in previous radiotherapy fields
- Previous incomplete excision with conventional surgery
- Size of lesions (especially if >2 cm diameter)
- Immunosuppression
- Genetic syndromes (e.g. Gorlin–Goltz syndrome, xeroderma pigmentosum)
- Environmental exposures (e.g. arsenic)

The above is predicated on guidelines such as those issued by the BSDS. *Figures 29.1–29.4* represent a typical case of a classical micronodular BCC that would satisfy many of the criteria above.

Recurrent tumours may predispose to atypical growth patterns due to fibrosis from previous irradiation and/or scarring from excision. Certain anatomical areas may also encourage lateral growth patterns along

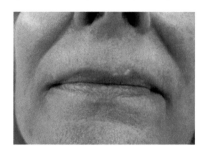

Figure 29.1 Biopsy-confirmed micronodular basal cell carcinoma (BCC) with clinically indistinct margins in a critical anatomical location.

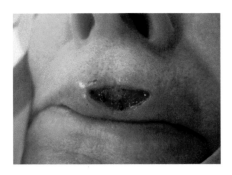

Figure 29.2 Resultant Mohs micrographic surgery defect is small but arguably challenging to repair given the loss of a reasonable length of vermilion with preservation of the cutaneous portion of the lip.

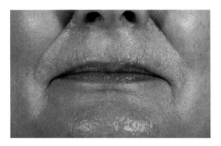

Figure 29.3 Repair at 2 months, achieved with lateral advancement flaps of vermilion combined with V-Y advancement from oral mucosa to maintain lip length.

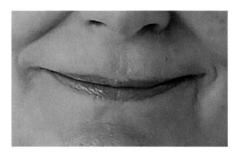

Figure 29.4 Repair at 18 months with seamless blending of mucosal advancement flap with remainder of vermilion.

deeper tissue (e.g. cartilage invasion in the pinna) that results in a 'tip of the iceberg' effect, causing operators to underestimate excision margins in conventional surgery. The so-called 'H-zone' of the face is the anatomical subsite that should give surgeons pause for thought to consider a discussion of MMS as a treatment option.

With regards to histological subtype, it is telling that micronodular BCC positive tumour margins have been shown to be as high as 18.6% on conventional excision, and in one study of morpheaform BCCs, spread was on average 7.2 mm from the clinically apparent tumour. While MMS use is well established in non-melanoma skin cancer (NMSC), its use in invasive and *in situ* melanoma is less frequent, not least due to the difficulty in identifying melanocytes in frozen sections without additional stains, increasing processing times. MMS can achieve superior margin control in rare tumour types, however (e.g. DFSP, AFX, etc.).

Preoperative investigations

There are few absolute contraindications to MMS. The main reasons revolve around existing multiple medical comorbidities or patients who are non-compliant due to dementia. Some giant neglected BCCs may not be suitable for MMS where tumour clearance is unlikely to be achievable and the morbidity resulting from the surgery is likely to be detrimental to the patient.

Patients do need to have a sufficient level of compliance to tolerate a staged procedure that may be many hours in length as well as the potential requirement for delayed reconstruction.

In situations where a complex repair is anticipated with possible implications for function and/or cosmesis, the authors have found a pre-ablative surgery appointment with the reconstructive surgeon to be beneficial. This enables a realistic discussion with the patient of likely reconstructive techniques that may be employed, the need for staged repairs (e.g. interpolated paramedian forehead flaps ± cartilage grafts), likely outcomes and the potential for complications that may be encountered. It will also enable the patient to develop a rapport with the reconstructive surgeon who may assume principal care of the patient postoperatively and during follow-up.

It should be noted, however, that exact dimensions may be difficult to anticipate as highlighted in *Figures 29.5* and *29.6*, where ablative surgical defects following multiple stages during the Mohs surgery are arguably more extensive than could first be anticipated, crossing multiple facial subunits.

Where extensive defects are anticipated, consideration should be given to ensuring that the option is

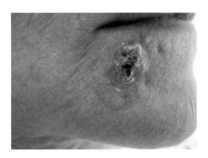

Figure 29.5 Biopsy-confirmed micronodular basal cell carcinoma (BCC) which was present for many years untreated, demonstrating clinically indistinct margins in a facial subunit with potential functional implications from distortion of the lower lip, oral sphincter (orbicularis oris) and buccal commissure.

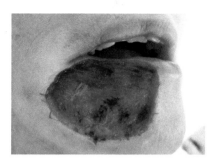

Figure 29.6 Mohs ablative defect of patient in Figure 29.5. While continuity of the orbicularis oris is maintained, there has been tissue loss extending into the medial cheek and vermilion, making reconstruction challenging. It would have been easy to underestimate the extent of the tumour and conventional excision would have almost certainly yielded involved margins.

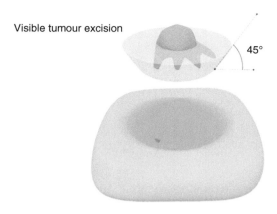

Figure 29.7 Removal of visible tumour with curettage or surgical blade.

available to the patient for repair under general anaesthesia. Such patients may also have developed some degree of 'fatigue' from repeated stages of Mohs surgery under local anaesthesia in the preceding days. This will involve planning ahead to secure a theatre session within an appropriate time frame of the ablative Mohs surgery (no longer than 7 days within the authors' practice) and ensuring that the patient has had a full preoperative assessment with any necessary investigations to facilitate the option of general anaesthesia if warranted.

STEPWISE OPERATIVE TECHNIQUE

Patients undergoing Mohs surgery are almost invariably treated using local anaesthesia due to the potential for multiple cycles being required and lengthy treatment sessions, although rarely sedation may be used in some centres. In our centre, we use 1% lidocaine, with adrenaline 1: 200 000, ensuring the safe dose limits for anaesthetic toxicity are not exceeded. For larger tumours, we rely on tumescent anaesthesia by diluting the local anaesthetic with normal saline. Some centres also use a combination with bupivacaine to achieve longer lasting anaesthesia.

The process involves the following steps:

- The patient is prepped with a suitable antiseptic solution and draped. Local anaesthetic is infiltrated
- Curettage or a surgical blade is used to remove the bulk of the tumour (*Figure 29.7*)
- Visible tumour excision is performed with a 2 mm margin of normal skin with orientation marked with superficial scalpel incisions ('hash marks'). Excision is done as a 'saucer' with inwardly bevelled incisions at the margins at 45° angle to the skin
- A temporary dressing is applied
- The specimen is divided and inked with various coloured dyes for orientation

- The specimen is flattened and frozen in 5–7 μm horizontal sections created and examined microscopically, with sections subdivided in specimens small enough to fit on a glass slide. These subdivisions are delineated with numbers and oriented with the use of coloured dye (*Figure 29.8*)

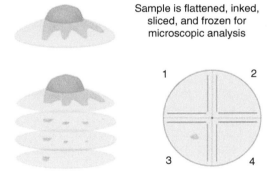

Figure 29.8 Preparation of the specimen and delineation of subdivisions.

- Positive tumour margins are marked on a mapping diagram (*Figure 29.9*)
- Further tissue samples are taken in corresponding tumour positive area(s) as delineated by the map, with augmentation of local anaesthesia if required
- This process is repeated until negative margins are obtained

The residual defect is then repaired with an appropriate reconstructive method. The Mohs surgeon themselves may undertake the repair or elect to engage the services of a colleague to facilitate more complex surgical repairs (e.g. specialists in oral and maxillofacial surgery, plastic surgery, ophthalmology/oculoplastics or otorhinolaryngology). Separate operators enable the Mohs ablative surgeon to concentrate on obtaining

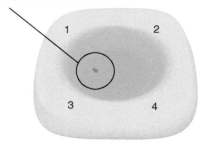

Mapping diagram identifies where further samples will be taken from

1   2

3   4

Figure 29.9 Mapping diagram preparation.

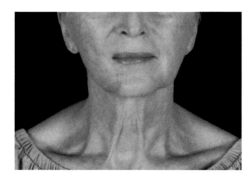

Figure 29.10 Patient from Figure 29.5 with repair at 6 months postoperatively. Repair utilised a lateral advancement flap from the ipsilateral cheek with excision of standing cone deformity from the nasolabial sulcus, blending the resultant scar with a normal anatomical structure. The lower lip was restored with a mucosal advancement flap over the intact orbicularis oris muscle.

clear margins and allow the reconstructive surgeon to operate safe in the knowledge that tumour clearance has been achieved.

In the head and neck region, repairs can be critical in terms of the importance of both cosmetic outcome and functional implications. Substandard repairs may invite complications including eyelid retraction and/or ectropion, oral incompetence and distortion of the nose with issues such as alar asymmetry due to retraction, contour abnormality and valve compromise.

POSTOPERATIVE CARE AND RECOVERY

In the authors' practice, if the Mohs surgeon is able to undertake the repair at the same sitting, then this is provided with further augmentation of local anaesthesia as required. If the complexity and/or size of the defect warrants a more complex repair, then availability of the reconstructive surgeon may enable repair at the same sitting. More frequently, this is done at a separate sitting within 7 days of the ablative surgery. In the intervening time period, the patient is given a course of oral flucloxacillin 500 mgs qds PO (erythromycin is substituted in penicillin allergy) and a dressing applied comprising a non-adherent layer (e.g., Jelonet® or Mepitel®), Sorbisan® or Kaltostat® is also applied to promote haemostasis, with an overlying occlusive dressing securely affixed to minimise the risk of bleeding and infection.

Within the authors' practice, clinical photographs are securely sent by the Mohs surgeon to the reconstructive surgeon on the day of the ablative surgery to enable final planning of the repair and/or further communication with the patient in advance of the reconstruction. As highlighted previously, multiple facial subunits may be involved and *Figure 29.10* exemplifies a repair that required a combination of techniques to achieve reconstruction with minimal distortion of anatomy, hence reducing the potential for functional and cosmetic deficits.

It should be noted that longer delays to reconstruction and composite defects involving more than one

facial subunit have been shown to correlate significantly with complication rates in Mohs surgery reconstruction.

Patients having local flap repairs are instructed to avoid exertion for at least 48 hours following reconstructive surgery, as well as keeping the wound dry and applying topical chloramphenicol 1.0% ointment. Suture removal for facial subunits is recommended within 5–7 days postoperatively. Graft recipient sites are inspected at 7–10 days, with further dressings selected based on healing at this point. The value of nursing staff with a special interest in wound management and tissue viability cannot be overstated.

POSSIBLE COMPLICATIONS AND HOW TO DEAL WITH THEM

Complications are similar to those encountered in any local anaesthetic dermatological surgery including (but not limited to): scarring; hypertrophic or keloid scarring; bleeding; bruising; flap or graft failure; alteration in sensation (including temporary or permanent numbness and/or neuropathic pain); and infection.

The key complication to avoid is patient dissatisfaction. Contracture from scarring may have cosmetic and functional implications as previously highlighted dependent on the facial subunit(s) involved. *Figures 29.11* and *29.12* demonstrate an unanticipated ablative defect involving the entire cheek subunit, which required a cervicofacial flap repair. Despite careful planning and execution, subsequent ectropion required further corrective revision surgery.

The most important consideration at the outset is to have an informed and prepared patient following a full and frank discussion (preferably with visual aids and written information) by the Mohs surgeon and separate reconstructive surgeon where warranted.

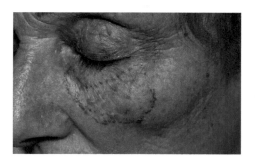

Figure 29.11 Preoperative clinical photograph of a poorly defined biopsy-confirmed infiltrative basal cell carcinoma of the left medial cheek.

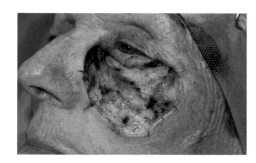

Figure 29.12 Post-Mohs ablative defect for lesion in Figure 29.11, which was much larger than anticipated requiring a large cervicofacial flap.

TOP TIPS AND HAZARDS

- Assessing expectations at the outset may inform reconstructive technique choice (e.g. a single stage nasolabial flap may be quicker, but a staged interpolated paramedian forehead flap is likely to more accurately recreate the nasofacial sulcus and contour of anatomical subunits).

- Reconstructions near the eyelid demand good periosteal suspension sutures to avoid ectropion, and perioral lesions demand a discussion at the outset of preserving the continuity of the oral sphincter to retain function at the cost of microstomia (e.g. Abbe-Estlander flaps, Karapandzic) weighed against other options such as a radial forearm free flap with palmaris longus tendon transfer.

- While it may be tempting to revise reconstructions early, time will often settle many issues including lymphoedema and visually apparent scarring (provided the contour is correct and scars are carefully placed).

- The reconstructive surgeon should have a range of different options available for refining results including (but not limited to) dermabrasion, steroid injections, laser resurfacing, fat transfer, camouflage make-up and scar revisions.

ACKNOWLEDGEMENT

With thanks to Cole Panayides for the accompanying illustrations.

FURTHER READING

Berens AM, Akkina SR, Patel SA. Complications in facial Mohs defect reconstruction. *Curr Opin Otolaryngol Head Neck Surg* 2017;**25**:258–64.

British Association of Dermatologists. *Service Guidance and Standards for Mohs Micrographic Surgery.* Available online at: https://www.bad.org.uk/shared/get-file.ashx?itemtype=document&id=6346.

Chen ELA, Srivastava D, Nijhawan RI. Mohs micrographic surgery: development, technique, and applications in cutaneous malignancies. *Semin Plast Surg* 2018;**32**:60–6.

Patel SA, Liu JJ, Murakami CS et al. Complication rates in delayed reconstruction of the head and neck after Mohs micrographic surgery. *JAMA Facial Plast Surg* 2016;**18**:340–6.

Wain RAJ, Tehrani H. The plastic and reconstructive Mohs surgery service. *J Plast Reconstr Aesthet Surg* 2014;**67**:331–5.

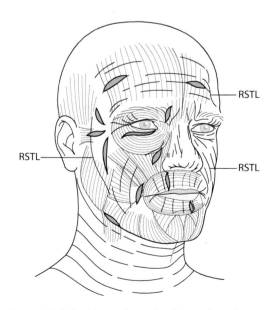

Chapter 30

Principles of Wound Repair and Harvesting Skin, Bone and Cartilage

Robert Isaac, Rabindra P. Singh, Peter A. Brennan

INDICATIONS

Surgeons are often faced with a plethora of wounds requiring differing forms of repair and reconstruction. This can be even more challenging in the head and neck where obvious deformity can have profound implications on a patient's quality of life. A comprehensive understanding of wound healing physiology is required to achieve the optimum outcome for the patient.

When considering reconstructing a wound, a surgeon must consider from the most basic of strategies, allowing the wound to heal via secondary intention, through to the most complex reconstructive method: free tissue transfer. This approach is commonly considered the reconstructive ladder. Each of the options within the reconstructive ladder have advantages and disadvantages (*Table 30.1*).

A firm grasp of the reconstructive ladder will always give a surgeon a 'fail-safe' option should a more complex method fail. For example, should a radial forearm free flap to the submental region fail, then a regional flap, for example in the form of a pectoralis major, can always be considered as a backup.

SURGICAL TECHNIQUE

Closure tension is the amount of stress per unit area along the edges of the wound. Wounds with excessive tension will result in widening of the subsequent scar and potential distortion of facial features such as the eyelid and upper lip. This will result in a conspicuous postoperative result.

Therefore, surgeons attempt to place their incisions using so-called 'lines of maximum extensibility'. These are areas of skin that are more extensible due to elastic fibres, allowing for reduced tension across the wound in a particular vector.

Perpendicular to lines of maximum extensibility are relaxed skin tension lines (RSTL). Lines of tension in skin were first identified by Dupuytren, and later referred to as relaxed skin tension lines by Borges. Relaxed skin tension lines arise from the orientation of collagen fibres. Placing incisions within RSTLs results in wound closure tension parallel to lines of maximum extensibility, thus minimising closure tension, resulting in a finer scar (*Figure 30.1*).

It is not uncommon for RSTLs to be used interchangeably with another term, 'Langer's Lines.' These are often used by surgeons to explain the same rationale; however, Langer's Lines were originally described as cleavage lines in cadavers. They were never intended to be used as locations for ideal surgical incisions.

The face is divided into a number of aesthetic regions, each sharing common characteristics such as colour, texture, thickness, hair growth etc. The boundaries of such aesthetic regions are determined by underlying attachment to the facial skeleton and musculature. Placing incisions in these boundaries can result in the scar being camouflaged.

DIRECT SKIN CLOSURE

This is best achieved using an elliptical incision placed in or as close to parallel as possible to the RSTLs in

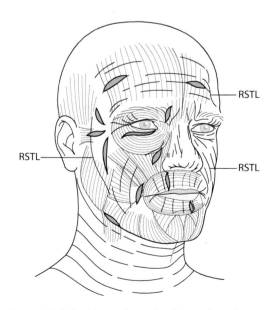

Figure 30.1 Incisions along the lines of tension, as shown, create narrow scars. Crossing these lines produces a broad ugly scar. These tension lines are even more important in the facial region.

TABLE 30.1 Reconstructive ladder options

Procedure	Advantages	Disadvantages
Allow wound to heal by secondary intention	• Simplest strategy requiring no reconstructive element • Harnesses body's natural healing potential	• Limited to wound beds that will allow for secondary intention • Takes longer to heal • Requires intensive wound management, e.g. dressings • Highly vulnerable to hypertrophic scarring and contracture
Direct closure	• Incision lines can be kept along the lines of natural tension, improving aesthetic outcome • Using local skin from the same aesthetic zone	• Limited defects only, as closure will create excessive tension leading to wound breakdown and infection
Skin graft – full thickness	• Large area of skin can be covered • Better aesthetics, in terms of thickness of the graft and aesthetic skin match than split skin but not as good as local flap	• Problems of a donor site, produces a second area of scarring • Poor skin colour and thickness match • Takes 10–14 days to heal
Skin graft – split skin	• Almost limitless amount of skin in terms of the head and neck	• Very poor skin texture and thickness match • Painful donor site • Both sites take 10–14 days to heal • Significant wound contracture – up to 20%
Local flap	• Allows much larger lesions to be closed • Skin has similar qualities as defect region, e.g. thickness, skin tone etc. • Usually can be raised from the same aesthetic zone	• Unlikely that all the skin incisions will run along natural tension lines • If only part of aesthetic zone is missing, it is sometimes better to remove entire zone
Regional flap	• No delay in healing • Retains its own blood supply negating the need for microvascular anastomosis • Robust technique	• Can result in donor site morbidity • Can result in deformity along path of pedicle
Skin – free tissue transfer	• Large area • No delay in healing • Usually possible to get the correct thickness	• Long surgical procedure • Poor colour and texture match

areas that have enough laxity to allow for direct closure. This can be tested preoperatively by 'pinching' the area.

Ideally a 3:1 length to width ratio is used, which can be marked preoperatively. Shelving should be avoided with an incision placed perpendicular to the skin; however, local undermining of the surrounding tissue can help to achieve tension-free closure (*Figure 30.2*).

One would think that the best means of closing a wound would be to approximate the wound edges together precisely. However, when the wound heals, the edges of the scar widen. Instead everting the wound edge will compensate for the spreading of the wound, resulting in a finer scar.

LOCAL AND REGIONAL FLAP CLOSURE

Unlike a skin graft, which is transferred to another region without a direct vascular supply, a flap is a segment of tissue with an established blood supply. Flaps can be considered as local, where the flap is taken from tissues adjacent to the defect, or regional, where the flap is obtained from a site distant to the head and neck, but where its blood supply is able to tolerate movement into the defect without compromise.

Nowadays with the number of units providing free tissue transfer, the use of regional flaps is becoming less common. Despite this, having a regional flap in mind can be an important fail-safe should the primary reconstruction fail.

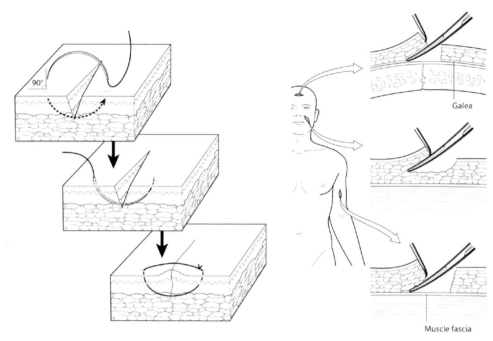

Figure 30.2 Undermining of the tissues should be in the subcutaneous level and only about 1 cm distance. Sharp dissection is better but may induce more bleeding than blunt dissection. Suturing with resultant skin eversion is imperative.

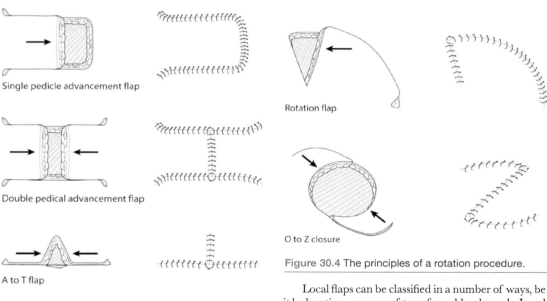

Single pedicle advancement flap

Double pedical advancement flap

A to T flap

Burow's triangle flap

Figure 30.3 The principles of an advancement procedure.

Rotation flap

O to Z closure

Figure 30.4 The principles of a rotation procedure.

Local flaps can be classified in a number of ways, be it by location, manner of transfer or blood supply. Local flaps are classified as being 'random pattern' where the blood supply is from the subdermal plexus, or 'axial', based on a named underlying vessel.

The local flap can be either 'advanced' or 'rotated' into the defect (see *Figures 30.3–30.5*). Some also consider the transposition flap as a separate category, but this is usually a variation of rotation and/or advancement (*Figure 30.6*).

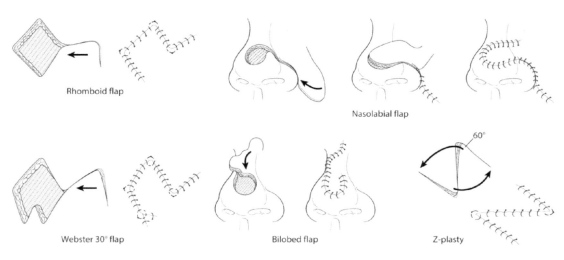

Figure 30.5 Different examples of rotation procedures.

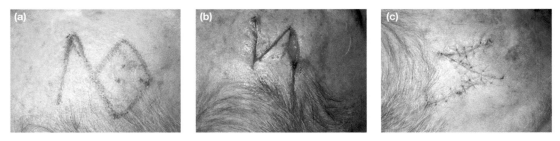

Figure 30.6 Transposition flap in the right temple area showing (a) marking, (b) flap raised and (c) postoperative appearance.

SKIN GRAFTING

A graft is tissue that is mobilised from one part of the body devoid of a blood supply and placed in another part of the body where it will need to acquire one.

The two types of skin graft are full-thickness, also known as Wolfe graft, and split-thickness grafts. Full-thickness skin grafts contain all of the dermis and its appendages, whereas split-thickness skin grafts contain varying levels of dermis (*Figure 30.7*).

Largely, the survival of a skin graft is dependent on its initial ability to receive nutrients from the underlying wound bed, prior to the revascularisation.

Skin graft success is based on three stages:

- *Plasmatic imbibition (first 24–48 hours)*: prior to establishing a new blood supply, the graft requires 'nourishment' from fluid movement from the underlying wound bed. This is principally reliant on diffusion and as such, the space between graft and wound bed must be kept to a minimum to prevent any barriers

- *Inosculation*: from 48 hours, capillary buds from the underlying wound bed begin to make contact with vessels within the graft
- *Revascularisation*: formal connections between graft and recipient blood vessels are established. The graft is revascularised

Failure rates of skin grafts have been documented at between 2% and 30%. Skin graft failure is typically down to one of three main mechanisms:

- Haematoma: affecting initial plasmatic imbibition
- Shearing forces: preventing the realignment of blood vessels between wound bed and skin graft
- Infection

It is therefore common practice to prepare the recipient site before application of an occlusive, sterile dressing. This is often bathed in an antimicrobial liquid prior to being secured with sutures or clips to limit space and movement between the graft and wound bed while also preventing potential infectious agents entering the wound.

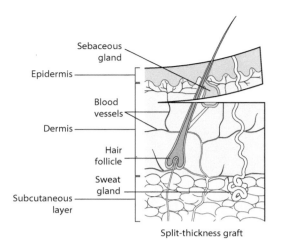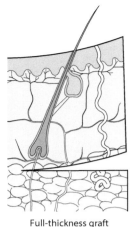

Split-thickness graft   Full-thickness graft

Figure 30.7 The differences between split- and full-thickness grafts.

Full-thickness graft

When deciding on a donor site, the surgeon must consider these key points:

- Prospective donor site is sufficiently lax to provide enough skin and achieve primary closure
- Good colour and thickness match
- Following harvesting of the skin graft, the patient should not be left with an obvious scar

The following donor sites are frequently used (*Figure 30.8*):

- *Root of the neck*: this can often provide up to 4–6 cm grafts, and can be hidden in a skin crease and the scar can be covered by clothing. The skin is thinner than that of the abdomen
- *Post-auricular*: the biggest issue with this site is the limited size of graft that can be obtained (usually no more than 2–3 cm in width). The scar is hidden and the colour match can be good. It can sometimes cause the pinna to be pulled back. It is not easily seen. The skin is thin with good colour match
- *Pre-auricular*: this provides a good colour and texture match for the facial skin but as with the post-auricular harvest site, is limited by width

- *Abdomen*: a large graft can usually be taken from the lower abdomen and hidden in the underwear line. These grafts are particularly good for larger defects

Technique

The graft can be harvested under local or general anaesthesia. Often a template can be made to represent the defect. This template can be used to mark the donor site as an exact replica of the primary defect. It is then excised as an ellipse to enable primary closure. The two end parts can be subsequently removed.

The skin is excised in to the underlying subdermis with a scalpel. The harvested graft should be defatted using scissors and the donor site should be closed in a two-layer technique (*Figures 30.9* and *30.10*).

Prior to insetting the graft at the defect, it is important to have meticulous haemostasis allowing intimate contact between the skin graft and wound bed. Some surgeons insert small stab incisions into the graft to allow for ventilation and prevention of build-up of a seroma or haematoma between the graft and wound bed. The graft is then secured in place with fine resorbable sutures and an occlusive, antimicrobial dressing is applied (as described above).

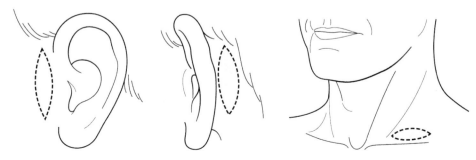

Figure 30.8 Good sites for full-thickness grafts.

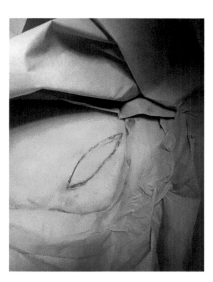

Figure 30.9 The abdomen is a good donor site for full-thickness skin grafts. They are often taken as an ellipse of tissue in the underwear line. There is often an excess of tissue in this area making primary closure straightforward.

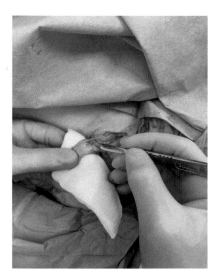

Figure 30.10 The graft is excised in the subdermis. If necessary, it can then be further defatted or thinned.

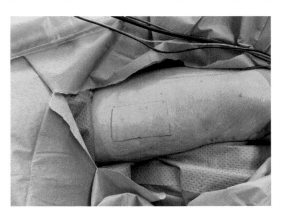

Figure 30.11 The lateral thigh is routinely used to provide a split-thickness skin graft. The leg is prepped; once the defect size is measured, it is drawn as a rough template at the prospective donor site.

Postoperative management

The grafted recipient site should ideally be left undisturbed for 10–14 days. During this time the patient is instructed to monitor the dressings for any evidence of haematoma, active bleeding or infection. Following this, the dressing can be removed and the recipient site can be cleaned of any excess tissue or debris.

Split-thickness skin grafts

As split-thickness skin grafts only remove part of the dermis, they heal by re-epithelialisation. As such, any part of the skin is a potential donor site! That being said, donor sites can heal with hyper/hypopigmentation and indeed scarring and this should limit the choice of donor site. Ideally a flat surface which is not too visible and has adequate dimension is chosen. This is often from the lateral aspects of the upper thigh or upper (non-dominant) arm (*Figure 30.11*).

Technique

The thinner the graft, the more likely it will form a blood supply but the greater the potential for contraction. Traditionally, the skin was harvested with a conventional handheld instrument (Humby knife); nowadays it is more common to use a dermatome (*Figures 30.12 and 30.13*).

The dermatome blade can be set to a particular thickness, producing a graft of universal, equal thickness.

The skin and dermatome should be well lubricated, with liquid paraffin or chlorhexidine-based solutions frequently chosen. A flat board should be advanced just in front of the dermatome to ensure a flat surface is presented to the blade (*Figure 30.14*).

Meshing of the graft can increase the size of the graft by about 30%, but in most cases is merely used to create small perforations allowing ventilation and escape of potential haematoma or seroma.

Once the graft has been obtained, it is transferred to the defect site and inset with resorbable sutures. Following this, again an occlusive, antimicrobial dressing is secured in place with non-resorbable sutures or staples.

Postoperative management

The donor site can be painful but this must be anticipated and prevented. A commonly used technique is

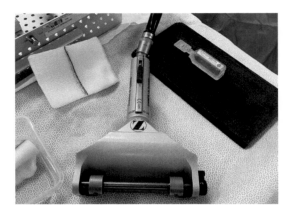

Figure 30.12 A dermatome provides a graft of even, consistent thickness.

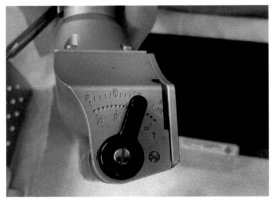

Figure 30.13 Usually on such a dermatome, the thickness of skin achieved can be set by a dial mechanism.

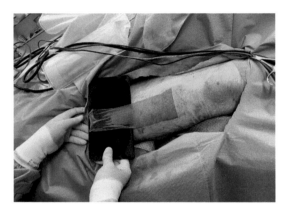

Figure 30.14 A flat board is advanced in front of a well-lubricated surface of skin, allowing the dermatome to glide across the dermis. Here you can see the split-thickness skin graft reflected on itself on to the board. The next step is dividing it, with scissors from the underlying free edge of skin.

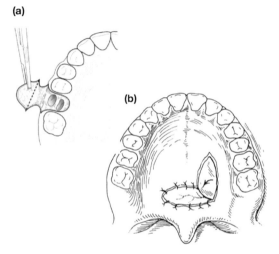

Figure 30.15 (a) Lateral advancement flap for closure of an oroantral fistula. In this case, the periosteum is cut gently to give much greater laxity to the overlying mucosa enabling closure. (b) Palatal transposition flap based on the greater palatine artery can be raised to close a palatal defect.

to apply an alginate-soaked dressing impregnated with long-acting local anaesthetic, such as 0.5% bupivicaine. Regular systemic analgesia is also useful.

The wound should be left untouched for 14 days, after which the occlusive dressing can be removed. In the interim period, the patient is again advised to monitor for evidence of haematoma, active bleed or signs of infection.

ORAL MUCOSAL FLAPS

As with commonly used skin flaps, mucosal flaps can be directly closed, or be taken as local rotational and advancement flaps. As with skin flaps, excessive tension will reduce the blood supply and lead to dehiscence. Therefore, the flap length/width ratio should be no more than about 4:1.

Like local flaps in the skin, mucosal flaps can either be random pattern or axial pattern. In reality, the only non-muscle flap with a true axial element is based on the greater palatine vessels, the rest are random pattern flaps (e.g. the buccal advancement flap used to close oroantral communications) (*Figure 30.15*).

Unlike skin, the local anatomical variations of the mucosa demand special attention. It is most important that attached mucosa is attached to the gingiva of the teeth so flaps must be designed to ensure that the mucogingival junction is maintained. When this is not possible, a free full-thickness attached mucosal graft is harvested, usually from the palate. This can be achieved using a microdermatome.

NON-VASCULARISED BONE HARVESTING

Bone grafting can be achieved from four sources, which are listed in *Chapter 10 (p. 68)*. Autogenous grafts are considered the gold standard as they possess all three characteristics, which aid in new bone formation:

- *Osteogenesis*: obtain cells such as osteoblasts that can actively produce bone in their new environment
- *Osteoinduction*: obtain growth factors capable of recruiting host cells from surrounding tissues that can deposit new bone
- *Osteoconduction*: provide a scaffold-like structure which can facilitate ingrowth of new vessels, bony deposition and remodelling

Like skin grafts, during an initial period of inflammation, grafts must survive on nutrients from the surrounding wound bed prior to revascularisation. It is therefore essential that the graft is placed in a highly vascular region, absent of infection.

Following this initial inflammatory period, osteoid and new bone are laid down by viable cells within the graft. This is known as the proliferative stage.

The bone graft does not 'survive' once transplanted. While acting as a scaffold for osteoid deposition, it provides growth factors to stimulate angiogenesis and osteoblast recruitment and is resorbed by osteoclasts. New bone is laid down while existing bone is resorbed. This is the remodelling stage and can take months to years to complete.

Autogenous bone grafts can be cortical, cancellous or particulate. Cortical bone takes longer to resorb than cancellous or particulate bone and because of its structural integrity can be used as block grafts. Cortical bone, however, has reduced osteogenic properties and takes longer to revascularise than particulate or cancellous bone, which contain large spaces for blood vessel ingrowth.

Indications

Due to the increasing role of microvascular techniques, certainly in the developed world, widespread use of non-vascularised bone grafts is not as common as it once was. There are, however, several indications where non-vascularised bone grafts are useful:

- Alveolar bone defects in cleft lip and palate
- Small defects in the jaws, whereby the defect is surrounded by bone walls (*Figure 30.16*)
- Small bone defects in which an implant is to be placed
- Post-traumatic grafting, e.g. orbital defects
- Secondary jaw reconstruction of small continuity defects, where fragments have been stabilised by bone plates

Common donor sites

A few sites are commonly used for bone harvest (see *Table 30.2*).

Surgical techniques

Cranium

Bone may be harvested at the time of bicoronal flap or from an incision made over the parietal bone prominence taking care to avoid damaging hair follicles (*Figure 30.17*).

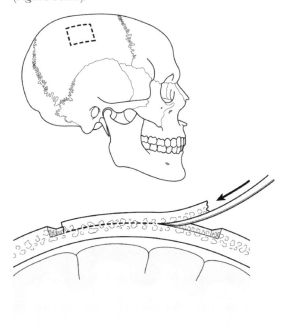

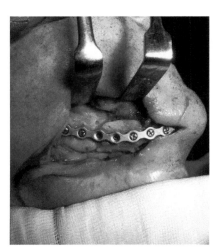

Figure 30.16 Iliac crest bone graft for small mandibular defect.

Figure 30.17 A groove is scored through the outer table and the outer table is removed with fine chisels.

TABLE 30.2 Common donor sites

Site	Indications and disadvantages
Cranium, outer cortical plate	Hard stable bone, scar normally hidden in the hair. Difficult to carve and manipulate. Reported risk of precipitating intracranial bleeding. Small volume.
Rib with or without costal cartilage	Small volume, very soft but pliable bone. With the cartilage in 30% of cases harvested in young children, it will continue to grow. Small risk of chest complications, especially in the elderly, pneumothorax and chest infection. Can be painful.
	In young females, the harvesting may, if too high, damage breast development
Iliac crest	Yields large volumes of bone (especially with the posterior approach), it has an unobtrusive scar. While it is very painful, unless a trephine is used, it has few significant side effects. Damage to the lateral cutaneous nerve of the thigh should be easy to avoid, but it does happen and is a significant problem. Fractures of the iliac crest can occur. The posterior approach is much less frequently used as it is necessary to rotate the patient prevent synchronous surgery to the mouth and bone harvest.
Tibia	This is a trephine approach which yields small volumes but is ideal for alveolar defects. Few complications and little pain, but unrewarding in elderly patients as the bone is replaced by fat and blood.
Intraoral	See *Chapter 10, Bone Augmentation Techniques in Oral Implantology*

The incision is down to bone, and the periosteum is elevated. The outline of the bone graft is cut in the outer table with an oscillating or ultrasonic saw, fissure burs or small curved chisels. The outer plate is then raised with osteotomes. While parietal bone is used most commonly due to its inherent thickness, it may be helpful to obtain a preoperative computed tomography (CT) to ensure adequate bone volume.

Alternatively, when working concomitantly with neurosurgeons, particularly when a craniotomy is performed, the inner table can be harvested and used, prior to re-siting the bony segment in its existing site.

As the bone is very rigid and hard, it has to be fashioned with cuts and bending forceps to the desired shape. It may be necessary to grind the bone to produce small fragments to pack around the main graft and produce a smooth contour at the recipient site.

Closure usually requires a small vacuum drain and should be in layers.

Rib

Refer to *Chapter 52* for the rib harvesting technique.

Iliac crest

An anterior approach is most commonly utilised. Access to the posterior iliac spine does yield larger volumes of bone; however, it requires intraoperative turning of the patient.

For an anterior approach, the incision is outlined after having marked the anterior superior iliac spine (ASIS) (*Figure 30.18*). The approach is deepened through the soft tissues (*Figure 30.19*) and down to the iliac crest (*Figure 30.20*).

Once down to bone, either the lateral or medial tissues should be elevated depending on which surface is to be harvested. On most occasions, it will be the

medial side as less muscle stripping is needed and it is less painful. The bone cuts should be made so that most of the crest remains intact with at least 1 cm of anterior iliac spine left untouched. This prevents weakness and subsequent fracture.

Harvest is then achieved by elevating the crest and hinging it laterally, so allowing access to the cancellous bone, before being returned once harvest is complete. In some circumstances, if only a thin piece of bone is needed, two-thirds of the crest can be preserved and a

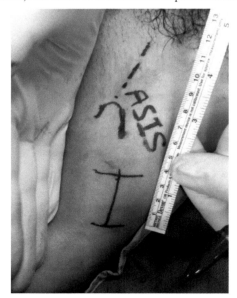

Figure 30.18 Incision marked for iliac bone harvest on the left side. The anterior superior iliac spine (ASIS) is shown. For orientation the groin in superiorly and the umbilicus is under the green marking pen.

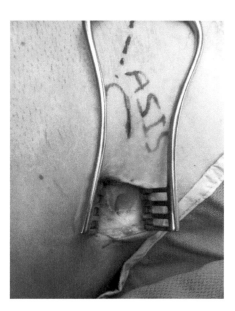

Figure 30.19 Dissection through the overlying muscles.

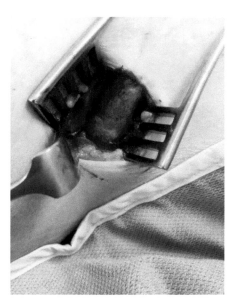

Figure 30.20 Exposure of the iliac crest with muscle and periosteal stripping.

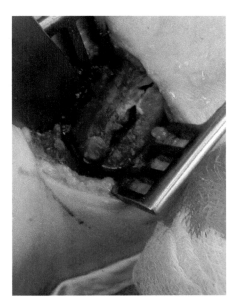

Figure 30.21 Bone cuts have been made using saws and the medial part of the crest can be removed using an osteotome. It is important to protect the medial structures when completing the bone cuts.

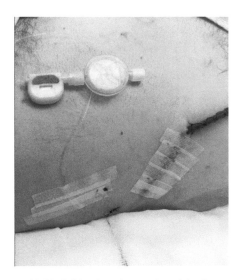

Figure 30.22 Epidural catheter placed in the wound for instillation of regular local anaesthesia to reduce postoperative pain.

thin slice of medial bone removed (*Figure 30.21*). The iliac crest if temporarily hinged laterally, should be kept attached to periosteum to preserve the blood supply and stability to the replaced crest.

Supplementary fixation is not normally needed. Prior to closure, an epidural catheter should be placed to allow infusion of long-acting local anaesthetic for the first 24 hours for analgesia (*Figure 30.22*).

If the periosteum and muscle are tightly approximated, this seems to reduce the haematoma by tamponade action. It may be helpful to place the suction drain just subcutaneously to avoid a haematoma. Bone wax should be avoided as this produces a foreign body reaction often requiring further exploration of the wound.

The process can be made less painful by a trephining technique. A small 1-cm stab incision is made on to

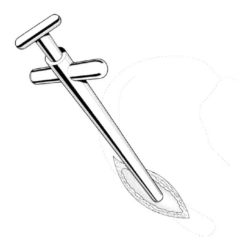

Figure 30.23 A core of cortical cancellous bone can be extracted using a trephine via a small stab incision.

the anterior crest and a trephine is directed posteriorly/inferiorly. This produces a core of cortical cancellous bone but a much smaller volume than an open procedure (*Figure 30.23*).

Postoperatively, temporary gait disturbances are not uncommon. The patient is advised not to fully weight-bear in the first week post-surgery, with a full return to normal exercise not considered before week 6. The patient should also be warned of potential cutaneous paraesthesia of the thigh and while minimal, the presence of a scar at the donor site.

Tibia

The proximal tibia offers a good volume of bone, comparable with that of an anterior approach to the iliac crest. It is relatively simple and has low morbidity.

An incision is placed laterally on the proximal tibia at Gerdy's tubercle. Here there are no underlying structures of concern and an incision can be made through skin, subcutaneous tissue and iliotibial tract onto underlying periosteum.

Either the bone can be trephined, or a small opening through cortical bone can be made with a fissure bur. Cores of cortical cancellous bone can be harvested in a medial and inferior direction away from inadvertently entering the joint, or in children, away from the epiphyseal growth centre (*Figure 30.24*).

Closure is normally a single layer. Post closure, the leg is wrapped with a pressure dressing. The patient is advised to begin mobilisation, but instructed to avoid full weight-bearing for a few days and a return to strenuous exercise for up to 6 weeks.

Intraoral sites

The use of intraoral donor sites for bone grafting is commonly used in implant surgery where prosthetic-guided bone augmentation is employed. The use of local sites limits morbidity and allows the surgeon to obtain small volumes of easily accessible bone (refer to *Chapter 10* for intraoral bone harvesting techniques).

Guided bone regeneration

This is sometimes employed in prosthetic-guided bone augmentation. It is based on the principle that bone-growing cells take longer to populate the defect and as such, a barrier, usually made of polytetrafluoro-ethylene (PTFE) or collagen based, is used to prevent ingrowth of soft tissue cells. This barrier is secured over the defect site and is either later removed or resorbs.

Recipient bed preparation

It is common practice to create multiple perforations in the cortex of the defect, to allow host growth factors

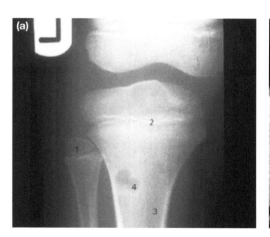
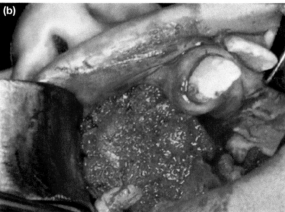

Figure 30.24 (a) 1, Head of fibula, which can be easily palpated, below the epiphysis; 2, epiphysis; 3, the trephine should not enter the shaft; 4 entry site. (b) The tibial graft easily fills this cleft alveolar defect.

to expedite neovascularisation and bone deposition. Some authors have advocated the role of additional platelet-rich plasma, derived from the patient's platelets to enhance angiogenesis and subsequent healing.

Cartilage grafts

There are several frequently used sites as outlined in *Table 30.3*.

Costochondral cartilage

Refer to '*Harvesting Technique*' in *Chapter 52*.

Ear

There are three sites: the small concave conchal bowl area, the longer curved area between the helix and antihelix and the tragus itself. The site is infiltrated with local anaesthetic for pain relief and to aid the dissection. The flap is raised in a subperichondral plane and the clean cartilage surface exposed. All sites are approached anteriorly, although they can be harvested from behind if prevention of a visible scar is essential. The skin flaps are sutured in one layer and a compression dressing with tie-over sutures placed to prevent haematoma formation.

Nasal septum

After infiltration with local anaesthetic, two approaches can be used. Traditionally, a small curved anterior incision is made on one side of the septum. An alternative is to make a high anterior intraoral incision around the nasal spine. This has the advantage of picking up the septal cartilage low down on the palatal shelf and the stripping of the mucoperiosteum is significantly simpler

TABLE 30.3 Frequently used sites for cartilage grafts

Site	Advantages and disadvantages
Rib	Can be harvested with bone
	Good bulk, but limited length
	May 'grow' in children
	Painful
Ear	Small area, and thin
	Not 'flat'
	Painful
Nasal septum	Invisible scar
	Flat
	Good size, but thin
	Few complications

and easier than the traditional approach. Stripping of the mucoperiosteum is the difficult part of the procedure and a sharp dissector is essential, to ensure no perforations of the mucosa occur. If a perforation does occur in both surfaces, a permanent fistula is likely to create an irritating whistling sound on breathing. Once the mucoperiosteum has been raised on the operative side, an incision is made through the cartilage and stripping commenced on the contralateral side. The septum can then be excised and harvested. If the nose is not to 'collapse', a horizontal and anterior vertical strut of cartilage about 5 mm in width must be preserved (*Figures 30.25–30.27*).

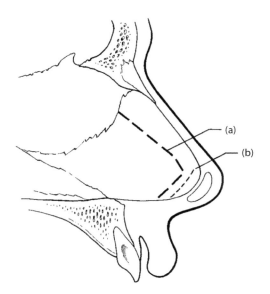

Figure 30.25 Right lateral view of nasal septum to show (a) mucosal cut anteriorly and (b) septal cut a few millimetres posterior to this.

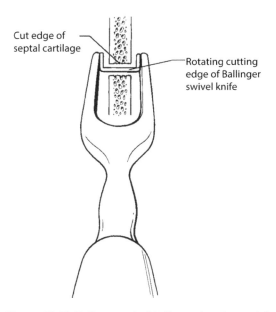

Figure 30.26 Ballinger swivel knife cutting the septal cartilage.

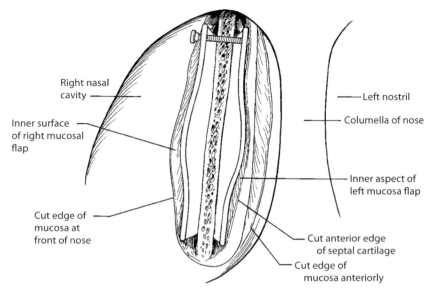

Right nasal cavity

Inner surface of right mucosal flap

Cut edge of mucosa at front of nose

Left nostril

Columella of nose

Inner aspect of left mucosa flap

Cut anterior edge of septal cartilage

Cut edge of mucosa anteriorly

Figure 30.27 View of the cut surface of the septal cartilage from the front through the right nostril after retraction of the mucoperichondrial flaps with a Killian's speculum.

Closure is in a single layer and supplemented by through-and-through mattress sutures to prevent haematoma formation. Sometimes, bilateral packs are placed to prevent haematoma formation but, while a traditional approach, its value in producing compression in the right place is doubtful.

FURTHER READING

Brennan PA, Mahadevan V, Evans BT. *Clinical Head and Neck Anatomy for Surgeons*. Boca Raton, FL: CRC Press; 2015.

Brennan PA, Standring SM, Wiseman SM. *Gray's Surgical Anatomy*. Oxford: Elsevier; 2020.

Fonseca RJ. *Oral and Maxillofacial Surgery*, Third Edition. Elsevier; 2018.

Ilankovan V, Ethunandan M, Seah T. *Local Flaps in Facial Reconstruction. A Defect Based Approach*. New York, NY: Springer; 2015.

TOP TIPS AND HAZARDS

- Incisions should always be placed in or as near to RSTLs as possible.
- Aim for eversion of the skin edge on closure. This will allow for contraction and prevent widening of the scar.
- Meticulous technique and haemostasis, and a two-layer closure is essential for the best results.
- When replacing skin in the facial region, the donor skin or skin flap should ideally be from the same aesthetic zone.
- A split-thickness skin graft should be no thicker than 0.2 mm (the thickness of a size no. 15 scalpel).
- Full-thickness skin grafts should be raised in the subdermis from a donor site amenable to primary closure.
- When harvesting a parietal calvarial bone graft, a preoperative CT scan can be invaluable in determining the thickness of bone that can be safely obtained.
- There are many sites for harvesting non-vascularised grafts but the iliac crest and proximal tibia provide a good volume of bone with low morbidity at the donor site.
- For prosthesis-guided implant placement, where possible, intraoral bone harvest can result in adequate bone volumes with limited additional morbidity.

Bailey & Love's Essential Operations Bailey & Love's Essential Operations
Bailey & Love's Essential Operations Bailey & Love's Essential Operations
Bailey & Love's Essential Operations Bailey & Love's Essential Operations

PART 5 | Reconstructive surgery

Chapter

31

Local and Pedicled Orofacial Flaps

Ashleigh Weyh, Majid Rezaei, Rui Fernandes

INTRODUCTION

Reconstruction of orofacial defects is a true reconstructive challenge as there is the need to re-establish both esthetics and function, while operating in a complex anatomical region. The selected list of local and pedicle flaps is in no way meant to be comprehensive, but instead representative of some of the most common and useful flaps when reconstructing both simple and complex orofacial defects.

Ultimately, flap selection is based on careful patient analysis of the defect location, size, depth, status of the recipient bed, as well as patient comorbidities, especially a history of smoking or previous radiation. As there is a large array of flaps to choose from, it is generally best to start with the simplest local flap, and then move up the reconstruction ladder as needed based on what is needed to achieve the best functional and cosmetic result with the least morbidity.

LOCAL FLAPS

Palatal flap

Principle

Technically simple and predictable, and it can be raised as an axial (palatal island) or random flap

(rotation-advancement flap). As an axial flap, up to 75% of the palatal mucosa can be used, to close defects up to 16 cm^2 in size. As a random flap, it is most suitable for oroantral communications, as it has less reach due to a less reliable blood supply.

Anatomy

The palatal mucosa is very adherent to the underlying periosteum. The rich anastomotic network with the nasopalatine artery anterior and the greater palatine artery posterior courses through the mucosa, submucosa and periosteum, allowing for the palate to be raised as a random flap, even with greater palatine ligation.

Procedure

For the palatal island-axial flap (*Figure 31.1*), a posteriorly based horseshoe incision is made, with medial incision near the palatal midline, and lateral incision approximately 5 mm from the gingival margins. Subperiosteal dissection is carried out anterior to posterior.

To increase reach, palatine neurovascular bundle can be freed from the foramen to increase the arch of rotation.

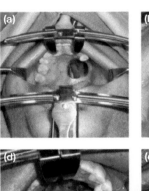
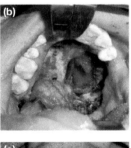
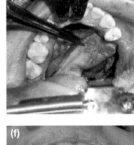
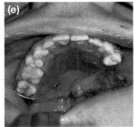
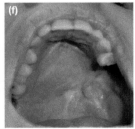

Figure 31.1 Palatal flap. (a) Patient after resection of palatal lesion with underlying bone margin. (b) Elevation of palatal flap based off right greater palatine artery. (c) Reach of flap. (d) Insetting of the palatal flap. (e) Use of a palatal splint to assist in healing of the flap and to cover exposed bone. (f) Final healing of repaired palatal defect.

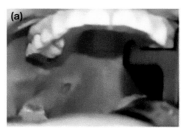
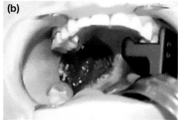
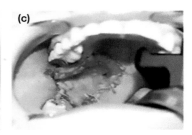

Figure 31.2 Buccal fat pad flap. (a) Patient with a polymorphous low-grade adenocarcinoma of soft palate. (b) Resulting defect after resection of palatal mucosa and Brown I maxillectomy. (c) Defect repaired with buccal fat pad.

Pitfalls

Donor site palatal bone is often left denuded, which causes patient discomfort due to slow re-epithelialization of the denuded palatal bone. This can be avoided by raising the flap submucosally, using the superficial layer to cover the donor site, and a separate submucosal flap to repair the defect.

Buccal fat pad

Principle

A simple and reliable flap due to its location and rich blood supply, especially for repairing oroantral fistulas or smaller Brown type I maxillectomy defects. Intraoral epithelialization of this flap occurs within 3–4 weeks.

Anatomy

It is composed of a main body and four extensions (lobes): temporal, buccal, pterygoid and pterygopalatine. When properly dissected, the fat pad provides a 6 × 5 × 3 cm graft. The highly vascularized fat pad is supplied by the maxillary artery, and superficial and deep temporal arteries.

Procedure

A 2–3 cm mucosal incision is made ≥2 cm inferior to Stensen's duct, through the buccinator (*Figure 31.2*). Blunt dissection and mild traction via tissue forceps is used to assist the pad as it herniates out of this opening. This prevents injury to the capsule overlying the fat, while preserving blood supply and maintaining volume.

The herniated pad is stretched over the defect and sutured through the capsule to the periphery of the defect.

Pitfalls

The flap can undergo necrosis or dehiscence, especially if the capsule is torn from mishandling. Tension-free closure and use of a nasogastric tube postoperatively can be used to prevent dehiscence when appropriate.

Paramedian forehead flap

Principle

The main use of the paramedian flap is to reconstruct partial to total nasal defects, but can be used to reconstruct any area within its arc of rotation. This flap provides excellent color, thickness and texture match to surrounding skin. However, the main drawback is the need for multiple staged surgery, spanning over the course of several weeks.

Anatomy

The blood supply is based on the supratrochlear vessels. The artery is located just above the pericranium as it emerges from its foramen caudally, but as one travels towards the hairline the vessel branches are in a more subcutaneous plane.

Procedure

Stage one: The supratrochlear artery is marked (Doppler can assist with design). The pedicle is centered over the artery, with a width of 1.5 cm, while pedicle length is determined by the size and location of the defect.

Elevation of the flap begins subperiosteally or in a subgaleal plane at the most superior aspect, traveling caudal until approximately 1 cm superior to the brow, to protect the vascular pedicle. From here, dissection then must continue above the periosteum (*Figure 31.3*).

The flap is inset from most caudal to cephalad, where the most superior portion is not sutured into the skin due to the skin and vascular pedicle.

The forehead defect is closed inferior to superior, and if primary closure is not possible then it can be left to heal by secondary intention.

Stage two: The flap must heal for no less than 3 weeks to develop collateral circulation, before sectioning the pedicle. If there is any question about collateral blood supply prior to amputation, the pedicle can be constricted with a rubber band for a few minutes to evaluate blood flow and color.

Pitfalls

If unable to close the resulting forehead during stage one, later scar revision may be needed.

Cervicofacial flap

Principle

A cheek rotational advancement flap (also known as a Mustardé flap) that is well suited for the defects

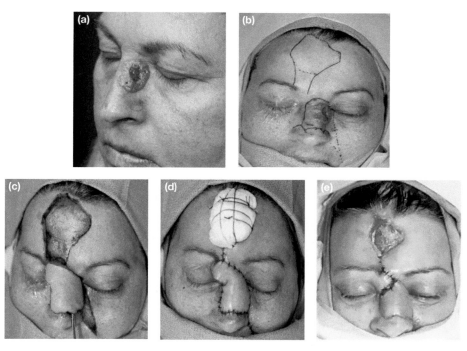

Figure 31.3 Paramedian forehead flap. (a) Preoperative photo. (b) Planned resection of lateral nasal lesion and planned paramedian forehead flap. (c) Raised paramedian flap and testing inset for adequate reach. (d) Closure of flap with forehead defect left to heal by secondary intention due to inability to close. (e) Second-stage surgery takedown. Note forehead defect will require closure via skin grafting or local tissue rearrangement in a third-staged surgery.

of lower lid and medial or lateral cheek regions. The major advantages are excellent color and skin texture match.

Anatomy

The flap is usually raised subcutaneously, as the blood supply depends on a rich subdermal plexus of vessels. However, a deep plane sub-superficial musculoaponeurotic system (SMAS) elevation has also been recommended, especially for smokers, which gives the flap an axial blood supply, utilizing the superficial temporal artery for a posteriorly based flap, or the facial/submental arteries for an anteriorly based flap.

Procedure

The expected defect is marked and the flap design is outlined (anteriorly versus posteriorly based) (*Figure 31.4*). The flap design could be extended anteriorly toward the lateral canthal region and superiorly along the hairline. The marking also includes the pre- and post-auricular area toward the hairline behind the ear similar to the rhytidectomy approach. It then continues through the neck, along the anterior border of the trapezius muscle.

The flap is elevated subcutaneously in a supra-SMAS plane, although dissection should continue underneath the platysma in the neck. Elevation

continues until adequate rotation/advancement is obtained and the defect is closed primarily without tension.

Pitfalls

Distal flap margin necrosis and hematoma formation.

Temporal artery posterior auricular skin flap (TAPAS flap)

Principle

A non-hair-bearing fasciocutaneous flap, that may also be raised as a free flap, for reconstruction of small to medium sized defects of the face and oral cavity, as well as the ear. It provides an ultrathin skin flap with good skin color and texture match. It is reported that a skin paddle can be raised as large as 70×70 mm^2, and its arc of rotation allows reconstruction of almost all of the ipsilateral face.

Anatomy

This flap utilizes the posterior auricular skin based on the superior auricular branch of the superficial temporal artery. The flap can be designed as chimeric to also bring superficial temporal fascia, or vascularized cartilage from the inferior portion of the concha.

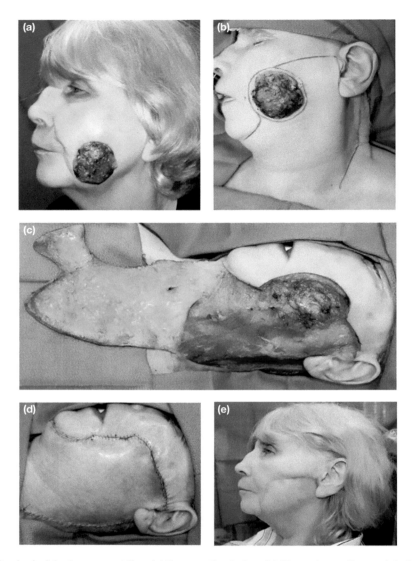

Figure 31.4 Cervicofacial advancement flap. (a) Preoperative lesion. (b) Planned resection and design for cervico-facial advancement flap. (c) Flap has been raised. (d) Inset and suturing of the flap. (e) Late postoperative photo.

Procedure

The skin paddle is centered over the retroauricular sulcus, where the anterior border can be extended anteriorly onto the pinna, and posterior to the hairline (*Figure 31.5*).

The flap is elevated in a supra-perichondrial plane beginning at the lobule inferiorly, working towards the root of the helix superiorly.

Pitfalls

The superior auricular artery may be congenitally absent, thus mapping the pedicle with Doppler prior to elevation is recommended.

PEDICLED FLAPS

Supraclavicular flap

Principle

A thin and pliable, axial, fasciocutaneous flap used for reconstruction of stomal, mandible, intra-oral, parotid, neck, skull base and facial skin defects. Advantages include minimal donor site morbidity, reliable pedicle, good color match and texture, and ease of harvest. It may also be used in the multiply operated and vessel-depleted neck. The amount of tissue available for transfer and flap length is limited to what can be harvested while still allowing for primary closure of the donor site.

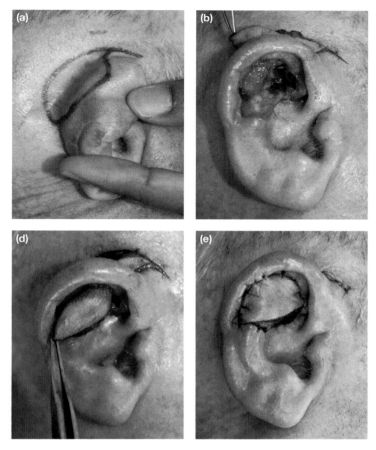
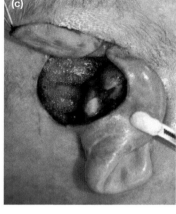

Figure 31.5 Temporal artery posterior auricular skin (TAPAS) flap. (a) Marking of skin for TAPAS flap. (b) Skin defect upper third of ear. (c) Fully raised TAPAS flap and its reach. (d) Insetting of flap. (e) Final closure.

This flap is contraindicated in the case of prior level V neck dissection and concern for prior disruption of the transverse cervical or supraclavicular artery.

Anatomy

The main blood supply (axial) is the supraclavicular artery, a branch of the transverse cervical artery. The artery can be found in a triangle formed by the posterior border of the sternocleidomastoid muscle, the external jugular vein and the clavicle. The artery is usually found 3 cm above the clavicle. The diameter of the artery is 1.5 mm. The harvestable skin area ranges from 10–16 cm wide to 22–30 cm long.

Procedure

The shape of the defect is transferred to the shoulder directly over the angiosome of the supraclavicular artery, identifying the main pedicle with a Doppler (*Figure 31.6*). A pinch test determines the width of the flap while allowing primary closure.

The elevation of the flap begins from distal to proximal in a suprafascial or subfascial plane until the supraclavicular vascular pedicle is identified. Subfascial dissection around the clavicle and then skeletonization

of the pedicle to its takeoff from the transverse cervical artery will improve arc of rotation.

Flap inset with connection to the neck scar rather than tunneling is recommended to avoid constriction of the pedicle. Proximal flap may be de-epithelialized if needed.

Pitfalls

Large visible scar at donor site, and can result in some neck constriction.

Submental artery island flap

Principle

Despite having reliable pedicle, good color match and well-hidden scar, wide acceptance has been slow due to difficult dissection of the pedicle and concern of oncologic safety in cancer patients.

Anatomy

This flap is an axial fasciocutaneous flap based on submental artery which takes off 5–6 cm from the origin of the facial artery with a mean diameter of 1.7 mm. Cutaneous perforators pierce the platysma muscle and

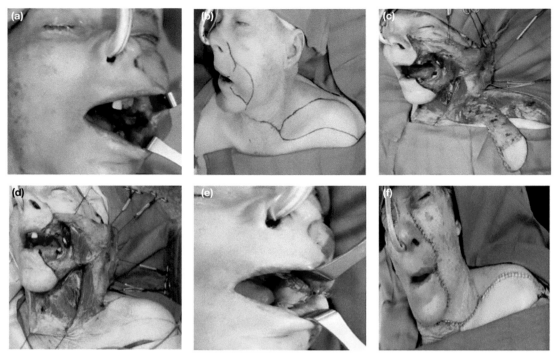

Figure 31.6 Supraclavicular flap. (a) Buccal mucosa squamous cell carcinoma prior to resection. (b) Proposed supraclavicular flap and resection margin of malignancy. (c, d) Completed resection, neck dissection and raised supraclavicular skin flap with pedicle. (e) Inset of the skin paddle to repair buccal defect. (f) Final closure.

merge into the subdermal plexus and anastomose with contralateral artery. The harvested flap could be, from angle to angle, as wide as 7–8 cm with a length of 17–18 cm. Pedicle length is 5–8 cm with an excellent arch of rotation. The submental artery traverses deep to the anterior belly of digastric muscle in 70% of cases.

Procedure

A pinch test is used to determine available skin, while being able to primarily close the donor site.

Skin/subcutaneous tissue is incised, and dissection continues over the fascia of the contralateral anterior belly of digastric muscle. Dissection is then extended over the mylohyoid muscle, followed by ipsilateral digastric muscle (*Figure 31.7*).

Attachment of the muscle to inferior border of mandible is detached, and anterior belly is included in the flap and sectioned at the intermediate tendon. Submental vessels are identified and skeletonized to their takeoff from facial vessels. The submandibular gland is usually removed at this point.

Reach can be improved by dividing the facial vessels distal to the submental vessels, or by dividing the posterior belly of the digastric and skeletonizing the vessels to the external carotid and internal jugular vein.

The flap is tunneled subcutaneously or intraorally depending on the location of the defect.

Pitfalls

Tedious pedicle dissection, oncologic safety issues and contraindication in metastatic neck involvement.

POSTOPERATIVE CONSIDERATIONS

The postoperative course of local and pedicled flaps is typically less tenuous than free flaps, and often patients can be discharged home the same day. Flaps can be monitored by simple clinical observation. Most complications result from poor planning, causing excessive tension across the flap, which then causes a myriad of problems. First, wound edges can simply undergo dehiscence causing poor esthetics and scarring. Excess tension can also cause pull, distorting adjacent anatomy which can result in a function deficit such as lagophthalmos, or unesthetic asymmetries. Tension as well as poor technique and flap design can cause flap ischemia or necrosis. Another complication to avoid is hemorrhage/hematoma, thus proper preoperative medical management and achieving hemostasis before leaving the operating room are both imperative.

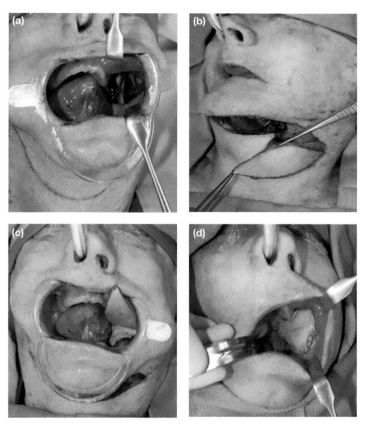

Figure 31.7 Submental island flap. (a) Intraoral defect of buccal mucosa. (b) Raised skin flaps. (c) Insetting of submental flap. (d) Final closure.

TOP TIPS AND HAZARDS

- For pedicled flaps it is always best to 'measure twice and cut once' to obtain appropriate reach. It is better to elevate a longer flap that can be closed without tension.

- Use surrounding tissues when possible, replacing like with like, to obtain a better match of color and texture.

- Do not be afraid to debulk and revise flaps.

- Follow patients long term to observe how surgical choices mature with time.

FURTHER READING

Al Shetawi AH, Quimby A, Fernandes R. The cervico-facial flap in cheek reconstruction: a guide for flap design. *J Oral Maxillofac Surg* 2017;**75**:2708.e1-2708. e6.

Cheng A, Bui T. Submental island flap. *Oral Maxillofac Surg Clin North Am* 2014;**26**:371–9.

Fernandes R. *Local and Regional Flaps in Head and Neck Reconstruction, A Practical Approach.* Wiley Blackwell; 2014

Ganry L, Ettinger KS, Rougier G, Qassemyar Q, Fernandes RP. Revisiting the temporal artery posterior auricular skin flap with an anatomical basis stepwise pedicle dissection for use in targeted facial subunit reconstruction. *Head Neck* 2020;**42**:3153–60.

Ramirez CA, Fernandes RP. The supraclavicular artery island and trapezius myocutaneous flaps in head and neck reconstruction. *Oral Maxillofac Surg Clin North Am* 2014;**26**:411–20.

Chapter 32 | Lip Reconstruction

Montey Garg, Kunmi Fasanmade, Brian Bisase

INTRODUCTION

Lip reconstruction can be a challenging task for any reconstructive surgeon. Most of the modern techniques of reconstruction of full-thickness defects of lip are derivations of methods described in the 19th century. Interestingly, Susruta's descriptions of lip reconstruction in the Indian Sanskrit writings date back to at least 1000 BC.

Lips have multiple motor functions including facial expressions, articulation of speech, deglutition, whistling and kissing. The sensory functions of the lip are also important and include temperature, touch and pain. Cosmetically, it is the principal feature of the lower face. Be it for facial trauma or lip cancer, restoration of normal form and function is key to a successful lip reconstruction.

SURGICAL ANATOMY

The anatomy of the lips includes three layers: skin, orbicularis oris muscle and mucosa. The vermilion is formed of non-keratinising mucosa; the 'white line' is where the skin meets the vermilion. Alignment of this zone is the initial and one of the most important steps in lip skin closure, as even a minor discrepancy can stand out.

The blood supply includes the superior and inferior labial arteries, which are branches of the facial artery (*Figure 32.1*). They course deep to the mucosal surface of the lip. The motor nerve supply of the lips is from the facial nerve, through the buccal and marginal mandibular branches. Innervation for sensation is from the trigeminal nerve, through the infraorbital nerve (upper lip) and the mental nerve (lower lip). Wide excision of cancer in the lip frequently requires full-thickness excision to optimise clearance of the disease and improve survival.

INDICATIONS

Defects related to oncological resection, trauma, burns and congenital deformities are all indications for lip reconstruction. A vast majority of cases of lip cancer involve the lower lip due to a higher level of ultraviolet light exposure compared with the upper lip.

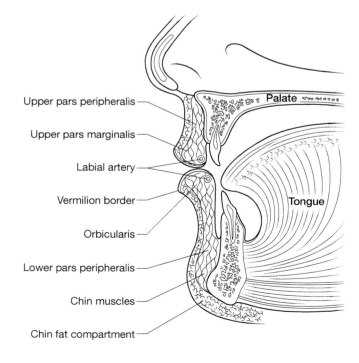

Figure 32.1 Lip anatomy.

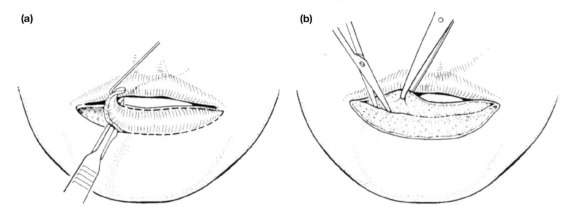

Figure 32.2 (a) The vermilion is excised with a No. 11 blade and (b) mucosal flap raised with scissors.

OPERATIVE TECHNIQUES

Lip reconstruction may be required for vermilion only, cutaneous (partial-thickness) or full-thickness defects. It should be borne in mind that no single technique will be applicable to every patient and a tailored reconstruction based on the defect is needed to restore the form and function of the lips.

Vermilion defects

The vermilion may be affected by actinic damage resulting in dysplasia or superficially invasive carcinoma, and the entire vermilion may be affected necessitating vermilionectomy. This can be achieved by CO_2 laser excision or a surgical excision. The preferred method of reconstruction following a surgical excision of the vermilion is by advancing the labial mucosa, which is redraped over the underlying orbicularis musculature. The technique is described below.

- In an appropriately consented and anaesthetised patient, mark the site to be excised prior to injecting any local anaesthesia
- Stretch the lower lip using skin hooks placed in the commissure
- A no.11 or no.15 blade is used to transfix the width of the vermilion starting at one end
- The blade is advanced to the opposite commissure (*Figure 32.2a*)
- The depth of resection will depend on the depth of the lesion
- Closure of the defect is by local advancement of the mucosa (*Figure 32.2b*)

Oral mucosa is undermined to the depth of the sulcus to allow tension-free advancement to reconstruct the vermilion.

The potential complications of this method include thinning of the lip as a result of scar contracture, excessive lip fullness from overadvancement and colour mismatch.

If a CO_2 laser is used, then the area can be left to granulate.

If more bulk is required for reconstruction, a tongue flap can be used (*Figure 32.3*). The technique is described below.

- A 5-mm thick 'bucket handle' bipedicled flap is raised from the dorsal tongue (*Figure 32.3a*)
- The dorsal tongue defect is closed primarily
- The bucket handle is sutured to the lip and remains attached (*Figure 32.3b*)
- Surgical separation is performed in 2–3 weeks

Other techniques of vermilion reconstruction include a mucosal V-Y advancement flap, cross-lip mucosal flaps and the facial artery musculo-mucosal (FAMM) flap. In addition, small vermilion lesions can be excised as an 'ellipse' and closed primarily. Incisions should be placed in the radially oriented relaxed skin tension lines for ease of closure and good cosmesis.

Cutaneous (partial-thickness) defects

Partial-thickness defects of the upper or lower lip can either be closed primarily or with local flaps. In these local flaps, the underlying facial musculature remains intact and only the skin and subcutaneous tissue are mobilised.

Various techniques of closure of such defects include linear closure, 'O-T' flap (*Figure 32.4*), 'V-Y' advancement local flap, 'M' plasty at margin, transposition flap, crescentic advancement and, rarely, skin grafts. It is important to bear in mind that any transposition flap from outside the lip subunits brings in non-hair-bearing skin to the lip defect to ensure a better cosmetic outcome.

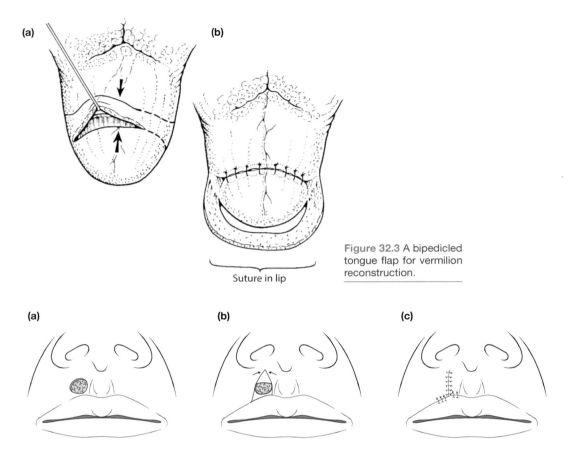

Figure 32.3 A bipedicled tongue flap for vermilion reconstruction.

Suture in lip

Figure 32.4 O-T advancement flap. (a) Right upper lip defect. (b) Standard O-T design. Arrows show the vector of advancement. (c) Postoperative result.

Full-thickness defects

Full-thickness defects of the lip can be divided into less than one-third of lip resection, one-third to two-thirds of lip resection and greater than two-thirds of lip resection. The reconstructive options may be tailored according to the extent of the defect.

Defects requiring less than one-third of the lip reconstructed

V excision with primary closure is considered adequate in most full-thickness defects encompassing up to one third of the lower lip. To avoid crossing the mentolabial groove, a V resection is selected for smaller defects and W resection for larger defects. The surgical technique is described below.

- Appropriately position the patient, prepare the site with an aseptic solution, and mark the margin of the planned excision
- Decide on the type of reconstruction and draw this at or around the excision

- Options include V excision with primary closure, V with pentagonal closure or a W-shaped excision with primary closure (*Figure 32.5*)
- The W-shaped excision may be used to avoid crossing the mentolabial crease and to allow for larger defects to be closed primarily
- Administer adequate local anaesthesia (e.g. 2% lignocaine with 1:80 000 adrenaline) with bilateral mental nerve blocks and local infiltration of the incision/excision line
- Using a No. 15 or No. 11 scalpel blade, excise the lesion along the marked lines and orientate the specimen for pathology
- Obtain meticulous haemostasis using bipolar cautery, or monopolar if safe to do so. Pay particular attention to the labial artery
- The vermilion border must be realigned meticulously to avoid malalignment. It is sometimes advisable to do this first and ensure that it is correct
- This should be followed by a careful three-layer closure, including the oral mucosa, the orbicularis oris muscle, and the overlying skin in individual layers

(a) (b) (c)

(d) (e)

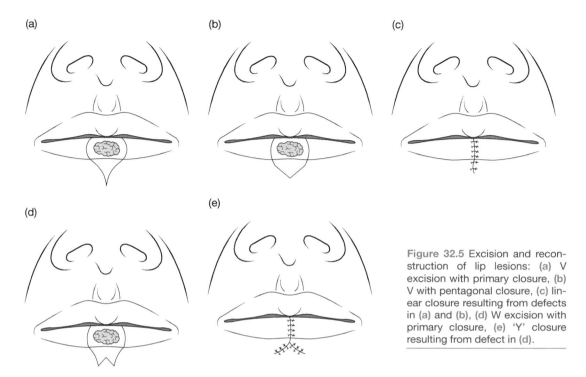

Figure 32.5 Excision and reconstruction of lip lesions: **(a)** V excision with primary closure, **(b)** V with pentagonal closure, **(c)** linear closure resulting from defects in **(a)** and **(b)**, **(d)** W excision with primary closure, **(e)** 'Y' closure resulting from defect in **(d)**.

For oral mucosa closure, 4-0 or 5-0 Vicryl Rapide™ (Ethicon) can be used. For muscle-to-muscle closure, 3-0 Vicryl, and for deep subcutaneous skin, 4-0 Vicryl Rapide can be used. For skin and superior mucosa just beyond the vermilion, 6-0 nylon sutures can be used. For surface cutaneous dressings on non-hair-bearing skin, we employ Steri-Strips and brown tape, but we use Vaseline or a protective spray (such as Opsite) on hair-bearing surfaces.

Defects requiring one-third to two-thirds of the lip reconstructed

Defects encompassing between one-third and two-thirds of the lip require alternative techniques such as the Staircase technique (progressive horizontal distances that involve half of the defect width) and McGregor variation of the fan flap. Both techniques are described below.

Staircase technique. A full-thickness horizontal incision is extended from the inferior defect margin in one or both directions for a unilateral (*Figure 32.6d*) or bilateral flap (*Figure 32.6a–c*), respectively.

- Each line of incision is of equal length
- The line follows the submental crease
- The mucosa is left intact
- Partial-thickness rectangular excisions of skin and subcutaneous tissue are made below each step and the skin flaps are undermined laterally
- A Burow's triangle is excised at the bottom of the staircase
- Flap is advanced to close the defect

McGregor variation of the fan flap. This technique is useful for defects between one-third and two-thirds size which involve the lip commissure (*Figure 32.7*). The technique is described below.

- The tumour is excised as a square (*Figure 32.7a*)
- Two squares are designed as shown in Figure 32.7a. These are full-thickness flaps
- These are rotated into the defect with the commissure being the pivot point
- Primary closure of the remaining defect
- Local mucosal advancement to recreate the vermilion

Defects requiring two-thirds to total lip reconstruction

Defects greater than 60% of the lip usually require rotational flaps, using techniques such as those introduced by Abbe, Estlander, Bernard, Webster, Gillies or Karapandzic.

Abbe flap. The Abbe lip-switch transposition flap was described by Robert Abbe, an American surgeon, in 1898. Professor Pietro Sabbatini is credited as the originator of this flap described in 1838.

- Transposition of lip flap on a narrow pedicle based on the labial artery
- Designed as a rotation or lip-switch flap from the opposite lip and the labial artery is preserved on one side to serve as a pedicle of the interpolated flap

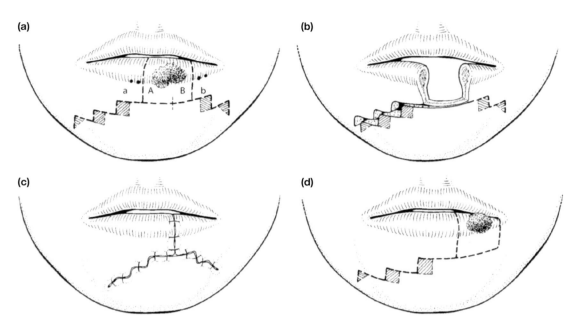

Figure 32.6 The Staircase technique. (a) Flap markings for a bilateral flap. (b) Flap raised and excess skin removed from shaded areas. (c) Closure. (d) Unilateral flap for lateral incision.

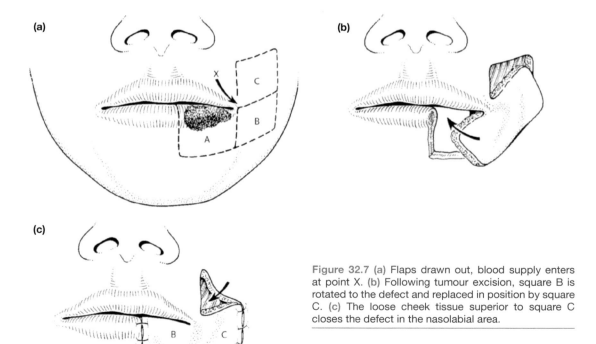

Figure 32.7 (a) Flaps drawn out, blood supply enters at point X. (b) Following tumour excision, square B is rotated to the defect and replaced in position by square C. (c) The loose cheek tissue superior to square C closes the defect in the nasolabial area.

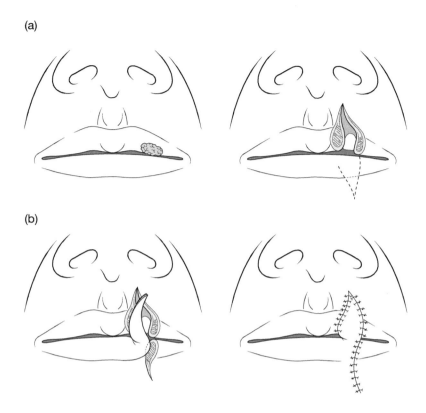

Figure 32.8 Abbe flap. (a) Flap designed at same height but half of the width of the defect. (b) 180° rotation of flap to insert into the opposing lip defect.

- Flap designed as same height but half of the width of the defect (*Figure 32.8a*)
- A full-thickness incision is made
- 180° rotation of the flap is needed to insert into the opposing lip defect, and closed in multiple layers (*Figure 32.8b*)
- Separation of the pedicle can be performed in 2–3 weeks

Estlander flap. In 1872, Estlander, a Finnish surgeon, described a commissural transposition flap.

- It is a one-stage procedure
- It repairs a defect involving the oral commissure of either lip
- It transfers a full-thickness lip flap around the commissure with a medially based pedicle containing the labial artery
- There is always resultant blunting of the oral commissure on the operated side and rarely a commissuroplasty may be required later (*Figure 32.9*)

Bernard–von Burow bilateral cheek advancement flap/Webster modification. Bernard and von Burow separately described horizontal bilateral cheek advancement flaps (*Figure 32.10*).

- These flaps recruit adjacent cheek skin to reconstruct total lip defects
- This requires excision of Burow's triangles or standing cutaneous deformity
- It does not maintain oral sphincter

In Webster's modification of this flap:

- Partial-thickness crescent triangles are excised from upper and lower cheeks rather than full-thickness triangles as in the Bernard–von Burow flap (*Figure 32.11*)
- Medial advancement of flaps to close the defect

Gillies 'fan' flap. Described in 1957, this is a rotation flap.

- Circumoral advancement with a vertical incision of the contralateral lip which is similar to the medial incision of the Estlander flap
- Flap is raised by marking a full-thickness incision that begins laterally, turns vertically and then turns back to the opposite lip
- Like the Estlander flap, there is blunting of the commissure
- There is denervation due to the vertical incision

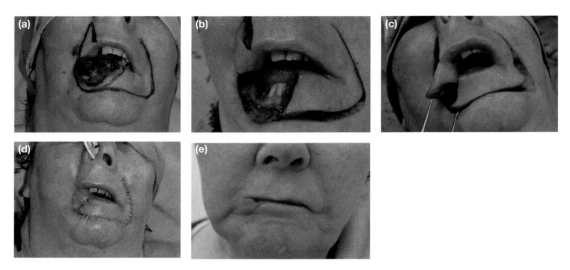

Figure 32.9 Estlander flap figures (a–e) showing reconstruction of a defect involving the right lip commissure. Also note Karapandzic flap raised on left side. (Courtesy of Rabindra P. Singh, University Hospital Southampton.)

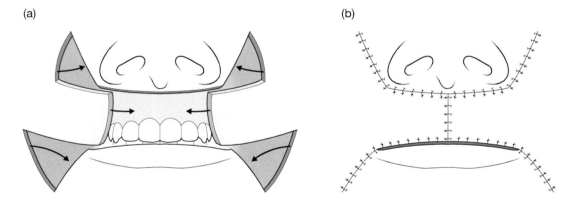

Figure 32.10 Bernard–von Burow bilateral cheek advancement flap.

and therefore a Karapandzic flap is preferred over Gillies fan flap

Karapandzic flap. This was described by Karapandzic in 1974. This rotation flap preserves the neurovascular structures entering the orbicularis oris. It is a single-stage flap with a relatively easy design and preserves oral competence, and therefore is preferred over Gillies fan flap.

- Mark the outline of the flap circumorally starting in the mental crease around commissure into the melolabial crease (*Figure 32.12a*)
- The width of the flap should equal the height of the defect

- Incision is made through skin and subcutaneous tissue
- The orbicularis oris is mobilised from perioral muscles
- Blunt dissection allows identification and preservation of the neurovascular structures
- Flaps are rotated, advanced and the perioral muscles are reattached (*Figure 32.12b*)
- Mucosa can remain intact or can be incised separately to get further advancement

Large composite defects of lip may require distant pedicled or free-flap reconstruction.

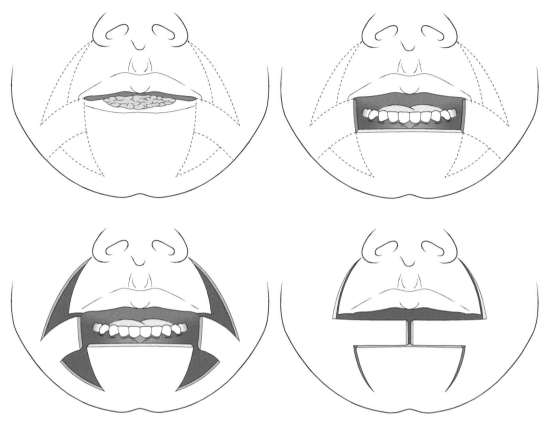

Figure 32.11 Webster bilateral cheek advancement flap.

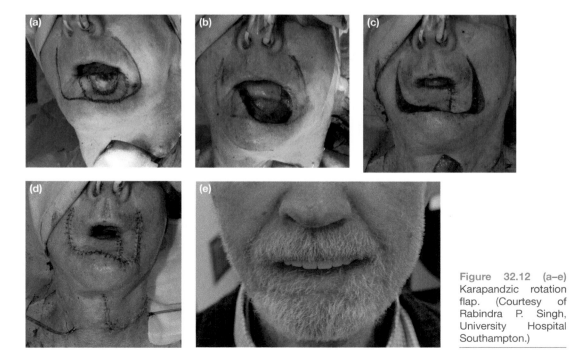

Figure 32.12 (a–e) Karapandzic rotation flap. (Courtesy of Rabindra P. Singh, University Hospital Southampton.)

POSTOPERATIVE CARE

Patients should be advised to keep the cutaneous aspect of the wound dry, rinse the oral side (with a chlorohexidine 0.2% or saltwater mouthwash) and minimise tension on the wound for the first 2–3 weeks (avoid excessive stretching of the lips, e.g. laughing).

Local flap viability should be monitored postoperatively prior to discharge. Depending on the local flap, some patients may require overnight stay.

Removal of sutures should be carried out at 7 days unless the patient has had previous radiotherapy or has any other potential wound-healing issues, such as long-term steroid therapy. For these patients, consider removal of sutures at 9–10 days.

After surface wounds (skin and mucosa) have healed, bimanual massage of the lip while the deeper wound matures should minimise deep scar tissue.

COMPLICATIONS

Complications include wound breakdown necessitating resuturing of wound, infections requiring antibiotics, microstomia requiring lip stretching or commissuroplasty and unaesthetic result requiring revision surgery.

TOP TIPS AND HAZARDS

- The skin vermilion junction should be aligned well as even a minor discrepancy may be very noticeable.
- The flap outline should be marked out well before injecting any local anaesthesia as lips become very swollen distorting the anatomy.
- Carefully select a flap which maintains lip competence and nerve function if possible.
- Always aim for meticulous three-layered closure for full-thickness defect to get optimum cosmetic results.

FURTHER READING

Coppitt G, Li DT, Burkey BB. Current concepts in lip reconstruction. *Curr Opin Otolaryngol Head Neck Surg* 2004;**12**:281–7.

Lubek J, Ord R. Lip reconstruction. *Oral Maxillofacial Surg Clin N Am* 2013;**25**:203–14.

Kolokythas A. *Lip Cancer Treatment and Reconstruction.* Springer; 2014

Larrabee YC, Moyer JS. Reconstruction of Mohs defects of the lips and chin. *Facial Plast Surg Clin N Am* 2017;**25**:427–42.

Matin MB, Dillon J. Lip reconstruction. *Oral Maxillofacial Surg Clin N Am* 2014;**26**:335–57.

Chapter
33
Pectoralis Major Flap

Rabindra P. Singh, Jean-Pierre Jeannon, Peter A. Brennan

INTRODUCTION

The pectoralis major flap, first described by Ariyan in 1979, has often been considered by many as the workhorse reconstructive option for a medium to large surgical defect of the head and neck. The popularity of the flap has, however, diminished in recent years due to continued advances in microvascular free tissue transfer techniques. Nevertheless, it remains a formidable fall-back option in many cases when free-flap surgery may not be feasible for several reasons, such as complex medical comorbidities or a vessel-depleted neck related to previous surgery or radiotherapy, and when a previous free-flap surgery has not been successful, requiring a salvage surgery.

The pectoralis major flap is an axial patterned flap which can be raised as a myocutaneous or a 'muscle only' flap depending on the characteristics of the recipient defect. The principle of raising this flap involves transposing the muscle on the axis of rotation of the pedicle, partially detaching and mobilising it from the muscle origins and insertions. This, therefore, limits its application as it has a finite reach depending on the pedicle length and mobilisation. In general, the upper height limitation of this flap is a tangent that runs from the tragus of the ear to the oral commissure.

The main recipient sites used for this flap are the anterior floor of mouth, oral tongue, oropharynx, lateral pharyngeal wall after laryngectomy and external neck skin where it may be particularly useful. The reconstruction of a segmental mandibular defect with this flap in conjunction with a reconstruction plate is not recommended due to the considerable possibility of poor healing and the risk of plate exposure. The excessive bulk of the pectoralis muscle and subcutaneous tissue often makes it unsuitable for many applications in the oral cavity and oropharynx, therefore a careful case selection is necessary. Donor site morbidity can be problematic in terms of cosmetic asymmetry of the anterior chest wall and deformity of the breast, especially in females. The large muscle pedicle may be visible in the neck, which may cause cosmetic concerns. In addition, the muscle contracts over time and may become ptotic which worsens the deformity and may contribute to a sump formation if used in the oral cavity. Despite these potential drawbacks, several advantages such as the ease of use, reliability, availability of a large amount of soft tissue and omission of need for microvascular

surgery mean that the pectoralis major flap remains a valuable tool in the reconstructive armamentarium of a head and neck surgeon.

SURGICAL ANATOMY

The pectoralis major muscle is a paired fan-shaped thick muscle on the anterior chest wall, originating from two sites: a clavicular head, from its sternal half, and a sternocostal head, extending from the sternum to the costal cartilages of the upper six ribs and sometimes up to the seventh costal cartilage. Both heads converge into a flat tendon that inserts into the lateral lip of the intertubercular sulcus of the humerus.

The main blood supply is from the branches of the thoraco-acromial artery (branch of the second part of axillary artery), which branches into a deltoid branch supplying the humeral head and a pectoral branch to supply the remainder of the muscle. The pectoral portion of the muscle also gets its blood supply from the lateral thoracic artery and perforators from the internal mammary artery. To allow for maximum mobilisation of the flap, often the smaller branches are sacrificed, and the flap is mainly based on the pectoral branch. When raised as a myocutaneous flap, the viability of skin is dependent on the perforators supplying the skin paddle. The larger the skin paddle design, the more the reliability as this may increase the number of the perforators captured within the flap itself.

STEPWISE OPERATIVE TECHNIQUE

Patient positioning and surface marking

The patient is positioned supine with the arm laid straight by the side or on a board abducted to 90°, the latter option may help define the muscle and may be useful for the less experienced surgeons. A note is made of the line from the medial tip of the coracoid process to the tip of the xiphisternum, and a vertical line is drawn inferiorly from the midpoint of the clavicle. This approximates to the surface markings of the vascular pedicle. We prefer a curvilinear 'defensive' incision superiorly extending into the angle of the deltopectoral groove to allow the option of a deltopectoral flap in the future if needed. This marking should avoid the skin territory that derives its blood supply from the 2nd and

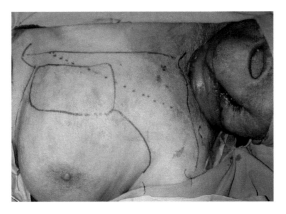

Figure 33.1 Skin paddle designed just above the level of the costal margin with a 'defensive' incision superiorly.

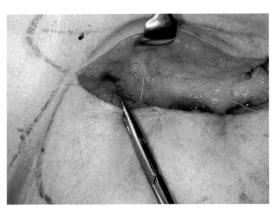

Figure 33.2 Initial incision down to the muscle. Several interrupted sutures are placed between the muscle and subcutaneous tissue to avoid damage to perforators due to shearing forces.

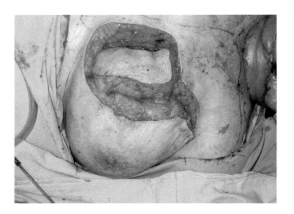

Figure 33.3 Flap completely incised around periphery with a defensive incision.

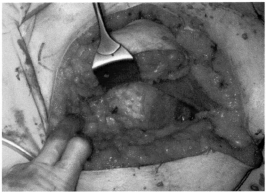

Figure 33.4 Skin flap raised laterally, and the lateral edge of the pectoralis major muscle is exposed.

3rd internal mammary artery perforators, which form the basis for a deltopectoral flap (*Figure 33.1*).

The skin paddle should be designed to be placed on the furthest distance possible for maximum reach. It should, however, not be marked beyond the costal margin to avoid inadvertently incorporating the fibres of the rectus abdominis muscle, and to achieve the maximum skin reliability. In females, for cosmesis, the pedicle can be orientated horizontally in a submammary position. This option does add to the complexity of the technique due to the need for the flap to be transferred from under the mammary gland tissue, and if not careful, may risk the skin reliability due to inadvertent damage to the perforators during tissue handling.

Incision and raising of flap

The skin paddle should be incised through subcutaneous tissue to the underlying muscle, with the incision slightly bevelled away from the paddle to increase the amount of subcutaneous tissue on the skin paddle, which may help improve its integrity. It is extremely important to take care and keep the skin island connected to the muscle and avoid shearing forces that might damage the perforator vessels entering the skin island. Some resorbable sutures should be placed to secure the skin paddle to the underlying muscle at this stage (*Figures 33.2* and *33.3*).

The skin flap is raised laterally over the pectoralis major muscle until its lateral edge is fully exposed (*Figure 33.4*). Dissection is then continued medially under the muscle to expose the main pedicle of the flap (*Figure 33.5*). The muscle edge is followed on inferiorly below the level of the skin paddle. The muscle is then cut at the inferior margin and the flap is raised from the chest wall in superior direction over a plane on the surface of the rib periosteum and fascia over the intercostal muscles. The authors find the harmonic scalpel useful

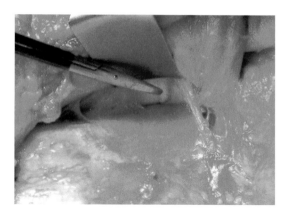

Figure 33.5 Dissection is continued medially under the muscle and the main pedicle is identified. Also note the lateral thoracic artery lateral to the main pedicle.

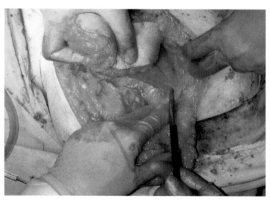

Figure 33.6 Flap is raised in cephalad direction. Humeral head of the muscle is divided under direct vision to mobilise the flap.

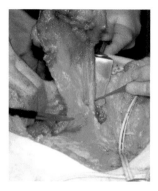

Figure 33.7 Pedicle moved back and forwards while dissection progresses on both medial and lateral surfaces.

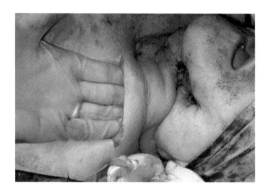

Figure 33.8 Wide tunnel created between the clavicle and skin for passage of the flap into the neck.

in dissecting the muscle tissue. During the dissection, perforators are encountered entering the muscle from the chest wall which should be cauterised or ligated appropriately.

At the midway point along the chest wall, pectoralis minor muscle is encountered, over which the dissection is continued, looking out for the vascular pedicle, which should be visible through the fascia on the deep surface of the pectoralis major muscle. At the lateral part of the dissection, the antecostal brachial nerve is identified and divided.

The muscle is divided at the sternal attachment and the dissection continued in a cephalad direction. Smaller branches of the blood vessels are encountered laterally, which are ligated and divided to improve flap mobilisation. The humeral head insertion is divided in the axilla, which will add considerable length to the flap (*Figure 33.6*). The narrower the flap stem at the superior end, the better the flap mobilisation; however, care must be taken to avoid injury to the vascular pedicle (*Figure 33.7*).

Creating skin tunnel and flap transfer into the neck

A skin flap tunnel is created between the clavicle and the skin to facilitate transfer of the flap to the defect. This is achieved by dissecting downwards from the neck in a subplatysmal plane and upwards from the chest in a subcutaneous plane. The space within this tunnel can be assessed by inserting at least four fingers of a hand, thereby ensuring that there will be no compression of the pedicle (*Figure 33.8*). Once the flap is fully mobilised, it should be gently delivered through the tunnel into the neck avoiding trauma to the skin island or twisting of the pedicle (*Figure 33.9*).

Flap inset and wound closure

The flap should be inset tension-free, and the defect closed in layers. The skin component can be utilised to re-surface two separate linings, such as the co-existing intra- and extraoral defect by de-epithelialising a bridge of tissue on the skin paddle (*Figure 33.10*).

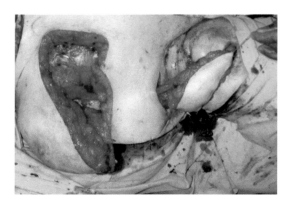

Figure 33.9 The flap is delivered into the neck.

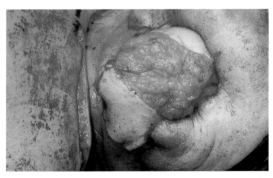

Figure 33.10 De-epithelialisation of the skin paddle to create a bi-paddled flap to resurface intra- and extraoral defects.

The donor site is closed primarily by undermining the skin flaps, and rarely is a problem as there is ample laxity of tissue in the region (*Figure 33.11*). Meticulous haemostasis is needed to prevent haematoma formation. Two suction drains are placed within the wound and kept in until the drain output drops below 30 mL over 24 hours. A seroma occurs on occasion, requiring the drain(s) to remain in place for longer.

POSTOPERATIVE CARE

It is important to avoid any compressive or occlusive dressings or tapes that might compromise the vascular flow in the pedicle. It is normal for the base of the neck to appear bulged out due to the rotation of the muscle, and this appearance should be appropriately handed over to the team at the care handover as this may be misinterpreted as a haematoma and a compression dressing inadvertently applied over the pedicle compromising the flap.

Frequent flap monitoring is not necessary and a clinical review three times a day should suffice. In the immediate postoperative phase, it is not uncommon to see a slightly hyperaemic skin paddle which usually settles with time. Unless there is an obvious sign of strangulation of the vascular pedicle at the point of flap rotation, no further intervention is required other than simple monitoring.

COMPLICATIONS

One of the more common complications of this flap is the partial or complete necrotic loss of skin paddle. This can be minimised by gentle tissue handling and avoiding the shearing forces that can damage the perforators entering the skin from the muscle. The pedicle may be damaged during flap elevation and should be regularly inspected as the dissection continues.

If there are concerns about the viability of the skin component intraoperatively, a 'muscle only' flap can be

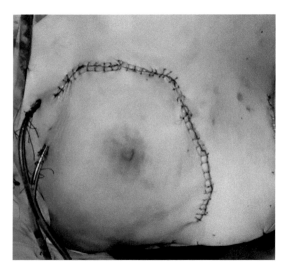

Figure 33.11 Wide undermining of the skin allows primary closure of the donor defect.

raised, and a split-thickness skin graft utilised to cover the muscle if used extraorally. This technique may also be useful when there are concerns of a bulky flap due to excessive subcutaneous tissue. If a skin paddle is lost intraorally, a simple debridement and excision of the necrotic tissue will allow mucosalisation of the muscle surface.

Early postoperative bleeding from the perforator vessels can be problematic; hence a meticulous haemostasis is important prior to wound closure. Significant haematoma or seroma may require incision and drainage. The muscle lying over the clavicle may be misdiagnosed as a haematoma, therefore if there is any clinical ambiguity, imaging should be considered to aid diagnosis. Pneumothorax due to inadvertent deep dissection into the anterior chest cavity is a rare complication.

TOP TIPS AND HAZARDS

- Avoid extending the skin paddle beyond the costal margin or over the sternum to minimise the risk of skin component failure.

- Design a 'defensive' incision to preserve the option of a deltopectoral flap in the future.

- The narrower the muscle tissue around the base of the pedicle, the better the flap mobilisation. However, one must take care not to damage the vascular pedicle.

- Split-thickness skin graft over the muscle can be utilised if there are concerns with the excessively bulky subcutaneous tissue or a dubious viability of the skin paddle.

FURTHER READING

Ariyan, S. The pectoralis major myocutaneous flap. A versatile flap for reconstruction in the head and neck. *Plast Reconstr Surg* 1979;**63**:73–81.

Bussu F, Gallus R, Navach V. Contemporary role of pectoralis major regional flaps in head and neck surgery. *Acta Otorhinolaryngol Ital* 2014;**34**:327–41.

Gabrysz-Forget F, Tabet P, Rahal A et al. Free versus pedicled flaps for reconstruction of head and neck cancer defects: a systematic review. *J Otolaryngol Head Neck Surg* 2019;**48**:13.

Chapter 34

Principles of Microvascular Surgery

Cyrus J. Kerawala, Francesco M. G. Riva

INTRODUCTION

Within the head and neck, microsurgical reconstruction is employed when other options such as local or distant flaps are deemed inappropriate. Although microsurgery is widespread, it is not the first choice in the reconstructive ladder and may not be the best solution for all defects. However, it offers the widest range of possibilities for complex reconstruction.

INDICATIONS

- Replacement of vital structures, e.g. glossectomy defect
- Obliteration of cavities, e.g. maxillectomy defect
- Bone reconstruction, e.g. segmental mandibulectomy
- Replacement of muscle and nerve, e.g. facial re-animation
- Alimentary tract reconstruction, e.g. after laryngopharyngectomy

CONTRAINDICATIONS

Microsurgical transfers can be long and technically demanding operations and emergency re-intervention may be necessary. Contraindications for this type of procedure include medical illnesses that preclude the ability to tolerate prolonged anaesthesia. Advanced age is not necessarily a contraindication, nor is a potentially severe medical problem so long as it is well controlled.

PREOPERATIVE WORKUP

A comprehensive history and physical examination are mandatory, as is close liaison with anaesthetists and intensivists. Preoptimisation of patients may be advantageous. Many patients will have already undergone imaging for their primary disease, but additional investigations may be appropriate, e.g. angiography.

Selection of donor site

Decision making is critical to success. Flap selection is based on a combination of factors including tissue type, pedicle length, flap reliability and donor-site morbidity.

The microsurgeon should be familiar with the majority of available options. Although inevitably some will be used more than others, ultimately each defect should be reconstructed on its own merit.

Within the head and neck, most reconstructions can be comfortably undertaken with these flaps:

- Radial forearm (RFFF)
- Anterolateral thigh (ALT)
- Lateral arm
- Rectus abdominis
- Latissimus dorsi
- Fibular
- Deep circumflex iliac artery (DCIA)
- Scapular/parascapular
- Jejunum
- Gracilis
- Medial sural artery perforator (MSAP)

The above can be divided into three groups: soft tissue flaps, hard tissue flaps and combinations. The choice of soft tissue flap depends on the volume of the defect. The body habitus of the patient in part determines bulk although variation in operating technique may overcome this (e.g. intraoperative thinning of ALT).

MICROSURGICAL PRINCIPLES

An alternative reconstruction should always be considered as a 'lifeboat'. Recipient vessel location should be planned out considering potential zones of injury (e.g. previous radiotherapy). Two-team operating should be employed wherever possible to minimise the length of the operation and ensure that a well-rested surgeon is available for the more technically challenging aspects of surgery.

The overall plan should be discussed with the anaesthetist including details of the length of procedure and required positioning of the patient. The patient should be adequately hydrated with a good central venous pressure and their core temperature should be maintained to avoid vasospasm. If hypotensive anaesthesia is adopted at any stage, it should be reversed prior to microsurgery. Good control of mean blood pressure output during revascularisation can be crucial, especially in the case of previous radiotherapy treatment with poor recipient arterial flow.

Physical exertion, alcohol and caffeine should be avoided for at least 24 hours in individuals prone to tremor. Short breaks are advised to minimise waning

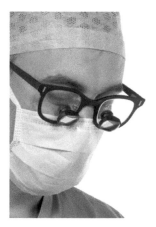

Figure 34.1 Binocular loupes.

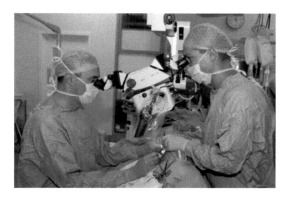

Figure 34.2 Double-headed operating microscope.

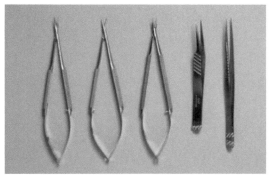

Figure 34.3 Microvascular instruments.

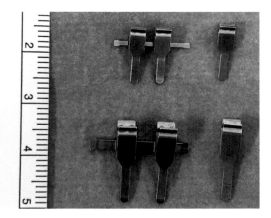

Figure 34.4 Vessel clamps and twin approximators.

performance. Both microsurgeon and assistant should feel physically comfortable, with appropriate seating and microscope and table ergonomically positioned.

Optical systems

Magnifying ocular loupes

Loupes are often more convenient than the microscope for preliminary dissection. Simple models magnify up to 1.8× whereas more sophisticated ones can provide up to 4× magnification (*Figure 34.1*). Loupes with higher magnifications have smaller fields of vision and depth of focus. Expanded-field models are available, although with heavier optics.

Operating microscope

The operating microscope has many advantages in providing magnification and illumination. A double-headed operating microscope with the surgeon and assistant at opposite sides is essential for head and neck reconstruction (*Figure 34.2*). Coaxial illumination is important to avoid shadows. Zoom systems can be operated by either a foot or finger. A good-quality built-in camera can be of help for teaching reasons and also provides the scrub nurse with the ability to keep pace with the surgical steps. A well-trained scrub

nurse can be of great help in reducing surgical time and minimising the need for operating surgeons to look away from the microscope eyepieces.

Instrumentation

Most microsurgical procedures can be performed with a simple, basic set (*Figure 34.3*).

- Jeweller's or watchmaker's forceps (hereafter called microsurgical forceps)
- Vessel dilators: these are microsurgical forceps rounded and polished at the tip
- Needle holders: spring-loaded handles with either round or flat grip
- Dissecting scissors: spring handled with short or long curved blades
- Adventitia scissors: identical to dissecting scissors but have straight blades
- Vessel clamps (*Figure 34.4*): spring-loaded varieties are available for arteries and veins
- Double-approximator clamps of varying sizes to aid anastomosis
- Instrument case: a metal-lined case with rubber spigots to avoid instrument damage

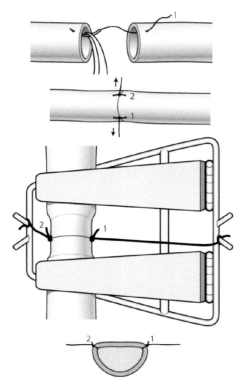

Figure 34.5 Triangulation method of vessel approximation.

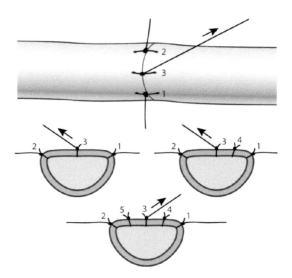

Figure 34.6 Completion of front wall co-optation.

At least two sets of microvascular instruments should always be available in case of emergencies. Regular demagnetisation is necessary.

Super micro set

With the increased demand for super microvascular procedures, started with lymphatic anastomosis and perforator to perforator anastomosis, super micro sets have appeared on the market. Although these procedures are not standard for all microsurgeons, they are becoming more common and a smaller set of instruments can be of help for particularly challenging anastomosis for vessels of 1 mm diameter and below.

BASIC ANASTOMOTIC TECHNIQUE
Essentials for a patent anastomosis

- Meticulous, atraumatic dissection of vessels with ligation, avoiding thermic injury
- The vessel wall must be free from atherosclerotic plaques, spontaneous intima dissection or, in case of veins, adjacent valve flaps
- Adequate blood flow at the recipient artery prior to anastomosis
- Anastomoses should be completed without tension, employing vein grafts as necessary

- Overhanging adventitia should be removed and sutures placed without trauma to the intima. Lumen should be irrigated with heparinised solutions (100 U/mL) prior to the anastomosis. In case of a tear in the intima or any damage, there should always be a very low threshold for trimming the damaged part and repeating the whole anastomosis. In trained hands this will only add 15–20 minutes to the ischaemic time and will dramatically reduce the risk of thrombosis

End-to-end anastomosis techniques

The technique most commonly taught is the joining of vessels end-to-end using a triangulation method whereby two stay sutures are inserted 120° apart so that when they are placed under tension the front wall of the anastomosis is stretched laterally (*Figure 34.5*). As a result, the back wall tends to fall away and is less likely to be picked up inadvertently. In the clinical situation, this is not always possible and many prefer two sutures at 180° or the suturing of one wall at a time from 0° to 180°.

The wall is then sutured using square or reef knots that must lie flat against the anastomosis line so that the threads do not project into the vessel lumen (*Figure 34.6*). Two or more co-optation sutures are then placed between the stay sutures before the vessel is rotated through 180°. The anastomosis should be critically appraised before the back wall is closed (*Figure 34.7*).

In certain circumstances (e.g. where there are short vessel stumps) it can be challenging to rotate vessels through 180° to provide access to the back wall. In these settings the posterior wall can be sutured first paying special attention not to trap the tails of the sutures inside the lumen.

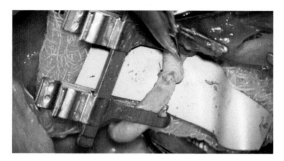

Figure 34.7 Critically appraise rotated vessel before back wall closure.

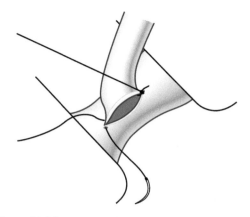

Figure 34.8 Stay sutures in end-to-side anastomosis.

The venous anastomosis is performed in an identical manner to the artery but can be technically more demanding because the absence of a substantial tunica medial means the vein wall collapses easily. Minimal adventitial stripping is recommended. Overuse of irrigation should also be avoided as it tends to strip the adventitia.

Once the anastomosis is complete, the clamps are released and blood flow observed under magnification.

Pulsatile bleeding requires placement of further sutures.

End-to-side anastomosis technique

The arteriotomy or venotomy in the recipient vessel must match the size of the vessel to be anastomosed. The adventitia around the intended site should be carefully removed so as not to protrude into the lumen. Stay sutures are initially placed at the proximal and distal ends of the arteriotomy or venotomy (*Figure 34.8*). Secondary co-optation sutures are then inserted along the anastomosis line with either the front or back wall being closed first depending on operator preference (*Figure 34.9*).

Size discrepancy

Discrepancy in vessel size can be solved by 45° diagonal (*Figure 34.10*) or a fish-mouth anastomosis (*Figure 34.11*).

For both arterial and venous anastomoses, it can be useful to adopt a combined stitching technique for the last two or three (or more) stitches on each wall. This means passing the needle and the thread in a continuous fashion and then tying and cutting each stitch one by one. This permits a good view into the lumen up to and including the last stitch (*Figure 34.12*).

Assessment of suture lines

The most common errors in technique include:

- Stitches are too tight/loose
- Too many or too few sutures
- Suture holes are not equidistant from the edge
- Uneven spacing between sutures
- Inversion of tissue edges

Microsurgical couplers

Some surgeons prefer microvascular anastomotic couplers to hand-sewn anastomosis. The coupler is a mechanical implantable device comprising an interlocking ring-pin design. Its use is most established in the end-to-end anastomosis of veins.

In recent year, Doppler probes integrated into couplers have become available.

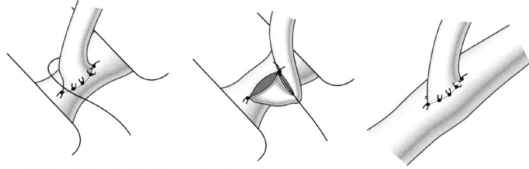

Figure 34.9 Completion of end-to-side anastomosis.

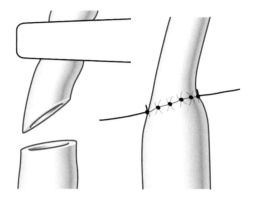

Figure 34.10 Diagonal transection of vessel.

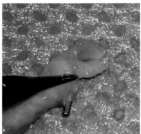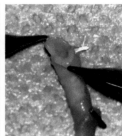

Figure 34.11 Fish-mouth technique.

Patency test

Anastomotic patency can be assessed in a variety of ways. Arterial patency is indicated by well-dilated vessels with expansile pulsation. The empty and refilled patency test ('milking') is traumatic and should be performed as gently and infrequently as possible. Ultimately, anastomotic patency can be assessed by a return of colour and capillary refill to the revascularised tissue.

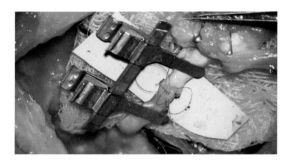

Figure 34.12 Combined stitching technique.

POSTOPERATIVE CARE

Staff must be familiar with flap monitoring and the general care of the microsurgery patient. A hyperdynamic circulation with adequate hydration, filling pressures, urine output and body temperature should be the aim. Anticoagulation may be used depending on preference, although as a standard prophylactic tinzaparine is usually sufficient.

Free flap monitoring is also dependent on preferences. The criterion standard remains careful and regular clinical examination of the flap (colour, skin turgor, refill, etc.). The use of needle test should be avoided whenever possible as this can lead to a widely bruised skin paddle and more confusion regarding flap assessment. Further details on flap monitoring can be read in *Chapter 35*.

If a vascular compromise is suspected, immediate measures should be taken as follows:

- General assessment of the patient (e.g. exclusion of hypotension)
- Repositioning of the patient to relieve possible pedicle compromise
- Exclusion of haematoma
- In the absence of haematoma, release of the vacuum on any relevant drain in case the pedicle is in contact with the drain holes
- Removal of compressive dressings or tight sutures
- Removal of straps from around the neck (e.g. tracheostomy tapes and oxygen mask straps)

If such simple manoeuvres are not successful, immediate re-exploration is critical so long as the patient's general condition allows it.

COMPLICATIONS

Microsurgical operations are by their very nature physiologically traumatic for the patient. Informed consent is mandatory and should include detailed discussions with appropriate warnings to include the following:

- Bleeding, with possible transfusion
- Donor and recipient site infection
- Morbidity specific to the free flap
- Potential need for emergency reoperation
- Flap loss
- Possible revisionary operations (e.g. flap thinning)

RECIPIENT VESSEL SELECTION

The delivery of blood into and out of the flap depends on meticulous harvesting, careful preparation of the recipient vasculature and meticulous anastomosis. Care must also be paid to the geometry of the pedicle to prevent tension and kinking.

General considerations

Recipient vessel selection is one of the most critical steps for a successful outcome as it greatly facilitates the process of revascularisation. Vessels should be selected and isolated prior to flap division to minimise the ischaemic period. The flap should be only partially inset prior to the anastomosis so that any tension in the vascular pedicle can be appreciated. This reduces the ischaemic time, allows any potential bleeding sources to be identified on the flap after revascularisation and provides a longer period of observation of the anastomoses prior to closure of the neck.

Aside from availability, several other factors must be considered when selecting recipient vessels. The choice of vessel is in part limited by the site of the defect and particular flap employed (e.g. length of pedicle). The presence of a previous ipsilateral radical neck dissection may limit the availability of recipient vessels. Advanced age and previous irradiation may also lead to atherosclerosis.

RECIPIENT ARTERY SELECTION

The main sources of arteries are branches of the external carotid artery and the thyrocervical trunk. Because of their proximity to defects, the upper branches of the former are the most commonly employed. However, the thyrocervical trunk and in particular its transverse cervical artery (TCA) is almost always preserved following neck dissections and provides a useful alternative. The TCA can be traced for a significant distance underneath the trapezius muscle and transposed into the mid portion of the neck. This vessel is far less prone to atherosclerosis and usually lies outside the area of most intense radiation therapy. Other options can include superficial temporal vessels, occipital artery and internal mammary system.

RECIPIENT VEIN SELECTION

There are three primary recipient veins in the neck. While the internal jugular vein or its immediate branches serve as an excellent outflow, the external jugular and transverse cervical veins are alternatives. The anterior jugular vein should be avoided as its drainage is at risk in case of a tracheostomy. The cephalic vein may be used as a source of vein grafts or can be used as a recipient if traced into the arm and transposed over the clavicle.

TOP TIPS AND HAZARDS

- For the novice microvascular surgeon *in vitro* practice is essential either in a dry lab or a wet lab.
- The microsurgeon should be well rested prior to the operation and comfortable throughout it.
- Flaps used should reflect anatomical and functional considerations rather than the surgeon's favourite.
- The surgeon should be critical about every suture placed. If they are not satisfied, that suture should be replaced.
- The surgeon should be critical about the completed anastomosis. It is far better to repeat an anastomosis during the time of primary surgery than return to it once vascular compromise is apparent hours later.
- Recipient artery and vein selection is fundamental.

FURTHER READING

Bozikov K, Arnez ZM. Factors predicting free flap complications in head and neck reconstruction. *J Plast Reconstr Aesthet Surg* 2006;**59**:737–42.

Bui DT, Cordeiro PG, Hu QY, Disa JJ, Pusic A, Mehrara BJ. Free flap reexploration: indications, treatment, and outcomes in 1193 free flaps. *Plast Reconstr Surg* 2007;**119**:2092–100.

Chalian AA, Anderson TD, Weinstein GS, Weber RS. Internal jugular vein versus external jugular vein anastomosis: implications for successful free tissue transfer. *Head Neck* 2001;**23**:475–8.

Chang EI, Zhang H, Skoracki RJ, Yu P, Hanasono MM. Defining an algorithm to guide salvage of a failing free flap in head and neck reconstruction. *Plast Reconstr Surg* 2014;**134**:12–13.

Okazaki M, Asato H, Takushima A, Sarukawa S, Nakatsuka T, Yamada A, Harii K. Analysis of salvage treatments following the failure of free flap transfer caused by vascular thrombosis in reconstruction for head and neck cancer. *Plast Reconstr Surg* 2007;**119**:1223–32.

Bailey & Love's Essential Operations Bailey & Love's Essential Operations
Bailey & Love's Essential Operations Bailey & Love's Essential Operations
Bailey & Love's Essential Operations Bailey & Love's Essential Operations

PART 5 | Reconstructive surgery

Chapter 35

Flap Monitoring Techniques in Free-Flap Surgery

Kaveh Shakib, Rabindra P. Singh

INTRODUCTION

Over the past four decades, free tissue transfer has evolved into a reliable tool for immediate reconstruction following ablative surgery for head and neck tumours. The success of free flap depends on continuous arterial inflow and venous outflow through the patent microvascular anastomoses until neovascularisation is established at the recipient wound bed. Multiple large series have documented overall flap success rates of greater than 95%. This improvement has in part been attributed to improved postoperative care and monitoring typically in an intensive care unit (ITU) or a high dependency unit (HDU). In broad terms, the benefits of planned admission to a high care unit include cardiopulmonary support and monitoring including optimal sedation and analgesia control, airway support and management, close monitoring of free flaps, and optimal nurse to patient ratio. These reasons are not mutually exclusive, and the physiological status of the patient has a major influence on the viability of the transferred tissue. The survival of the flap will depend on satisfactory control of blood pressure, oxygen levels and oxygen delivery to the flap.

The first part of this chapter will focus on general initial care of the patient and the latter half will focus on contemporary specific techniques in free-flap monitoring.

GENERAL CARDIOPULMONARY SUPPORT AND MONITORING

Lines

To optimise both body systems support and monitoring, patients typically have the following lines established perioperatively and arrive in ITU or HDU with a nasogastric or gastrostomy feeding tube, large gauge peripheral access, arterial line, urinary catheter, and often a tracheostomy tube and central line.

Positioning of the patient

The patient should be nursed at a 30–45° head-up position. This position will improve ventilation and thus oxygenation by reducing the ventilation–perfusion mismatch and reduce swelling. The patient's head should be kept in a neutral position or slightly turned to the side of the anastomosis to eliminate any tension on the microvascular anastomosis. During the early postoperative period, extreme movement of the neck should be avoided.

Blood pressure and cardiac output control

The goal is to maintain a mean arterial pressure (MAP) of 70 mmHg or over, guided by continuous invasive blood pressure monitoring. The preservation of a good perfusion pressure with wide pulse pressure is essential for regional autoregulation of blood flow and flap survival.

Hypotension is usually secondary to hypovolaemia or vasodilation and should be treated appropriately. The use and choice of inotropes is still open to debate and are best avoided in hypovolaemic patients. Systemic phenylephrine has been shown to increase the MAP with no adverse effect on the free flap blood flow. When required, it is the choice of inotrope at the authors' unit, where the flap success rates are over 99%. Conversely, gross hypertension should be avoided, which may cause bleeding and damage to the vascular anastomosis of the flap. β-Blockers are best avoided as they can lead to peripheral vasoconstriction. Central venous pressure (CVP) reflects cardiac filling pressures and can be manipulated to increase cardiac output. Modest hypervolaemia reduces sympathetic vascular tone and dilates the supply vessels to the flap. An increase in the trend of CVP above the control measurement can enhance the cardiac output, and produce skin and muscle vasodilatation.

Urine output

Urine output greater than 0.5 mL/kg/hour should be maintained with appropriate fluid management. Diuretics are contraindicated because volume depletion may compromise flap survival.

Haematocrit

Isovolaemic haemodilution to a haematocrit of 30% improves blood flow by reducing viscosity, reducing reperfusion injury in muscle, and increasing the number of patent capillaries. This level of haematocrit is established by keeping the haemoglobin levels in the range of 8–10 g/dL.

Free Flap and Donor Site Observation Guidelines

If any of the following observations are marked 'Yes', the surgical team must be notified immediately.

Signs of Venous congestion

- Tense/ Bouncy flap   Yes ☐   No ☐
- Easily visible capillary refill (first 2 days) Yes ☐   No ☐
- Bleeding from Flap margin   Yes ☐   No ☐
- Loss (or change of) doppler signal   Yes ☐   No ☐
- Dusky/Bluish/mottled colour   Yes ☐   No ☐

- Prompt dark bleeding on needle prick test (*only to be performed by surgeons involved in surgery*)   Yes ☐   No ☐

Signs of Arterial compromise

- Loss (or change) of doppler signal   Yes ☐   No ☐
- Cold flap (extra-oral)   Yes ☐   No ☐

- No bleeding on needle prick test (*only to be performed by surgeons involved in surgery*)   Yes ☐   No ☐

Donor Arm and Leg Observation (Radial forearm and Fibula flaps)

At the time of the flap observation, please assess donor arm or leg for signs of ischaemia:

- Low SO_2 Yes ☐   No ☐
- Warm fingers or toes   Yes ☐   No ☐
- Capillary refill <3 secs   Yes ☐   No ☐
- Able to move fingers or toes   Yes ☐   No ☐

Frequency of Flap Observation

- Hourly immediately post op
- Day 1- hourly
- Day 2- hourly
- Day 3- 3 hourly
- Day 4 onwards- three times daily
- Day 7- Implantable Doppler wire out

Review flap observation frequency in case of flap compromise or return to theatre.

Figure 35.1 An example of flap and donor site monitoring. (Department of OMFS, University Hospital Southampton, UK.)

Temperature control

The patient must not feel cold, and the temperature should be maintained over 36.5°C. A fall in skin temperature can reflect hypovolaemia and vasoconstriction. Hypothermia may lead to a raised haematocrit and plasma viscosity, and aggregation of red blood cells and platelets, which may reduce the microcirculatory blood flow in the flap.

FLAP MONITORING

The flap is closely monitored in the early postoperative period to detect any signs of vascular compromise so that a clinical decision to re-explore the anastomosis can be made without delay. The success rate of flap salvage is inversely related to the period of onset of flap ischaemia and its clinical recognition. Once tissue ischaemia occurs, there is a finite amount of time after which the microvasculature is irreversibly damaged and the 'no re-flow' phenomenon takes place. The consequences of losing a free flap are, at best, a prolonged hospital stay and delayed recovery and, at worst, significant patient morbidity and even mortality with significant healthcare financial cost.

Venous congestion is the most common cause of flap failure. An increased risk is noted between 24 and 72 hours postoperatively. Less commonly, an arterial occlusion may cause flap failure with an increased risk in the first 24 hours postoperatively.

A myriad of techniques varying in complexity and sophistication have been used in flap monitoring. There is a general lack of high-quality evidence in the effectiveness of various methods, and units may differ in their practice of flap monitoring. Most units rely on simple clinical observation or a combination of techniques. Free flaps in the head and neck region present with their own challenges compared with free flaps elsewhere in the body. Many flaps are used for oral cavity and oropharyngeal mucosal reconstruction, which may be difficult to visualise and clinical judgement may be difficult in relation to flap surface temperature and tissue turgor. Some flaps are 'buried' with no external skin surface visible, which precludes any clinical observation. If possible, an attempt should be made to exteriorise a small component of the flap to allow clinical observation in buried flaps. For jejunal flaps, a nasendoscopy may be considered specifically looking for colour of flap and peristalsis.

Clinical monitoring

Clinical assessment is regarded as the most reliable monitoring tool. However, it is a subjective and labour-intensive method, which depends on the expertise of the observer and ambient lighting. Interpretation of the clinical findings can be difficult, even for the most experienced observer. A change in the status of the flap normally mandates a return to the operating room to try to salvage the flap by correcting the problems with the vein or artery.

Clinical monitoring includes the assessment of flap colour, turgor or consistency, surface temperature and capillary refill time as well as some other specific signs of venous or arterial compromise as shown in an example of flap monitoring protocol (*Figure 35.1*).

Colour

The colour of the flap should be similar to the skin colour of the patient (*Figure 35.2*). It should be stressed that most flaps, especially intraorally, will appear a little pale when compared with normal oral mucosa. A dusky or a blue flap is a congested flap signifying venous obstruction. There may be bleeding from the flap edges in venous compromise. Assessment of colour changes in flaps with dark skin can be difficult. Although venous compromise of a free flap may manifest as an abrupt colour change, it is usually an insidious process lasting for 1–2 hours, causing clinical uncertainty and frustration. Availability of a digital photo of the flap immediately postoperatively may provide an invaluable baseline against which to measure any evolving changes.

Turgor

Flap should feel soft to palpation. Any oedema or tension may indicate kinking or obstruction of the vascular pedicle, or formation of haematoma deep to the flap and can be a sign of impending flap failure.

Surface temperature

A healthy flap should be of a similar temperature to that of the surrounding normal tissue and a cool flap may be an indicator of arterial insufficiency. It is useful in the monitoring of extraoral flaps; however, the sensitivity of this observation for intraoral flaps has been questioned as the flap usually assumes the core temperature of the oral cavity and any subtle changes are difficult to detect.

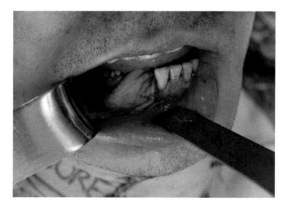

Figure 35.2 Osteocutaneous fibula flap for reconstruction of right mandible defect. Note the flap colour matching the patient skin colour immediately postoperatively.

Capillary refill time

This is assessed by applying gentle pressure on the flap for 3 seconds. A refill time of 3–5 seconds should be considered 'normal'; however, frequently it may be difficult to observe refill immediately postoperatively. A brisk refill may indicate early venous congestion. A prolonged, more than 6 seconds, or no refill may indicate an arterial occlusion.

Needle stick test

A needle stick or scratching of skin surface of the flap can assist in assessing the flap circulation. If there is no bleeding, the problem lies at the inflow. Rapid exit of dark red blood is indicative of venous congestion. This test is not routinely performed due to risk of damaging the vascular pedicle and causing bruising. If indicated, it should be performed by the surgical team involved in the insetting of the flap who will be aware of the location of the vascular pedicle.

Doppler flowmetry

Hand-held pulse Doppler assessment is a simple and rapid method of objectively monitoring blood flow. The probe is placed on the skin overlying the pedicle and the characteristic arterial noise and sound of venous outflow is heard. The limitation of this method is a high false-positive rate due to the Doppler signal of adjacent vessels being mistaken for that of the pedicle. It may be helpful to mark the pedicle (with indelible marking or suture) immediately postoperatively by the surgeons to guide the probe placement.

Monitoring frequency

The optimum frequency of clinical assessment of flap remains elusive. Although there are no data to support specific observational timings, there is a general consensus that frequent monitoring in the early postoperative phase allows for early detection and improved salvage rate. There may be a wide variation in the frequency of flap observation. An example of frequency of flap monitoring is shown in *Figure 35.1* (University Hospital Southampton, UK). An hourly observation is recommended at least for the first 2 postoperative days when the likelihood of flap compromise is the highest. There is little evidence to support continued frequent flap monitoring after the first 4 days.

A flap observation chart provides an instant visual record of any underlying trend. Due to the subjectivity of such observations, at the shift changeover, the nursing observers should agree on baseline flap observations against which any observed changes in colour, capillary refill time, consistency and temperature can be measured.

Innovations in flap monitoring

A plethora of innovative non-invasive and invasive monitoring techniques have been described but none

has become widely accepted or available. The overall quality of evidence in their efficacy in clinical use is poor and cost/benefit analyses extremely rare. Interpretation of results may be difficult requiring staff training and the excessive equipment costs have restricted their use. Some of the methods are briefly described below.

Implantable Doppler monitoring

This technique, which is the authors' routine flap monitoring method of choice, uses high-frequency pulsed ultrasound providing real-time monitoring of the blood flow into or away from the flap. The Cook–Swartz model uses a 20 MHz ultrasonic Doppler crystal on a small silicone cuff, which is wrapped around the vessel and sutured or liga-clipped to itself. The wire is then attached to a battery or mains powered portable unit that gives audio and visual signal to indicate flow signal (*Figures 35.3* and *35.4*). There is a variation in practice in terms of choice of vessel (artery or vein) for the cuff to be placed onto. A probe implanted on an artery will detect the cessation of arterial flow immediately; however, the arterial signal will persist for several hours in the case of venous thrombosis, which may give a false reassurance to the observer. On the other hand, a probe on the vein will detect cessation of venous

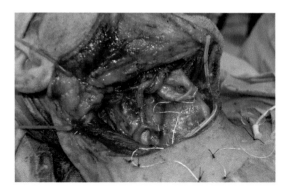

Figure 35.3 Cook Medical implantable Doppler placed on artery. Wire connected to the silicone cuff is connected to a portable audiovisual monitor. Also note a suction drain *in situ*.

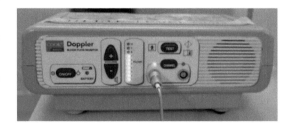

Figure 35.4 The battery or mains-operated portable monitor demonstrating continuous visual (and audio) Doppler signal.

outflow immediately and any compromise on arterial flow is also immediately reflected on the venous outflow signal. It is the authors' preference to place a probe on the artery, mainly because the venous Doppler signal can be variable and a false-positive signal may lead to an unnecessary trip to the theatre for exploration of the anastomosis. It is also easier to detect the signs of venous congestion clinically.

The electrode wire is removed at day 7 postoperatively by which time the cuff is sufficiently adherent to the vessel and the vessel is safely adherent to the surrounding tissue. The electrode is designed to separate from the cuff with a gentle tug of 50 g force. If excessive resistance is experienced, the tugging should be abandoned, and the removal attempted again in the next few days.

Laser Doppler flowmetry

This method relies on measuring the blood flow using the Doppler shift of laser light. Helium neon laser has been used which relies on reflectivity of light by the red blood cells and detects the frequency shift between the transmitted and reflected light directly proportional to the velocity of capillary blood flow.

Surface and invasive temperature monitoring

Two types of surface temperature monitors, thermoelectric thermometers and infrared thermometry, have been described which measure differential temperatures at two points in time. A reduction of greater than 1.8°C has been reported as indicative of an ischaemic event. Intraoral flaps may not lose significant heat even in the event of compromised blood flow, which is a major limitation of this method in head and neck free flaps. An implantable thermocouple probe applied to the inflow artery may pick up the drop in temperature that results from reduced blood flow because of venous or arterial thrombosis.

Oxygen tension/oxygen partial pressure monitoring

This method of assessing the tissue oxygen tension measures cellular oxygen availability. The PaO_2 microcatheter probe (e.g. flexible Clark-type probe) is placed within the tissue (muscle or subcutaneous fat), which continuously measures the oxygen partial pressure and is displayed on a self-calibrating monitor. Any compromise in blood flow to the flap is reflected as reduction in oxygen partial pressure.

Microdialysis

The microdialysis method detects ischaemia indicated by measurements such as very low glucose level, rising lactate concentration and high lactate/pyruvate ratio. A double lumen microdialysis catheter with a dialysis membrane is placed within the subcutaneous or muscle tissue of the flap. The fluid that diffuses through the membrane is analysed for various parameters mentioned above. The results are recorded as curves and numeric values on the bedside monitor.

Donor site monitoring

Donor site should also be monitored at the time of the monitoring of flap during the early postoperative period. In the case of free flaps such as radial forearm and fibula flaps, the donor limb should be monitored for signs of ischaemia which may occur secondary to compartment syndrome. An oxygen saturation (SO_2) probe can be placed on fingers or toes of the donor limb for continuous monitoring of tissue perfusion. The digits should be checked for warmth and capillary refill (see *Figure 35.1*).

FURTHER READING

Abdel-Galil K, Mitchell D. Postoperative monitoring of microsurgical free tissue transfers for head and neck reconstruction: a systematic review of current techniques – part I. Non-invasive techniques. *Br J Oral Maxillofac Surg* 2009;**47**:351–5.

Abdel-Galil K, Mitchell D. Postoperative monitoring of microsurgical free-tissue transfers for head and neck reconstruction: a systematic review of current techniques – part II. Invasive techniques. *Br J Oral Maxillofac Surg* 2009;**47**:438–42.

Shen AY, Lonie S, Lim K, Farthing H, Hunter-Smith DJ, Rozen WM. Free flap monitoring, salvage, and failure timing: a systematic review. *J Reconstr Microsurg* 2021;**37**:300–8.

Chapter
36

Radial Forearm Flap

Jeremy McMahon, Giovanni Diana, Craig Wales, Ewen Thomson

INTRODUCTION

The fasciocutaneous radial forearm free flap (RFFF) has been a frequently deployed option for head and neck reconstructive surgeons for four decades. The RFFF provides a moderate area of the thinnest and most pliable lining of all the fasciocutaneous flap donor sites. The harvest is technically straightforward, provides a long vascular pedicle (>10 cm) in most configurations, with large calibre radial artery and veins (communicating and cephalic) for anastomosis. Simultaneous flap raising with head and neck ablative surgery is widely practised. The late donor site morbidity is acceptable. This flap is associated with the lowest failure rate (1.9%) in our experience. These characteristics account for the enduring importance of the RFFF in head and neck reconstruction.

CONTRAINDICATIONS

There are few absolute contraindications except for those rare individuals who have an inadequate collateral arterial supply to the hand. Patients with Raynaud's disease and scleroderma may be at increased risk of hand ischaemia. Previous surgery to the forearm, including distal radius fracture repair, are regarded as relative contraindications.

PREOPERATIVE ASSESSMENT

A modified Allen test is performed to ensure adequate collateral circulation with careful inspection of the thumb and index finger. Where the Allen test is equivocal, or where clinical concern persists despite a satisfactory Allen test, imaging evaluation is indicated. Unfortunately, there is no consensus on the optimal imaging modality. This could be CT or MR angiography, duplex ultrasonography evaluation or digital plethysmography. Hyperspectral imaging may prove to be an alternative. Where further evaluation, in the presence of an equivocal Allen test, indicates a forearm flap harvest may well be safe, it is prudent practice to perform a 'cutdown' exposure onto the distal radial artery prior to tourniquet inflation. The radial artery is occluded with a vascular clamp and the hand inspected with particular reference to thumb and index finger, supplemented by pulse oximetry. If this appears satisfactory, a small arteriotomy is performed distal to the clamp and retrograde bleeding is confirmed. In the presence of a well-perfused hand, and back bleeding, it is reasonable to proceed with flap harvest.

SURGICAL ANATOMY

Arterial supply

The arterial supply of the fasciocutaneous forearm flap relies on perforator vessels from the radial artery as it lies in the lateral intermuscular septum. Proximal perforators may be musculocutaneous, piercing brachioradialis or septocutaneous lying between brachioradialis and pronator teres muscles (*Figure 36.1*). In the distal forearm, the perforators are given off as the vessel passes between brachioradialis and flexor carpi radialis muscles/tendons where the radial artery lies on flexor pollicis longus muscle. The cutaneous perforators of both the radial and ulnar arteries are smaller and more numerous in the distal forearm, with roughly equal numbers of radial and ulnar cutaneous perforators and a watershed on the volar aspect halfway between the two source vessels. The cutaneous vessels at this watershed link with each other. The vessels form longitudinal linked vascular systems running parallel with the source (radial and ulnar) arteries. Studies of the perforator anatomy of the distal forearm reveal a greater concentration of perforators in the zone closer to the insertion of pronator teres than distally but there will be at least one relatively large perforator within 2 cm of the radial styloid. Sources vary on the number of distal radial perforator vessels present, with a range of 6–15.

A proximal skin paddle can be raised, and we have deployed this occasionally when an external monitoring skin paddle has been desirable, or a bi-paddled flap with a short proximal pedicle applicable. The successful use of a proximal skin paddle as a perforator flap, with or without preservation of the radial artery, has been reported.

Extending the RFFF distal skin paddle dissection beyond the line of the ulnar artery, on the volar surface of the forearm, can result in marginal necrosis of this extension.

The superficial ulnar artery variation is of significance in forearm flap harvest. In this variant, the

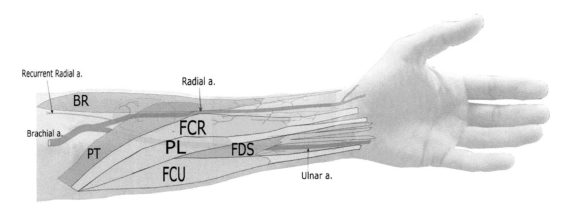

Figure 36.1 The arterial supply of the fasciocutaneous forearm flap. *Abbreviations*: BR, brachioradialis muscle; FCR, flexor carpi radialis; FCU, flexor carpi ulnaris; FDS, flexor digitorum superficialis; PL, palmaris longus; PT, pronator teres.

ulnar artery arises from the axillary or brachial artery, descending superficial to it and the median nerve. In the proximal forearm it remains superficial to the pronator teres muscle. Its superficial location makes it susceptible to inadvertent injury if not detected preoperatively. With an incidence of around 1 in 250, it is likely that high-volume surgeons will encounter this anomaly. A persistent median artery appears to be the most prevalent forearm vascular variation (4%). Identification preoperatively may be important where the persistent median artery contributes substantially to the perfusion of the distal forearm skin. McCormack et al. demonstrated a 4.3% incidence of radial artery variations and there have been a number of reports describing both unanticipated and preoperatively identified variants in the RFFF literature. A high origin of the radial artery appears to be the most common and does not influence the selection, or dissection, of the RFFF except that it is associated with absence of a cubital fossa communicating vein. Absence, and hypoplasia, of the radial artery are likely to be detected by careful clinical evaluation. Duplications of the radial artery, with a superficial dorsal antebrachial branch, or branch lying superficial and lateral, may be missed preoperatively and require an intraoperative determination of how best to proceed. It has been observed that the former variation has been associated with an absence of septocutaneous perforators from the radial artery itself.

Venous anatomy

The venous drainage of the forearm flap is via both a deep venae comitantes and a superficial venous system, which interconnect (*Figure 36.2*). It is apparent that either system can provide adequate venous egress in the majority. The interconnections between the superficial and deep venous systems are via communicating veins distally and at the cubital fossa, as well as at the microcirculatory level. The venous tributaries, running

into the radial venae comitantes via the lateral intermuscular septum, invariably accompany septal arterial vessels. The paired interconnecting venae comitantes of the radial artery have numerous valves, occurring at 1–3 cm intervals, which are more numerous than in the superficial veins. The valve arrangement appears to be orientated to prevent deep to superficial reflux. This might account for clinical observations noting congestion persisting for several hours when only the superficial venous system is anastomosed. However, extensive experience with reverse flow pedicled forearm flaps in hand reconstruction demonstrates that flow reversal reliably occurs. There may be an advantage in ensuring drainage from both venous systems with dual venous anastomosis.

The paired venae comitantes drain into a large communicating vein in the cubital fossa in the majority of forearms (reports vary from 68% to 98%). This fortuitous arrangement, allowing an exceptionally long venous pedicle, obviates the need for vein grafting in the majority of vessel depleted recipient defects. In most circumstances, however, the use of a single large cubital fossa vein creates undesirable pedicle redundancy in the neck and, potentially, an unfavourable disposition of either the cephalic (superficial) or deep system. It is the authors' usual practice to separate the systems and perform discrete anastomoses. In most patients, it is possible to drain one (usually the deep system via the communicating vein) into the internal jugular vein and the other (usually cephalic) into the external jugular vein. Flap venous insufficiency has been observed with internal jugular vein thrombosis and this provides the rationale for dual recipient drainage. Radial forearm free flaps are occasionally used for pharyngo-laryngeal reconstruction. The dual venous outflow tract allows bilateral drainage in the neck, which may provide protection against venous thrombosis associated with salivary leak.

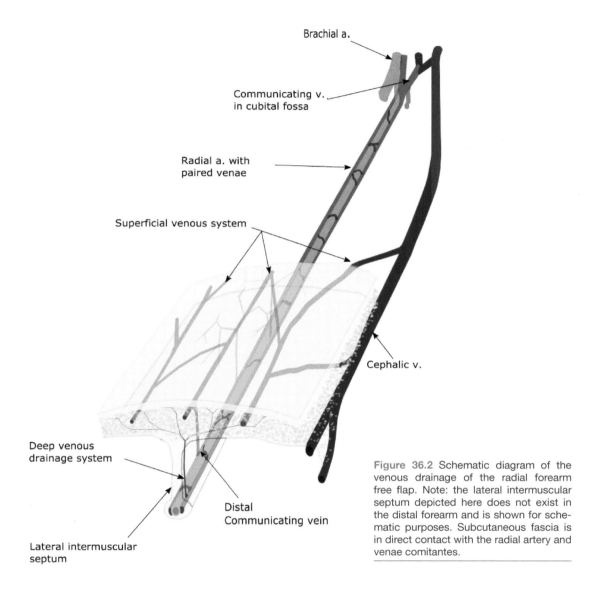

Brachial a.

Communicating v.
in cubital fossa

Radial a. with
paired venae

Superficial venous system

Cephalic v.

Deep venous
drainage system

Distal
Communicating vein

Lateral intermuscular
septum

Figure 36.2 Schematic diagram of the venous drainage of the radial forearm free flap. Note: the lateral intermuscular septum depicted here does not exist in the distal forearm and is shown for schematic purposes. Subcutaneous fascia is in direct contact with the radial artery and venae comitantes.

A body of literature advocates a suprafascial dissection of the distal skin paddle in raising the RFFF. Improved donor site wound healing with a reduction in tendon exposure is attributed. However, prospective studies have been unable to demonstrate a significant difference in donor site outcomes. Selection is therefore based on surgeon preference and experience. The anatomical basis for suprafascial dissection has been confirmed with perforators from the radial artery forming networks in the plane between the fascia and dermis. Eloquent technical descriptions of suprafascial forearm flap dissection are recommended reading. The reader is directed to descriptions by Wong et al. and Avery. The technique described here is subfascial (*Figure 36.3*).

Preparation and positioning

On admission, the selected forearm is inscribed with 'no needles' in surgical marker. Patients shower within 12 hours of surgery with particular attention to finger-nails.

A pneumatic tourniquet is preferred by the majority of, but not all, surgeons for forearm flap procedures. It is contraindicated in those with sickle cell disease and relatively so in those with a hypercoagulable state including history of thromboembolism. It is important to select the correct size (width: greater than half the arm diameter; length: cuff should overlap by 8–15 cm). Soft padding must completely cover the skin surface beneath the cuff. Current guidelines recommend that optimal cuff pressure should be based on the patient's

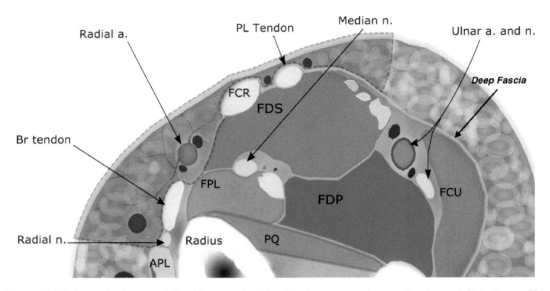

Figure 36.3 Schematic diagram of distal forearm depicting fasciocutaneous forearm flap harvest. Note the position of the small perforator vessels running in a plane above fascia and sending vertical branches to the dermal plexus. A suprafascial flap requires dissection above this plane and this is likely to be technique-sensitive. *Abbreviations*: APL, abductor pollicis longus; FCR, flexor carpi radialis tendon; FCU, flexor carpi ulnaris; FDP, flexor digitorum profundus; FDS, flexor digitorum superficialis; FPL, flexor pollicis longus; PQ, pronator quadratus.

systolic blood pressure or limb occlusion pressure. For patients with a pressure systolic (Ps) of 130 mmHg or less, add 40 to preoperative Ps; for those with a systolic pressure above this, add 60 mmHg. We do not employ exsanguination. Filled vessels facilitate a precise dissection and haemostasis. Inflation time should be kept to a minimum. The surgeon is notified when tourniquet time reaches 90 minutes (60 minutes in the paediatric population), and the tourniquet is released as soon as practicable after that time. Experienced surgeons will perform this procedure in 60 minutes comfortably. The arm is abducted to 70° with forearm supination and supported with an arm board attached to the operating table.

SURGICAL PROCEDURE

After skin preparation, sterile drapes are applied which leave exposed the entire hand, forearm and arm to a point 2.5 cm above the cubital fossa skin crease. The precise dimensions and configuration of the flap required are determined with the resection team and marked on the forearm.

The precise sequencing of operative steps outlined is not intended to be proscriptive and will be varied by surgeons depending on experience and preference.

Step 1: Dissection of cephalic vein and superficial radial nerve

Dissection proceeds on the radial aspect of the cephalic vein, proximal to the planned skin paddle, down to deep

fascia (*Figure 36.4*). This dissection is carried distally ligating tributaries from the extensor aspect and staying above investing fascia as far distally as appropriate, preserving superficial tributaries coming from the distal

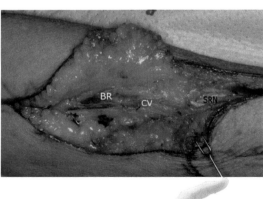

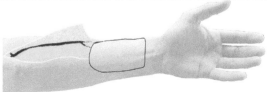

Figure 36.4 The proximal forearm incision is made from cubital fossa to the proximal limit of the outlined skin paddle. The initial dissection can proceed along the ulnar or radial aspect. *Abbreviations*: BR, brachioradialis muscle; CV, cephalic vein; SRN, superficial radial nerve.

fasciocutaneous component. The cephalic vein is then ligated towards the distal end of the skin paddle but will usually lie beyond the radial edge of the skin paddle. It will remain connected to it by subcutaneous fat and draining tributaries. The cephalic vein is then dissected free in its portion proximal to the distal skin paddle up to the cubital fossa and the large communicating vein identified. The lateral (antebrachial) cutaneous nerve of the forearm runs in close proximity to the cephalic vein and is incorporated if a sensate flap is planned. The superficial part of the radial nerve is identified as

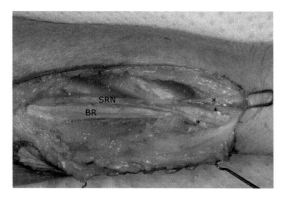

Figure 36.5 On the radial and extensor aspect of distal skin paddle the dissection is suprafascial lifting the cephalic vein off deep fascia over abductor pollicis longus and extensor pollicis brevis. *Abbreviations*: BR, brachioradialis muscle; SRN, superficial radial nerve. *Branches of radial nerve. Note that the most volar branch approaches the radial artery crossing the radial styloid.

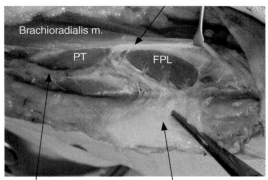

Radial a + venae comitantes   The radial aspect of the skin paddle is retracted. Note the small septocutaneous perforator (pointer) is closely applied to the fascia in the intermuscular septum

Figure 36.6 Dissection of brachioradialis aspect of intermuscular septum. *Abbreviations*: PT, pronator teres muscle; FPL, flexor pollicis longus muscle.

it emerges on the extensor aspect of the brachioradialis tendon. It is dissected free of fascia and will be found to divide into two to three branches; the most volar of which will run towards the distal radial pedicle. With nerve hook traction this is carefully separated from investing fascia to preserve sensation to the dorsal aspect of the first web space. Deep fascia is then incised at the flexor edge of brachioradialis muscle (*Figure 36.5*). If a proximal skin paddle is planned, the incision through deep fascia will be further on the radial aspect.

Step 2: Dissection of brachioradialis aspect of intermuscular septum

Starting in the proximal forearm, the brachioradialis muscle is retracted and dissection proceeds around its volar border onto its ulnar aspect (*Figure 36.6*). In this proximal location one or more large perforators will be seen as well as large muscular branches. Those coming off the radial pedicle will be ligated. It is advisable to use ligaclips or ligatures on nearly all branches off the radial pedicle. Bleeding from arterial side branches secured only with bipolar diathermy is common and can be a source of postoperative haematoma at the recipient site. The radial artery and venae comitantes will be visible as will the radial nerve. It is important to keep the dissection on the deep aspect of brachioradialis muscle to prevent inadvertent injury to small septocutaneous vessels. As the dissection progresses distally, traction is maintained displacing brachioradialis and the dissection is subfascial plane on its deep aspect in the zone of the distal skin paddle. This ensures capture of all available small perforators supplying skin. Having completed the radial dissection of the lateral intermuscular septum, a row of perforators is visible as they are given off to pronator quadratus, periosteum of the distal radius, flexor pollicis longus, radial nerve, pronator teres and flexor digitorum superficialis. These are ligated and divided or can be cauterised using bioplar diathermy ensuring this is done away from the main pedicle.

Step 3: Dissection of ulnar aspect of skin paddle and lateral intermuscular septum

The ulnar skin incision is now completed and dissection proceeds down to deep fascia, ligating superficial veins except those already dissected and draining into the cephalic system (*Figure 36.7*). These are ligated and divided.

A series of muscular branches arises from the ulnar aspect of the pedicle and contributes to the supply for the muscles of the superficial and intermediate groups of forearm muscles (*Figure 36.8*).

Figure 36.9 highlights the location (pointer) of the septocutaneous vessel immediately above fascia of the lateral intermuscular septum. *Figure 36.10* shows the flap immediately prior to division of the radial artery and venae comitantes at the wrist.

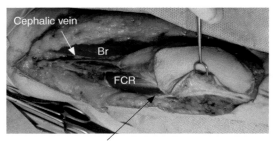

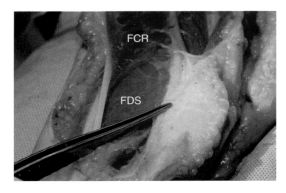

Figure 36.7 Dissection of ulnar aspect of skin paddle and lateral intermuscular septum. *Abbreviations*: Br, brachioradialis muscle; FCR, flexor carpi radialis muscle.

Figure 36.9 Note the location (pointer) of the septocutaneous vessel immediately above fascia of the lateral intermuscular septum. *Abbreviations*: FCR, flexor carpi radialis; FDS, flexor digitorum superficialis.

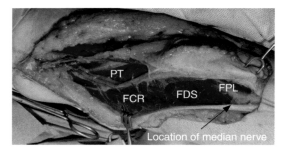

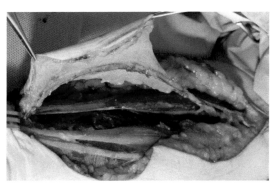

Figure 36.8 Muscular branches from the ulnar aspect of the pedicle. *Abbreviations*: FCR, flexor carpi radialis; FDS, flexor digitorum superficialis; FPL, flexor pollicis longus; PT, pronator teres.

Figure 36.10 Flap immediately prior to division of radial artery and venae comitantes at wrist (photo taken from ulnar aspect). Note the small titanium vascular clips on the side branches and the completed dissection of the lateral intermuscular septum (note that this is a right forearm dissection).

Step 4: Dissection of cubital fossa

Figure 36.11 shows dissection of the cubital fossa, with vascular pedicle of flap.

Step 5: Flap disconnection

The anaesthetic team is informed 5 minutes before tourniquet deflation. Time of deflation is noted. Perfusion of the entire hand and then flap is checked immediately. The wound is irrigated with warm saline and any bleeding points secured. We try to time flap harvest to be complete approximately 20 minutes prior to completion of the head and neck procedure. It seems prudent to allow an adequate reperfusion time prior to a further ischaemic insult.

After confirmation of pulsatile arterial flow in a suitable recipient artery and isolation of an appropriate recipient vein(s), the radial artery is clamped and time noted. After division, the radial artery is ligated with a transfixion suture distal to the radial recurrent branch, the veins ligated and divided, and the flap is handed off to the head and neck set.

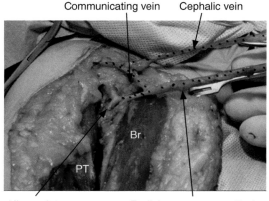

Figure 36.11 Dissection of the cubital fossa. *Abbreviations*: Br, brachioradialis; PT, pronator teres.

Prior to inset the radial artery is cannulated and irrigated with a warm solution of heparinised saline (10 IU/mL) until the venous effluent runs clear. Subjective assessment of resistance to flow is noted. The flap skin paddle is then partially inset. Having completed this the radial artery is again cannulated and irrigated with warm heparinised saline. Lack of flow from the venous system or subjective increased resistance implies a conformational problem with the pedicle. This must be resolved prior to completing anastomoses. It will be necessary to dissect a minimum of 3–4 cm of radial artery from the venae comitantes to achieve adequate separation of arterial inflow and venous egress.

Step 6: Closure of donor defect

A skin graft is applied to the donor defect and secured with resorbable sutures and a silicone sheet with a 'tie-over' liquid paraffin-impregnated sponge dressing applied. No measurable improvement in graft take or tendon exposure has been demonstrated with negative pressure wound therapy. Purse-string suture to the distal defect to reduce its size, volar slab application with wrist in mild dorsiflexion, and suturing muscle over tendon are all practices employed in the past in our patient series but now largely abandoned due to absence of perceptible benefit.

COMPLICATIONS

Partial graft loss with tendon exposure occurs in up to 20% of procedures. The average number of dressings to achieve complete healing in this circumstance is in excess of 50 and takes approximately 6 weeks.

The superficial part of the radial nerve is dissected with the donor site located distally. Furthermore, the lateral (antebrachial) cutaneous nerve of the forearm is often incorporated in the flap dissection where the cephalic vein is included. A third of patients will experience one or more of scar contracture, altered sensation or chronic pain. Cold intolerance is reported in up to 10%, and aesthetic concerns are a consideration with women reporting less satisfaction than men. It requires 24 months for patient-reported function to return to pre-surgery levels and there is a small, but persistent, decrease in hand grip strength.

The loss of a major source artery to the hand is a consideration. Acute ischaemia associated with harvest of a RFFF has been reported on four occasions to our knowledge. Careful preoperative evaluation is likely to identify the potential for acute ischaemia in most, but not all, patients. Teams should be equipped and prepared to perform immediate revascularisation whenever performing this procedure. The elderly, and patients with atheromatous disease, may merit imaging assessment in addition to those with an equivocal Allen test.

TOP TIPS AND HAZARDS

- The fasciocutaneous radial forearm remains an essential procedure in the repertoire of reconstructive head and neck surgeons.
- It is arguably the most straightforward of all free flaps to raise and deploy in the head and neck region.
- It does involve loss of a major source artery which can have rare, but important, ischaemic consequences.
- Delayed healing with tendon exposure will occur in a significant minority of patients and relatively minor long-term adverse functional consequences are prevalent.

FURTHER READING

Avery C. Prospective study of the septocutaneous radial free flap and suprafascial donor site. *Br J Oral Maxillofac Surg* 2007;**45**:611–16.

Matthews JLK, Alolabi N, Farrkhyar F, Voineskos SH. One versus 2 venous anastomoses in free flap surgery: a systematic review and meta-analysis. *Plast Surg* 2018;**26**:91–8.

McCormack LJ, Cauldwell EW, Anson BJ. Brachial and antebrachial arterial patterns; a study of 750 extremities. *Surg Gynecol Obstet* 1953;**96**:43–54.

Timmons MJ. The vascular basis of the radial forearm flap. *Plast Reconstr Surg* 1986;**77**:80–92.

Wong C-H, Lin J-Y, Wei F-C. The bottom-up approach to the suprafascial harvest of the radial forearm flap. *Am J Surg* 2008;**196**:e60–e64.

Chapter
37
Fibular Flap
Peter A. Brennan, Mark Singh

INTRODUCTION

The fibula is a long slender triangular-shaped bone that is said to have two functions: ankle joint stability and microvascular reconstruction of bony defects. It is mainly composed of cortical bone, giving it great stability. The advantages of the fibula are that it offers an abundant supply of tubed bi-cortical bone, which is useful for reconstruction of long segmental defects across the midline – 25 cm or more of bone can be harvested. There is usually little morbidity at the donor site, and it is highly reliable with a 95% success rate (when used, the skin paddle component is reported to be less reliable). It is also possible to harvest the fibula simultaneously with the tumour resection as no change in the patient's position is required. Bone height is the main potential disadvantage, especially when reconstructing the dentate mandible. To overcome this problem, the osteotomised fibula can be folded back onto itself while maintaining intact soft tissue and periosteum on one side ('double barrelling'). Distraction osteogenesis, followed by implant placement, can also give a very good result (*Figure 37.1*). It is usual to leave the flap for several months before distraction, to allow bony union with the recipient bed and enable the fixation plates to be removed.

HISTORICAL DEVELOPMENT

The first vascularised fibula flap transfer was used for ulnar reconstruction by Ueba in 1974. Taylor et al. subsequently reported free fibula transfer for two tibial defects. Chen and Yan were the first to report an osteo-cutaneous fibula flap in 1983. Hidalgo reported its use in mandibular reconstruction in 1989.

VASCULAR ANATOMY

The fibula is supplied by periosteal branches of the peroneal artery, and by an endosteal vessel which directly enters the bone at the middle third/distal third junction. The peroneal artery arises from the tibio-peroneal trunk and runs between the chevron-shaped fibres of tibialis posterior and flexor hallucis longus (FHL), running close to the fibula, along its deep surface. The vascular pedicle is relatively short (approximately 6 cm), but it can be made longer by harvesting the fibula more proximally than that required for the reconstruction – following detachment of the flap, the

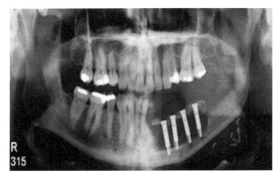

Figure 37.1 Implants placed in a recently distracted fibula.

pedicle is dissected free from this excess bone, which is subsequently discarded.

Between two and six cutaneous perforator vessels emerge from the peroneal artery. They pass posterior to the fibula and may be myocutaneous (perforating FHL and/or soleus) or septocutaneous. A paddle of skin can be harvested with the main bone flap. There is anatomical variation in location, course, size and number of these cutaneous perforators according to anatomical studies and various clinical reports. Yu et al. performed a live study on 80 consecutive fibula flaps looking at perforator patterns. They found two discrete groups of perforators located proximally and distally. If the fibula was divided into quarters, the clinically useful perforators (distal) were located over the third quarter. In 51% of cases, there were two or more perforators approximately 1.5 cm posterior to the line connecting the fibula head to the lateral malleolus. Surprisingly, they also found that over 90% of the perforators were septocutaneous. The most reliable region for harvesting the skin paddle was found to be 8–12 cm above the ankle – an area corresponding to the third quarter of the fibula. To facilitate identification of the cutaneous perforators, preoperative mapping using a handheld Doppler probe is advisable.

There are a number of important anatomical variations of the lower limb arterial supply, which need to be known (*Figure 37.2*). The normal arterial supply is found in 88%. The mainstay vascular assessment preoperatively is by computed tomography angiogram (CTA) or magnetic resonance angiography (MRA). These two are becoming widely used, especially because

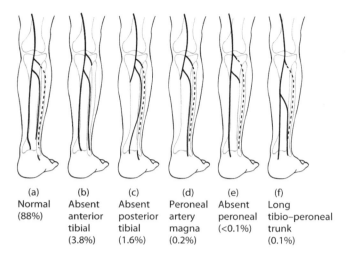

(a)
Normal
(88%)

(b)
Absent
anterior
tibial
(3.8%)

(c)
Absent
posterior
tibial
(1.6%)

(d)
Peroneal
artery
magna
(0.2%)

(e)
Absent
peroneal
(<0.1%)

(f)
Long
tibio–peroneal
trunk
(0.1%)

Figure 37.2 Anatomical variations of the lower limb arterial supply.

they avoid arterial puncture and its associated complications. Vascular assessment is mandatory before harvesting a fibula flap to exclude congenital peroneal artery anomalies. These include a dominant peroneal artery (0.2% of patients) or congenital absence of the peroneal vessels (less than 0.1%). Most anomalies are unilateral so it is sensible to obtain bilateral imaging.

Modern practice is for specialised radiologists to report on these assessments. Surgeons too, should be able to visualise the anatomy on the scans and not rely solely on the radiology reports. If there is any doubt regarding the collateral supply of the foot, balloon occlusion of the proximal peroneal artery could be requested to assess the dependence of the foot on the blood supply provided by the peroneal. The alternative is to use the other side or choose a different bone flap.

It should be noted that in the authors' experience there can be a discrepancy in the length of the pedicle depending on which leg is chosen. This is due to variations in the length of the tibio-peroneal trunk. This is shown in *Figure 37.3*.

Peripheral vascular disease and limb oedema are signs that harvest may be unnecessarily complicated and so other alternatives should be sought. Foot loss following this procedure has been reported in the literature.

CLINICAL USE OF FIBULA FLAP IN MAXILLOFACIAL SURGERY

In maxillofacial surgery, the fibula flap is mainly used for primary or secondary reconstruction of extensive mandibular and maxillary bone defects. When greater depth of bone is required in large mandibular defects, it may be possible to fold the bone back on itself (double barrelling) or perform interval distraction osteogenesis.

Fibula anatomy can allow us to raise solely a soft tissue flap based on the same pedicle. This can be very useful especially if one wants to avoid the complications

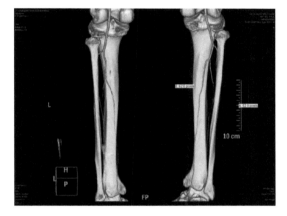

Figure 37.3 Computed tomography angiogram showing the longer tibio-peroneal trunk on the left side, resulting in a shorter pedicle length.

concerning the donor site of the radial forearm. The anterolateral thigh flap has been suggested as an alternative to the radial forearm flap, but this can be difficult if the patient is not thin and can lead to quite a bulky flap. Wolff et al. published their series of 30 peroneal perforator flaps which details the procedure.

When considering implant placement, there are some operators who prefer to place implants when the bone flap is raised due to easy access and advances in computer-assisted planning. This also allows time for the implants to osseointegrate, especially if it is likely that radiotherapy may be part of treatment. However, surgeons need to be mindful of the sequelae of this type of surgery, which include trismus and lower bite force. Trismus will make the second stage very difficult due to lack of space/height and operators may find there is no place for future teeth. Lower bite forces generated due to the surgery also raise the question of whether the

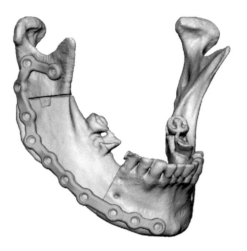

Figure 37.4 Computer-assisted design showing plate to span the defect. To aid with resection, cutting guides can also be made. Bone thickness can also be provided to assist with screw selection.

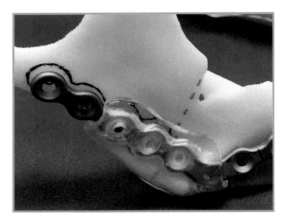

Figure 37.5 Transparent locator placed on mandible to assist with placement of holes for reconstruction plate. Dotted red line to assist planning resection.

patient will require dentition in future. Lastly, it should be appreciated that in many instances, the fibula is placed too low to allow for adequate dental rehabilitation and if the placement of fibula or implant deviates even minimally from the computer-assisted plan then this may become non-restorable.

PLANNING

With the advent of computer-assisted design and computer-assisted manufacture (CAD–CAM) technology and rapid prototyping modelling (RPM), surgical planning for fibula flaps has evolved to a very precise procedure. The advantages have been well documented to improve outcomes and save operative time (*Figure 37.4*).

Manufacture of three-dimensional (3D) models allows the ablative surgeon, with the assistance of the maxillofacial technician, to perform model surgery to assess the shape and size of the defect. This then gives the surgeon a chance to plan for complex shapes such as a mandibular resection involving body, angle and ramus or the anterior mandible (*Figures 37.5* and *37.6*). Knowing the shape of the defect allows for reconstructive plates to be pre-bent, 3D printed or milled, which saves time at operation and improves accuracy at restoring form. The plates can be made with locators so the operator can reproduce their placement from the lab to the theatre. Maintaining spatial relationships ensures improved outcomes.

From a reconstructive point of view, the same technology can be used to reproduce the donor fibula. The fibula can then be assessed for the quality of bone to help produce stents to guide osteotomy cuts and even implant placement (*Figure 37.7*).

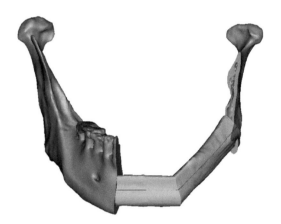

Figure 37.6 Computer design for planned fibula left mandible. The green and yellow sections are the same fibula segment after being osteotomised.

SURGICAL TECHNIQUE

The fully anaesthetised patient is placed on their back, and the leg is flexed at both the hip and knee joint and brought into a prone position for better access to the lateral and posterior aspect of the calf. We have described a simple triangular-shaped padded device that when placed under the knee, greatly facilitates this position. It can be easily constructed by a competent dental technician as follows:

1   The entire lower extremity is prepared with antiseptic solution, and the foot is enclosed in a sterile drape. Both authors do not routinely use a tourniquet for flap harvest. If a tourniquet is preferred, this should be inflated to over 300 mmHg, and should be released after a maximum of 2 hours to prevent re-perfusion injury. The fibula head and

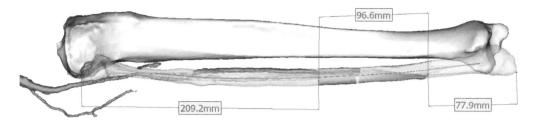

Figure 37.7 Planning on fibula for case in *Figure 37.8*. Shows length of segment and where osteotomy cut. Guides can be provided to assist with this.

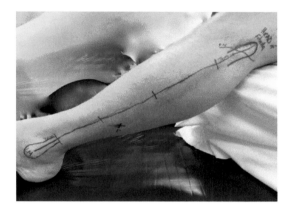

Figure 37.8 Surface markings.

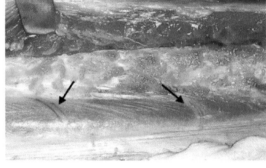

Figure 37.9 Two perforators can be seen emerging posterior to the fibula (arrows).

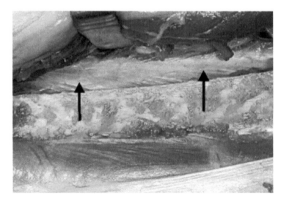

Figure 37.10 White interosseous membrane (arrows).

lateral malleolus (as constant anatomical landmarks) are identified and marked. A line drawn between the two is the surface marking of the posterior intercrural septum (one of the approaches to the lateral fibula – the other being via the anterior crural septum).

2   For a bone-only fibula graft, a skin incision is made along this line, in the middle to distal one-third of the palpable bone. Superiorly, the incision should not pass too close to the fibula head, for risk of subsequent damage to the common peroneal nerve. Inferiorly, at least 6–7 cm of bone should be left to maintain ankle joint stability (*Figure 37.8*). When a skin paddle is required, the initial linear incision can be modified and placed more anteriorly than the line marked in Step 1. Once the skin flaps have been raised and the perforator(s) identified emerging from the posterior surface of the fibula (*Figure 37.9*), the skin paddle can be marked and raised centred on these perforators. As previously mentioned, a Doppler probe can also be used to mark the perforator sites.

3   The skin and subcutaneous fat is raised from the underlying muscle fascia using sharp dissection. The posterior crural septum will come into view, appearing as a white line directly over the lateral aspect of the fibula. Posteriorly soleus is identified, and peroneus longus and brevis with their longitudinally running muscle fibres are retracted anteriorly. The septum can then be followed onto the bone.

4   Peroneus longus and brevis are detached from the lateral surface of the fibula using sharp dissection. The dissection passes anteriorly, along the whole length of the incision in a broad front, with detachment of the anterior crural septum, extensor digitorum longus and FHL. The safest way to do this is with sharp dissection, staying close to the bone but leaving a small cuff of muscle attached to it.

5   A thick white membrane (the interosseus membrane) will be encountered next (*Figure 37.10*).

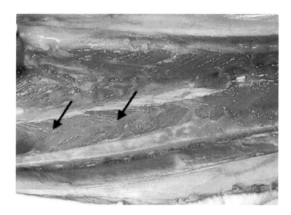

Figure 37.11 Chevron arrangement of the tibialis posterior muscle fibres.

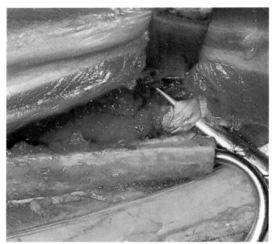

Figure 37.12 Identification of the distal pedicle.

The anterior tibial artery and vein and the deep peroneal nerve are sometimes visible lying between this membrane and the underside of the tibialis anterior muscle. This vascular pedicle is retracted and the membrane is incised along its length using a pair of sharp scissors which are opened and slid along the membrane from proximal to distal (or vice versa) at a distance of about 1 cm from the fibula.

6   Attention should now be paid to the fibula bone cuts. The periosteum at the proposed bone cuts is incised. An instrument (such as a McDonald or Howarth retractor) is gently passed around the deep surface of the fibula in a subperiosteal plane to protect the underlying pedicle. The bone cuts (both proximal and distal) are performed with an oscillating saw. Some surgeons complete the cuts with an osteotome. The fibula should now be carefully retracted laterally using bone clamps. This procedure gives greater access to the peroneal vessels. When a longer pedicle is required, the amount of bone harvested can be increased by making a more proximal bone cut. The pedicle can be dissected free from this bone (and the latter discarded by making a further bone cut at the required length) once the flap is detached.

7   Gentle lateral traction of the fibula reveals the chevron-shaped fibres of tibialis posterior (*Figure 37.11*). The next stage depends on operator preference. Most surgeons will dissect through tibialis posterior at the distal bone cut site, using sharp and blunt dissection and staying close to the fibula (it is usual to leave 1 cm or so of tibialis posterior attached to the fibula). The peroneal vessels (artery and two accompanying veins) will readily come into view (*Figure 37.12*), and can be ligated and divided, thereby allowing the bone to be further retracted laterally. Others prefer to expose the length of the pedicle by dissecting along the length of tibialis posterior using sharp and blunt

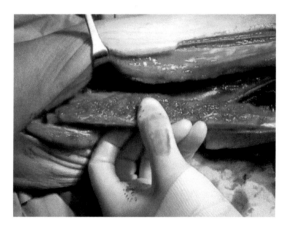

Figure 37.13 Flap is retracted laterally to aid dissection proximally.

dissection. The advantage of the former method (and that preferred by the authors) is that the peroneal artery can be identified early, and followed up the fibula, in a manner not dissimilar to following the facial nerve during a parotidectomy – the overlying tibialis posterior can be lifted off the pedicle and safely cut.

8   If skin is required, the skin incision around the paddle is now completed (see Step 2). It is sensible to include a cuff of both FHL and soleus when completing this part of the dissection to include as many perforating muscular branches as possible. The laterally retracted fibula flap can be moved from side to side, to ensure that this is done from both sides (laterally and medially), thereby reducing any chance of damage to either the main pedicle (*Figure 37.13*) or these perforators. As the skin and muscle paddle are released, it is wise to temporarily

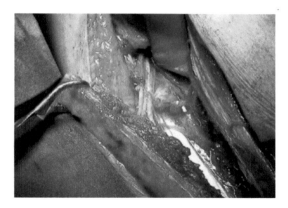

Figure 37.14 Proximal vascular pedicle after completed dissection and prior to vessel ligation.

suture the paddle to the muscle cuff attached to the fibula to reduce the chance of shearing.

9 As more of the tibialis posterior is released, the flap can be retracted further laterally (*Figure 37.14*), revealing FHL and the posterior intermuscular septum. The FHL is released from the fibula, taking care to ensure that the pedicle is not damaged during this procedure. Several perforating vessels arise from the peroneal artery and enter the FHL, and if care is taken, these can be identified and dealt with before they are cut. The posterior tibial vessels are found more medially and should be left undisturbed.

10 Finally, any remaining muscle attachments are released from the fibula. Once the flap has been raised, it can be 'rested' in a heparinised saline-soaked gauze swap and temporarily placed back in the wound with the pedicle still running until it is needed for the reconstruction. When finally tying off the artery, a transfixation suture as well as conventional ligation ensures that the divided vessel will not inadvertently start bleeding postoperatively.

11 If osteotomies are needed to allow the fibula to satisfactorily fit the defect, these can be performed from the lateral aspect of the bone after the pedicle has been divided. Before these osteotomy cuts are made, the soft tissues and periosteum at the proposed bone cuts are carefully stripped off using sharp dissection and subsequently protected using a periosteal retractor. The cuts can be made with an oscillating saw on a sterile table, and completed with an osteotome. With the advent of modern imaging and software, it is possible to accurately plan the osteotomy cuts in three dimensions, and to perform these cuts while the flap is still attached

on the peroneal pedicle. The flap is secured at the recipient site using the surgeons' choice of fixation (either a reconstruction plate or multiple 2-mm miniplates). As already mentioned, the pedicle is sharply dissected off any excess bone to increase its length.

12 The wound is closed in layers by carefully suturing muscle groups together. A suction drain is also placed. When a skin paddle has been harvested, the defect is closed with either a full- or split-thickness skin graft. The latter can be taken from the thigh of the same leg, preferably using a powered dermatome.

13 At the end of the procedure it is prudent to check the distal pulses with a Doppler and document this in the notes.

14 For the first few days, the donor limb should be gently elevated on a pillow to reduce dependency and swelling.

15 Patients should mobilise early, initially with partial weight-bearing. Ankle and foot movements are encouraged. Skin grafts should be managed in the conventional way. When patients are slow to mobilise, low molecular weight heparin prophylaxis should be considered.

TOP TIPS AND HAZARDS

- Careful preoperative assessment with imaging is recommended (either angiography, CTA or MRA).
- Correct leg positioning with adequate stabilisation facilitates access.
- Surgical landmarks: mark the fibula head and lateral malleolus and draw a line between them. Leave at least 7 cm of bone proximally and distally to maintain ankle joint stability and prevent damage to the common peroneal nerve.
- Always dissect on a broad front, and leave a small cuff of muscle attached to the bone.
- Identify cutaneous perforators early if a skin paddle is to be used (they emerge posterior to the fibula).
- Place a retractor subperiosteally during proximal and distal bone cuts to prevent pedicle damage.
- The pedicle is always lateral to the tibial nerve in the posterior compartment.
- Proximal venae comitantes can be quite voluminous and fragile, so dissection should proceed with caution.
- Include a generous muscle cuff (FHL and soleus) when a skin paddle is raised.

ACKNOWLEDGEMENT

The authors would kindly like to thank Nicholas Connolly, IMPT, Gloucester Royal Hospital, UK, for his contribution to this chapter.

FURTHER READING

Chen ZW, Yan W. The study and clinical application of the osteocutaneous flap of fibula. *Microsurgery* 1983;**4**:11–16.

Hidalgo DA. Fibula free flap: a new method of mandible reconstruction. *Plast Reconstr Surg* 1989;**84**:71–9.

Taylor GI, Miller GDH, Ham FJ. The free vascularized bone graft. *Plast Reconstr Surg* 1975;**55**:533–44.

Wolff K, Bauer F, Wylie J, Stimmer H, Hölzle F, Kesting M. Peroneal perforator flap for intraoral reconstruction. *Br J Oral Maxillofac Surg* 2012;**50**:25–9.

Yu P, Chang E, Hanasono M. Design of a reliable skin paddle for the fibula osteocutaneous flap: Perforator anatomy revisited. *Plast Reconstr Surg* 2011;**128**:440–6.

Chapter
38

Anterolateral Thigh Flap

Rabindra P. Singh

INTRODUCTION

First described by Song et al. in 1984, the anterolateral thigh (ALT) flap has become one of the most popular free flaps in head and neck reconstructive surgery. It is a relatively easy flap to raise with proven reliability and is indicated for coverage of various soft tissue defects, particularly useful for large tongue and scalp, composite parotid resection defects as well as maxillary obturation and tubed flaps for laryngeal reconstruction. It may be raised as a chimeric flap with multiple skin paddles based on individual perforator vessels, or a vastus lateralis muscle as a separate component. The pedicle length and the vessel size are almost always generous with the average pedicle length of 12 cm and mean arterial and venous size of 2–4 mm. If the skin paddle is based on a distal perforator, a very long pedicle length is possible; however, the extent of tissue dissection will be greater. The width of the skin paddle depends on the laxity of local tissue, which should be tested by pinching the skin with fingers, and the appropriate size skin paddle designed allowing for primary closure of the defect. If needed, a skin graft is possible for the harvest site defect; however, it is not recommended because of possible poor cosmetic outcome.

The thickness of skin paddle may be a problem in obese patients, which can be a contraindication for raising this flap in this group of patients, especially relevant in the Western population. Some authors have described radical thinning of the flap leaving 3–4 mm thickness, except around the perforators; however, there is a risk of damage to perforators, compromising the reliability of the flap. Therefore, this should only be undertaken by clinicians with considerable experience in this technique.

SURGICAL ANATOMY

This operative technique chapter assumes that the reader is familiar with the basic knowledge of branches of profunda femoris artery and the orientation of quadriceps muscle of the thigh and in particular the rectus femoris and vastus lateralis muscle. The vascular supply of the flap is from the descending branch of the lateral circumflex femoral artery (LCFA), which runs along the septum between the rectus femoris and vastus lateralis muscles (*Figure 38.1*). The artery is accompanied by two venae comitantes that may or may not form a confluence. The ALT flap is a perforator flap, which

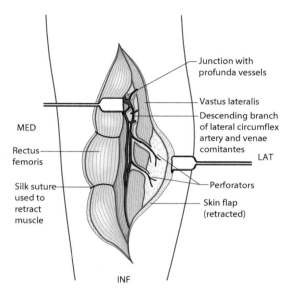

Figure 38.1 A schematic diagram of a left leg anterolateral thigh flap based on the descending branch of the lateral circumflex artery running along the septum between the rectus femoris and vastus lateralis muscles. *Abbreviations*: MED, medial; LAT, lateral.

means that it is based on a perforator vessel originating from an axial vessel, passing through various structural elements of the body besides interstitial connective tissue and fat before reaching the subcutaneous fat layer.

In 80–90% of the cases, the perforators take an intermuscular course (myocutaneous), with the rest being septocutaneous, where the perforator has a direct course to the skin through the intermuscular septum piercing into the fascia lata without passing through the vastus lateralis muscle. The dissection of perforators is straightforward in the latter case, whereas muscle dissection is required for the myocutaneous course. There may be a variation in the pattern of cutaneous perforators arising from the main pedicle. Most commonly (90%), the cutaneous perforators arise from the descending branch of the LCFA, whereas in 5–10% of the cases, the perforators originate from the transverse branch of the LCFA. In the latter variation, the perforators take a long intermuscular course to the transverse branch of the LCFA. In the third group of patients (1–5%), the cutaneous perforators arise directly from the profunda femoris and take a myocutaneous course through the rectus femoris and vastus lateralis muscle. In this variation, the vessels are usually of very small size and unsuitable for flap harvest.

PREOPERATIVE CONSIDERATIONS

A handheld Doppler may be useful to mark out the location of the perforators prior to skin incision. However, it has a positive predictive value of only 65%, therefore should only be used as a guide. Inability to locate a suitable Doppler signal must not be a reason to abandon the chosen leg for flap harvest. One may, however, select the leg with the best Doppler signal. A vast majority of patients (96%) have usable perforators. The patients should be consented for harvesting the flap from the alternative leg or an alternative flap altogether in case of failure to find the suitable perforator.

High magnification surgical loupes are recommended for raising this flap as this will help to identify small perforators.

STEPWISE OPERATIVE TECHNIQUE

The patient should be positioned supine without any sandbags under the hip or splinting of the leg. A pneumatic compression device can be placed on the lower leg. Ideally, all monitoring lines should be placed in a different limb.

A line is drawn between the anterior superior iliac spine (ASIS) and the superior border of the patella. As a guide, a 4 cm diameter circle is drawn at a point midway along this line, and a 10 MHz handheld Doppler probe is used to identify perforators lateral to this line. The most common site for finding the perforators is suggested to be the inferolateral aspect of this circle; however, it may not always be the case (*Figure 38.2*).

The skin paddle is designed with the medial border at least 1.5 cm from the line drawn from ASIS to patella. This is important because the misplaced first incision may damage the perforator and may render the leg unsuitable for ALT flap. The lateral border of the skin paddle is marked later once the perforators are located and chosen for the flap.

The draping of the surgical site should leave the ASIS and the knee fully exposed. An incision is made full length along the medial border of the skin paddle

with the knife angled slightly away from the paddle, avoiding undermining of the skin paddle and damaging the perforators. The incision is deepened to the fascia and then cut through it to expose the rectus femoris muscle.

Several artery clips are placed on the fascial edge of the skin paddle and a gentle retraction applied laterally as the dissection continues at subfascial level carefully looking for perforators entering the skin paddle through fascia lata. One must not rush this step of the operation as it is easy to damage the fine perforators if not careful. There may be more than one perforator present which may be included in the skin paddle; however, a single vessel is adequate for skin paddle perfusion. In general, the largest appearing perforator closest to the centre of the skin paddle is selected (*Figure 38.3*).

At this point, the main pedicle, descending branch of LCFA, is identified in the septum between rectus femoris and vastus lateralis muscles (*Figure 38.4*). It may sometimes be a little tricky for the inexperienced surgeon to differentiate between the rectus femoris muscle and vastus lateralis muscle. The rectus femoris muscle is readily identified by its bipinnate muscle fibre orientation and its insertion into the patella centrally.

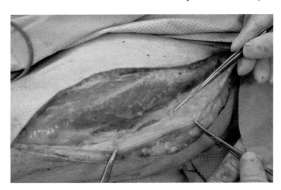

Figure 38.3 Subfascial dissection laterally to identify perforator entering the fascia. Note artery clips placed on the fascia to facilitate gentle retraction. Note bipinnate orientation of rectus femoris muscle.

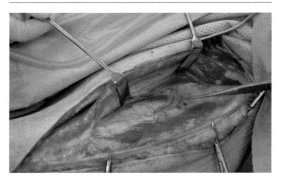

Figure 38.4 The main pedicle is identified in the septum between the rectus femoris and vastus lateralis muscles.

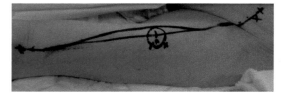

Figure 38.2 A line is drawn from the anterior superior iliac spine to the superolateral border of the patella. A handheld Doppler is used to identify perforators.

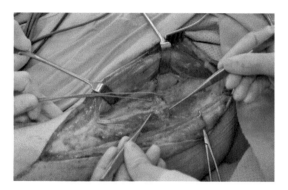

Figure 38.5 Intramuscular dissection of the perforator towards the main pedicle.

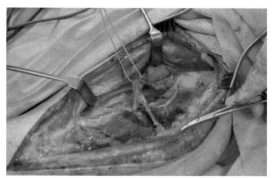

Figure 38.6 The perforator is dissected free of the muscle, and the dissection continues to free up the main pedicle superiorly.

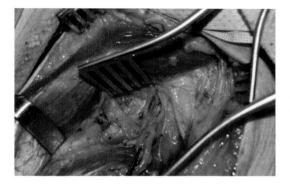

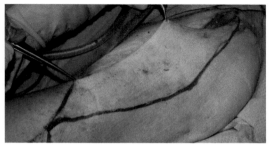

Figure 38.8 The lateral skin incision is marked safely below the level of the perforator.

Figure 38.7 A self-retainer deep in the muscle improves the surgical access greatly and allows dissection of the pedicle superiorly.

The chosen perforator(s) may be myocutaneous or septocutaneous in their course. The perforator vessel is carefully dissected free towards the main pedicle through muscle or fascia. Vascular slings may be useful in gently retracting the vessel to facilitate dissection (*Figures 38.5* and *38.6*). Side branches from the perforators should be coagulated with a bipolar diathermy or ligated with metal clips, particularly if close to the perforator. It may be a safer practice to leave a cuff of muscle around the myocutaneous perforator to make the dissection less hazardous.

The pedicle (artery and accompanying venae comitantes) is then dissected free from the junction with the perforator superiorly up to the point of its branching from the lateral circumflex artery. If a reasonable size and length of pedicle is evident as the dissection progresses superiorly, there may not be a need to continue dissecting to the entire length. A self-retainer placed under the muscle superiorly will improve access to facilitate this part of the dissection (*Figure 38.7*).

During the dissection, several branching arteries and veins will be encountered and will require cauterisation or ligation. Branches of the femoral nerve run

alongside the pedicle and will have to be dissected out. Smaller branches of the femoral nerve may have to be sacrificed if their dissection puts the pedicle at undue risk.

A sheet of vastus lateralis muscle can be harvested if needed. If the muscle is included in the flap, the myocutaneous perforating vessel may not need to be freed up separately if the surgeon is certain that the perforating vessel does lead to the main pedicle. The muscle is usually 1.5–2.5 cm thick and 6–10 cm in width. Although sheets of muscle greater than 10 cm in length inevitably have at least one perforator, smaller lengths of muscle can be raised by identifying muscular perforators coming off laterally from the pedicle into the muscle.

The distal end of the main pedicle beyond the point of branching of the perforator vessel is ligated and divided.

Once the main pedicle and the perforator(s) have been fully dissected out, the lateral extent of the skin flap can be marked out (*Figure 38.8*). The perforator need not be centrally based but should be determined by the shape of the recipient defect. However, if placed close towards the centre, then that may allow flexibility at the flap insetting stage when part of the flap may have to be excised to fit into the defect. It is extremely important to take care to avoid damage to the perforator while making the lateral flap incision by repeatedly checking the position of the perforator entry point in relation to the progressing skin incision. The author places one of their fingers below the level of the perforator entry point as the skin incision is progressed safely. Once the skin paddle incision is complete, the skin edges should be checked to ensure that there are bleeding points confirming the viability of the skin paddle. This now completes the raising of the flap (*Figure 38.9*).

If the recipient defect site is not ready for flap detachment, the flap should be sutured or stapled to the superior wound margins with pedicle under no tension, while waiting for flap detachment.

The detachment of the flap is straightforward with artery and venae separated free from each other and appropriate size metal clips placed before division. A skin staple or a suture can be placed on the skin edge to mark the perforator, which may help with flap insetting later.

The donor site closure is recommended as soon as the flap is detached because a prolonged delay may lead to difficulty closing the defect because of swelling and oedema of tissue that may ensue. A thorough haemostasis is achieved, and a suction drain is placed along the course of the pedicle with the muscle tacked over gently with few 2-0 resorbable sutures. The skin is closed in layers with subcuticular 3-0 resorbable skin sutures (*Figure 38.10*). The flaps of 8–10 cm width can be closed primarily depending on the laxity of the tissue. A non-adhesive dressing is placed over the incision line followed by a cotton padding and a tight crepe bandage.

POSTOPERATIVE CARE

The donor leg should be elevated on a single pillow supporting the knee from underneath. It is the author's practice to always monitor the donor limb with an oxygen saturation probe placed on the toe to detect any ischaemic complications, which is, however, extremely rare in this flap. The specifics of flap monitoring are described in *Chapter 35*.

COMPLICATIONS

Flap-related complications are rare in the harvesting of the ALT flap. In the author's experience, this is an extremely reliable flap with an exceptionally low morbidity rate. If there is damage to the perforator vessel intraoperatively and there are no alternative perforators available, the flap may have to be abandoned for an alternative leg or a different flap. If this

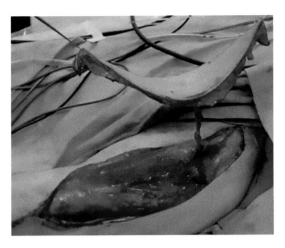

Figure 38.9 The flap is fully raised and ready for detachment.

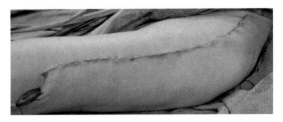

Figure 38.10 The donor site is closed primarily with resorbable sutures.

occurs at a late stage, then depending on the recipient defect, a decision may have to be made to take the flap with the muscle component alone. For a cutaneous defect, a split-thickness skin graft can be raised and utilised to cover the muscle. For defects such as tongue, some authors have reported vastus lateralis muscle-only flap with reasonable results.

A common complication of this flap is the formation of a seroma postoperatively. Occasionally, the drain output may not settle and continue to extrude large amounts of drainage. If this occurs, the drain should be removed, and a tight pressing dressing should be applied to the thigh. Repeated aspiration of the seroma every several days may be required; however, the aspiration should not be carried out too frequently as this will only lead to quick refilling of the seroma.

If a large part of muscle has been harvested, there may be a weak extension of the knee. Gait disturbances are rare but may take several months to resolve if several femoral nerve branches have been sacrificed. Thigh numbness may be demonstrated objectively; however, it is usually of little or no concern to patients.

TOP TIPS AND HAZARDS

- It is important that the patients are consented for raising the ALT flap from the alternative leg or a different flap altogether in case of failure to locate suitable perforators.

- Preoperative handheld Doppler assessment may not be entirely reliable. It is therefore particularly important to take time and carefully look for perforators intraoperatively as the skin paddle is retracted laterally at subfascial plane.

- The rectus femoris muscle can be identified by its bipinnate muscle orientation and its insertion centrally into the patella.

- A single perforator is adequate for skin paddle perfusion; therefore, one should not waste time by dissecting multiple perforator vessels unless intending to harvest a chimeric flap with multiple components.

- It may be safer to dissect the perforators with a cuff of muscle around them especially in case of fine vessels.

- The skin closure should commence as soon as possible after the flap is detached to avoid swelling and oedema, which may make it difficult to achieve a primary closure.

FURTHER READING

Wolff KD, Hölzle F. Anterolateral thigh/Vastus lateralis flap. In: *Raising of Microvascular Flaps – A Systematic Approach*, 2nd edition. Springer; 2011:39–63.

Song YG, Chen GZ, Song Y. The free thigh flap: a new free flap concept based on the septocutaneous artery. *Br J Plast Surg* 1984;**37**:149–59.

Urken ML, Cheney ML, Blackwell KE et al. Anterolateral thigh free flap. In: *Atlas of Regional and Free Flaps for Head and Neck Reconstruction*, 2nd edition. Wolters Kluwer; 2011:234–49.

Bailey & Love's Essential Operations Bailey & Love's Essential Operations
Bailey & Love's Essential Operations Bailey & Love's Essential Operations
Bailey & Love's Essential Operations Bailey & Love's Essential Operations

PART 5 | Reconstructive surgery

Chapter

39

Deep Circumflex Iliac Artery (DCIA) Flap

Colin MacIver

The vascularised iliac crest free flap is a highly versatile free flap for head and neck reconstruction. It provides the best bone stock for orofacial reconstruction, allowing adequate quality and quantity of bone for mandible or maxillary reconstruction and oral rehabilitation with dental implants. It can be raised as a bone-only flap but is commonly raised as a bone and muscle flap utilising the internal oblique muscle for soft tissue coverage. It can also be raised with an overlying skin paddle. The traditional bone–muscle–skin flap often produces a bulky soft tissue component. Although technically more demanding, raising the skin paddle as a perforator flap, allowing it to be used as a chimeric flap, produces a thin skin paddle with independent movement to the bone.

The blood supply is from the deep circumflex iliac artery (DCIA) (a branch of the external iliac artery) and its venae comitantes (which drain into the saphenous vein, then into the femoral vein). The artery is 1.7–4 mm and the vein 2–7 mm in diameter. In most cases, there is a single artery and vein. It divides into a deep branch supplying the ilium and lower transversalis, and an ascending branch supplying the muscles of the abdominal wall. Occasionally, separate pedicles for the DCIA and ascending branches are found. In this situation it is important to raise the flap on both pedicles and anastomose both sets of vessels to ensure viability of the flap.

The flap can be raised from a superior or inferior approach. The superior approach, using location of the distal ascending branch of the pedicle on the undersurface of the internal oblique muscle, is considered the safer and more straightforward approach by the author. The inferior approach has two options. The first approach is subinguinal. The femoral vessels are isolated below the inguinal ligament, and the deep circumflex iliac vessels are identified by upward retraction of the inguinal ligament. The second, transinguinal approach involves identification and retraction of either the spermatic cord or the round ligament and dissection through the transversus abdominus to expose the external iliac vessels.

The patient should be warned of postoperative pain and altered sensation of the anterior thigh, and that gait may be abnormal for 3 months.

INDICATIONS

The flap can be used for reconstruction of segmental mandibular defects (*Figure 39.1*), particularly in dentate patients. It can also be used for reconstruction of maxillary defects that extend outside the maxillary alveolus. The flap can be raised with a skin paddle that can cover skin defects resulting from both maxillary and mandibular pathology. When there is a large intraoral soft tissue and bony defect after resection of mandible and adjacent soft tissue pathology, the DCIA with a skin paddle can be used to reconstruct the mandible, with the skin paddle and internal oblique muscle used to reconstruct the tongue and floor of mouth. If the soft tissue defect requires more complex reconstruction, a DCIA in combination with another soft tissue free flap may provide a more optimal solution.

The ipsilateral hip should be used for optimal placement of the vascular pedicle in mandibular or maxillary reconstruction. In the mandible, the curvature of the iliac crest can provide an ideal lower border, angle

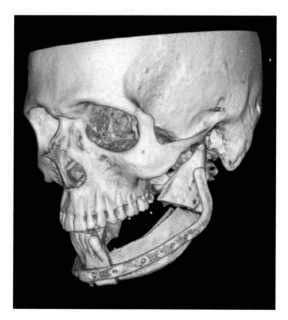

Figure 39.1 Left mandible reconstruction with left deep circumflex iliac artery free flap and custom-made plate.

or symphysis; this is best utilised using preoperative 3D planning (*Figure 39.2*) and intraoperative guided surgery. In midline defects, the flap should be raised ipsilaterally to the side where the pedicle is to be anastomosed. Using the ipsilateral side in the maxilla gives optimal pedicle orientation and bone-to-bone apposition. As much length as possible should be preserved on the recipient vessels for maxillary reconstruction.

Contraindications to using a DCIA include a previous iliac crest graft, an inguinal hernia repair or previous abdominal surgery within the surgical field. Patients with gait problems are not good candidates for this procedure in either limb. Obesity does make flap raising more challenging but is not a contraindication.

PREOPERATIVE CONSIDERATIONS

The surgical site should be checked for scars and evidence of previous surgery. A handheld Doppler can be used to locate perforators and aid skin paddle placement when a skin paddle is to be used. Most perforators lie 5–11 cm posterior to the anterior superior iliac spine (ASIS), in 8% they are absent. 3D-planning and 3D-printed guides can be used for intraoperative templates for accurate bone harvest and optimal pedicle length.

SURGICAL TECHNIQUE

Positioning the patient

With the patient supine, a sandbag is placed beneath the hip. Skin preparation should be from the midline to the posterior axillary line medially to laterally and from the costal margin to the thigh below the greater trochanter. A line is drawn from the pubic symphysis to a point 1 cm above the ASIS and continues 1 cm above and parallel with the iliac crest to the posterior axillary line (*Figure 39.3*). If a skin paddle is to be harvested, it should be marked out following perforator location with a Doppler probe.

Incision

Along the length of the incision, the skin and fat are incised through Scarpa's and Camper's fasciae to the external oblique muscle, the fibres of which run in a downwards and forwards direction. The external oblique muscle should be incised in the direction of its fibres and dissected off the underlying internal oblique muscle along the full length of the wound. The internal oblique muscle fibres are oriented downwards and backwards. The lower edge of the muscle should be dissected downwards over the iliac crest and detached from the outer table of the ilium.

Perforating vessels should be identified coming through external oblique and preserved if a skin paddle is to be raised. A cuff of at least 1 cm should be left around the perforators when they are being dissected out to protect their integrity.

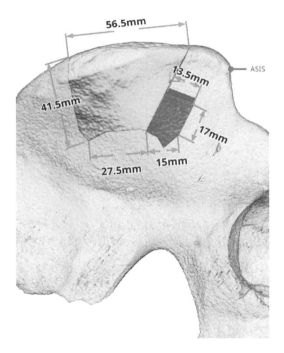

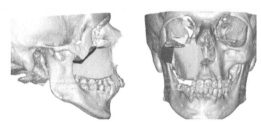

Figure 39.2 Three-dimensional plan for right maxillary reconstruction with a right deep circumflex iliac artery free flap.

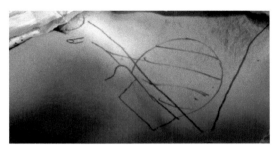

Figure 39.3 Skin markings showing location of pubic symphysis, inguinal ligament, iliac crest and anterior superior iliac spine and costal margin. Bone flap outline with internal oblique muscle cuff marked on skin as well as a line 1 cm above the iliac crest that will be the incision line for the harvesting procedure.

The remainder of the chapter will describe the DCIA being raised with vascularised iliac crest and internal oblique muscle without a skin paddle, which is the most commonly used version of this flap.

Raising the muscle flap

Once the internal oblique has been exposed, the extent of muscle for harvest should be marked out with ink. In mandibular reconstruction, the iliac crest can be used as the lower border, and the amount of muscle to be harvested should be able to wrap around the full height of the harvested ilium. In the rare event that there is only an ascending branch of the DCIA, the flap will have to rely on the periosteal supply from this vessel and preserving a small muscle cuff will maintain the integrity of the ascending branch (*Figure 39.4*).

An incision should be made at the superolateral aspect of internal oblique and onto the transversalis muscle. The internal oblique should be raised together with the transversalis fascia on its deep surface. The distal end of the ascending branch of the DCIA vessels can be located at the superolateral aspect of the transversalis fascia. Dissection continues along the length of the ascending pedicle separating the internal oblique muscle/transversalis fascia flap from transversalis muscle. The ascending branch is usually a single large pedicle but may have small branches, which should be preserved. Less commonly, it is made up of small tributaries that run from the DCIA pedicle directly to the muscle from the iliac crest. Raising the transversalis fascia together with the internal oblique muscle will provide a safe and viable flap (*Figure 39.5*).

Dissection of the pedicle

As the dissection proceeds inferiorly, the ascending branch joins the DCIA pedicle to form the conjoined DCIA pedicle. Dissection of the ascending branch beyond the ASIS should be carried out with caution to avoid inadvertent damage to the DCIA. Once the DCIA main pedicle is identified, it is dissected carefully down to the iliac vessels. Exposing the pedicle along its length ensures flap harvest with full visualisation of the pedicle. The large deep muscular branches running off the pedicle can be divided once the flap is mobilised. Retrograde dissection from the junction of the DCIA and ascending pedicle to the ilium allows location of the pedicle relative to the height of the ilium to be established and ensures safe bone harvest. Maintaining a cuff of 2–3 cm of iliacus under the pedicle medial to the iliac crest ensures safety of the pedicle when the bone is harvested. The lateral cutaneous nerve of the thigh will be identified 2–3 cm medial to the ASIS and can be dissected from the pedicle if possible.

Bone harvesting

Bone harvest is determined by two factors: quantity of bone required and pedicle length. Around 16 cm

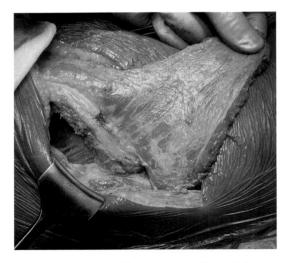

Figure 39.4 Internal oblique muscle cuff on a left deep circumflex iliac artery flap. The external oblique has been stripped from iliac crest and retracted laterally exposing the lateral border of the ilium.

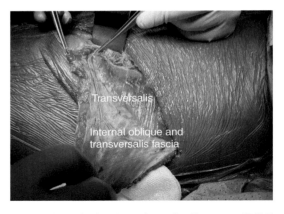

Figure 39.5 Left side deep circumflex iliac artery (DCIA) flap with internal oblique muscle cuff raised with the ascending DCIA pedicle exposed on the transversalis fascia overlying the internal oblique muscle.

of bone can be harvested but the more bone that is required, the shorter the pedicle length. Preserving ASIS will increase the pedicle length. If ASIS is to be preserved, at least 3 cm of ilium must be preserved to avoid fracture. It is important to consider the area of reconstruction in relation to bone quantity required and pedicle length. Mandibular reconstruction does not usually pose a problem with pedicle length, but maxillary reconstruction will require a longer pedicle to reach the recipient vessels in the neck.

Bone cuts are made with a saw or piezo. The anterior and posterior cuts are made from the lateral side of the ilium. The pedicle should be protected by making a pocket between the periosteum and bone on

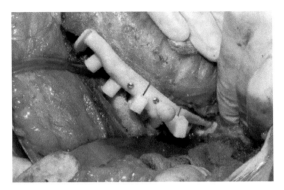

Figure 39.6 Left deep circumflex iliac artery free flap being raised with a 3D cutting guide *in situ*. The soft tissue lateral to the guide restricts access to make the lower bone cut from the lateral side of the ilium with the guide in place.

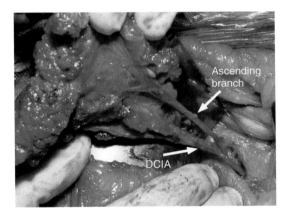

Figure 39.7 A right deep circumflex iliac artery (DCIA) free flap demonstrating the relationship of the ascending DCIA and conjoined DCIA pedicle.

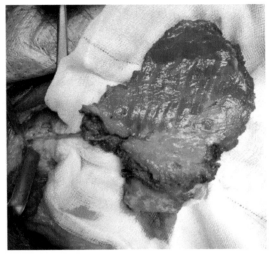

Figure 39.8 A left deep circumflex iliac artery free flap still attached to the iliac vessels. The flap offers a large volume of bone and soft tissue available with the internal oblique muscle.

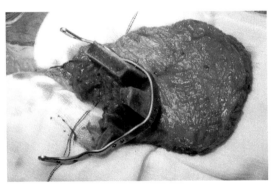

Figure 39.9 Left deep circumflex iliac artery free flap attached to the iliac vessels having had osteotomies completed and custom-made plate fitted.

the medial side of the iliac bone and placing a narrow retractor to protect the pedicle. The lower cut is most easily performed from a medial approach inside the pelvis. A cutting guide placed on the lateral side of the iliac bone makes the lower cut more challenging as the cut is on the outer surface of the ilium and the soft tissue restricts access (*Figure 39.6*). This should be considered in the 3D-planning and guide design.

The pedicle should always be protected when bone cuts are being made (*Figure 39.7*). When the cuts are complete, the bone can be mobilised with gentle digital pressure or a Smith's spreader. It should be carefully handled out of the pelvis, and the pedicle carefully dissected from the ASIS region (*Figure 39.8*).

If using guided surgery, osteotomy cuts can be completed, and the custom-made plate attached to the flap while the pedicle remains attached to the iliac vessels (*Figure 39.9*). This ensures viability of the flap after the osteotomy cuts have been made and will reduce time during inset.

Closure of the donor site and pedicle division

Haemostasis should be achieved and a haemostatic agent (e.g. bone wax) should be placed over the trabecular bone of the cut ilium. The pedicle should be carefully dissected down to the iliac vessels. Any side branches should be ligated and the flap mobilised to allow visualisation of the pedicle on all sides. Marking the orientation of the pedicle with dots of ink is a useful way to avoid twisting the pedicle when it is inset, particularly if it passes through a tunnel, for example, in maxillary reconstruction. The pedicle should be divided as close to the iliac vessels as possible to maximise pedicle length.

The closure technique of the donor site is of particular importance to avoid long-term morbidity.

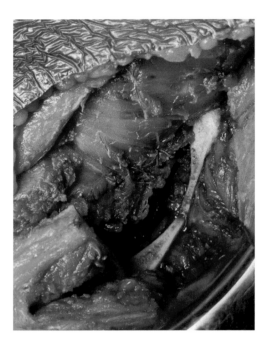

Figure 39.10 The cut ilium with bone wax over the cut surface and the iliacus muscle cut end closed directly to the cut end of transversalis muscle.

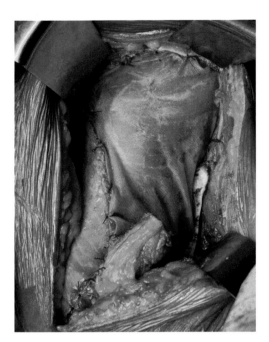

Figure 39.11 A mesh repair of the defect created by harvesting the deep circumflex iliac artery with a large internal oblique muscle cuff. The mesh can be attached to the cut end of the ilium by drilling holes in the bone and suturing the mesh to the holes as seen here.

The abdomen should be closed in layers. The cut ends of the iliacus and transversalis can be closed primarily (*Figure 39.10*).

An infusion catheter for local anaesthesia infusion should be placed over the repaired muscles and brought through the skin inferior to the incision. The defect created from the harvest of internal oblique can be repaired with a hernia repair mesh sutured tension-free to the cut end of internal oblique. It can be attached to the defect in the ilium by drilling holes in the inner table of the bone and suturing the lower end of the mesh (*Figure 39.11*).

The medial end of internal oblique can be closed primarily. A suction drain should be placed over this layer and taken through the skin adjacent to the wound infusion catheter. External oblique and skin can be closed primarily in layers. A sterile dressing can be placed over the wound and should remain undisturbed for at least 72 hours. Primary closure is usually possible even with large skin paddles.

Insetting and anastomosis

If a 3D guide has been used, then very little adjustment will be needed prior to inset. If osteotomies are required, a table should be set up to use as a work bench beside the patient. Care should be taken to preserve viable segments of bone and maintain periosteal attachment. Opening osteotomies can be performed by cutting the outer table and crest and green sticking the

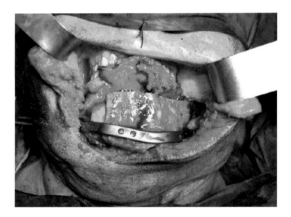

Figure 39.12 A left-sided mandible defect reconstructed with a left-sided deep circumflex iliac artery flap and custom-made plate. The internal oblique muscle can be seen at the upper border of the bone ready to wrap over the newly created mandible for soft tissue reconstruction. Dental implants that were placed using a custom-made guide can be seen on the upper border of the bone.

inner table. Plates and screws should be used for fixation (*Figure 39.12*). Gaps in osteotomy cuts can be filled with bone chips. The muscle or skin should be sutured to the mucosa to provide a watertight seal.

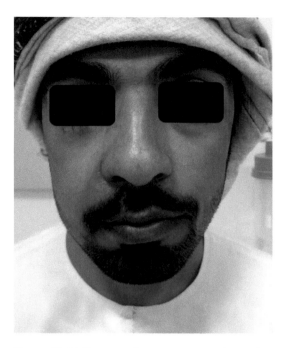

Figure 39.13 Postoperative appearance of a patient reconstructed with a deep circumflex iliac artery free flap following a right maxillectomy.

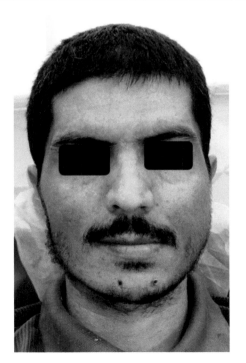

Figure 39.14 Postoperative appearance of a patient who had left mandible reconstruction with a left deep circumflex iliac artery free flap following a ballistic injury with tissue loss.

The anastomosis should be performed under no tension. The vessels are usually a good match for the facial, superficial temporal or superior thyroid vessels. Ensuring the patient has had preoperative low molecular weight heparin, maintaining a systolic blood pressure of greater than 100 mmHg and the use of papaverine will help prevent spasm in the artery and optimise flow.

In the initial postoperative period the flap may appear bulky but the muscle will mucosalise and shrink back within the first 2–3 months (*Figures 39.13* and *39.14*).

POSTOPERATIVE CARE

Monitoring of the flap can be done with visual inspection of the skin or muscle and a flap observation chart. A handheld Doppler probe, implantable Doppler if fitted intraoperatively or indocyanine green can also be used to monitor flow integrity. Further details on flap monitoring are given in *Chapter 35*.

The abdomen should be inspected daily. Patients should be mobilised on day 1 postoperatively and actively managed with a mobilisation regime during their hospital stay. Pain management should be optimal to allow adequate mobilisation.

COMPLICATIONS

Intraoperative

The delicate pedicle is susceptible to damage – wide exposure, visualisation of the pedicle, gentle handling and protecting the vessels during osteotomies minimise vessel trauma.

Inadvertent damage can be caused to the pedicle due to separate take-off of DCIA and ascending pedicles. It is important to ensure both DCIA and ascending branches are identified before ligating any branches.

There can be inadequate bone harvest or pedicle length; however, 3D-planning and 3D-guides can be used to ensure accurate bone harvest and pedicle length.

Postoperative

To prevent vascular compromise due to external pressure, avoid pressure on the delicate pedicle from face masks or ties.

There can be avulsion of ASIS; however, ensuring an adequate amount of bone remains under ASIS will reduce this risk.

Closure of the donor site is extremely important. To reduce complications such as donor site dehiscence or bulge of abdominal wall, haemostasis and mesh repair can be used.

Gait problems can be reduced with optimal postoperative analgesia, early mobilisation and an exercise regime supervised by a physiotherapist.

TOP TIPS AND HAZARDS

- The muscle contracts when cut, so ensure enough muscle is harvested for soft tissue reconstruction.
- To lengthen the pedicle, harvest bone as far back along the iliac crest as possible.
- If ASIS is to be preserved, ensure enough bone is preserved to prevent spontaneous avulsion of ASIS on mobilisation.
- Do not underestimate the time, complex nature and importance of carefully closing the donor site defect. Medium- and long-term morbidity can be avoided by attention to detail in planning, harvest and closure.

FURTHER READING

Bergeron L, Tang M, Morris SF. The anatomical basis of the deep circumflex iliac artery perforator flap with iliac crest. *Plast Reconstr Surg* 2007;**120**:252–8.

Brown JS. Deep circumflex iliac artery free flap with internal oblique muscle as a new method of immediate reconstruction of maxillectomy defect. *Head Neck* 1996;**18**:412–21.

Kimata Y, Uchiyama K, Sakuraba M et al. Deep circumflex iliac perforator flap with iliac crest for mandibular reconstruction. *Br J Plast Surg* 2001;**54**:487–90.

van Gemert JT, van Es RJ, Rosenberg AJ et al. Free vascularized flaps for reconstruction of the mandible: complications, success, and dental rehabilitation. *J Oral Maxillofac Surg* 2012;**70**:1692–8.

Zheng HP, Zhuang YH, Zhang ZM et al. Modified deep iliac circumflex osteocutaneous flap for extremity reconstruction: anatomical study and clinical application. *J Plast Reconstr Aesthet Surg* 2013;**66**:1256–62.

Chapter 40

Scapular Flap

Ralph W. Gilbert

INTRODUCTION

The current standard of care for mandibular and maxillary reconstruction is virtually planned bone reconstruction. Several donor sites are available for these types of reconstructions including the osteocutaneous fibular transfer, the deep circumflex iliac artery (DCIA) transfer of the iliac crest and the free scapular bone flaps. The scapula has two potential donor options, the standard lateral border transfer based on the bone perforator arising from the circumflex scapular vessels and the angular tip of scapular flap based on the angular branch of the thoracodorsal system.

This chapter will describe the basic technique of harvest and potential applications of the angular tip of scapular flap in head and neck (H&N) reconstruction.

HISTORY

The scapular flap was first described by dos Santos in 1980. This flap, based on the circumflex branch of the subscapular artery, had the unique advantages of limited donor site morbidity and a variety of chimeric options for soft tissue and skin reconstruction. The flap design, which harvested the lateral border of the scapula, had the limitation of a relatively short pedicle and somewhat limited skin mobility relative to bone transfer. In 1991, Coleman described the use of the 'bipedicled scapular flap', which later became popularised as the angular tip of scapula flap. The past two decades have seen a rapid expansion in the use of the angular tip of scapula flap based on the available pedicle length (up to 12–15 cm) and the possibility of multiple chimeric skin paddles based on the thoracodorsal artery and its venae comitantes. Currently, the angular tip of scapula is most widely used for maxilla reconstruction, either placed horizontally or vertically, and for mandibular reconstruction where it can used to reconstruct defects of up to 10 cm. The tip of scapula has a cartilaginous tip, which can be used to advantage in vertical ramus reconstructions when the condyle of the mandible has been resected.

SURGICAL ANATOMY

To successfully harvest this flap, a detailed understanding of the subscapular system and its variations is essential. The subscapular artery arises from the axillary artery high in the axilla. As it descends, it has two major branches: the circumflex scapular artery and its venae comitantes, and the thoracodorsal artery and venae comitantes. The circumflex branch passes between the teres major and minor and provides a nutrient bone branch to the upper one-third of the scapula and cutaneous perforators to the skin of the back overlying in the scapula. The thoracodorsal branch descends on the deep surface of the latissimus dorsi muscle accompanied by the nerve to latissimus, and just prior to entering the muscle splits to provide the blood supply to the serratus anterior muscle. The angular branch usually arises from the thoracodorsal artery just prior to the branch to serratus (usually 50% of the size of the serratus branch). The branch to the tip of the scapula will always pass deep to the serratus branch along the lateral edge of the scapula. Numerous variations of this vasculature may occur, including the angular branch arising from the serratus branch (usually very close to the take-off of the serratus branch from the thoracodorsal) as well as a very proximal branch arising 2–3 cm after the circumflex branch. The artery and venae usually have some small branches that will supply the posterior portion of the serratus muscle.

Based on injection studies, the angular branch supplies the distal 6 cm of the tip of scapula and the medial portion of the tip. Surgical experience would suggest that up to 10 cm of bone can be reliably harvested.

PREOPERATIVE CONSIDERATIONS

Planning harvest of the angular tip of scapula is usually relatively straightforward. Specific contraindications include:

- Previous thoracotomy or axillary incision
- Limited range of motion of the shoulder (patients must be able to abduct passively to 90°) to allow proximal dissection of the pedicle
- Morbid obesity is a relative contraindication, excessive axillary fat or fat distributions into the axilla can make the pedicle dissection technically difficult

SURGICAL TECHNIQUE

Positioning

There are several potential patient positions for harvesting this flap. Numerous authors and surgeons

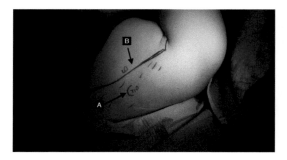

Figure 40.1 Incision location, patient positioned partially rotated to the right. A, scapular tip; B, incision posterior axillary line.

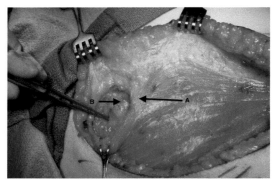

Figure 40.2 Initial dissection. The anterior border of the latissimus dorsi muscle is visualised (A). A space is created between the serratus anterior (B) and the latissimus dorsi muscle.

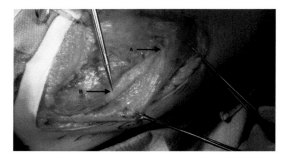

Figure 40.3 After mobilising the latissimus dorsi muscle, the following structures are visualised: the pedicle to latissimus dorsi (A) and the scapular tip (B).

have recommended a supported lateral position for the harvest. Unfortunately, this approach makes it impossible to harvest the flap without repositioning the patient after ablative procedures. We have adopted a single position for the H&N ablative surgery and flap harvest. The patient is placed in the supine position on a 'beanbag', which, when deflated, maintains the position of the patient. We rotate the patient 15–20° from supine and hold them in position with the 'beanbag'. The patient is then draped in the usual fashion with the arm draped freely to allow rotation of the arm during the harvest (*Figure 40.1*). The patient is rotated in the long axis of the surgical bed towards the flap harvest side for the performance of the ablative procedure and then rotated in the opposite direction for flap harvest and closure. Great care must be taken to secure and pad the patient to the bed as their position may shift during the rotations.

Incision planning

There are several potential incision designs dependent on the nature of the skin flap required. In a bone-only harvest, we usually design an incision placed in the posterior axillary line which angles along the anterior edge of the latissimus muscle tendon towards the axilla. The inferior extent of the incision will be 5–10 cm below the inferior border of the tip of the scapula.

Stepwise operative technique

The incision is made (usually with monopolar cautery) down to the enveloping fascia of the latissimus dorsi muscle. Posterior skin flap elevation occurs along the length of the muscle and incision until approximately the medial 10 cm of flap is visible (this allows reflection of the muscle for visualisation of the pedicle and the scapula).

Starting over the lower one-third of the latissimus dorsi muscle, the lateral border of the muscle is mobilised away from the serratus anterior (distal mobilisation to avoid injury to the thoracodorsal pedicle). The space between the latissimus dorsi muscle and the serratus

anterior is developed bluntly or with sharp dissection when adherent (*Figure 40.2*). The thoracodorsal branches to the serratus anterior are identified and followed retrograde to the thoracodorsal origin where the pedicle to the latissimus dorsi is identified (*Figure 40.3*) along with the nerve to latissimus dorsi. The remainder of the latissimus dorsi lateral border is reflected posteriorly to reveal the pedicle as it passes superiorly.

The nerve to latissimus dorsi and the pedicle are followed proximally and dissected out of the axillary fat. At this point the dissection and visualisation are made much easier with external rotation of the arm along with some abduction of the shoulder. Great care must be taken to cauterise or clip small perforators as blood in the wound will make the dissection more difficult. Dissection is continued up to the circumflex branch. No branches should be divided until the operative surgeon has identified the angular branch with certainty. The course and take-off of the angular branch is variable and can easily be divided if not experienced with this flap.

Once the angular branch is identified, the branch to serratus (assuming a proximal angular take-off) can

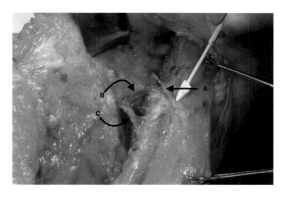

Figure 40.4 The vascular anatomy of this dissection is visualised. The nerve and artery to latissimus dorsi (A) are visualised. The branch to serratus anterior (B) is seen arising from the thoracodorsal artery. In this patient, the angular branch (C) arises from the branch to serratus anterior.

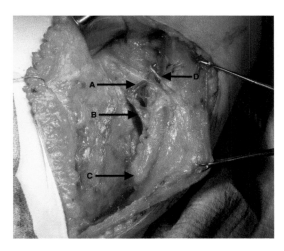

Figure 40.5 Overview of the entire dissection; branch to serratus anterior (A), angular branch (B), scapular tip (C), nerve and pedicle to latissimus dorsi (D).

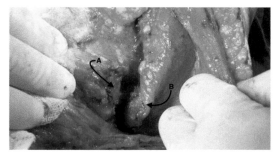

Figure 40.6 Division of the serratus anterior from the tip of the scapula; serratus anterior (A), tip of scapula (B).

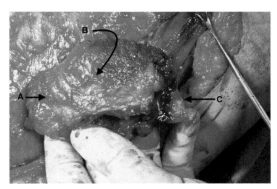

Figure 40.7 Harvested scapular tip. In this patient, this is being used for maxillary reconstruction with large cuff of teres major muscle (B), scapular tip (A) and osteotomy through the lateral crest and blade portion of the scapula (C).

be divided along with the branches to the latissimus dorsi. The pedicle is fully mobilised from the lateral border of the scapula to the subscapular origin. The thoracodorsal nerve should be preserved in the majority of dissections.

With the vascular anatomy fully exposed (*Figures 40.4* and *40.5*), the latissimus dorsi is separated from the teres major. The serratus anterior is detached from the medial edge of scapula (*Figure 40.6*) with the monopolar cautery (this will free the scapula posteriorly making the bone cuts technically easier).

In mandibular reconstructions, we usually leave a small cuff of teres major attached, whereas in maxillary reconstructions where the muscle is required for volume filling or for horizontal palate reconstruction, we take a large portion of the teres muscle. Once the teres mobilisation is completed, we measure the length of bone required on the lateral border from the tip of the scapula. We then use a 'Cobb elevator' to dissect the remaining teres major posteriorly to allow visualisation of the osteotomies.

Once the length of bone required is established, we make a transverse cut through the lateral border of the scapula towards the blade portion of the scapula. Once completed the saw is rotated 90° and a vertical cut medial to the tip of the scapula is performed, completing the osteotomies (*Figure 40.7*).

Muscular attachments are divided medially to free the bone flap. Once the viability of the flap is assured (bleeding from the serratus attachment site), the proximal pedicle can be ligated and transferred to the back table.

Significant blood loss can occur as the osteotomies are performed and meticulous haemostasis is required prior to closure.

The serratus muscle is re-attached to the remnant lateral border of the scapula or sewn to the remaining teres major (dependant on reconstruction required) with at least a No. 1 braided suture. Repairing this muscle is critical to avoid scapular winging. Depending on the flap harvest (bone only versus composite flap), we place one or two suction drains.

POSTOPERATIVE CARE AND RECOVERY

The major issue for patients with this donor site is perioperative pain in the shoulder. We routinely provide patients with regional anaesthetic blockade and patient-controlled analgesia. Shoulder mobilisation (passive movement) begins on postoperative day 2, with active movement and physiotherapy beginning on day 5. In our practice as compared to other bone donor sites, this site appears to be the least morbid and most-easily tolerated, a clear advantage of this donor site in the elderly and patients with other comorbidities.

POSSIBLE COMPLICATIONS AND MANAGEMENT

Brachial plexus traction injury

Excessive external rotation and abduction of the arm during bone harvest can result in a traction injury to the brachial plexus. We have seen a few patients with transient paraesthesia and weakness in wrist extension. Prolonged and aggressive abduction should be avoided in the fully paralysed patient.

Frozen shoulder

Inadequate pain management and poor postoperative physiotherapy can result in patients avoiding the use of the operative arm, resulting in significant shoulder disability. Early mobilisation and aggressive physiotherapy can be extremely helpful.

> **TOP TIPS AND HAZARDS**
>
> • *Patient positioning:* avoid the lateral position for harvest, repositioning a patient during the procedure is extremely time consuming and potentially hazardous. Harvest this flap in the supine position with rotation.
>
> • *Know the anatomy:* as in all flap dissections, the anatomy of this flap must be understood and the potential variations in the take-off of the angular branch understood. Do not divide any branches from the thoracodorsal artery until you have clearly visualised the angular branch.
>
> • *Carefully re-attach the serratus anterior:* to avoid significant scapular winging and shoulder instability, carefully re-attach the serratus to the teres major and/or scapular border.

FURTHER READING

Clark JR, Vesely M, Gilbert R. Scapular angle osteomyogenous flap in postmaxillectomy reconstruction: defect, reconstruction, shoulder function, and harvest technique. *Head Neck* 2008;**30**:10–20.

Coleman JJ, 3rd, Sultan MR. The bipedicled osteocutaneous scapula flap: a new subscapular system free flap. *Plast Reconstr Surg* 1991;**87**:682–92.

dos Santos LF. The vascular anatomy and dissection of the free scapular flap. *Plast Reconstr Surg* 1984;**73**:599–604.

Miles BA, Gilbert RW. Maxillary reconstruction with the scapular angle osteomyogenous free flap. *Arch Otolaryngol Head Neck Surg* 2011;**137**:1130–5.

Seneviratne S, Duong C, Taylor GI. The angular branch of the thoracodorsal artery and its blood supply to the inferior angle of the scapula: an anatomical study. *Plast Reconstr Surg* 1999;**104**:85–8.

Bailey & Love's Essential Operations Bailey & Love's Essential Operations
Bailey & Love's Essential Operations Bailey & Love's Essential Operations
Bailey & Love's Essential Operations Bailey & Love's Essential Operations

PART 5 | Reconstructive surgery

Chapter 41

Rectus Abdominis Flap

Joshua E. Lubek

INTRODUCTION

The rectus abdominis free flap is a versatile myocutaneous flap based on the deep inferior epigastric artery and its associated venae comitantes. The flap was first described by Drever in 1977 as the 'epigastric island flap', and later adapted for breast reconstruction. Credit is also given to Mathes and Bostwick for their use in abdominal wall reconstruction during that same year.

The flap has been well described for its use in the reconstruction of large-volume soft tissue defects of the head and neck, including subtotal glossectomy, orbital exenteration (*Figure 41.1*) and large cutaneous facial defects. General advantages include a large caliber artery and associated venae comitantes (2–4 mm), long pedicle length (8–10 cm), consistent anatomy and a two-team approach. A large skin paddle with adequate bulk can be provided with minimal donor site morbidity. The flap can also be harvested based solely on the perforating vessels traversing the rectus muscle within the periumbilical region. Although donor site morbidities such as hernia, abdominal wall bulging and pain are generally considered to be of a low risk, the option to use a muscle-sparing skin and subcutaneous DIEP (deep inferior epigastric artery perforator) flap for the avoidance of such complications can be utilized.

SURGICAL ANATOMY

The rectus abdominis muscle is a strap-like vertical muscle, approximately 30 cm in length by 6 cm in width, originating from the symphysis pubis and inserts

into the 5th, 6th and 7th costal cartilage along with the xiphoid process. The muscle is enveloped by a tough rectus sheath, formed by the fascia of the three abdominal wall muscles (external/internal oblique and the transversalis abdominis muscles) originating at the linea semilunaris. The aponeurosis in the midline adjoining the two rectus muscles is known as the linea alba. The rectus sheath splits into an anterior and posterior sheath to surround the rectus abdominis muscle. The posterior rectus sheath ends abruptly at the arcuate line at the level of the anterior superior iliac spine bilaterally. Below this line there only exists an anterior rectus sheath, and deep to the rectus muscle is a thin layer of tissue through which the preperitoneal fat is easily identified.

The dual vascular supply to the rectus abdominis muscle is based on the deep superior and inferior epigastric arteries. Rectus flaps for head and neck reconstruction are largely based on the deep inferior epigastric vessels due to increased pedicle length, larger vessel caliber, anatomic reliability due to skin vasculature based on the musculocutaneous perforators from the inferior epigastric vessels and anterograde venous outflow of the flap.

The deep inferior epigastric artery is a large caliber vessel (3–4 mm diameter) that travels on the deep surface of the rectus abdominis muscle. The vessel splits into two main branches as it courses the undersurface of the muscle greater than 50% of the time. From the point that the artery exits the muscle at the level of the arcuate line traveling inferiorly for approximately 8–10 cm it inserts into the medial aspect of the external iliac artery. Paired venae comitantes accompanying

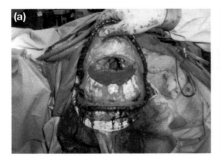
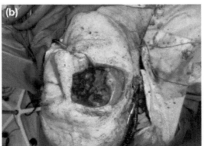
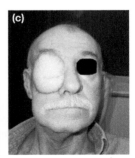

Figure 41.1 (a) Squamous carcinoma of the orbit and ethmoid sinuses requiring orbital exenteration and craniofacial resection. Communication with the neurocranium depicted. (b) Squamous carcinoma of the orbit and ethmoid sinuses requiring orbital exenteration and craniofacial resection. Orbital defect depicted. (c) Reconstructed craniofacial resection/orbital exenteration with a rectus abdominis free flap.

the artery will commonly form into a single larger caliber vein (greater than 60%) and enter the external iliac vein.

The perforators to the skin are most often (80%) situated in a 3–5 cm area surrounding umbilicus. These perforators are quite robust (average diameter greater than 0.5 mm). The perforators identified at the level of the umbilicus and inferiorly are supplied by the deep inferior epigastric vessels forming the basis of the rectus abdominis/DIEP flap for head and neck reconstruction.

Innervation to the rectus abdominis muscle and its overlying skin is supplied by the lower six thoracic ventral rami and exiting T6–T12 thoracic nerves (7–11th intercostal nerves and subcostal nerve). The nerves travel between the transversus abdominis and the internal oblique muscle and enter the rectus muscle on the posterior aspect, ultimately piercing the anterior rectus sheath to supply the overlying skin via the cutaneous branches.

PREOPERATIVE CONSIDERATIONS

- For use with large soft tissue defects of the head and neck (i.e. subtotal/total glossectomy, orbital exenteration, skull base coverage and cutaneous facial defects)
- Flap bulk and dissection may be more difficult in the obese patient
- Contraindicated in those patients with previous abdominal wall hernia repair
- The contralateral rectus abdominis flap can be harvested in those patients requiring a gastrostomy tube

OPERATIVE TECHNIQUE

Flap design

The skin paddle of the flap can be oriented in a vertical (VRAM) or transverse (TRAM) orientation to the underlying rectus muscle based on the highly consistent perforators from the deep inferior epigastric artery surrounding the umbilicus (*Figure 41.2*). The flap can be extended in an oblique fashion from the periumbilical area toward the ipsilateral lower costal margin. Total width of flap harvest is generally guided by the ability for primary closure; however, a skin paddle measuring up to 12 × 30 cm can be harvested (especially in the transverse direction). Elevation of the skin paddle in the transverse direction will allow for less muscle to be harvested for a less bulky flap. Disadvantages of the TRAM orientation include a shortened pedicle length and the need to preserve the umbilicus. Although not necessary, the perforators can be identified using a handheld surface Doppler. During dissection, only the ipsilateral perforating vessels need to be preserved to ensure viability of the flap.

Landmarks to be identified include the umbilicus, xiphoid process, the inferior costal margin, pubic tubercle, anterior superior iliac spine bilaterally and the iliofemoral pulse at the level of the inguinal ligament (origin of the deep inferior epigastric vessels).

Rectus abdominis myocutaneous flap

After noting the appropriate landmarks and designing the skin paddle, the skin and subcutaneous tissue are incised and dissected from the lateral aspect until the fascia overlying the external oblique muscle is encountered.

Continuing in a medial direction, the linea semilunaris is identified and the flap is gently elevated toward the midline, watching carefully for the periumbilical perforators originating through the rectus muscle and supplying the overlying skin and subcutaneous tissue.

The anterior rectus sheath is incised laterally to the perforator vessels in a vertical direction identifying the underlying lateral border of the rectus muscle. Incision of the anterior rectus sheath is performed in a transverse direction ensuring an adequate safe distance both superiorly and inferiorly from the perforator vessels until the linea alba is encountered.

The skin paddle is circumferentially completed on its medial aspect stopping at the linea alba at the midline. The superficial surface of the rectus muscle is also exposed inferiorly below the level of the skin paddle and the perforator vessels. Suturing of the subcutaneous tissue to the underlying muscle with a resorbable suture can help to avoid any risk of shearing of the perforators from the overlying subcutaneous tissue.

The rectus muscle is divided superiorly identifying the posterior rectus sheath. The distal end of the pedicle will be encountered superiorly and ligated with silk ties or hemoclips.

The flap can be raised in an inferior direction, keeping the posterior rectus sheath intact. The linea alba will be incised in the midline, as one continues to identify the medial border of the rectus muscle, elevating the myocutaneous flap off the posterior rectus sheath. Care must be taken not to enter the umbilicus and to protect the ipsilateral periumbilical perforators.

The pedicle can be easily identified on the undersurface of the rectus muscle. The rectus muscle will be divided inferiorly staying above the level of the arcuate line, all the while protecting the pedicle of the deep inferior epigastric artery (*Figure 41.3*) and its venae comitantes.

The vascular pedicle can be dissected with instrument or gentle finger dissection as it traverses over the preperitoneal fat/fascia traveling into the inguinal region to join the external iliac vessels.

Below the arcuate line, the anterior rectus fascia should be closed with a non-resorbable suture to avoid the risk of hernia or abdominal bulge. If there is loss of integrity of the anterior rectus sheath below the arcuate line, it should be repaired with a synthetic or resorbable

A – Transverse rectus abdominis flap design
B – Vertical rectus abdominis flap design
C – Extended oblique rectus abdominis flap design

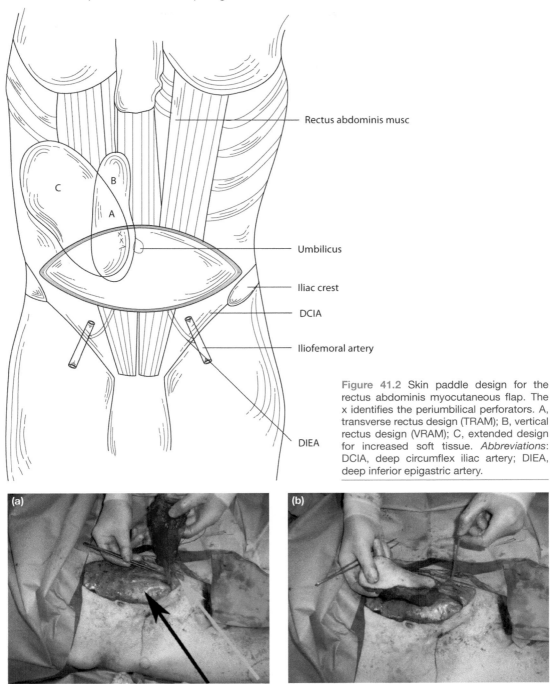

Rectus abdominis musc

Umbilicus

Iliac crest

DCIA

Iliofemoral artery

DIEA

Figure 41.2 Skin paddle design for the rectus abdominis myocutaneous flap. The x identifies the periumbilical perforators. A, transverse rectus design (TRAM); B, vertical rectus design (VRAM); C, extended design for increased soft tissue. *Abbreviations*: DCIA, deep circumflex iliac artery; DIEA, deep inferior epigastric artery.

(a)

(b)

Figure 41.3 (a) Harvest of the rectus abdominis myocutaneous free flap. Blue arrow: the superficial epigastric vessels which do not need to be preserved but can also perfuse and provide venous flap drainage. Instrument pointing to the pedicle of the deep inferior epigastric vessels. Black arrow: the distal extent of the posterior rectus sheath. Line drawn on the abdomen demarcates the arcuate line. (b) Harvest of the rectus abdominis myocutaneous flap. Vessel loop around the superficial epigastric vessels.

mesh sutured to the wound margins. Above this line, the posterior rectus sheath is usually strong enough so that closure of the anterior sheath is not necessary, especially if it will result in a tight abdominal wall closure or if one wants to avoid the risk, albeit low, of mesh infection. Any violation of the posterior rectus sheath with exposure of the peritoneum should be repaired with a non-resorbable suture and/or mesh closure once identified.

Closure of the subcutaneous tissue and skin is usually quite easily done without the need for tissue undermining. A suction drain should be placed to help minimize the risk of hematoma or seroma formation.

POSTOPERATIVE CARE AND RECOVERY

Standard free-flap monitoring should be performed per specific surgical unit protocol with intensive flap monitoring for the first 72 hours following surgery. Methods of monitoring include assessment of arterial and venous Doppler signal, flap color, temperature and quality of bleeding on scratch test. Various methods of anticoagulation (i.e. aspirin, heparin, dextran) are also surgeon specific; however, there is very little level I evidence to suggest their clinical efficacy.

An abdominal binder may be used for added patient comfort and avoidance of heavy lifting should be followed for approximately 2 months to avoid the risk of hernia or wound dehiscence. Although the peritoneum is generally not violated during harvest of the rectus abdominis flap, bowel sounds should be assessed prior to starting a diet due to the risk of ileus. Perioperative antibiotics should be administered per standard protocols generally for a period ranging from 24 to 48 hours postoperatively. Early mobilization is useful to help prevent the risk of pneumonia and deep venous thrombosis (*Figure 41.4*).

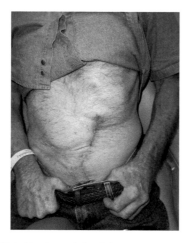

Figure 41.4 Rectus abdominis myocutaneous flap donor site postoperatively.

COMPLICATIONS

Complications can be divided into both medical and surgical issues. Donor site wound infection is low and ranges from 3% without a mesh to 5% with a mesh. Surgical wound infections should be treated with appropriate antibiotic and drainage. Infected mesh will need to be removed and active wound care may be required. Drains can be removed early with risk of seroma and hematoma formation ranging up to 8%.

Postoperative atelectasis/pulmonary complications can occur because of pain associated from the dissection of the abdominal wall muscles or because of a tight abdominal wall closure.

Ileus should be managed with gastric decompression, bowel rest and nutritional support.

TOP TIPS AND HAZARDS

- Previous ventral hernia or significant abdominal surgery involving the ipsilateral side is a contraindication to flap harvest.
- Widening of the paired rectus muscles at the midline (widened linea alba) secondary to previous surgery or abdominal wall weakness can cause the cutaneous perforators to appear more laterally positioned. Only perforating vessels lateral to the linea semilunaris can be safely ligated.
- DIEP flap can be harvested with a small cuff of muscle (especially if multiple perforators harvested) to protect the cutaneous perforators and avoid vessel kinking or twisting.
- The rectus abdominis flap may be too bulky in the morbidly obese patient.
- TRAM (transverse flap) allows for a more aesthetic closure.
- Avoid elevating the flap below arcuate line to avoid risk of abdominal bulge and hernia.

FURTHER READING

Drever JM. The epigastric island flap. *Plast Reconstr Surg* 1977;**59**:343–6.

Mathes SJ, Bostwick J. A rectus abdominis myocutaneous flap to reconstruct abdominal wall defects. *Br J Plast Surg* 1977;**30**:282–3.

Nakatsuka T, Harii K, Asato H et al. Analytic review of 2372 free flap transfers for head and neck reconstruction following cancer resection. *J Reconstr Microsurg* 2003;**19**:363–8.

Urken ML, Turk JB, Weinberg H, Vickery C, Biller HF. The rectus abdominis free flap in head and neck reconstruction. *Otolaryngol Head Neck Surg* 1991;**117**:857–66.

Woodworth BA, Gillespie MB, Day, T, Kline RM. Muscle-sparing abdominal free flaps in head and neck reconstruction. *Head Neck* 2006;**28**:802–7.

Chapter
42

Latissimus Dorsi Flap

Frank Hölzle, Anna Bock

INTRODUCTION

The latissimus dorsi flap was described by Tansini as the first pedicled musculocutaneous flap in 1896. It was used for reconstruction of a post-mastectomy defect in 1912 by D'Este, and the first utilisation in the reconstruction of a head and neck defect was reported by Quillen in 1978. Shortly thereafter, in 1979, Watson et al. reported the first successful microvascular transfer of a free latissimus dorsi flap and exploited a wide variety of applications.

The latissimus dorsi has several indications in the head and neck region as a pedicled or as a free microvascular flap. As a pedicled flap, it is indicated for defects in the neck, skull base, lower and middle face region. As a microvascular flap, it can be used anywhere in the body if a donor and recipient vessel can be identified (*Figure 42.1*).

In most cases, the flap is raised as a musculocutaneous flap. Compared with other flaps, the latissimus dorsi flap provides a large amount of tissue and a moderate amount of adipose tissue between muscle and skin, therefore it is particularly suitable for deep and large defects. In case of a through-and-through defect of the oral cavity, the flap offers the possibility to be raised with two skin paddles. If a functional reconstruction is required, that is, the tongue or the face, an additional inclusion and anastomosis of the thoracodorsal nerve is possible, although its value is debated. Further variations include the osteo-myocutaneous flap, with inclusion of a rib or the tip of the scapula, or the musculo-subcutaneous flap, for contour augmentations. When reconstructing the scalp, a pure muscle flap can be used, which provides an even larger surface area than the musculocutaneous flap. Also, a combination of a muscle with a musculocutaneous part can be used to cover extended defects. In this case, the area of raw muscle can be covered with a split- or a full-thickness skin graft simultaneously or in a delayed surgery after a few days of granulation. The advantage of this 'fan flap' is the ability to cover extended defects and retain the possibility of primary closure of the donor site.

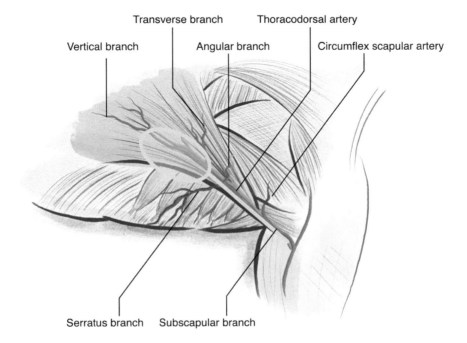

Figure 42.1 Vascular supply to the latissimus dorsi muscle and standard flap design.

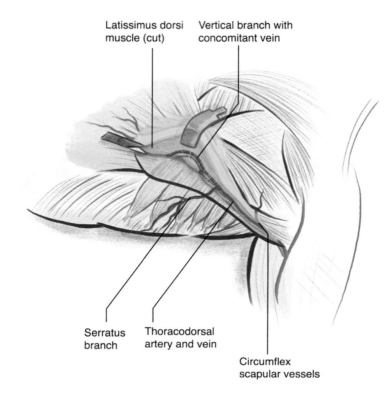

Figure 42.2 Relation of the vascular pedicle and its side branches after incision of the skin and elevation of the anterior muscle rim.

The major advantage of the latissimus dorsi flap is the predictable vascular anatomy with long and high-calibre vessels, which are rarely affected by atherosclerosis. In addition, the flap offers a high density of myocutaneous perforators to the overlying skin and low donor site morbidity.

ESSENTIAL SURGICAL ANATOMY

The latissimus dorsi muscle is a planar muscle that originates from the lower thoracic, lumbar and sacral vertebrae and the iliac crest, and inserts into the crista tuberculi minoris humeri of the humerus. The cranial and lateral part of the muscle are nourished by the thoracodorsal artery. Only the mediodistal muscle part is supplied by the adjacent segmental intercostal vessels.

The thoracodorsal artery is a terminal branch of the subscapular artery, which in turn arises from the axillary artery. In 5% of cases, the thoracodorsal artery arises directly from the axillary artery. Therefore, depending on the anatomical variation, the vascular pedicle of the latissimus dorsi flap is 6–16 cm long. The second terminal branch of the subscapular artery is the

circumflex scapular artery, which runs dorsally to the lateral edge of the scapular. The thoracodorsal artery runs caudally and enters directly from the bottom into the muscle at the vascular hilum. Before penetrating the muscle, the artery gives off branches running anteriorly to the serratus anterior muscle and the anterolateral chest wall. In addition, on its extramuscular course, proximal to the serratus branch, the pedicle gives off another branch to the tip of the scapula (*Figure 42.2*).

In 98% of cases, the thoracodorsal artery is accompanied by a single vein. Analogous to the course of the vessels, the motor thoracodorsal nerve runs intra- and extramuscularly. In the pedicle, the vein is lateral to artery and the motor nerve runs between the vessels.

Intramuscularly, the thoracodorsal artery divides into two to three main branches. This is important for the design of the flap as each of these branches can supply an autonomous piece of composite tissue. To locate the main branches, a Doppler sonography, diaphanoscopy or simple palpation can be used. Two main branches can be identified, one parallel to the lateral border of the muscle and the other parallel to the cranial muscle rim.

PREOPERATIVE CONSIDERATIONS

The patient can be positioned on a lateral decubitus or a prone position for flap harvest. The prone position requires re-preparation and re-draping, therefore in most cases the lateral decubitus position is preferred. A pad should be placed between the shoulder and neck on the contralateral side to prevent the clavicle causing an impingement on the brachial plexus. On the ipsilateral side, the arm must be included in the operating field to allow its free movement. In this preferred operating position, it must be recognised that it is difficult to raise the flap simultaneously with the tumour resection in the head and neck area.

The latissimus dorsi flap offers a high degree of variability for the flap design over the whole proximal two-thirds of the muscle. In all cases, the anterior border of the skin paddle should not exceed the edge of the muscle to ensure safe perfusion of the skin paddle. In addition, to protect the vertical branch running 1.5–3 cm away from the anterior border, a 4–5 cm broad strip of muscle should be integrated into the flap design (*Figure 42.3*).

If primary wound closure of the donor site is intended, which usually is the case, the width of the flap is limited to 10 cm depending on the laxity of the local tissue. The maximal length of the skin paddle is 20–22 cm.

STEPWISE OPERATIVE TECHNIQUE

After positioning of the patient, the anatomical landmarks and the planned incision line are drawn (*Figure 42.4*).

The skin is incised along the anterior border of skin paddle into the axilla. The incision is continued through the subcutaneous fatty tissue until muscle fibres appear and the anterior rim of the latissimus dorsi muscle is identified.

Next, the branch of thoracodorsal artery that supplies the serratus anterior muscle is located. Tracing the branch proximally, it leads to the vascular pedicle of the flap. Alternatively, the vascular pedicle can be identified by palpating the pulsation underneath the proximal muscle rim.

By elevation and retraction of the anterior muscle rim, the vascular pedicle can be dissected in cranial direction. The second side branch, which runs to the inferior angle of the scapula, should appear. To obtain the maximum pedicle length, it is possible to dissect the pedicle up to the circumflex scapula vessels. The neurovascular hilum, where the thoracodorsal vessel enters the muscle at its undersurface, is about 2–4 cm distal to the serratus branch (*Figure 42.5*).

A vessel loop should be placed around the neurovascular pedicle inferior to the side branches. The

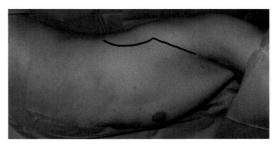
Figure 42.4 Positioning of the patient and the planned incision line.

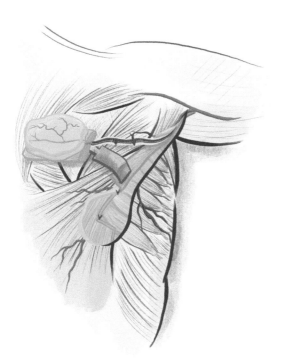
Figure 42.3 Raised flap before ligating the pedicle, demonstrating the density of perforators.

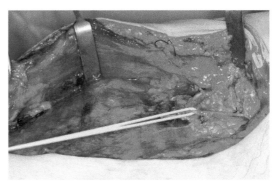
Figure 42.5 Identification of the vascular pedicle and elevation of the anterior muscle rim. The serratus branch has already been ligated.

latissimus dorsi muscle is undermined by blunt dissection. A careful haemostasis must be performed, where segmental branches of intercostal arteries supply the latissimus dorsi muscle.

Next, the complete skin paddle is circumscribed to the muscle fascia. Stay sutures should be placed from the skin to the muscle to prevent an injury to the perforator vessels. The muscle needs to be elevated to perform a transection of muscle fibres along the inferior pole of the flap. Along the anterior border of the flap no transection is needed as it corresponds to the anterior muscle border.

Further undermining, the posterior part of the latissimus dorsi muscle is undermined and elevated. The fibro-fatty tissue between latissimus and serratus muscle must be divided.

This is followed by incising along the posterior border of the flap. To prevent an injury of the neurovascular pedicle, it can slightly be retracted from the muscle to reveal its exact position (*Figure 42.6*).

Finishing the circumscription cranially, a strip of muscle is left between the neurovascular hilum and the cranial border of the skin paddle.

The transverse branch can then be transected, shortly after the bifurcation of thoracodorsal vessel at the cranial flap pole. Also, the side branches to the serratus muscle and inferior angle of scapula (angular branch) need to be dissected. The flap is ready for microvascular transfer or transposition as pedicled flap.

When used as a free flap, the vessels are ligated at the proximal end. The pedicle can be dissected into the subscapular system to achieve maximum vessel size (*Figures 42.7–42.9*).

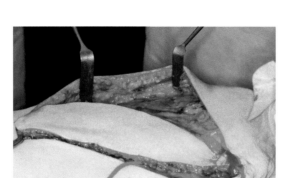

Figure 42.6 Complete circumscription of the skin paddle.

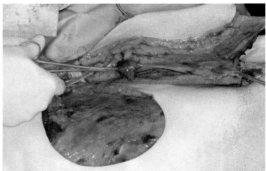

Figure 42.7 Completely raised flap before ligating the pedicle.

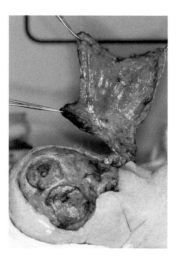

Figure 42.8 After the anastomosis has been performed successfully, the skin island and the muscle, in this case of a fan flap, is sutured over the enormous defect with resected dura on the posterior part of the scalp in the desired position.

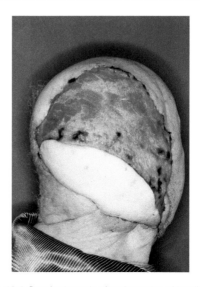

Figure 42.9 Surgical result after 3 weeks of healing and granulation. The muscle is now ready to be covered with a split- or full-thickness skin graft.

When used as a pedicle flap, a tunnel between the pectoralis major and minor muscles and at the muscular insertion of the pectoralis major at the clavicle must be prepared. After passing the flap through the tunnel, the flap can be placed at the desired position.

At the donor site, meticulous haemostasis should follow. Then, a drain is placed before the wound is closed in layers.

POSTOPERATIVE CARE AND RECOVERY

When the output is low, the drain can be removed (usually after 2 days). Depending on the wound tension, the cutaneous sutures should be left in place for 10 days. Alternatively, skin stapling can also be used.

COMPLICATIONS

Raising of the latissimus dorsi flap harbours the usual risks of surgical complications, that is, bleeding, haematoma, seroma, infection and tissue necrosis. Management should be directed accordingly.

Regardless of whether a pedicled or a free flap is used, twisting or kinking of the pedicle must be prevented to ensure a good circulation and survival of the flap. Free flaps additionally carry the risk of a microvascular failure.

Due to the partial loss of the latissimus muscle, there may be a negative impact on activities such as swimming and skiing. In case of an injury or dissection of the accessory nerve during the neck dissection, the stability of the shoulder can be affected. In both cases, intensive physiotherapy is recommended for recovery of at least some of the function.

TOP TIPS AND HAZARDS

- The latissimus dorsi flap can be raised as a pedicled flap or as a free flap.
- Due to the relatively constant vascular anatomy of the pedicle and the perforators, the latissimus dorsi flap is a reliable and a safe flap.
- The skin paddle should be placed over the anterior edge of the latissimus dorsi with flap axis running 4–5 cm dorsal to the anterior edge.
- The serratus branch helps to clearly identify the thoracodorsal artery and therefore should not be transected too early during dissection.
- A subsequent atrophy of the muscle component has to be taken into account when used for facial contour augmentation to prevent unfavourable secondary volume loss.
- The contralateral brachial plexus might be damaged when positioning for operation.
- The positioning of the patient can make it difficult to raise the flap simultaneously to the tumour resection in the head and neck area.
- An injury of the perforator vessels is possible when separation occurs through the subcutaneous fatty tissue and the muscle. Suturing of the skin paddle to the muscle early on will prevent this.

FURTHER READING

Bartlett SP, May JW, Jr, Yaremchuck MJ. The latissimus dorsi muscle: a fresh cadaver study of the primary neurovascular pedicle. *Plast Reconstr Surg* 1981;**67**:631–6.

Hölzle F, Riediger D, Ehrenfeld M. Mikrochirurgische Transplantate. In: Hausamen JE, Machtens E, Reuther JF, Eufinger H, Kübler A, Schliephake H. *Mund-, Kiefer- und Gesichtschirurgie.* Springer; 2012:672–6.

Quillen CG. Latissimus dorsi myocutaneous flaps in head and neck reconstruction. *Plast Reconstr Surg* 1979;**63**:664–70.

Watson JS, Craig RD, Orton CI. The free latissimus dorsi myocutaneous flap. *Plast Reconstr Surg* 1979;**64**:299–305.

Wolff KD, Hölzle F. *Raising of Microvascular Flaps: A Systematic Approach.* Springer; 2018.

Chapter 43

Acute and Delayed Dynamic Facial Reanimation

Jan S. Enzler, Adriaan O. Grobbelaar

INTRODUCTION

Facial paralysis may originate from a broad list of acquired or congenital aetiologies ranging from an isolated single branch palsy to a complete bilateral palsy. Operative concepts and techniques should be adapted to the underlying cause of the palsy and the affected branches. The other important aspects of management include the duration of facial palsy, remaining muscle functionality and patient's age. The treatment must be tailored specifically to the needs of each patient.

PREOPERATIVE PLANNING

Indications

The approach to the management of any patient with facial paralysis should be based on subunits: forehead, eyes, and mid- and lower face (including neck).

In an elderly patient, the facial asymmetry at rest may be obvious and static treatment options alone may yield the desired outcome. This will not, however, provide any dynamic facial mimic function.

In the younger population, the armamentarium of viable options may need to be much broader, with a focus towards restoring a dynamic facial function.

Timing

Timing of surgery will vary greatly depending on the aetiology of the facial palsy and age of the patient. Acute facial nerve injuries (i.e. soft tissue trauma with facial nerve branch transection) should be treated promptly (within 72 hours) because of the likely significant shrinkage and retraction of the nerve ends after 72 hours, hence making it very difficult to correctly identify the nerve.

In cases of closed facial nerve injuries (i.e. blunt facial trauma) as well as idiopathic facial paralysis (Bell's palsy), observation for spontaneous recovery of facial nerve function is warranted. Serial electromyography (EMG) may provide helpful information on recovery and decision making on repair.

Patients requiring a free functional muscle transfer can be divided into four groups with varying treatment options:

- *Patients under 18 years:* two-stage procedure with a cross-facial nerve graft followed by a free muscle transfer 6–12 months later. The first stage is normally performed at around 4 years of age to enable the second stage to be completed by the time the child goes to school
- *Patients aged 18–40 years:* a one-stage procedure can be performed utilising a muscle with a long nerve (e.g. the latissimus dorsi or gracilis muscle). The length of the nerve allows reach to the contralateral face and therefore the procedure requires only one neurorrhaphy. This is not possible in children due to different anatomical proportions
- *Patients aged over 40 years:* a single-stage free muscle transfer with a neurorrhaphy typically to the masseter nerve. The masseteric nerve is preferred because it is a much more powerful motor nerve than either a cross-facial nerve graft or a buccal branch of the facial nerve
- *Patients over 65–70 years:* mostly static facial nerve reconstruction

OPERATIVE TECHNIQUE

Direct facial nerve repair

The facial nerve can be damaged at different levels and the determination of the exact location of injury is important for decision making. The nerve injury locations can be categorised into: distal to the masseter muscle, proximal to the masseter muscle, around the mastoid or in the skull base. For acute facial nerve injuries with adequate length for a tension-free neurorrhaphy, a direct neurorrhaphy should be performed. Loupe magnification or an operating microscope is normally used. Epineural sutures with 10-0 or 11-0 suture material are performed for direct facial nerve repair.

Nerve grafts

If the facial nerve continuity is interrupted and adequate length for a tension-free direct neurorrhaphy is not available, nerve grafts should be considered.

Options include autologous and decellularised nerve grafts. Classic autologous donor nerves include the sural nerve or the great auricular nerve. The authors prefer to use the sural nerve harvested with an

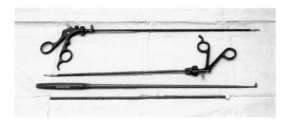

Figure 43.1 The endoscopic nerve harvesting set.

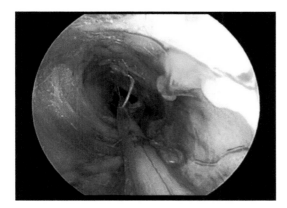

Figure 43.2 Intraoperative endoscopic view of the sural nerve harvesting process.

endoscopic-assisted technique to minimise donor site morbidity. This also allows control of the side branches of the sural nerve. An overview of the endoscopic nerve harvesting set, as well as an intraoperative photograph, is provided in *Figures 43.1* and *43.2*.

Recently, decellularised nerve grafts have been described for repair of segmental deficits of the facial nerve. These offer the benefit of avoiding donor site morbidity and are available off the shelf. However, major drawbacks include the excessive costs and that the potential for re-innervation is reduced with increased graft length and thickness.

Nerve transfers

If the proximal ipsilateral nerve stump is unavailable (i.e. after tumour resection) but the distal stump(s) are present, a nerve transfer procedure can be considered. The masseteric nerve is one of the best options to perform a coaptation to the distal stump. However, it is recommended to choose wisely which part of the face should be reanimated. If one attempts to use a single nerve transfer for all the facial nerve branches, the rate for synkinesis will increase. The eyelid can be effectively treated with static options; therefore, it is recommended that the buccal and/or the marginal mandibular branch are selected for nerve coaptations for restoration of dynamic function.

Selective neurolysis (modified selective neurectomy)

Synkinesis is a frequent long-term complication of facial nerve paralysis. Selective neurolysis, as described by Azizzadeh et al., can be helpful. Nerve branches that innervate the facial muscles they are supposed to innervate are preserved, while the nerve branches that are responsible for synkinesis are identified and are deactivated by selective neurectomy.

Functional muscle transfers

Regional functional muscle transfers offer an option for dynamic facial reanimation without the use of free functional muscle transfers. Commonly used muscles are the temporalis and masseter muscles. One of the drawbacks, however, is temporal hollowing following temporalis transfer. In 1997, Labbé described and modified this procedure now known as the lengthening temporalis myoplasty. It involves an osteotomy of the zygomatic arch and detaching of the temporalis muscle insertion at the coronoid process. This part will then have to be inserted and attached to the modiolus to allow for a dynamic smile. Drawbacks of the Labbé procedure are the short length of the muscle and that neuronal plasticity is required to allow for a dynamic smile.

Free muscle transfers

Free muscle transfers can be considered as the gold standard for facial reanimation. Uni- or bilateral free muscle transfers may be indicated. Several factors must be considered preoperatively:

- If the contralateral facial nerve is functioning, then a cross-facial nerve graft can be used to power the free muscle transfer (two-stage procedure)
- In bilateral facial palsy cases (e.g. Moebius syndrome), the contralateral facial nerve option is not possible
- Decision making on the choice of the procedure is based on patient's age

For patients younger than 18 years, a two-stage procedure with a cross-facial nerve graft and a free muscle transfer 6–12 months later is considered to be the best option.

Figure 43.3 shows the setup for the second-stage surgery after the cross-facial nerve grafts are performed. It is important to mark the facial nerve grafts to ensure that the neurorrhaphies are made to the correct branches. The facial artery and vein as well as the superficial temporal vessels are prepared.

Figure 43.4 shows a young patient with a facial palsy on the left side before the operation. The postoperative result is shown in *Figures 43.5* and *43.6*. *Figures 43.7* and *43.8* show pre- and postoperatively a patient with Moebius syndrome with a bilateral facial paralysis.

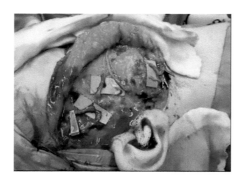

Figure 43.3 Setup for the second-stage surgery after the cross-facial nerve grafts are performed.

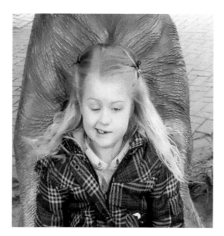

Figure 43.4 Preoperative view of a young patient with a facial palsy on the left side.

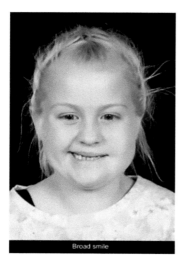

Figure 43.5 One-year postoperative result after facial reanimation on the left side.

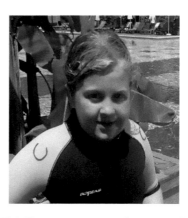

Figure 43.6 Five-year postoperative result after facial reanimation on the left side.

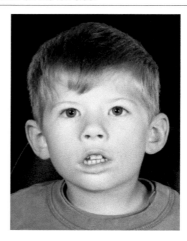

Figure 43.7 Preoperative view of a young patient with Moebius syndrome with bilateral facial paralysis.

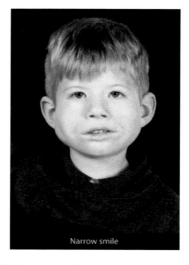

Figure 43.8 Postoperative view of a young patient with Moebius syndrome with bilateral facial paralysis.

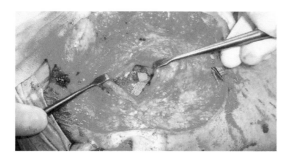

Figure 43.9 Dissected masseteric nerve ready for neurorrhaphy.

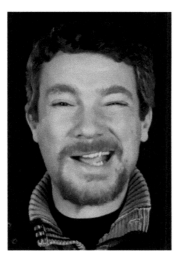

Figure 43.10 A middle-aged patient with a right facial palsy is shown preoperatively.

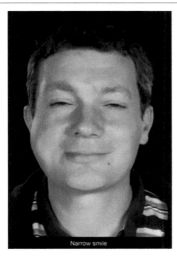

Figure 43.11 Postoperative result after dynamic facial reanimation with a free functional segmental latissimus dorsi flap to the contralateral buccal branch of the facial nerve.

For the age group 18–40 years, a direct one-stage procedure is usually preferred. This involves exploration of the most distal buccal facial nerve branch on the functioning side. The motor nerve of the free muscle flap is then tunnelled to the contralateral side to allow for a neurorrhaphy. Therefore, flaps with a long motor nerve are selected for this technique, most commonly the gracilis and latissimus dorsi muscle flaps.

Patients over 40 years are candidates for a single-stage free muscle transfer with a neurorrhaphy typically to the masseteric nerve. It is powerful enough to provide motor function to the transferred free muscle also in patients over 40 years. A downside of the masseteric nerve is that mime therapy is needed to allow for a spontaneous smile. The preparation of the masseteric nerve is performed as described by Zuker (Zuker's point, see *Further Reading*). *Figure 43.9* shows the dissected masseteric nerve ready for neurorrhaphy. The masseteric nerve is the donor nerve of choice in patients with bilateral facial paralysis.

It is important to note that unless a facial nerve either with or without a cross-facial nerve graft is used to power a functional muscle transfer, a spontaneous smile in response to emotion may not be possible in all cases. Intensive mime therapy is always required.

Figures 43.10 and *43.11* show pre- and postoperative views of a patient with a right facial palsy after dynamic facial reanimation.

Common donor muscle options include the gracilis, the latissimus dorsi or a pectoralis minor muscle. The gracilis muscle is easy to harvest and has a long motor nerve. Drawbacks are that the muscle is unidirectional and that there is no tendon to facilitate the insertion onto the facial structures. The latissimus dorsi and the pectoralis minor muscle on the other hand are fan-shaped muscles with a good tendon component for insertion. The latissimus dorsi muscle can be harvested as a segmental flap, therefore reducing donor site morbidity significantly. The thoracodorsal nerve divides into two branches, allowing harvesting of the muscle flap on one branch while preserving the other branch, which will continue to innervate the rest of the muscle.

The pectoralis minor muscle has similar advantages regarding shape and the availability of tendon as well as being less bulky. It is the authors' first choice for two-stage reconstruction. The downsides include the inconsistent vascular pedicle, a short donor nerve and a more challenging harvesting procedure. It can be accessed through an axillary incision (*Figure 43.12*). In *Figure 43.13*, the vascular pedicle as well as the pectoral nerve can be seen.

For bilateral facial palsy cases, the pectoralis minor muscle is not an option because the motor nerve is too short for a neurorrhaphy to the masseteric nerve. Hence, the options for bilateral cases are the (segmental) latissimus dorsi and the gracilis muscle.

Dynamic facial reanimation with free functional muscle transfers is not limited to smile recreation.

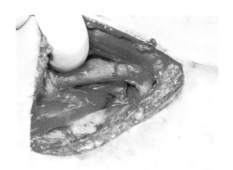

Figure 43.12 Access to the pectoralis muscles through an incision in the axilla.

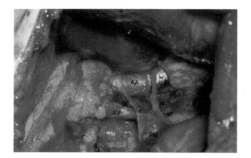

Figure 43.13 View of the vascular pedicle as well as the pectoral nerves.

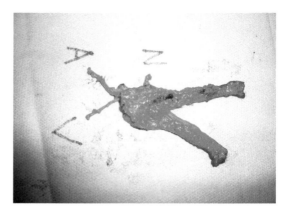

Figure 43.14 Free functional platysma flap with its vascular pedicle and motor nerve (cervical branch of facial nerve).

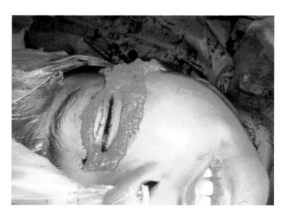

Figure 43.15 Division of the platysma muscle into two slips to mimic the orbicularis oculi muscle.

While static procedures are reliable options for eye closure, spontaneous blink cannot be restored with these methods. The use of a free functional platysma muscle transfer in conjunction with a cross-facial nerve graft as a two-stage procedure has been described for restoration of a spontaneous blink, thereby allowing for an ideal protection of the cornea. While it is a technically challenging procedure and only suited for younger patients (under 18 years), the results and benefits are rewarding. The muscle flap with its vascular pedicle and motor nerve is outlined in *Figure 43.14*. The platysma muscle is divided into two slips (*Figure 43.15*). The platysma flap is then placed below the orbicularis oculi muscle and vascular anastomosis as well as the neurorrhaphy are performed under the operating microscope to the superficial temporal vessels and the previously prepared cross-facial nerve graft.

Static facial nerve reconstruction

For elderly patients, the goal should be to recreate facial symmetry at rest. Several options are available, depending on the affected area.

Management of the brow and forehead

Frequently, sagging of the brow on the affected side and compensatory movement of the forehead on the

contralateral side are encountered. As a non-surgical option to achieve better forehead symmetry, the contra-lateral frontalis muscle can be chemo-denervated with Botulinum Toxin A injection.

The surgical options for the affected brow include a brow-lift, either directly or endoscopically. Direct brow-lift incisions include brow, bi-coronal or mid-forehead approaches. The direct brow-lift with the incision placed above the brow is a straightforward and effective way to address a brow ptosis. An elliptical excision of redundant tissue is planned, and skin as well as frontalis muscle are excised to achieve symmetry. The orbicularis oculi muscle can be fixed to the periosteum for increased durability of the lift.

Management of the eye

Protection of the cornea with good eye closure is one of the main goals in facial reanimation. Standard statical options include placement of a weight (gold weight or platinum chain) in the upper lid. Test weights can be attached to the upper lid with tape to decide how much weight is needed. Most commonly 1–1.2 g will suffice. The platinum chain is attached to the tarsal plate and two-layered closure of the orbicularis oculi and the skin is performed (*Figure 43.16*).

Due to the paralysis of the orbicularis oculi muscle, the lower lid will also be affected, and an ectropion is frequently a consequence of this. This can be addressed by a lateral tarsorrhaphy, as described by McLaughlin, where the posterior lamella of the upper lid (tarsal plate and conjunctiva) and an identical area of the anterior lamella of the lower lid (skin and muscle) are excised. The resulting denuded areas are overlapped and sutured.

Additional procedures such as palmaris longus slings, tarsal strip procedures and conchal grafts may also be used to support the atrophic lower eyelid and correct the ectropion if indicated.

Management of the midface and mouth

Drooping of the midface and the corner of the mouth on the affected side are consequences of a longer standing facial palsy and skin laxity. The patients may be affected by the appearance, as well as experiencing drooling and impaired speech.

A reliable option to treat this is the use of an autologous fascia lata graft. The graft is harvested through two separate horizontal incisions on the lateral thigh. A large enough piece of fascia should be taken to afterwards allow for division into three distal slips for insertion at the midline of the upper as well as the lower lip and at the modiolus. A facelift-type incision and elevation of the facial skin will allow placement of the fascia graft in the cheek. Additional incisions in the midline of the upper and the lower lip will have to be made to allow placement of the fascia lata slips. The orbicularis oris muscle will allow for fixation of the slips with non-resorbable sutures. The fascia lata graft should be sutured in with enough tension to compensate for potential future stretching of the graft. An illustration of a fascia lata graft can be seen in *Figure 43.17*.

Figures 43.18 and *43.19* show pre- and post-operative views of a patient who underwent tensor fascia lata insertion.

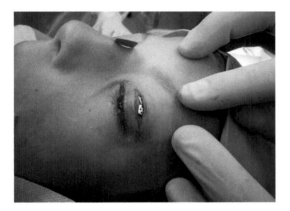

Figure 43.16 View of a platinum chain in the upper lid to allow for closure of the eyelid.

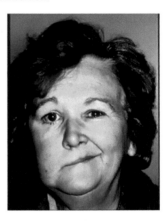

Figure 43.18 Preoperative view of a patient with right facial paralysis before static facial nerve reconstruction.

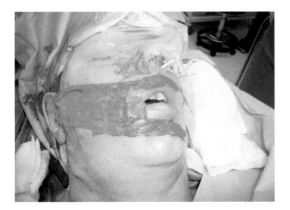

Figure 43.17 Fascia lata graft divided into three slips ready for insertion into the face.

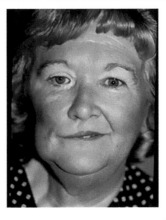

Figure 43.19 Postoperative view after static facial nerve reconstruction with a tensor fascia lata sling.

POSTOPERATIVE CARE AND RECOVERY

Other than smaller operations, facial reanimation procedures are mostly performed under general anaesthesia as an in-patient procedure. Broad spectrum perioperative antibiotics are routinely given to prevent infections, especially if foreign material or grafts are used.

A facial compression dressing is applied to prevent hematoma formation while still allowing flap perfusion. The dressing is removed on the first postoperative day. Drains are removed according to their output.

Pneumatic compression stockings are worn until the patient mobilises. No medical thrombosis prophylaxis (i.e. heparin) is administered.

Physiotherapy with stretching of the transferred muscle is started 4 weeks postoperatively, once the wound healing is deemed satisfactory. Active physiotherapy/mime therapy with exercises specifically for the transferred muscle can be started and intensified once the muscle starts to show movement to optimise function, symmetry and brain plasticity where a non-facial motor nerve has been used.

POSSIBLE COMPLICATIONS

Complications can be classified as acute or delayed and as general or specific with regard to the free muscle flap transfer. General complications such as bleeding, hematoma, wound infection and wound breakdown can occur.

Specific complications related to the transfer of the free flap include flap necrosis due to insufficient vascularisation or failure of muscle re-innervation.

Acute complications are mostly related to bleeding or wound infection. Delayed complications occur weeks to months after the operation and may exhibit non-existing or insufficient muscle action.

TOP TIPS AND HAZARDS

- Treatment options vary depending on patient age. Free muscle transfer procedures are generally performed only in younger patients. Patients over 65 typically require a static facial reconstruction.
- As a guideline, the masseteric nerve can be found 3 cm anterior to the tragus and 1 cm inferior to the zygomatic arch, described as Zuker's point.
- For dynamic facial reanimation, a pectoralis minor or a segmental latissimus dorsi muscle is favoured due to their fan-shaped geometry and their tendon.
- Active physiotherapy/mime therapy can greatly improve symmetry and function of the transferred muscle.

FURTHER READING

Azizzadeh B, Irvine LE, Diels J, et al. Modified selective neurectomy for the treatment of post-facial paralysis synkinesis. *Plast Reconstr Surg* 2019;**143**:1483–96.

Borschel GH, Kawamura DH, Kasukurthi R, et al. The motor nerve to the masseter muscle: an anatomic and histomorphometric study to facilitate its use in facial reanimation. *J Plast Reconstr Aesthet Surg* 2012;**65**:363–6.

Leckenby J, Butler D, Grobbelaar A. The axillary approach to raising the latissimus dorsi free flap for facial re-animation: a descriptive surgical technique. *Arch Plast Surg* 2015;**42**:73–7.

Leckenby JI, Ghali S, Butler DP, Grobbelaar AO. Reanimation of the brow and eye in facial paralysis: review of the literature and personal algorithmic approach. *J Plast Reconstr Aesthet Surg* 2015;**68**:603–14.

Leckenby JI, Harrison DH, Grobbelaar AO. Static support in the facial palsy patient: a case series of 51 patients using tensor fascia lata slings as the sole treatment for correcting the position of the mouth. *J Plast Reconstr Aesthet Surg* 2014;**67**:350–7.

Chapter 44

Submandibular, Sublingual and Minor Salivary Gland Surgery

Panayiotis A. Kyzas, Leandros-Vassilios Vassiliou

BACKGROUND

The indications for surgery for the submandibular, sublingual and minor salivary glands can be categorised into four groups: neoplasia, infection, sialolithiasis and pseudocysts.

The submandibular gland gives rise to around 10% of all salivary gland tumours; half are malignant, and of the remainder that are benign, almost all are pleomorphic adenomas. Tumours of the sublingual gland are very rare, but almost all are malignant. Finally, 10% of all salivary gland tumours arise in minor salivary glands, and about 50% are malignant.

Sialadenitis means 'infection of a salivary gland' and, in the context of the chapter, is almost unique to the submandibular salivary gland. The aetiology is obstruction due to a calculus (stone-sialolithiasis), in most cases. Sialadenitis can be acute (which is treated non-surgically, with antibiotics and rehydration) or chronic, which usually leads to an atrophic/non-functional submandibular gland. Finally, pseudocysts are formed by extravasation of saliva, most commonly from a minor salivary gland (mucoceles) or the sublingual gland (ranulas).

PREOPERATIVE WORK-UP: INVESTIGATIONS

A simple occlusal radiograph, in conjunction with an orthopantomogram (to exclude dental pathology) is the appropriate first line investigation, as most submandibular sialoliths are calcified. The size and the exact position of the calculus can be accurately investigated with an ultrasound scan. A sialogram is very useful once a sialolith has been ruled out and is valuable when investigating chronic sialadenitis.

When a neoplastic mass is present in the submandibular gland, the sublingual gland or a minor salivary gland, cross-sectional imaging is indicated. A magnetic resonance imaging (MRI) neck is adequate for benign neoplasms, whereas the full staging protocol for head and neck cancer (MRI neck, computed tomography (CT) thorax) must be utilised in malignant neoplasms.

Histological investigation of salivary neoplasms has been a subject of historical debate. However, the current gold standard is an ultrasound (US)-guided fine needle aspiration (FNA) (with or without cytospin/cellblock) for submandibular gland neoplasms or a US-core biopsy if the initial FNA is inadequate. For the sublingual gland and the minor salivary glands, an open biopsy is the investigation of choice (this can be an excisional biopsy for very small minor salivary gland lesions; it will often be the only treatment required). As almost all sublingual gland neoplasms are malignant, an incisional biopsy will confirm the histology and allow resection planning.

SURGICAL PROCEDURES OF THE SUBMANDIBULAR GLAND

Submandibular gland excision

The technique described below refers to excision of the gland for benign disease (benign neoplasms, chronic sialadenitis, sialolithiasis). When it comes to malignant disease, the gland is removed en bloc, as part of the neck dissection (if one is indicated). The submandibular gland occupies much of the contents of level Ib of the neck. Clearance of level Ib (submandibular triangle) is often the only treatment required for early-stage (T1/T2) low-grade malignant tumours of the submandibular gland.

Technique

The procedure is performed under general anaesthesia, with the patient supine with moderate neck extension. Skin infiltration with tumescent solution helps haemostasis and outlines tissue planes with hydrodissection. Despite previous teaching about placement of the skin incision to protect the marginal mandibular branch of the facial nerve, surgeons can be assured that the skin incision is completely irrelevant to injuring this nerve, as it runs in a much deeper anatomical plane. One should therefore place the skin incision in a suitable skin crease close to the submandibular gland. The skin incision does not need to be longer than 4–5 cm. However, it is important to emphasise the need for supra-platysma skin dissection (in the same concept as a facelift) prior to platysma incision. This allows easier retraction, better access and reduces the risk of traction injury

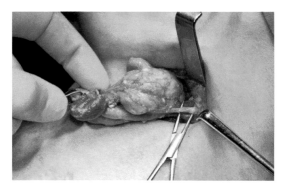

Figure 44.1 Dissection, control and ligation of the proximal facial artery (at the 5 o'clock position for this LEFT submandibular gland).

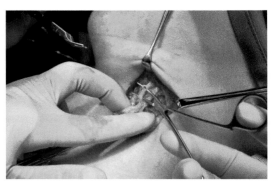

Figure 44.2 Dissection, control and ligation of the distal facial vessels, prior to crossing the lower border of the mandible.

to the marginal branch. Following this manoeuvre, the platysma is incised, usually 3 cm below the lower border of the mandible. This reveals the investing layer of the cervical fascia, that hosts, in its deep surface, the marginal branch of the facial nerve. This fascia is carefully divided, under direct visualisation and loupes magnification. Following that, dissection continues at the level of the gland; the fascia is retracted upwards, and this protects the marginal branch. The submandibular gland can be conceptualised as floating in loose connective tissue but anchored in place at four points: the proximal facial vessels at the posterior belly of the digastric, the distal facial vessels towards the lower border of the mandible, the duct and the attachment of the lingual nerve at the submandibular parasympathetic ganglion. Therefore, excision of the gland requires control and division at those four points. Once the anterior surface of the gland is revealed, the gland is held with Allis forceps and lifted upwards. The proximal facial vessels are identified at the posterior belly of the digastric (5 o'clock on the LEFT, 7 o'clock on the RIGHT), controlled and ligated (*Figure 44.1*).

The intraglandular course of the facial artery is variable but also irrelevant in the context of the procedure. Once the proximal facial vessels are controlled and ligated, the surgeon dissects the superolateral aspect of the gland and identifies the distal part of the facial vessels, prior to crossing the lower border of the mandible; these are dissected, controlled, ligated and divided (*Figure 44.2*).

At this stage, the anterior pole of the superficial lobe of the gland is retracted posteriorly, the submental vessels are controlled and the groove between the superficial and deep lobes of the gland is revealed. The posterior border of the mylohyoid lies within this groove. The muscle is freed retracted forward and upward with a Langenbeck retractor. This allows mobilisation of the deep lobe of the gland. Downwards pulling reveals the U-shaped lingual nerve and its attachment to the gland via the parasympathetic fibres to the submandibular

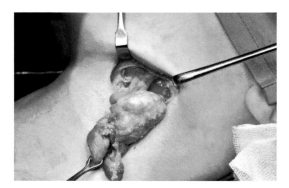

Figure 44.3 Dissection and separation of the submandibular gland from the lingual nerve at the ganglion.

ganglion. These fibres are carefully released allowing the lingual nerve to spring upwards (*Figure 44.3*).

The final step is to control, ligate and divide the submandibular duct. Following removal of the gland, one should ensure that the hypoglossal nerve (which is found at a deeper level at the submandibular triangle) is intact. The wound is then closed meticulously in layers. A drain is not required as the blood supply to the gland is exclusively from the facial vessels, and, similarly to hemithyroidectomy, research evidence suggests that drains do not reduce the risk of haematoma.

Provided that dissection stays 'on the gland', the risk of injury to the hypoglossal nerve during this procedure is negligible. The same holds true for the risk of permanent damage to the marginal mandibular branch of the facial nerve, although temporary neuropraxia due to traction cannot be excluded. The main nerve at risk during submandibular gland excision is the lingual, due to direct connection (and the need to separate it) with the gland. Careful traction and meticulous dissection minimise the risk of prolonged tongue paraesthesia.

Removal of sialolith

If the size and location of the stone permits, an endoscopic basket retrieval of the sialolith should be attempted (see *Chapter 45*). When this is not possible, open surgery is needed. This is easier to perform when the stone lies within the lumen of the duct distal (anterior) to the point where the duct crosses the lingual nerve. This procedure can safely be carried out under local anaesthetic in a minor op setting.

Technique

Following local anaesthesia, the stone is palpated and assessed for mobility. For mobile sialoliths, traditional teaching suggests passing a stay suture into the floor of the mouth around the duct proximal to the stone, to prevent it from being displaced backwards. In our experience, this is very rarely needed. The mucosal incision is made along the line of the duct overlying the stone. The duct is encountered and opened in a fashion parallel to its course. The stone is seen, mobilised and released with careful dissection with a fine mosquito. Once the sialolith has been removed, cloudy mucinous saliva will often follow from the duct proximally. The duct is then gently irrigated with sterile saline and the floor of the mouth mucosa is loosely approximated with two to three resorbable sutures. No attempt should be made to close the duct as this would result in scarring and stricture formation leading to further obstruction.

For stones located more proximal (i.e. closer to the hilum of the gland), one should consider the risk of damage to the lingual nerve; it may be wise to remove the submandibular gland together with the stone from an external approach. If, however, stone removal is indicated, the procedure is usually carried out under general anaesthesia. The mucosal incision is performed at the posterolateral floor of the mouth. Care must be taken to retract and protect the sublingual gland and the lingual nerve (which at that point has crossed and passes immediately deep to the gland). The submandibular duct and the hilum of the gland are elevated with the application of upwards pressure through the neck by the assistant. The duct is then opened, and the stone retrieved, as previously described. Closure follows the same principles. This procedure is nowadays rarely performed, as the risk of traction injury to the lingual nerve, especially at the hilum, where it firmly connects to the gland via the parasympathetic ganglion, is significant. It is safer to remove the gland and the stone in a controlled fashion via a neck approach.

Sublingual gland excision

The sublingual gland needs to be removed in cases of ranulas and neoplasms. As almost all of the sublingual salivary gland neoplasms are malignant, the gland excision is part of the overall ablative plan. This involves, as a minimum, en bloc resection of floor of mouth mucosa (superior margin), mylohyoid muscle (gland bed, deep margin) and ventral tongue (medial margin). Therefore, this procedure is very different from a simple gland excision and follows the principles addressed in *Chapter 25*. Here, we discuss the simplest form of sublingual gland excision, for benign disease (almost always ranula, rarely chronic sialadenitis).

Technique

Two structures are very important during this procedure: the Wharton's duct and the lingual nerve. The operation is performed under general anaesthesia. Infiltration with local anaesthetic with adrenaline helps with vasoconstriction and haemostasis. The mucosal incision is made parallel and lateral to the submandibular salivary gland duct and runs from anteriorly towards the first lower molar. At that area, the lingual nerve crosses the duct and is at risk of injury – due caution is needed. If the gland is removed for a ranula, one might need to aspirate the contents or open the sac, especially for very large lesions. However, preserving the pseudocyst wall intact sometimes aids dissection. The first aim of the procedure is to identify the submandibular gland duct, separate it from the sublingual gland and protect it by retracting it medially. We find the use of fine bipolar diathermy to be invaluable for this part, as it ensures bloodless and fine separation of the duct without injuring it. Following this, the lingual nerve can be identified and protected, as it runs deep to the lingual aspect of the operating field. The gland is then gently mobilised from its muscular (mylohyoid) bed and removed. If the ranula is of the plunging form, care must be taken to ensure complete removal of the neck component; external digital pressure at the chin by the assistant usually helps. Haemostasis is paramount in these cases, as small branches of the emissary lingual veins, if not adequately controlled, can retract deep and bleed later, giving rise to sublingual haematoma and potential airway compromise. For that reason, the overlying floor of mouth mucosa is loosely sutured with three to four resorbable stitches.

Special considerations for sublingual and submandibular gland tumours

Some malignant salivary gland neoplasms have a high neurotropic potential and tend to spread very early along the course of named nerves. The classic didactic example is the adenoid cystic carcinoma, although other high-grade salivary neoplasms exhibit similar behaviour. It is therefore crucial to plan the ablative resection in a way that includes an adequate margin on the main nerves that might be involved. For sublingual and submandibular gland tumours the main nerve is the lingual, although in some advanced cases of submandibular gland adenoid cystic carcinoma, the hypoglossal nerve can also be involved.

Preoperative assessment with an MRI scan can highlight perineural spread (*Table 44.1*) and guide the extent of the nerve resection required. Sometimes this needs to extend at the level of the lingula, and beyond, significantly more posterior to the primary tumour side. Planning for an access procedure and use of intraoperative frozen sections might be required.

The location of small intraglandular T1–T2 submandibular gland adenoid cystic carcinomas is crucial. Tumours located near the hilum of the gland, where the lingual nerve is close and tethered to the gland, require a low threshold of sacrificing the nerve. More early peripheral tumours can safely be addressed without lingual nerve excision.

TABLE 44.1 Points of caution in submandibular and sublingual gland tumours

Importance of histology (biopsy)	Adenoid cystic carcinoma High-grade tumours with perineural invasion
Importance of imaging	MRI – perineural spread MRI and/or US – location of small submandibular tumours

SURGERY OF THE MINOR SALIVARY GLANDS

Minor salivary gland biopsy

A lower lip salivary gland biopsy is sometimes needed to confirm the diagnosis of Sjögren's syndrome. This is a relatively easy procedure and is performed under local anaesthetic in a minor op setting. The incision is performed in the inner aspect of the lip. The mucosa is excised horizontally, and the lip is then everted with the assistant's finger. This reveals the lower lip minor salivary glands and allows careful dissection and removal of an adequate number of glands (usually three). It is prudent to remove all the glands that can be seen, as not doing so risks the development of a future mucocele. Following that, haemostasis is obtained on the muscle bed and the wound is closed with resorbable sutures.

Small minor salivary gland tumours have a 50% chance of being malignant. In general terms, if a lesion is small enough to allow an excisional biopsy and primary mucosal closure, this is the diagnostic method of choice. If the results confirm a benign neoplasm, then the excisional biopsy was the treatment in most of the cases. If the biopsy shows malignancy, then further surgery is needed; the biopsy scar is included in the re-resection. Advances in US techniques and special intraoral US probes have recently allowed performance of US-guided intraoral FNAs for equivocal minor salivary gland tumours; this should be considered where available.

Palatal minor salivary gland surgery

Palatal minor salivary glands can give rise to several pathologies. These include acute necrotising sialometaplasia, adenoid cystic carcinoma, squamous cell carcinoma and pleomorphic adenoma, to name a few. The management of these conditions differs significantly, ranging from doing nothing (necrotising sialometaplasia) to extensive compartmental maxillectomy and skull base resection (advanced adenoid cystic carcinoma). It is imperative to know exactly what the pathology is, therefore an open biopsy of palatal lesions is required. Treatment for malignant minor salivary gland tumours of the palate involves the various forms of maxillectomy discussed in *Chapter 25*. We discuss here the procedure to excise benign neoplasms.

Technique

Most of the cases requiring this approach are pleomorphic adenomas. The procedure is usually performed under general anaesthetic. Infiltration with local anaesthetic with adrenaline aids haemostasis. The mucosal incision is performed to a clinically healthy-looking margin with a Colorado needle on a cutting diathermy. The mucosal incision is deepened down to bone and the periosteum is stripped under the tumour with a periosteal elevator. Rarely, benign tumours fenestrate into the floor of the nose or the maxillary sinus; care must be taken to gently free them without rupture or spillage. The defect may be left to heal by secondary intention, although protecting it with a cover plate is the usual standard of practice. The plate should be retained for 2 weeks, by which time the area will be granulating.

TOP TIPS AND HAZARDS

- Careful selection of sialoliths that can be removed via basket retrieval; size and location are of paramount importance.
- The four anchoring points during submandibular gland excision are the proximal and distal facial vessels, the lingual nerve and the submandibular duct.
- Almost all sublingual gland neoplasms are malignant.
- Lingual nerve resection might be needed in neurotropic malignant submandibular and/or sublingual gland tumours.
- Preoperative biopsy of a palatal minor salivary gland tumour is essential.

FURTHER READING

Bradley PJ, Ferris RL. Surgery for malignant sublingual and minor salivary gland neoplasms. *Adv Otorhinolaryngol* 2016;**78**:113–9.

Carlson ER, Schlieve T. Salivary gland malignancies. *Oral Maxillofac Surg Clin North Am* 2019;**31**:125–44.

Lombardi D, McGurk M, Vander Poorten V et al. Surgical treatment of salivary malignant tumors. *Oral Oncol* 2017;**65**:102–13.

Witt RL, Iro H, Koch M, McGurk M et al. Minimally invasive options for salivary calculi. *Laryngoscope* 2012;**122**:1306–11.

Chapter 45

Management of Salivary Stones and Strictures with Minimally Invasive Techniques

Simon C. Harvey, Jacqueline Brown, Michael P. Escudier

SALIVARY OBSTRUCTIVE DISEASE

Blockage of the salivary duct is characterised by pain and swelling of the affected gland during gustatory stimulation – a sign known as 'mealtime syndrome'. Swellings can arise rapidly and take hours to subside. Some patients may report a short-lasting electric shock-like symptom ('first bite syndrome') when eating – this may be a sign of pathology, but also can be entirely normal.

Salivary gland obstruction may be due to either extraductal or intraductal causes. Intraductal causes are far more common and include salivary calculi and duct stenoses. A large series of patients with obstructive symptoms showed physical obstruction in 64% of cases; 73% had salivary calculi and 23% had a stricture as the primary obstruction. Conversely, endoscopic investigation of sialadenitis by Koch et al. showed stenosis to be more common and revealed only 20% were due to calculi obstruction. Stones (calculi) are more commonly found in the submandibular gland than in the parotid gland, probably due to duct anatomy and saliva composition. There is no gender predilection. Strictures are far more common in the parotid glands, in women, in those above 40 years of age, and around 7% of patients have bilateral strictures. Mucous plugging is concurrent with both stones and strictures, causing transient duct blockage.

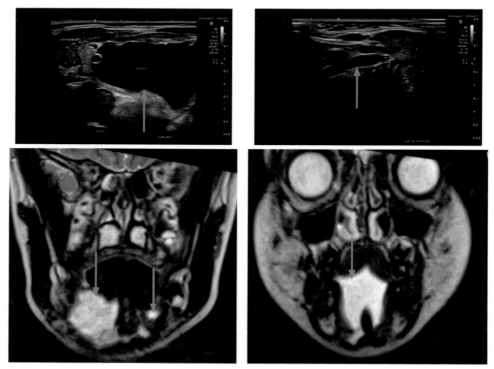

Figure 45.1 Extraductal causes of obstruction. Top row: ultrasound; bottom row: coronal magnetic resonance imaging. Blue arrow: right-sided ranula. Red arrow: dilated left submandibular duct.

Salivary obstruction				
Adult E08	Modality	Dose	Recommendation	Comment
	US	None	Indicated [B]	US (including with oral sialagogue if appropriate) is the first-line investigation to assess the presence, level and degree of obstruction, its cause (e.g. stone or stricture) and associated parenchymal changes.
	XR	☢	Indicated only in specific circumstances [B]	Mandibular anterior occlusal XR can be useful including if US has revealed submandibular/sublingual ductal dilatation but no calculus (anterior stones can be obscured by the mandible on US).
	CT/Cone beam CT (CBCT)	☢ - ☢☢	Indicated only in specific circumstances [B]	Non contrast CT or CBCT where available are superior to radiographs to detect and measure salivary calculi.
	Fluoroscopic sialography	☢☢	Indicated only in specific circumstances [B]	Fluoroscopic sialography is the gold standard imaging test for ductal evaluation. It is performed in patients with ductal dilatation on US, and in those without ductal dilatation but persistent symptoms suggestive of obstruction (e.g. peri prandial gland swelling). Besides diagnosis, it can assess suitability for minimally invasive treatments, and be therapeutic (duct washout). Fluoroscopic stone removal and sialoplasty may be performed in specific circumstances where expertise is available.
	MR sialography	None	Indicated only in specific circumstances [B]	MR sialography is an alternative to fluoroscopic sialography where available.
	CT/CBCT sialography	☢ - ☢☢	Indicated only in specific circumstances [B]	CT or cone beam sialography are alternatives to fluoroscopic sialography where available.

Figure 45.2 Royal College of Radiologists (RCR) iRefer (www.irefer.org.uk) guidance for imaging salivary obstruction. (Reproduced for this publication with permission, not for reproduction elsewhere.)

Extraductal causes of obstruction include invasion from a tumour, pressure from a benign lesion (such as a ranula) or side effects from surgery (*Figure 45.1*).

Both stones and strictures may cause decreased salivary flow, which can leave the patient prone to ascending sialadenitis. Amoxicillin is widely prescribed for bacterial infections, despite poor expression in saliva. A systematic review has shown that cephalosporins (e.g. cefuroxime) and fluoroquinolones (ciprofloxacin) display superior pharmacokinetics in saliva and cover the spectrum of all bacteria implicated in sialadenitis.

MANAGEMENT OF STONES

Sialolithiasis accounts for approximately 50% of major salivary gland disease. The incidence of symptomatic sialolithiasis is between 27.5 and 59 cases per million population per year.

A salivary calculus usually results in mechanical obstruction of the salivary duct. Stones are likely to originate around shed ductal cells acting as a condensation nucleus in a hypersaturated solution of calcium and magnesium. Such microscopic stones are usually shed spontaneously. Retained stones grow at approximately 1 mm diameter per year by precipitation of further minerals, demonstrating a concentric ring pattern. Stones may move throughout the ductal system or become wedged/attached to a duct wall.

Stones larger than the ostium (2 mm) may block the duct, causing symptoms such as mealtime syndrome.

Symptomatic stones usually require treatment. Until recently, this necessitated open surgery; sialadenectomy was frequently offered, despite its attendant risks.

Minimally invasive non-surgical techniques for removal of salivary calculi have been developed predicated on salivary glands having significant reparative potential. Scintigraphic studies before and after submandibular calculus removal have shown that gland function can recover.

Diagnosis of stones

High-resolution ultrasound is indicated first for salivary obstruction. Stones are seen as highly echogenic with posterior shadow. Sialography remains part of the Royal College of Radiologists' guidelines (https://www.irefer.org.uk) (*Figure 45.2*) as the most sensitive method for detecting small intraductal salivary stones and strictures (*Figure 45.3*). Stones are seen as a filling defect on sialogram. Its role has been extended into interventional radiological techniques in the salivary ducts to treat ductal obstruction. Lower occlusal radiographs are useful for distally placed submandibular duct stones (*Figure 45.4*).

MR sialography is possible where conventional sialography is contraindicated, offering a non-ionising technique, although more expensive and not dynamic. Heavily T2-weighted sequences without contrast are preferred, following sialogogue stimulation. Stones are seen as a filling defect (*Figure 45.5*). Cone beam computed tomography (CBCT) of the mandible may find incidental stones (*Figure 45.6*).

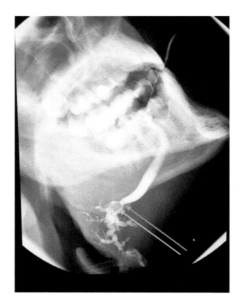

Figure 45.3 Point stricture (orange arrow) and proximal stone (white arrow).

Radiology-guided basket retrieval (fluoroscopy or ultrasound)

Radiology-guided treatment has become one of several new minimally invasive techniques to avoid surgery, developing from other areas of intervention.

Case selection for basket retrieval

Stones within the main parotid and submandibular ducts are amenable to extraction using a basket, but this technique is unsuitable for deep stones in the submandibular genu or hilum of either gland. Stone mobility on the preoperative sialogram is a good prognostic factor. Importantly, only sialography allows assessment of duct width distally, from a stone to the duct orifice. This is crucially important if the stone is to be withdrawn down the duct, as there must not be too great a mismatch between the size of stone and the duct.

Stones greater than 7 mm may not be suitable for basket extraction 'whole'. In addition, it would be sensible to avoid extraction of stones more than 25% greater in width than the width of the narrowest section of the distal salivary duct. If a large stone is captured but is too large to be withdrawn down the relatively narrow duct, then the basket will become impacted and will almost

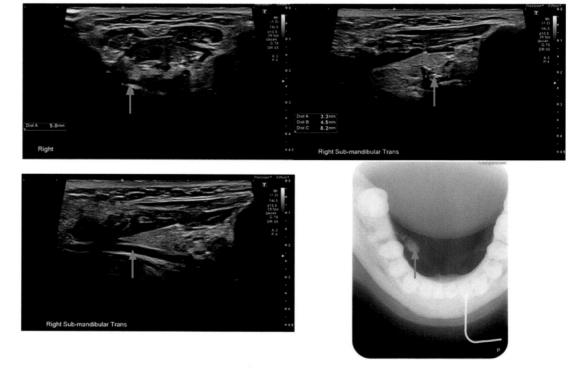

Figure 45.4 Ultrasound and lower occlusal radiograph showing obstructive anterior/distal calculus (red arrows) and proximal dilation (blue arrow).

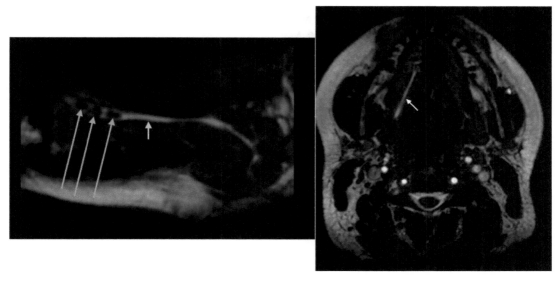

Figure 45.5 Heavily T2-weighted magnetic resonance images. The orange arrows indicate three stones in the anterior/distal right submandibular duct, and the white arrows show mild proximal dilation.

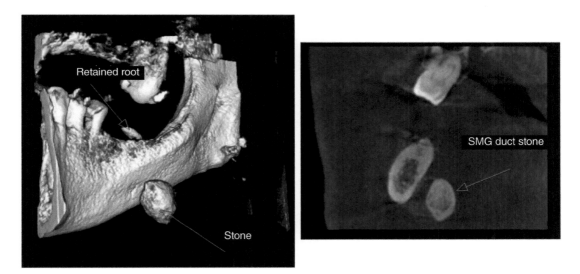

Retained root

Stone

SMG duct stone

Figure 45.6 Cone beam computed tomography of the mandible, with arrows indicating incidental SMG stone.

certainly require surgical release. This is an important complication, which can be avoided with appropriate treatment planning. Larger and very proximal stones may be treated first by lithotripsy (see '*Intraductal Fragmentation*' or '*Extracorporeal Shockwave Lithotripsy*') to break down the stone into more manageable pieces. If a stricture is identified distal to the stone to be removed, then balloon ductoplasty (see '*Radiologically Guided Balloon Dilation*') will be required to dilate this area of duct stenosis prior to stone extraction.

The technique for stone removal from the parotid and submandibular ducts using a Dormia basket technique (*Figures 45.7* and *45.8*) under fluoroscopic x-ray guidance, or ultrasound guidance, and local anaesthesia is a relatively simple procedure with a high success rate and low morbidity. Following treatment planning, on the basis of clinical examination and preoperative imaging, the patient is anaesthetised:

● *Parotid gland anaesthesia technique*: infiltrating the cheek around the Stenson's duct papilla with 2%

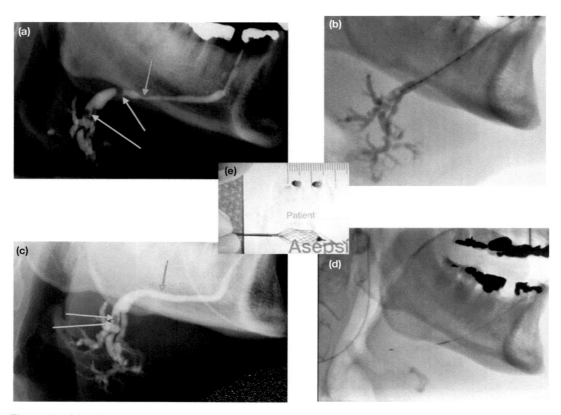

Figure 45.7 (a) White arrows indicate two filling defects (stones), and orange arrow indicates short diffuse stricture in the proximal third. (b) Balloon dilated in stricture. (c) Orange arrow shows the stricture now dilated, and white arrows show the stones remaining in the hilum. (d) Basket to retrieve stones. (e) Extracted stones and basket.

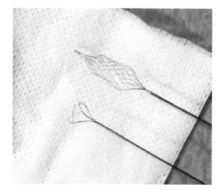

Figure 45.8 Dormia baskets.

lignocaine and instilling local anaesthetic into the parotid duct to create some topical anaesthesia of the duct wall
- *Submandibular gland anaesthesia technique*: by infiltrating the floor of mouth coupled with a lingual nerve block

Fluoroscopy-guided basket retrieval technique

The duct orifice is dilated with Nettleship dilators or specialist Kolenda dilators until sufficient to receive a Dormia basket. The basket is inserted in the closed position and guided into position under imaging control. The catheter tip must normally pass beyond the stone, into the proximal salivary duct. Once in position, the basket is opened and withdrawn across the stone to capture it. This can be confirmed by imaging and assisted by bimanual manipulation. The stone is captured and withdrawn to the papilla, where a small papillotomy incision allows delivery of the stone. Immediate postoperative sialography can confirm the duct is free from stones and debris.

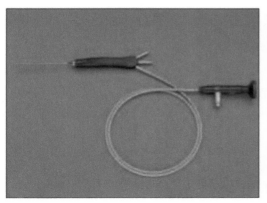
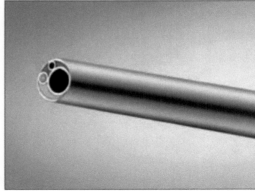
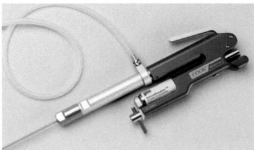
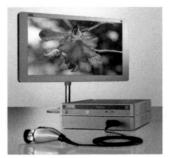

Figure 45.9 Rigid salivary endoscopes.

Endoscopic-guided basket retrieval

Progressively smaller, specialist rigid salivary endo-scopes have been developed, with diameters measuring between 0.8 and 2.1 mm in diameter (*Figure 45.9*).

Clinical and radiographic assessment of prospective cases is essential, as exclusion criteria for the technique include narrow ducts, ductal strictures and intraparenchymal location of stones. In addition, acute sialadenitis should be treated with antibiotics prior to intervention.

Endoscope stone retrieval technique

Surface anaesthesia is used, followed by infusion of the duct with lidocaine. After dilation of the ostium, the endoscope is introduced into the ductal system and progressed until the sialolith is identified. Irrigation both removes mobile debris and keeps the duct walls from collapsing. The stone is then removed using suction, basket or microforceps. If the stone is large, then fragmentation by microforceps or lithotripsy is required to facilitate its removal (see below). Postoperative antibiotics have been advocated.

In this technique, an overall success rate of more than 80% has been reported, although giving a 97% cure rate for stones smaller than 3 mm and 35% for those larger than 3 mm.

Intraductal fragmentation

Intracorporeal lithotripsy

If the stone is too large for extraction whole, it may be fragmented from within the duct. A lithotripsy probe is passed along the salivary duct, under endoscopic guidance, to lie adjacent to or in contact with the stone surface.

Electrohydraulic intracorporeal lithotripsy (Calci-tript; Storz Medical) successfully fragmented calculi in 60–70% cases, using a shock wave generated by a sparkover at the tip of a 600-μm probe applied 1 mm from the stone surface. Pneumoballistic lithotripsy includes LithoClast (Electro Medical Systems, Nyon, Switzerland) and StoneBreaker (Cook Medical) (*Figure 45.10*). This equipment uses a compressed air source to produce ballistic energy; the resultant shock waves are applied directly to the stone. Subsequent fragments are removed with a basket. Using a 2.1-mm endoscope, stone-free rates of up to 60–97.7% are reported.

Laser lithotripsy

The Rhodamine-6G-Dye-laser (595 nm; Lithoghost, Telemit-Company, Munchen, Germany) has proved

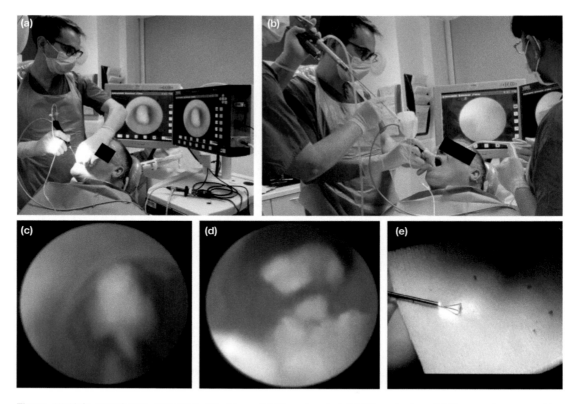

Figure 45.10 (a and b) Pneumoballistic lithotripsy. (c) Stone located. (d) Stone broken. (e) Fragments removed by basket. (Simon C. Harvey is the operating radiologist.)

among the most successful, with the added advantage of a novel spectroscopic feedback technique which analyses the reflected laser light to distinguish between calculi and soft tissue, so minimising damage to the duct. Complete removal of stones in 46% of cases after one to three treatment sessions are reported.

Extracorporeal shockwave lithotripsy

Following the successful introduction of lithotripsy for renal calculi in the 1980s, extracorporeal shockwave lithotripsy has been applied to the salivary glands, with the development of specialised machines (*Figure 45.11*). Current devices that generate the shock wave are either piezoelectric (Piezolith 2501; Richard Wolf, Knittlingen, Germany) or electromagnetic (Minilith; Storz Medical, Tagerwilen, Switzerland).

Patient selection

Developed selection criteria have led to this principally being used in management of fixed parotid stones. Pre-existing sialadenitis must be treated first.

Common, reversible complications include mild swelling of the gland (60–70%), self-limiting ductal haemorrhage (40–55%) and petechial skin

Extracorporeal shockwave lithotripsy technique

This is performed on an outpatient basis. After ultrasonographic localisation of the stone, shock waves are delivered to a maximum per visit (3000 piezoelectric, 7500 electromagnetic), requiring around three sessions.

Following successful fragmentation, pieces of calculus migrate distally and exit the duct either spontaneously or as a result of adjuvant measures (massage, sialogogues) or techniques (dilatation of ostium, papillotomy, endoscopic or basket retrieval).

haemorrhage (40–55%), while acute sialoadenitis is rare (1.5–5.7%).

In five published series of over 100 cases, the overall cure rates vary from 29–63%, whereas 56.7–100% are rendered stone- or symptom-free, with a better cure rate (34.2–69.3%) for parotid than for submandibular gland (29.0–41.1%) stones.

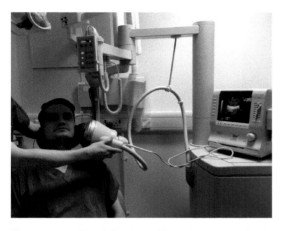

Figure 45.11 Specialised machines have been developed for application of extracorporeal shockwave lithotripsy to the salivary glands. (Simon C. Harvey is shown in photograph.)

MANAGEMENT OF STRICTURES

Salivary duct strictures probably develop secondary to previous duct wall inflammation, following the presence of a stone, local trauma or infection. Of the total, 75% are located in the main duct of the parotid gland, and strictures are more common in middle age

and in women. Strictures may be classified by imaging appearance, with single point, multiple point and diffuse patterns (*Figure 45.12*) described in addition to the location (proximal third, mid-third or distal third).

Koch classified strictures by visual endoscopic examination: type I, inflammatory 16%; type II, fibrous 18% (web like, <50% narrowing) and type III, fibrous high-grade 67% (>50% narrowing).

Diagnosis

Ultrasound imaging is the first choice, identifying gland parenchymal anomalies and dilated ducts. Sialogogue stimulation can highlight an enlarged, obstructed duct. Ultrasound may not be sufficient to image the stricture itself, although secondary signs are often helpful, such as proximal dilation, hypo-echoic, heterogenous gland texture.

Sialography is the gold standard for diagnosis of strictures, being the only imaging technique that shows the type, size and number of strictures accurately, and may be of therapeutic benefit. Fluoroscopic sialography is preferred, but if this is not viable, an MRI sialogram is acceptable.

Endoscopy is not considered a firstline diagnostic imaging technique, but is an option if sialography is not possible. However, if the scope cannot pass through a stricture, then the proximal disease cannot be examined.

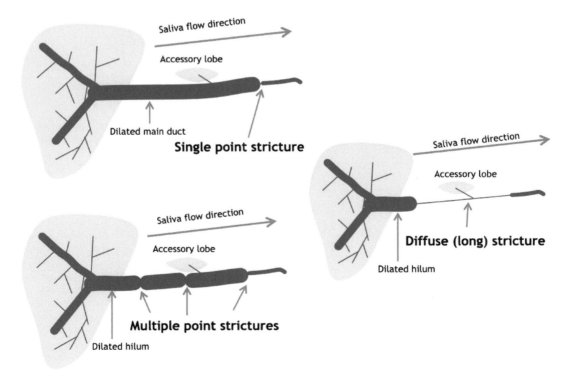

Figure 45.12 Classification of strictures as single point, multiple point or diffuse. (Illustration courtesy of Simon C. Harvey, used with permission.)

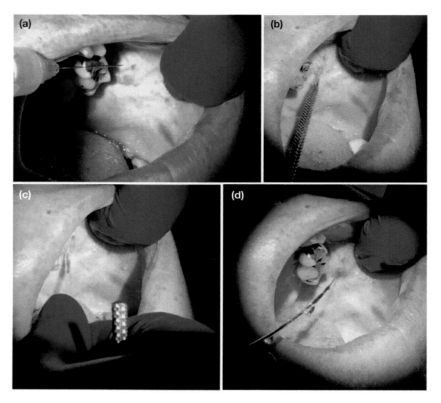

Figure 45.13 Radiologically guided balloon dilation prior to stone extraction. **(a)** Local anaesthetic delivered to papilla region. **(b)** Nettleship dilator to enlarge ostium. **(c)** Duct catheterised and contrast introduced. **(d)** Guide wire and balloon introduced.

Radiologically guided balloon dilation

This minimally invasive technique can dilate both primary strictures and those distal to a stone prior to stone extraction. Angioplasty balloons of between 2.5 and 4 mm diameter are suitable for dilation of parotid and submandibular ducts, respectively. The aim of the procedure is to dilate the duct to slightly greater than its normal calibre and to break the circumferential bands of fibrous tissue forming within the duct wall (*Figure 45.13*).

Endoscope dilation of stricture

The insertion of a blunt-ended sialendoscope allows the operator to visualise and advance to a stricture in the main extraglandular duct. At this point, a gentle tapping technique can be applied with the end of the endoscope to try and pass through the stricture. An alternative is to insert a stiff guidewire through the endoscope to try and break the stenotic tissue and release the stricture.

Radiologically guided balloon dilation technique

The patient is prepared as for stone extraction by administering a local anaesthetic and manual dilatation of the duct orifice with Nettleship dilator. A preoperative sialogram shows the character and position of the stricture(s). Immediately the balloon catheter is inserted into the duct. Lateral sialographic imaging is used to guide the balloon catheter into position along a guidewire, which is moved gently down the duct until passing through the most proximal area of strictured duct. The balloon is positioned centrally within the stricture and inflated fully. Tight stenosis may require several inflations. The balloon is then deflated and withdrawn forward to the next, more distal stricture if present. The procedure is repeated until all the stenoses are satisfactorily dilated. A postoperative sialogram (*Figure 45.14*) is used to check satisfactory duct calibre before the duct is finally irrigated.

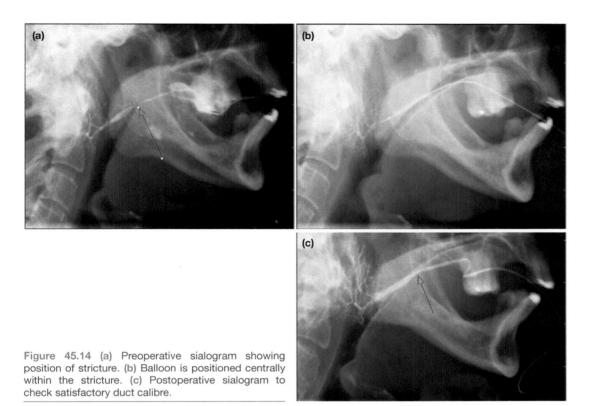

Figure 45.14 (a) Preoperative sialogram showing position of stricture. (b) Balloon is positioned centrally within the stricture. (c) Postoperative sialogram to check satisfactory duct calibre.

Stents

Stents have been trialled postoperatively for strictures in the distal duct. A stent consists of a 20–40-mm length, 3-mm diameter flexible polyethylene tube which has several extraductal 'anchors' designed to be sutured to the oral mucosa with non-resorbable sutures. The stent is left *in situ* for 2–3 weeks, aiming for epithelialisation around it. Complications include suture loss, with the free stent either coming into the oral cavity or passing into the ductal system requiring surgical removal. Stents are, however, not in widespread use due to limited data on value.

BOTULINUM TOXIN

Direct injection of botulinum toxin A into a salivary gland under ultrasound guidance (*Figure 45.15*) prevents saliva production for between 3 and 6 months. This is helpful in both sialorrhea and in symptomatic obstruction where minimally invasive techniques have failed to relieve obstruction, and where sialadenectomy is not desired. It is currently used off-licence for the latter purpose; consultant/specialist opinion is advised. Complications such as haematoma, postoperative pain and facial nerve weakness are rare, temporary and manageable in clinical practice.

Ultrasound-guided botulinum toxin injection technique

Anaesthesia is not usually required. 10–30 IU is injected into the parenchyma of each affected gland under ultrasound guidance, using not more than 100 IU total if multiple glands are to be treated. The procedure may need to be repeated, typically not more frequently than 16 weeks. The patients are encouraged not to stimulate the glands immediately post-injection.

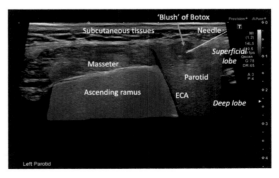

Figure 45.15 Direct injection of botulinum toxin A into a salivary gland under ultrasound guidance.

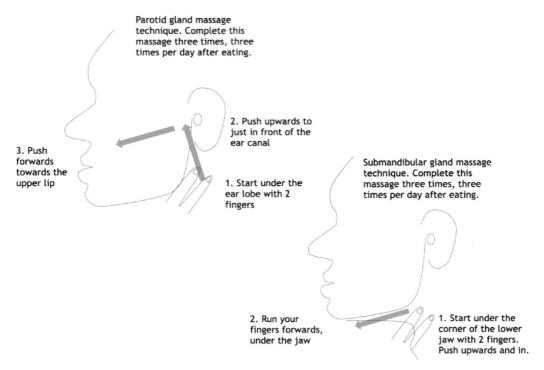

Figure 45.16 Following salivary intervention, the patient should perform self-massage to ensure that the operative site remains patent. (Illustration courtesy of Simon C. Harvey, used with permission.)

POSTOPERATIVE CARE AFTER MINIMALLY INVASIVE SALIVARY INTERVENTION

Following salivary intervention, the patient is advised to keep well hydrated, to stimulate the gland with sialogogues and self-massage to ensure that the operative site remains patent (*Figure 45.16*). Intervention is normally accompanied by some degree of local oedema, particularly following balloon ductoplasty. The patient should be counselled to expect local oedema causing temporary rebound mealtime swelling for several days. Postoperative antibiotic prophylaxis may be appropriate if infection is suspected. Local injection of steroid postoperatively and a short course of corticosteroids has anecdotally eased postoperative symptoms.

VALUE OF IMAGE-GUIDED TECHNIQUES

In our series of 252 salivary stones, successful clearance was achieved in 77% (194/252), partial clearance was achieved in 8.3% (some but not all stones removed) and in 14.7% (37/252) the procedure failed to remove the intended stone, primarily due to an immobile stone or inability to capture the stone from an unfavourable position within a secondary duct.

Balloon ductoplasty achieved elimination of duct strictures in 78.4% (152/194), whereas 11.8% (23/194) showed some residual stenosis on postoperative sialogram. The procedure was not successful in 5.2% (10/194), due to density of the stenosis preventing passage of the balloon.

TOP TIPS AND HAZARDS

- *Sialogram*:
  - If difficulty cannulating, dry the area thoroughly, and then massage the gland looking for a drop of saliva. If there is none, the ostium could be closed.
  - Duct ostia are usually symmetrical, look for the position on the ostium on the fleshy papilla on the normal side.
  - 'Tissuing'/extravasation of contrast can be seen during the first few frames of the sialogram – be ready to stop injection of the contrast quickly. It may feel sore and swollen for a few days but rarely causes serious issues.
- *Basket retrieval*:
  - Beware of multiple stones – they can impact unfavourably.
  - Beware of a narrow duct – always think how the stone can be delivered.
- *Balloon dilation*:
  - Postop pain can be significant so consider a long-lasting anaesthetic.
  - Occasionally the stretched duct swells so much the duct occludes – reassure the patient this will settle after a couple of days.
- *Botox*:
  - Ultrasound-guided botox offers a safe and comparable technique when compared with 'blind' injection.
  - Different brands have different potency assays so 'units' are not comparable.
  - It can take 2 weeks for the drug to take effect.

FURTHER READING

Brown JE, Drage NA, Escudier MP et al. Minimally invasive radiologically-guided intervention for the treatment of salivary calculi. *Cardiovasc Intervent Radiol* 2002;**25**:352–5.

Capaccio P, Ottaviani F, Manzo R et al. Extracorporeal lithotripsy for salivary calculi: a long-term clinical experience. *Laryngoscope* 2004;**114**:1069–73.

Marchal F, Dulguerov P. Sialolithiasis management: the state of the art. *Arch Otolaryngol Head Neck Surg* 2003;**129**:951–6.

McGurk M, Escudier MP, Brown JE. Modern management of salivary calculi. *Br J Surg* 2005;**92**:107–12.

Sigismund PE, Zenk J, Koch M et al. Nearly 3,000 salivary stones: some clinical and epidemiologic aspects. *Laryngoscope* 2015;**125**:1879–82.

<table>
<tr><td>

Chapter
46

</td><td>

Surgery of the Parotid Gland

Leandros-Vassilios Vassiliou, Panayiotis A. Kyzas

</td></tr>
</table>

INTRODUCTION

Over 80% of salivary gland neoplasms occur in the parotid gland, with approximately 80% representing benign neoplasms. The most common benign neoplasm of the parotid gland is the pleomorphic adenoma. Benign tumours can be treated either via extracapsular dissection (see *Chapter 47*) or superficial parotidectomy based on the operator's preference and patient factors.

The most common malignant tumour in the parotid gland is a metastasis from a head and neck skin cancer (squamous cell carcinomas [SCCs]), malignant melanomas or malignant adnexal tumours).

The most common primary parotid malignancies are mucoepidermoid carcinomas, followed by adenocarcinomas and adenoid cystic carcinomas.

PREOPERATIVE WORK-UP: INVESTIGATIONS

Parotid gland neoplasms, either benign or malignant, often present as firm, small, mobile and asymptomatic lumps. History and thorough examination of the head and neck and skin is important to rule out metastatic lymphadenopathy from a cutaneous carcinoma.

High-grade, biologically aggressive parotid gland malignant tumours present with rapid growth, pain, fixity to surrounding structures and/or skin tethering, ulceration and often concomitant cervical lymphadenopathy. Facial nerve weakness is a late-stage presentation or a sign of aggressive malignancy. Ultrasound-guided fine needle aspiration for cytological information comprises the first-line investigation. Magnetic resonance imaging (MRI) scan with contrast is nowadays routinely performed for parotid gland tumours. If there is a suspicion of malignancy, full staging computed tomography (CT) scans of the neck and thorax and a head and neck multidisciplinary team (MDT) discussion are required. Cytology through an ultrasound (US)-guided aspiration, although offering relatively high diagnostic value in distinguishing benign from malignant tumours, often is not sufficient to determine the exact diagnosis and an US-guided Tru-Cut biopsy is recommended.

SURGICAL ANATOMY

The parotid gland is separated by the plane of the facial nerve and its branches into a superficial and a deep lobe that occupies approximately 20% of the gland.

The key to performing a superficial parotidectomy is identification of the facial nerve trunk as it emerges from the sternomastoid foramen. Various anatomical landmarks have been suggested:

- The 'tragal pointer', a triangular edge of the cartilaginous external auditory meatus 'pointing' at the location of the nerve
- The posterior belly of the digastric muscle. Occasionally the nerve to posterior digastric (a branch of the facial nerve itself) can be identified and followed superiorly to the main trunk
- A palpable groove between the osseous external auditory meatus and the mastoid process leading to the stylomastoid foramen
- A branch of the posterior auricular artery most often is encountered just lateral to the facial nerve: following its ligation and division, the nerve is found almost immediately deep to it
- Retrograde dissection from a peripheral branch of the facial nerve: this is advised in previously operated or irradiated cases when the subsequent scarring or parenchymal fibrosis renders any dissection extremely difficult

The posterior belly of the digastric muscle is the most reliable starting point identifying the facial nerve trunk (*Figure 46.1*). All the other landmarks may not be consistent and are not directly associated to the course of the nerve.

SURGICAL PROCEDURES

Superficial parotidectomy

A superficial parotidectomy is the key operation involving the parotid gland. Most parotid neoplasms (benign, or low-grade malignant tumours) arise from the superficial lobe of the gland and therefore are excised with a superficial parotidectomy.

Very rarely, the tumours are located on the deep lobe of the parotid and therefore a different operation approach is required (discussed further in *Surgery for Deep Lobe Tumours*).

The operation is performed under general anaesthetic. Communication with the anaesthetist is important: a short-acting, or no muscle relaxant induction is preferred. If the patient is paralysed, the surgeon loses the ability to monitor face movements (twitching) when approaching the territory of the nerve.

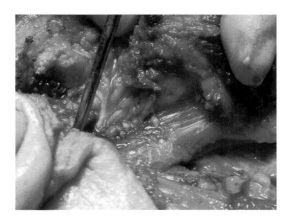

Figure 46.1 Identification of the facial nerve during superficial parotidectomy.

The patient is positioned supine with the head supported on a Rubens pillow and rotated towards the opposite direction. Overextension should be avoided. The table should be tilted slightly head-up.

A four-channel nerve monitor should be set up prior to prepping and draping of the patient.

Prior to preparing and draping the patient, the incision line is carefully drawn. The first pre-tragal crease is most popular; however, a more aesthetic incision may pass through the post-tragal region continuing around and behind the earlobe and in a lazy 'S' configuration. Caudally, this extends into an appropriate crease of the neck depending on the required level of exposure.

We advise infiltration of the subplatysmal and supra-SMAS planes using 1:200 000 diluted adrenaline. This induces vasoconstriction and temporary haemostasis and hydrodissection of the tissue planes.

A monopolar diathermy with a fine needle tip (Colorado needle) or a ceramic blade ensures bloodless dissection. The skin flap is raised in the plane of the pre-parotid fascia. This plane is easy to identify due to the white glistening appearance of the parotid fascia.

Caudally, the pre-parotid fascia and the associated denser SMAS blend with the insertion of the platysma muscle. The dissection continues in a subplatysmal plane and exposes the branches of the greater auricular nerve and the external jugular vein.

The anterior branch of the greater auricular nerve is usually divided and the dissection continues around the anterior edge of the sternocleidomastoid muscle (SCM) and by separating the parotid tail from the SCM until the spinal accessory nerves (SAN) and the posterior belly of the digastric are identified. The bulk of this containing the lower part of the parotid gland is mobilised forward, hence exposing more of the posterior belly of the digastric muscle. Currently, the tragus of the ear is exposed and the vascular plane immediately anterior to the ear tragus leading to the anterior wall of the cartilaginous ear canal is dissected.

As the dissection proceeds deeper, the join between the cartilaginous ear canal and the osseous part of the temporal bone is encountered. At this stage, the surgeon has performed a deep dissection cranially and caudally to the parotid gland bridging tissue that contains the facial nerve and its branches.

The next step is crucial and is the identification of the facial nerve trunk: the surgeon requests hypotensive anaesthesia, to minimise any bleeding. The posterior belly of the digastric is exposed. Immediately above its anterior superior border, blunt dissection of the parotid gland lobules is performed. The parotoid parenchyma is carefully dissected 'layer by layer' until the facial nerve is identified (*Figure 46.1*). The direction of the blunt fine instrument such as a fine artery clip or a non-ratchet clip is from posterior to anterior alongside the presumed course of the facial nerve. Then the thickness of every (bite) should be as such that with the separation of the dissector tips, the surgeon should be able to see through (this stage necessitates magnifying loupes). Any structure that appears solid white should be stimulated to check whether that triggers facial twitching or response from the monitor. When the dissectors approach the level of the nerve, an audible and visible trace will be detected by the facial monitor.

It is important to mention that the nerve originally emerges as a relatively narrow white structure. When the nerve is identified, the instrument is placed directly on the plane of the nerve (there is loose connective tissue separating the nerve from the parenchyma) and the tips are gently opened to allow mobilisation (and lifting of the parotid parenchyma) off the plane of the nerve. With this manoeuvre the nerve will be separated from the superficial lobe and in most cases the bifurcation of the facial nerve will be visualised. The nerve will start to appear as a flat structure, in comparison to its cylindrical state earlier in the process of dissection.

The dissection of the parotid parenchyma of the nerve continues. First, by dividing the tissues following the superior division of the nerve and moving caudally. Bipolar diathermy, ligature (Covidien) or harmonic scalpel (Ethicon) allow fast, safe and bloodless dissection. As the dissection proceeds anteriorly, gradually the superficial lobe of the gland is 'filleted' off the plane of the nerve.

The operation can be modified to remove part of the superficial parotid gland lobe (partial superficial parotidectomy) or its entirety (total superficial parotidectomy).

When this has been performed, the surgeon asks the anaesthetist to return the blood pressure to normal and perform a Valsalva manoeuvre to check the haemostasis. A vacuum drain is inserted and the closure is performed in layers.

Surgery for deep lobe tumours

Surgery for tumours arising in the deep lobe of the parotid gland can be divided into:

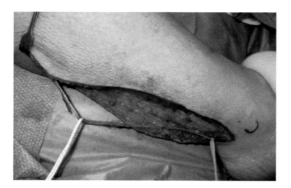

Figure 46.2 Sural nerve graft harvesting.

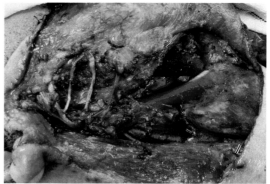

Figure 46.3 Primary facial nerve repair with sural nerve graft.

- Excision of tumours lateral to the mandibular ramus
- Tumours of the parapharyngeal space

Excision of deep lobe tumours lateral to the mandibular ramus (total conservative parotidectomy)

Tumours arising from the deep lobe of the parotid gland lateral to the mandibular ramus are essentially tumours of the deep superficial portion of the glandular parenchyma medial to the plane of the facial nerve. Only approximately 5–10% of parotid gland primary tumours arise on the deep portion of the gland, and of these quite a significant portion represent malignant tumours.

These tumours can be resected through the parotidectomy approach; however, as described previously, the nerve has to be carefully skeletonised to allow removal of all the parotid gland parenchyma, preserving only the facial nerve structure.

A malignant gland salivary tumour in this case is likely to involve the facial nerve. If the facial nerve is intact preoperatively, then resection of the tumour warrants sacrifice of all the facial nerve branches that are involved. A remedial repair with nerve cable grafts is required. Nerve cable grafts can be harvested from the great auricular or the sural nerve (*Figure 46.2*); antebranchial cutaneous, thoracodorsal or lateral vastus nerve can provide longer segments. The important aspect in this technique is to distinguish motor from sensory nerves and appropriately orientate the nerve graft (reverse the nerve graft if donor nerve is sensory). The nerve anastomosis is performed under the microscope with an epineural repair (*Figure 46.3*).

Tumours of the parapharyngeal space

The parapharyngeal space (PPS) is generally described as an inverted paramedial potential space with its base facing the skull base and its apex directed to the hyoid bone. The PPS is bound laterally by the mandibular ramus, medially by the buccopharyngeal fascia and the constrictor muscles of the pharynx. Division of the PPS is through the fascia running from the veli palatini muscles to the styloid process and its insertion into the pterygoid plate, into pre-styloid and post-styloid space. Tumours of the deep parotid gland extend into or arise from pre-styloid pharyngeal space. For the lip-split mandibulotomy, the anterior belly of the digastric muscle is divided. Further access techniques are described in *Chapter 25*.

Tumours in this area can be delivered through three different approaches depending on their size and exact site:

- Transcervical approach
- Transpharyngeal/transmandibular approach (lip-split mandibulotomy)
- Lateral skull base approach (lateral ramus mandibulotomy)

Transcervical approach for lower deep parotid lobe tumours medial to the ramus. A transcervical approach can be utilised that follows the initial steps and stages of the superficial parotidectomy. However, for access to the deep lobe after identification of the facial nerve and its lower division, the parotid superficial parenchyma including the lower branches of the facial nerve are retracted caudally. It is important to divide the posterior belly of the digastric and stylohyoid muscle. This releases the constriction and provides access to the parapharyngeal space by blunt dissection medial to the plane of the mandibular ramus and its attached medial pterygoid muscle. Benign tumours such as the most common pleomorphic adenoma have usually a plane of dissection around them and with careful blunt and finger dissection they can be delivered slowly and carefully through the neck.

Transpharyngeal/transmandibular approach surgical technique (lip-split mandibulotomy). A preoperative tracheostomy is advised.

The prep and drape of the patient is as described for the superficial parotidectomy; however, it is important to expose both sides of the neck and essentially drape the patient below the level of the clavicles. A curvilinear incision from the mastoid tip, through a neck crease to the chin is used. For a benign tumour, the first crease is suitable, otherwise, for a combined neck dissection, the second neck crease is preferred.

Various incisions have been described in the chin area: curved or zig-zagged to the midline. The depressor labii inferioris and/or mentalis muscles are to some degree disrupted if a circum-mental lip-split incision is preferred, therefore a z-type incision is a muscle-sparing technique and preferred. In principle, the incision is designed to be 'camouflaged' in the most appropriate existing creases/lines. For patients with a pronounced chin symphysis/cleft, a midline vertical incision is preferred.

The anterior belly of digastric and genioglossus muscles are attached in the midline and hence a mandibulectomy is performed in paramedial fashion to avoid torsion forces post fixation.

A subplatysma flap is elevated in a submandibular supracapsular plane of dissection to avoid injury of the marginal mandibular facial nerve branch. The lower soft tissues are divided into planes and the mandibular symphysis and parasymphysis on the site of the tumour are exposed subperiosteally. A mandibulectomy is usually performed between the canine and first premolar anterior to the mental foramen.

For dentate patients, two four-hole spaced plates are pre-adapted and the mandibulotomy is designed to cross through the midpoint of the plates.

For edentulous and atrophic mandibles, a reconstructive load-bearing plate with three holes and bicortical screws on each side is required. Carefully place the plates after contouring, appropriately orientated in separate ports, and ideally notch them to mark the orientation.

Various designs of mandibulotomy have been described; for those who prefer the stepped approach to improve mechanical interlinking of the mandible segments as well as increased bone-to-bone surface contact, a straight fashion osteotomy is acceptable. The mandibulotomy is performed with a reciprocating saw.

Lingually, an incision is made through the lingual sulcus and floor of mouth mucosa lateral to the sublingual gland. Deep, the mylohyoid muscle is divided using a harmonic scalpel, ligature or diathermy, until behind the posterior free edge of the mylohyoid muscle.

The lingual nerve will be identified crossing over from medially to the tongue. The nerve can be carefully retracted cephalad, and further dissection of the tissues medial to the plane of the medial pterygoid muscle is performed. The more that the tissues are mobilised the lateral aspect of the mandible post mandibulotomy is swung laterally, offering wider exposure of the PPS.

The tumour is then accessed and delivered. For benign tumours this is usually a vascular mainly parapharyngeal fat plane around the circumference of the tumour; however, the connection of the tumour with the rest of the submandibular gland will require sharp dissection from the parotid parenchyma laterally. It is important not to retract the tumour significantly medially as this may pull the facial nerve and result in inadvertent injury.

Following resection of the tumour, haemostasis is achieved, and oral closure is performed using interrupted sutures. Closure of the lower face wounds is performed in layers with careful approximation of the vermilion border.

Lateral skull base approach (lateral ramus mandibulotomy). Complex or malignant tumours of the PPS require lateral skull base surgery. Lateral ramus osteotomy with or without condylar disarticulation provides access to the PPS and infratemporal fossa (*Figure 46.4*).

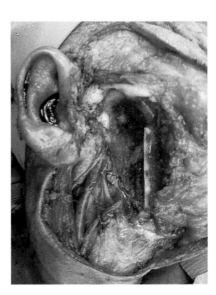

Figure 46.4 Ablative defect post-total radical parotidectomy.

TOP TIPS AND HAZARDS

- Surgery of the parotid gland is inherently linked with safeguarding the facial nerve.
- The best guide to identifying the facial nerve is careful dissection of the parenchyma superior to the posterior belly of the digastric approximately at the plane of the tympano-mastoid suture.
- In malignant parotid gland tumours, every effort must be undertaken to preserve a functional facial nerve; however, if there is a need to sacrifice the nerve, immediate nerve grafting is required.
- Parotid gland tumours may extend to complex anatomical spaces such as the parapharyngeal and infratemporal spaces, and advanced surgical approaches may be required for their resection.

FURTHER READING

Guntinas-Lichius O, Silver CE, Thielker J et al. Management of the facial nerve in parotid cancer: preservation or resection and reconstruction. *Eur Arch Otorhinolaryngol* 2018;**275**:2615–23.

McGurk M, Combes JG (eds). *Controversies in the Management of Salivary Gland Disease*, 2nd edn. Oxford: Oxford Academic; 2013.

Righini CA. Facial nerve identification during parotidectomy. *Eur Ann Otorhinolaryngol Head Neck Dis* 2012;**129**:214–19.

Sood S, McGurk M, Vaz F. Management of salivary gland tumours: United Kingdom National Multidisciplinary Guidelines. *J Laryngol Otol* 2016;**130**:S142–9.

Spiro RH, Huvos AG, Strong EW. Cancer of the parotid gland. A clinicopathologic study of 288 primary cases. *Am J Surg* 1975;**130**:452–9.

Bailey & Love's Essential Operations Bailey & Love's Essential Operations
Bailey & Love's Essential Operations Bailey & Love's Essential Operations
Bailey & Love's Essential Operations Bailey & Love's Essential Operations

PART 6 | Salivary gland and thyroid surgery

Chapter 47

Extracapsular Dissection

Rabindra P. Singh, Mark McGurk

PRINCIPLES OF JUSTIFICATION

Extracapsular dissection (ECD) is an example of the general move towards more minimally invasive procedures. The reputation for pleomorphic adenomas having a propensity to recur is largely undeserved. The reason for this is that in the 1930s, when the high incidence of recurrence was noticed, these lesions were thought to be hamartomas and not true neoplasms. They were called pathological adenomas. Consequently, it was an acceptable practice to enucleate these lesions after opening the capsule, in essence an intracapsular dissection. It was soon realised that a considerable number recurred. In response, several surgeons started to develop new techniques to deal with these parotid lumps. There was a second complementary reason for seeking new more reliable surgical techniques. This was the era of the true general surgeon who in one list may be doing an amputation, an abdominal procedure, a craniotomy, a thyroid and a small parotid lump. The operations taught in this era for the occasional surgeon were expansive (no small holes) with high morbidity but reliable. They needed a simple reliable operation for the general surgeon to safely remove a parotid lump. It proved to be a dissection of the facial nerve which cleaved the parotid into a superficial and a deep component. This operation gained added momentum with the seminal work of Patey and Thakray in 1958. The techniques of superficial parotidectomy (SP) and total conservative parotidectomy became the universal standards of care for what now has been shown is the wrong reason but with the correct result. The incidence of recurrence dropped with this change, thus reinforcing the intellectual and scientific bases of the incomplete tumour capsule which underpinned these techniques.

However, in the late 1940s, before the debate had been resolved in favour of superficial and total parotidectomies, general surgeon Alan Nicholson at the Christie Hospital, Manchester, UK, was continuing a local dissection technique which was incidentally used by Hamilton Bailey and others. By the late 1950s, when the debate was settled in favour of SP, Nicholson had 10 years of experience with the ECD technique without evidence of recurrence.

Consequently, he continued with this technique and was followed in turn by other surgeons both at Guy's Hospital, London, UK, and Erlangen, Germany, where over 1200 cases of benign parotid tumours have been treated by ECD. In reality, surgeons have been dissecting benign tumours in an extracapsular plane ever since the conservative parotidectomy technique was conceived because the tumour surface is in direct contact with one or more branches of the facial nerve in 60% of the cases. The evidence is now beginning to favour ECD as a viable and safe technique in the management of benign parotid tumours against the long-held views supporting more extensive traditional surgical techniques.

INDICATIONS

ECD is only appropriate for benign tumours of the parotid gland. It has no application in the submandibular gland because the morbidity of submandibular ECD and submandibular gland removal are the same. There is no facial nerve to complicate the issue. But the basic principle of a conservative extracapsular resection is applicable to pleomorphic adenomas at the junction of hard and soft palate.

Every effort should be taken to avoid inadvertent ECD of a salivary malignancy. This error of patient selection, which has probably delayed general acceptance of the technique of ECD, happens rarely and only occurs with very low-grade lesions masquerading as benign lumps. Clinically, it is difficult to discern these low-grade malignant tumours when they are small. Paradoxically, it is the small apparently benign parotid lumps that present a challenge, not the 2- or 3-cm diameter lesions. Also, small lumps are easily missed on fine needle aspiration so that normal benign tissue is sampled inadvertently. Therefore, small parotid tumours, those with symptoms or those with equivocal cytology should be approached with caution. There is a remarkably simple technique to accommodate the risk posed by these small 8–15-mm lesions. An ECD is undertaken but this time along a line drawn 5–10 mm peripheral to the margin of the tumour. A conventional parotidectomy is also an option. But the reality is that from an oncological perspective, most patients with malignant parotid lumps get adjuvant radiotherapy because of the proximity of the facial nerve.

The ideal lesion is a well-defined lump, 2–6 cm in diameter, in the superficial portion of the parotid gland, the circumference of which can be defined by palpation. With time and experience, most parotid lumps irrespective of their position are amenable to the ECD technique in its extended form.

STEPWISE OPERATIVE TECHNIQUE

Patient positioning and anaesthesia

The patient's neck is extended as it makes the parotid gland more prominent; this can be done by placing a small pack beneath the nape of neck. A nasal endotracheal tube is preferred because an oral tube, by opening the mouth, may make it difficult to draw the mandible forward which is necessary when the tumour is wedged between the ramus of the mandible and the mastoid process. The drapes are placed to leave the ipsilateral face exposed for facial twitching, which is the ultimate indicator of proximity to the facial nerve. Most surgeons use surgical loupes for this procedure.

If a paralysing agent is used, it should be short-acting as it is important that the patient is not paralysed during the surgery. Continuous nerve monitoring does no harm and is prudent to adopt.

Incision

The standard approach is a pre-auricular incision with cervical extension along a natural skin crease. But, with experience, the length of incision can be reduced and tailored to the individual lump.

It is useful to put superficial scratch marks on either side across this incision line to relocate the skin flap on closure.

Dissection

The skin is raised in a plane immediately superficial to the parotid fascia. This is a shining white plane, which is easy to identify and follow forward until the fibres of the platysma muscle are encountered.

The lobe of the ear should be freed from the mastoid process and both the skin flap, and the ear are retracted with sutures or retraction hooks. At this point, the great auricular nerve should be identified as it runs over the sternomastoid muscle. The nerve should be preserved if possible; however, it should not compromise oncological safety.

When the skin flap has been raised, the clinical features of the tumour are checked once again. If the lump is clearly mobile and there are no features of tethering to suggest malignancy, then ECD can proceed.

A new approach (extended ECD) that has transformed the approach to the parotid lump, especially those wedged between the mandible and mastoid or deep to the tail of the parotid, is to approach the procedure like an upper neck dissection. The posterior skin flap is developed to expose the sternomastoid muscle and a longitudinal incision is made along the anterior border of the muscle (1 cm from its edge). The fascia is lifted off the muscle and followed down its deep surface (*Figure 47.1*).

The parotid is quite a mobile structure when freed from the envelope of deep cervical facia encasing it. Once released from the sternomastoid, the crease below the parotid denotes the position of the posterior belly of digastric muscle – the friend to the head and neck surgeon. The gland should be freed from this muscle and the mastoid tip leading up to the pre-auricular dissection which has exposed the tragal pointer. Now the parotid can be lifted to expose lumps on its deep surface or rotated forward to bring lumps wedged between mastoid and mandible into view and to a more accessible position. The concept that the parotid gland is a mobile structure has never been appreciated because the nerve dissection technique requires a flat plain. But it revolutionises parotid surgery. Fingers can be placed either side of the parotid and the lump palpated to identify the best line of approach.

Once the lump is exposed, the periphery of the tumour closest to the parotid capsule is marked in ink and a cruciform incision drawn across the surface (*Figure 47.2*). It is particularly important that this incision extends for at least 1 cm beyond the tumour margin as it improves access to the tumour. Four artery clips are attached to the centre point (*Figure 47.3*) and used to provide upward tension while the parotid fascia is incised along the cruciform lines.

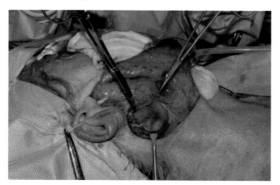

Figure 47.1 Fascia over the sternocleidomastoid muscle raised and followed deeper along its anterior border to allow manipulation of the parotid lump.

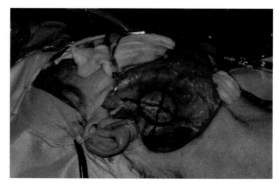

Figure 47.2 Parotid lump is defined and a cruciform incision extending at least 1 cm beyond the lump is marked out.

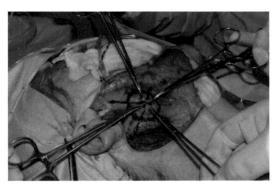

Figure 47.3 Four artery clips are placed onto the parotid fascia and retracted upward allowing a safe incision.

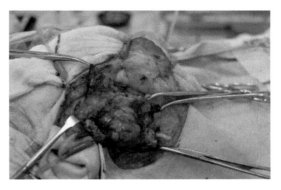

Figure 47.4 The artery clips are left attached to the parotid fascia and continually used as retractors as the dissection progresses around the parotid lump.

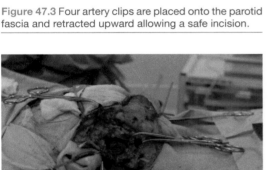

Figure 47.5 Careful dissection of the tumour avoiding retraction on the tumour itself, and facial nerve branch dissection as necessary.

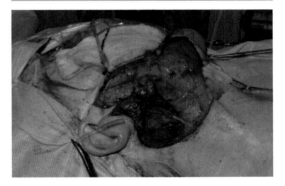

Figure 47.6 After the tumour is delivered, the parotid fascia is sutured back together with watertight closure. Blue discolouration due to surgical marking.

The key to ECD is finding a safe plane in which to dissect. This is done by drawing the normal parotid tissue away from the tumour revealing tissue planes 2–3 mm wide of the tumour capsule. The rule is that no instrument should be used to retract the tumour. If it no longer has a cushion of protective normal tissue, it can only be retracted by finger pressure, but retractors can be used to hold back the normal parotid tissue. The artery clips are left attached to the parotid fascia and continually used as retractors (*Figures 47.4* and *47.5*).

The process of dissection in the safe plane is identical to that used in SP when exposing the trunk of the facial nerve. The closed end of a blunt-tipped fine artery clip is pushed gently through thin sections of parotid tissue and opened with upward pressure to part the parotid tissue.

It is imperative that no tissue is cut without seeing the scissors through the fascia. In this way, a facial nerve branch is readily identifiable. If a branch of the facial nerve enters the surgical field, it is traced forward to reveal its position and if in close contact with the capsule is dissected from the tumour. Accuracy can be improved by using a facial nerve stimulator before cutting the tissue bridge between the scissor tips.

If the tumour arises in the deep lobe of the parotid gland, it can sometimes be dropped out by lifting the tail of the parotid without even seeing the facial nerve. But if the branches of the facial nerve are seen to be coursing over the lump, then all that is required is that the branches are freed off the tumour capsule and laid to the side while the ECD continues as normal. This situation is no different from that encountered in SP.

Another crucial point is to work slowly around the periphery of the tumour. If at any point the dissection becomes difficult, the surgeon should move to another area of the tumour.

It is not necessary to search for the facial nerve; an unseen nerve is a safe nerve. It is the dissection of the nerve and inadvertent trauma that produces facial nerve damage.

Once the tumour is delivered, the parotid fascia is re-approximated along the lines of the cruciform incision and closed with watertight resorbable sutures (*Figure 47.6*). This restores the contour of the cheek, eliminates any dead space within the parotid gland and the closed fascia and minimises the risk of Frey's syndrome. The skin flap is closed in two layers over a suction drain.

POSTOPERATIVE CARE

A light mastoid pressure dressing for 72 hours reduces the risk of sialocele to nearly zero. There are two options regarding surgical tissue exudate. The traditional method is the use of a suction drain which is kept in overnight and removed before discharge on the first postoperative day. The other is to wash the wound with haemostatic fluid and not use a drain at all. This has proved highly effective although a little expensive. It may facilitate discharge on the same day.

COMPLICATIONS
Tumour rupture

The risk of tumour rupture is the same as SP (1–3%). If such an event occurs, a clean sucker should be used to suction up any spilt tumour. The sucker should then be discarded. The tear in the tumour capsule should be closed with tissue glue in the first instance. Liga clips or sutures tend to aggravate the situation by making the tear even bigger.

It is unclear whether the operative field should be thoroughly washed with sterile water or not. If contamination is minimal, then the risk of recurrence is about 8% at 15 years. If gross contamination of the wound is encountered, then the risk of recurrence is increased, and the option of adjuvant radiotherapy should be discussed at the multidisciplinary meeting and indeed with the patient.

Haematomas

Meticulous haemostasis should be achieved throughout the procedure; small bleeding points should be identified with Valsalva manoeuvre and blood pressure returned to preoperative level.

Facial nerve injury

With ECD, the incidence of transient facial nerve injury is reduced from 30% to less than 10% and permanent damage is the same as SP (1–2%). The fundamental difference in technique is that in traditional surgery the threat of nerve injury drives the surgeon to find and proceed to a facial nerve dissection. In contrast, ECD is not a nerve dissection but a tumour dissection procedure. The management of facial nerve injury applies to all parotid surgery; the transected nerve should be repaired directly.

Sialocele

If it occurs, the incision line must not be reopened. It should be managed by regular needle aspiration, pressure dressings and salivary suppressants. Initially, it may require aspiration every 2 or 3 days but gradually the frequency will reduce and the sialocele will resolve spontaneously over 10 days. Persistent sialocele or salivary fistula may be treated with botulinum toxin injection.

Parotid duct injury

The transected parotid duct is treated the same for any type of parotid surgery. The duct should not be tied in the process of removing a benign parotid tumour unless it is absolutely essential. Tying the parotid duct increases the risk of sialocele formation.

Frey's syndrome

The incidence of Frey's syndrome is less than 1% following ECD because the re-approximated parotid fascia is a barrier to neural infiltration compared with the incidence of 38% with SP.

Neuroma

Traumatic neuromas are more common with SP than ECD. This is due to the limited exposure of the parotid gland with ECD; the greater auricular nerve can be avoided in the dissection in over 60% of cases.

Recurrence

The incidence of recurrent tumour following ECD is identical to that for SP, about 1–2% at 10 years. The median time to recurrence is 7 years.

TOP TIPS AND HAZARDS

- Beware of the small tumour; it may be low-grade malignancy.
- Retract the parotid away from the tumour not the opposite.
- Never use any retractors on the tumour.
- If you cannot see through the tissue do not cut it; if you always do this, especially if you use a nerve stimulator to identify a hidden branch, then the prospect of injuring a nerve branch is extremely low.
- Do not work in a hole, extend the cruciate incision if needed. If it is getting difficult at one site in the dissection, then stop and move around the tumour and come back later – it will be easier then.
- The Warthin's tumour is an ideal case for surgeons learning this procedure because it is not a true neoplasm, so fear of recurrence is absent and most Warthin's tumours lie in the tail of the parotid, well away from the facial nerve. Remember to release the parotid and rotate it forward.
- If during an ECD, the surgeon becomes uneasy with the surgical environment then the operation can be drawn to a close by re-approximating the cruciform incision with three or four simple sutures. The surgeon can revert to the SP. Nothing is lost in this approach.

ACKNOWLEDGEMENTS

We would like to thank Dr Paul Fernandes (University Hospital Southampton, UK) for kindly taking the photographs used in this chapter.

FURTHER READING

McGurk M, Thomas B, Renehan A. Extracapsular dissection for clinically benign parotid lumps: reduced morbidity without oncological compromise. *Br J Cancer* 2003;**89**:1610–13.

George KS, McGurk M. Extracapsular dissection – A minimal resection for benign parotid tumours. *Br J Oral Maxillofac Surg* 2011;**49**:451–4.

McGurk M, Combes J (eds.). *Controversies in the Management of Salivary Gland Disease*. Oxford, UK: Oxford University Press; 2013.

Foresta E, Torroni A, Di Nardo F, et al. Pleomorphic adenoma and benign parotid tumors: extracapsular dissection vs superficial parotidectomy – Review of literature and meta-analysis. *Oral Surg Oral Med Oral Pathol Oral Radiol* 2014;**117**:663–76.

Chapter 48

Thyroid and Parathyroid Surgery

Peyman Alam, Nathalie Higgs

INTRODUCTION

"Should the surgeon be so foolhardy to undertake it... every stroke of the knife will be followed by a torrent of blood and lucky it would be for him if his victim lived long enough for him to finish his horrid butchery. No honest and sensible surgeon would ever engage in it."

Samuel Gross, 1866

Once considered butchery, thyroid surgery has evolved tremendously, from a high-mortality procedure to a refined routine operation, with selected cases safely carried out as day surgery procedures.

Surgical excision of thyroid gland is frequently undertaken for confirmed cancerous lesions or histological diagnosis, symptomatic relief of pressure symptoms or acute management of thyrotoxicosis refractory to medical management.

This chapter describes standard thyroid lobectomy using lateral capsular dissection, which can be modified to total thyroidectomy by repeating the procedure on the opposite lobe of thyroid and removing the gland in continuity or individually by dividing the isthmus. In addition, we will describe minimally invasive open approach parathyroidectomy; however, there are other surgical techniques such as endoscopic, video-assisted or robotic surgery for both procedures. Finally, a brief description of the removal of a thyroglossal duct cyst (TGDC) is given.

THYROID ANATOMICAL CONSIDERATIONS

The thyroid gland is a horseshoe or butterfly shaped structure located in the central neck, anterior to the trachea to which it is attached firmly by condensation of investing fascia known as the suspensory ligament of Berry. It sits on the 2nd/4th tracheal ring, identified by the surface anatomy of cricoid cartilage and the suprasternal notch. The gland is composed of left and right lobes connected by an isthmus in the majority of cases. A small pyramidal lobe is present in up to 70% of the population giving rise to a small conical projection from the upper central isthmus. Another extension on the posterior aspect of each lobe is referred to as the tubercle of Zuckerkandl, the significance of which is explained later in the chapter. Under normal physiological

conditions, the lobes are pyramidal in shape and weigh 10–20 grams. Each lobe receives blood supply from the superior thyroid artery (STA) branch of the external carotid artery and inferior thyroid artery (ITA), which arise from the thyrocervical trunk. In 3–10% of the population, there is an additional artery known as the thyroid ima artery. This is usually a branch of the brachiocephalic trunk (but its origin can vary) running from the inferior aspect of the thyroid gland in the midline, which can be more prevalent in cases where the ITA is absent. Venous drainage is via superior and middle thyroid veins, which subsequently drain into the internal jugular vein as well as inferior thyroid veins which enter brachiocephalic or subclavian veins.

PREOPERATIVE PREPARATION

This comprises assessment and examination of the patient and appropriate investigations such as thyroid function test, ultrasound scan of thyroid as well as fine needle aspiration cytology if indicated. For large thyroid goitre with suspected retrosternal extension or malignant cases, computed tomography (CT) is also performed. We recommend a preoperative vocal cord check with fibreoptic laryngoscopy for selected patients, especially those with evidence of voice change and all thyroid malignancies, and a postoperative check for all patients. All our cases are discussed at thyroid/parathyroid multidisciplinary meetings preoperatively.

THYROIDECTOMY SURGICAL APPROACH

Most thyroid lobectomies are planned in patients who fulfil day surgery criteria and have not had any previous thyroid surgery as a day surgery procedure. If total thyroidectomy is planned, one may consider starting the operation from the side with known pathology. This approach is beneficial in case of any complication during surgery such as nerve injury where the operator might decide to terminate the procedure and therefore removal of the pathological tissue is ensured.

Positioning and skin incision

The patient lies on the operation table in the supine position with a shoulder bolster and a horseshoe head ring to allow adequate neck extension while maintaining head support (care must be taken while extending the neck in patients with a previous history of cervical spine injury/surgery or disease).

There are many data regarding use of intermittent or continuous intraoperative nerve monitoring (IONM), and although there is no consensus, we recommend intraoperative monitoring of the recurrent laryngeal nerve (RLN).

In addition to monitoring of the nerve, in the event of weak or lost signal, the operator will have the opportunity to decide whether to proceed or postpone contralateral side surgery.

The operator may stand on the ipsilateral or contralateral side to perform the procedure; however, while performing surgery from the contralateral side, care must be taken to avoid excessive medial retraction of the thyroid which can result in traction injury of the RLN. Tilting the operator table towards the operator could reduce this risk and improve visibility of the operation field.

Surface anatomy includes a transverse line midway between the cricoid and sternal notch, equidistant from the midline, using a skin crease if possible (*Figure 48.1*). The size of the skin incision is usually 3–6 cm but this can vary depending on the size of the thyroid to be excised or nature of the operation, such as the need for lateral neck dissection with or without tracheostomy. Local anaesthetic with adrenaline is administered subcutaneously. The incision is made through the skin using a no 10 or 15 blade exposing subcutaneous tissue where further incision can be done using cutting diathermy or other energy sources such as a harmonic scalpel.

It is important to incise the whole length of the platysma under the incision line to maximise exposure (platysma can be very thin or absent in the midline). Once the incision is complete, a subplatysmal skin flap is elevated up to the level of thyroid cartilage superiorly and sternal notch inferiorly (*Figure 48.2*). At this stage, anterior jugular veins can be encountered, which can be ligated if needed.

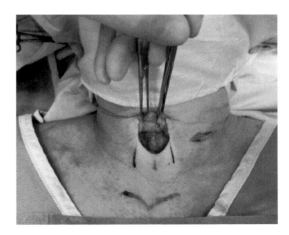

Figure 48.2 Raised superior subplatysmal flap.

Midline incision

Retracting skin flaps superiorly and inferiorly using retractors such as Joll or Langenbeck, an assistant can use toothed forceps to lift and retract the strap muscles laterally allowing midline incision through the cervical linea alba, the middle layer of the deep cervical fascia enclosing strap muscles thus exposing the thyroid gland (*Figure 48.3*). Different surgeons may prefer different instruments such as dissecting scissors, monopolar, bipolar or indeed other energy sources. In large thyroids, the strap muscles may need to be divided to improve access. In such situations, superior division of strap muscles is recommended if possible as the innervation of the muscles is more inferior. The muscle ends can be marked with silk sutures to help approximation at the end of the procedure. It is worth mentioning in some cases such as certain malignancies, a segment of the muscle/s might be left attached to the

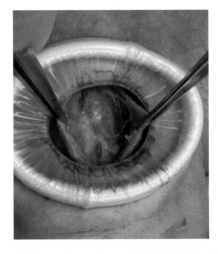

Figure 48.3 Lateral retraction of strap muscles fascia after midline incision, with Alexis retractor in place.

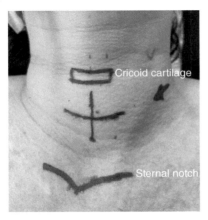

Figure 48.1 Surface anatomy.

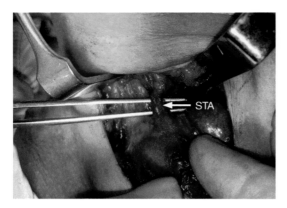

Figure 48.4 Superior thyroid artery (STA).

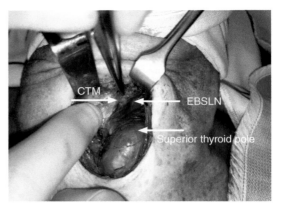

Figure 48.5 Avascular space between the cricothyroid muscle (CTM) and the medial aspect of the superior pole of the thyroid gland as a landmark for identification of the external branch of the superior laryngeal nerve (EBSLN).

thyroid capsule and excised. It is imperative that time is taken for haemostasis at every stage of the procedure, to allow unimpeded visualisation of the vital structures as well as to reduce the risk of delayed bleeding during the postoperative period.

Capsular dissection of thyroid lobe

The two strap muscles (sternohyoid-superficial and medial/sternothyroid-deep and medial) on the thyroid surface are identified and a pocket is created between the thyroid capsule and sternothyroid allowing Langenbeck retractors to retract the strap muscle laterally. Blunt dissection of fascia close to the thyroid capsule continues until the carotid sheath is visualised deep and laterally. The capsular dissection is done in a broad front in a caudocephalic direction. Using fingers to create a gentle counter tension by rotating the thyroid lobe towards the midline can ease identification and dissection of fascia over the thyroid capsule.. This step can be done with blunt dissection, bipolar diathermy, harmonic scalpel or gentle sweeping action pushing fascia away from the thyroid capsule using a pledget delicately to avoid bleeding from the injury to subcapsular blood vessels.

Identification of superior vascular pedicle

Identification of the superior thyroid artery and vein (STA/STV) is aided by retraction of the thyroid inferomedially and strap muscles laterally and superiorly. Once the superior pedicle is visualised, the artery vein can be ligated separately and then divided (*Figure 48.4*).

At this stage, care must be taken to avoid injury to the external branch of the superior laryngeal nerve (EBSLN), which supplies the cricothyroid muscle (CTM) aiding in lengthening of vocal folds.

The nerve can be visualised on the inferior pharyngeal constrictor muscle. Injury to the EBSLN can result in voice fatigue and have an adverse effect on

high-pitched voice, which can have a negative impact on quality of life especially for certain professionals.

Mossman et al. described the sternothyroid-laryngeal triangle as a landmark to identify the EBSLN boundaries, which are the retracted upper pole of thyroid laterally and inferiorly, sternothyroid muscle superiorly and thyroid cartilage and cricoid cartilage with overlying muscles medially.

Others described an avascular space between the CTM and medial aspect of the superior thyroid pole as a landmark for identification of EBSLN (*Figure 48.5*).

Mobilisation of the thyroid lobe

Once the superior pole of the thyroid is released, with medical and superior digital retraction of the thyroid, capsular dissection continues at the middle and inferior aspect of the thyroid. Middle thyroid veins are ligated or diathermied, allowing the gland to be mobilised. At all times, care must be taken to avoid traction injury to the RLN as the dissection continues, especially when the thyroid lobe is mobilised and exteriorised from the thyroid bed.

Identification of recurrent laryngeal nerve and preservation of parathyroid glands

The RLN is a branch of the vagus nerve that loops around the aortic arch on the left and the subclavian artery on the right, running parallel to a groove between the trachea and oesophagus, the tracheoesophageal groove (*Figure 48.6*). On the left, the RLN is close to the tracheoesophageal groove more inferiorly compared with the right side. Rare variations are non-recurrent laryngeal nerve (mostly on the right side) in less than 1% of population where the nerve enters the larynx directly without forming a loop, or reversal of RLN loops in

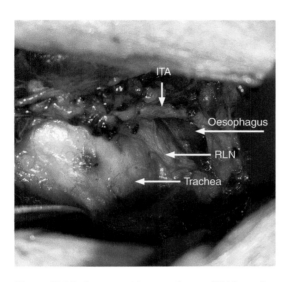

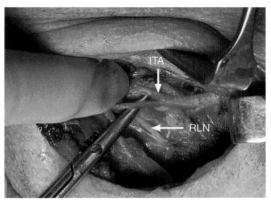

Figure 48.8 Recurrent laryngeal nerve (RLN) posterior to inferior thyroid artery (ITA) branches.

Figure 48.6 Left recurrent laryngeal nerve (RLN) running posterior to the inferior thyroid artery (ITA) in between the trachea and oesophagus.

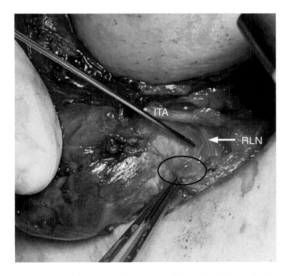

Figure 48.7 Medial retraction of the left lobe of the thyroid and recurrent laryngeal nerve (RLN) posterior to the inferior thyroid artery (ITA). The nerve stimulator is pointing at branching of RLN. The circle indicates a normal left lower pole parathyroid gland.

although there are reports suggesting penetration of the nerve through the ligament occasionally.

To identify the RLN, some recommend the RLN entry point to the larynx as a starting point (superior-to-inferior approach) in contrast to dissecting the nerve from the inferior pole of the thyroid moving superiorly. Veyseller et al. reported a lower rate of hypoparathyroidism using a superior-to inferior approach. However, we believe randomised controlled trials are needed to confirm superiority of one approach over another.

There are various reports about the relationship between the RLN and ITA and to avoid nerve injury, it is important for the operator to know that the nerve can run anterior, posterior or in between the branches of ITA (*Figure 48.8*).

Another common landmark for identification of RLN is the tubercle of Zuckerkandl, a posterior projection of the thyroid lobe which is mostly lateral to the nerve (*Figure 48.9*).

patients with right-sided aortic arch. Knowledge of such anatomical variations is important to minimise the risk of iatrogenic nerve injury. Many reports suggest that direct visualisation of the RLN during the procedure reduces the incidence of permanent nerve palsy. This approach not only allows identification and protection of the nerve but also makes the operator aware of the aforementioned anatomical variations (*Figure 48.7*).

Before entering the larynx inferior to cricoid cartilage, the RLN runs posterior to Berry's ligament

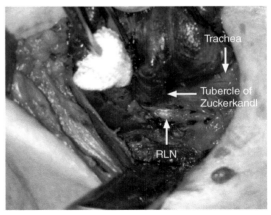

Figure 48.9 The tubercle of Zuckerkandl as a posterior projection of thyroid lobe (right), which is mostly lateral to the recurrent laryngeal nerve (RLN).

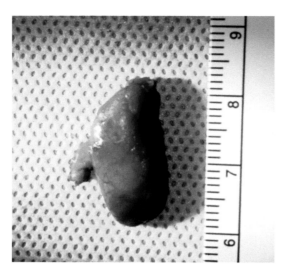

Figure 48.10 The excised parathyroid adenoma – note the smooth surface.

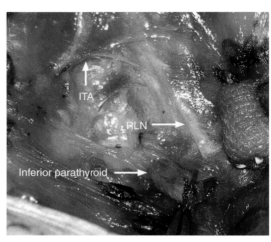

Figure 48.11 The right lower parathyroid gland anterior to the plane of the recurrent laryngeal nerve (RLN).

It is worth mentioning that medullary thyroid cancer (MTC) arises from parafollicular or calcitonin-producing C cells and as the tubercle of Zuckerkandl embryologically drives from the fourth branchial cleft, it has the highest concentration of C cells. Therefore, removal of the tubercle must be considered in total thyroidectomy for MTC.

Care must be taken to preserve parathyroid glands in thyroid surgery; therefore knowledge of anatomical location and variations of these glands is paramount.

These small endocrine glands are closely related to the posterior aspect of the thyroid gland and are responsible for maintaining calcium homeostasis. There are usually four in number: two on either side, one superior and one inferior. However, reports suggest occasional variations in number and location of the glands.

Unlike the thyroid gland or lymph node, parathyroid glands have a smooth surface with light-brown appearance (*Figure 48.10*).

The superior parathyroid glands are typically located lateral to the superior aspect of the thyroid gland, above the inferior thyroid artery and RLN junction and deep to the plane of the nerve. A superior parathyroid location is more predictable; however, as the glands share the same embryological origin as C cells of thyroid gland (fourth pharyngeal pouch), they can be occasionally located within the thyroid gland.

Inferior parathyroid glands, however, arise from the third pharyngeal pouch, similar to the thymus. They are usually located in close association with the inferior pole of the thyroid and inferior thyroid artery but more superficial to the plane of the RLN and more variable in location compared with superior parathyroid glands (*Figure 48.11*).

Both the superior and inferior parathyroid gland blood supplies are from the ITA; however, about 20% of superior glands and 10% of inferior glands receive their blood supply from the STA or other sources.

Removal of the thyroid gland

Once the RLN is identified and the integrity of the nerve confirmed by stimulation, blunt dissection continues and Berry's ligament and further fascial attachments between the thyroid and trachea are transacted using diathermy or harmonic scalpel. In thyroid lobectomy, the isthmus can be divided using ties or other energy sources. For total thyroidectomy, the procedure is repeated on the opposite side. Surgeons must always be aware of the thyroid ima artery. Once the thyroid gland is completely excised, it must be closely inspected for the possibility of capsular or subcapsular parathyroid gland/s. Surgeons must be aware of the possibility of extension of thyroid from isthmus, the pyramidal lobe also known as Lalouette's pyramid or even separate thyroid tissue in the thyrothymic tract, which is especially of significance in surgical management of thyroid malignancies.

Closure of the wound

A final check for haemostasis prior to closure is paramount. Temporary measures by the anaesthetic team such as the patient's head-down position, elevation of blood pressure above the patient's usual systolic pressure and the Valsalva manoeuvre could aid in identification of bleeding points which can then be stopped using bipolar diathermy. Absorbable haemostatic agents such as Surgicel or Floseal Haemostatic Matrix can be placed in the thyroid bed. We do not feel use of a drain is a substitute for careful haemostasis; however, suction drains are beneficial for large surgical defects. Closure is performed in layers, that is, repair of strap muscles in case of division if possible, midline vertical closure of straps fascia and horizontal platysma closure using absorbable suture. Skin can be closed meticulously using absorbable or non-absorbable sutures.

POSTOPERATIVE CARE

Monitoring for haematoma and airway obstruction is essential in patients who have had thyroid surgery. Bleeding or a large haematoma can become an acute airway risk and needs immediate decompression, therefore education of the team about such complications and immediate response is paramount. If such a complication arises, bedside opening of the surgical wound (superficial and deep sutures) can relieve the pressure and the patient should be considered for immediate return to the operating theatre for close inspection and haemostasis.

The patient should be carefully monitored for hypocalcaemia following total thyroidectomy or in hemithyroidectomy cases with previous history of contralateral thyroid surgery; if necessary appropriate calcium supplementation should be prescribed.

In addition to the common postoperative observations, in total thyroidectomy patients, thyroid replacement hormone should be commenced on the next postoperative day. It is important to know that some patients may develop hypothyroidism following hemithyroidectomy and therefore thyroid function should be checked should the patient become symptomatic.

COMPLICATIONS OF THYROID SURGERY

Thyroid surgery complications can be minimised provided careful patient assessment, appropriate investigations and meticulous surgery performed by skilled hands. *Table 48.1* summarises common and rare complications of this procedure.

Parathyroidectomy surgical approach

Most parathyroidectomies can be performed safely as a day case procedure unless the patient does not fit day surgery criteria such as those with complex underlying comorbidities. In more complex cases where multiple gland removal is planned and the patient's calcium level must be monitored, overnight stay is advisable.

Correct diagnosis of primary hyperparathyroidism, as accurate as possible localisation of the diseased gland/s and a multidisciplinary approach play an important role in successful parathyroid surgery and desirable outcome.

Before consideration for surgery, one must rule out other reversible causes for hyperparathyroidism such as secondary or tertiary hyperparathyroidism.

Localisation of diseased parathyroid/s

We routinely perform nuclear medicine (technetium Tc 99m sestamibi scintigraphy) followed by ultrasound scan. There are other imaging modalities for more challenging cases such as four-dimensional computed tomography (4DCT), single photon emission computed tomography/computed tomography (SPECT/CT), and even more invasive techniques like selective venous sampling. Some surgeons use a gamma probe for better localisation of the parathyroid gland/s and currently parathyroid autofluorescence techniques are gaining popularity.

Surgical steps

Preparation and patient positioning are similar to thyroidectomy as described. Low neck incision is approximately 2–3 cm with similar steps as with thyroidectomy for exposure of thyroid.

Based on location of parathyroid gland/s to be excised, limited capsular dissection of the thyroid gland allows anterior and medial rotation of the thyroid gland to visualise the surgical field (*Figure 48.12*). For some superior parathyroid gland explorations, very occasionally, STA needs to be divided for better mobilisation of the thyroid gland and improved access. Sometimes the enlarged parathyroid gland can be palpated and gentle dissection of fibrofatty tissue and meticulous haemostasis provides a clearer surgical field and easier identification of the diseased gland prior to excision. Once the parathyroid gland is identified, it can often be teased out using a peanut dissector.

One must remember the possibility of parathyroid glands in the thyroid capsular or subcapsular layer

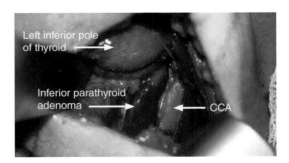

Figure 48.12 Left lower pole parathyroid adenoma posterior to the lower pole of the thyroid gland, medial to the common carotid artery (CCA).

TABLE 48.1 Complications of thyroid surgery

Complications	
Seroma, infection	Complications such as seroma, infection (1–2%) can be expected; however, meticulous surgical technique could minimise these risks
Postoperative bleeding and haematoma	This is a potentially life-threatening complication of thyroid surgery occurring in 0.1–4% (Abbas et al., 2001) and early recognition is paramount
RLN/EBSLN injury	Recurrent laryngeal nerve palsy (RLNP) is one of the most important complications of the procedure, with reported complication rates of permanent RLNP 0–3% and transient RLNP 5–8% (Hayward et al., 2013). Detailed knowledge of the RLN and its variations is essential to minimise such complications. Unilateral damage to the RLN results in hoarseness and loss of high-pitched voice, bilateral paralysis results in loss of voice, dyspnoea and upper airway obstruction. Injury to the EBSLN is relatively asymptomatic but inability to produce higher-pitched sounds can adversely affect certain professionals such as singers
Hypocalcaemia	Postoperative hypocalcaemia following total thyroidectomy is common and can be due to direct injury or inadvertent removal of the parathyroid glands. The reports suggest that incidence of temporary and permanent hypocalcaemia ranges from 3.15% to 64.25% and from 0% to 6.84%, respectively. Risk is higher in patients undergoing cancer surgery, likely because of the need for a more aggressive resection. Postoperative calcium and parathyroid hormone monitoring as well as a multidisciplinary approach can improve management of such complications
Rare complications	
Thyrotoxic storm	Intraoperative manipulation of the thyroid in patients with untreated Graves' disease or uncontrolled hyperthyroidism can result in thyroid storm during the operation or in the postoperative period, hence contraindication to perform such surgery in these patients. Tachycardia, hyperthermia, cardiac arrhythmias and increased sympathetic output are some of the manifestations and, if untreated, death can result. Therefore, careful preoperative assessment and multidisciplinary approach is crucial in such patients
Horner's syndrome	This rare complication can result from compression or stretching of cervical sympathetic chain due to haematoma or retractor tip, respectively. Reports also suggest ischaemia-induced damage caused by a lateral ligature on the inferior thyroid artery trunk may also result in such complication. Although 30% of patients may have full recovery, the majority have permanent damage or incomplete recovery
Conversion to tracheostomy	Tracheostomy is, on occasion, performed as a planned procedure as part of the thyroidectomy. This is most commonly needed in the case of large goitres with retrosternal extension, tracheal deviation or narrowing, pre-existing RLN damage, difficult intubation or advanced thyroid cancer. This can therefore be planned and the higher-risk patients made aware preoperatively
Death	Death as a result of thyroid surgery is exceedingly rare. Although postoperative haematoma and RLNP can be life-threatening, careful observation postoperatively reduces the risk of death. Increased risk of death is associated with large goitres and increasing age

(*Figure 48.13*), or indeed ectopic locations such as the retropharyngeal region or tracheoesophageal groove for superior glands and thymus and the anterior mediastinum region for inferior glands.

In more challenging cases such as multiple gland disease, intraoperative parathyroid hormone (PTH) assay can be considered. A decrease in PTH level by 50% from baseline level, approximately 10–15 minutes after excision of the gland can predict successful surgery.

In the event of inadvertent excision or devascularisation of a normal parathyroid gland, auto-transplantation of the gland can be considered. This procedure would involve cutting the gland in 1-mm slices and placing them in pockets created within sternocleidomastoid muscle. In case of multiple parathyroid gland disease where preservation of one or part of one gland is decided, auto-transplantation can be performed using brachioradialis muscle of the non-dominant hand. The reimplantation site can be marked using a non-absorbable suture or ligaclip for future identification of the gland if needed.

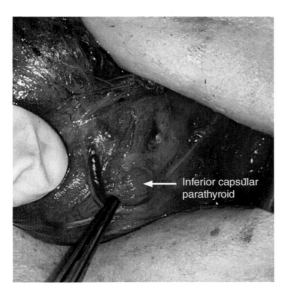

Figure 48.13 Parathyroid gland over capsule of the left lower pole of thyroid.

Protection and monitoring of RLN, haemostasis and closure are done in the same fashion as for thyroidectomy.

COMPLICATIONS OF PARATHYROID SURGERY

General complications are similar to thyroid surgery. Clean operation with meticulous homeostasis would reduce the risk of infection and bleeding to minimum. Identification of RLN in complex cases is beneficial in protection of the nerve as well as localisation of the parathyroid gland. In addition, some patients may suffer from persistent or recurrent hypercalcaemia due to failure to identify the diseased gland or involvement of diseased process in other remaining gland/s at later dates.

Thyroglossal duct cyst

Failure of involution of the thyroglossal duct after migration of thyroid tissue from the foramen caecum to its final position in the neck can result in the formation of thyroglossal duct cyst (TGDC), which is the most common congenital anomaly in the central neck. Although the majority are infrahyoid, they can present at the level of the hyoid bone or in the suprahyoid region. Diagnosis is usually made by clinical examination and ultrasonography. There are reports of carcinoma arising from the TGDC in 1% of cases. Operation to remove the TGDC, known as the Sistrunk procedure, involves transverse skin crease incision at the region of the cyst. Superior and inferior subplatysmal flaps are raised followed by separation of strap muscles to identify the cyst. The cyst is usually attached to the lower part of the body of the hyoid bone; therefore, excision should include the central portion of the body of the hyoid bone as well as the block of tissue up to the level of foramen caecum in continuity.

TOP TIPS AND HAZARDS

- Assess and document vocal cord mobility preoperatively for patients with voice change and thyroid malignancy and all postoperative cases.
- Capsular dissection of thyroid gland can reduce bleeding and risk of damage to recurrent laryngeal nerve and parathyroid glands.
- Excessive retraction of thyroid lobe during surgery can result in recurrent laryngeal nerve traction injury.

FURTHER READING

Abdelhamid A, Aspinall S. Intraoperative nerve monitoring in thyroid surgery: analysis of United Kingdom registry of endocrine and thyroid surgery database. *Br J Surg* 2021;**108**:182–7.

Qin Y, Sun W, Wang Z et al. A meta-analysis of risk factors for transient and permanent hypocalcemia after total thyroidectomy. *Front Oncol* 2021;**10**:614089.

Sheikh Z, Lingamanaicker V, Irune E et al. Introducing day case thyroid lobectomy at a tertiary head and neck centre. *Ann R Coll Surg Engl* 2021;**103**:499–503.

Steurer M, Passler C, Denk DM et al. Advantages of recurrent laryngeal nerve identification in thyroidectomy and parathyroidectomy and the importance of preoperative and postoperative laryngoscopic examination in more than 1000 nerves at risk. *Laryngoscope* 2002;**112**:124–33.

Yun JS, Lee YS, Jung JJ et al. The Zuckerkandl's tubercle: a useful anatomical landmark for detecting both the recurrent laryngeal nerve and the superior parathyroid during thyroid surgery. *Endocr J* 2008;**55**:925–30.

Bailey & Love's Essential Operations Bailey & Love's Essential Operations
PART 6 | Salivary gland and thyroid surgery
Bailey & Love's Essential Operations Bailey & Love's Essential Operations

Chapter

49

Orbital Decompression Surgery for Thyroid Eye Disease

Michael Perry, Vickie Lee

INTRODUCTION

Thyroid eye disease (TED) or Graves' orbitopathy (GO) is the most common inflammatory disorder of the orbit. It is usually disfiguring even in mild disease, and when severe can cause disabling double vision and sight-threatening corneal exposure/compressive optic neuropathy.

TED is a complex autoimmune condition, generally but not exclusively associated with Graves' disease (GD), with 40% of GD patients developing TED. Of TED patients, 85% have hyperthyroidism, 10% have hypothyroidism and 5% are euthyroid. TED affects up to 400 000 people in the UK, with an incidence of 16 per 100 000 females and 2.9 per 100 000 males.

Pathophysiology is not completely understood. Orbital fibroblasts play a key role in hyaluran deposition (causing enlargement and inflammation of the extraocular muscles) and adipogenesis. Orbital volume expansion then leads to proptosis.

TED is defined by disease severity and activity. The European Group on Graves' Orbitopathy classifies severity into mild, moderate, severe or sight-threatening. Older age, poor thyroid control, male gender and smoking are important risk factors for more severe disease.

Two phases of disease activity are commonly described: (1) an 'active' phase, which can last several months or years and (2) an 'inactive'/'burnt-out' phase, when inflammation and symptoms have resolved (*Figure 49.1*). However, patients are commonly left with residual disfigurement and dysfunction, especially in moderate, severe and sight-threatening disease.

Multidisciplinary management is essential. Patients must be made euthyroid to decrease eye disease volatility and stop smoking. Radio-iodine must be used with caution as this can precipitate or exacerbate eye disease. About one-third of patients require targeted TED management, usually with systemic immunosuppression (high-dose intravenous steroids, during acute stages). Second-line treatment with orbital radiotherapy and/or oral immunosuppressive agents can help to prevent relapse.

Medical treatment alone will not reverse proptosis, although a recent insulin-like growth factor 1 receptor (IGFR-1) antagonist teprotumumab (only available in the United States), shows some promise. Sight-threatening optic neuropathy occurs in about 5% of

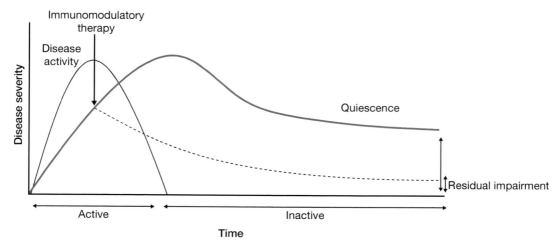

Figure 49.1 Natural progression in thyroid eye disease, and effects of therapy at different disease stages.

patients. This is believed to occur as a result of a compartment syndrome-type phenomenon, with pressure on the optic nerve or its vasculature from the orbital contents, notably the extraocular muscles. Thus, enlarged muscles on magnetic resonance imaging (MRI) and restricted motility are worrying features. Symptoms include reduced vision/colour vision, visual field defects, relative afferent pupillary defect (RAPD) and swelling of the optic disc. Without treatment, irreversible visual loss occurs in about one-third of cases.

SURGERY IN SIGHT-THREATENING TED

Vision-threatening optic neuropathy and severe corneal exposure require immediate intervention, usually commencing with high-dose intravenous methylprednisolone. If symptoms do not improve, surgery may be required. Patients with apical muscle crowding on MRI often benefit from deep apical medial wall decompression via an endoscopic approach, fenestrating the optic canal. This is usually undertaken by our ENT colleagues. This usually improves vision, but immunosuppressive treatment must be continued to control orbital inflammation and maintain improvement.

Rehabilitative surgery

Surgical management varies, depending on urgency, degree of proptosis and symptoms. In the inactive phase, a series of procedures may be undertaken in sequence to address residual proptosis, severe diplopia and deformities such as eyelid retraction. These should only be undertaken when the patient is in remission, is euthyroid and off all thyrotoxicosis treatment, or is post definitive treatment for hyperthyroidism. Systemic immunosuppression should be stopped for some time to ensure that TED is quiescent.

Orbital decompression surgery should be undertaken before extraocular muscle surgery and eyelid surgery. Decompression aims to reduce proptosis by fenestrating one or more orbital walls to allow backward displacement of the orbital contents. This can be followed by extraocular muscle surgery (strabismus surgery) for troublesome diplopia in the primary or reading positions. Double vision at extreme gaze is not amenable to primary strabismus surgery and can be accepted. Following muscle surgery or decompression, eyelid surgery (eyelid lowering, or blepharoplasty) may improve closure and appearance of the eyelids. It is prudent to leave at least 6 months between procedures to allow recovery and stabilisation of ocular balance.

Patients require careful counselling. Rehabilitative procedures often fail to restore pre-morbid appearances, and often several procedures are required. Relapse following decompression surgery is relatively rare, provided that risk factors have been optimised. Careful documentation of preoperative proptosis, ocular motility and any intraocular pathology is essential.

Patients with significant diplopia are likely to notice a significant change in their double vision that can be disabling. Anticoagulation treatments should ideally be stopped. In the UK, patients must inform the Driver and Vehicle Licensing Agency (DVLA) about any medical condition that could have an impact on their driving ability.

Specific complications to note include:

- Changed or development of double vision
- Haematoma
- Orbital apex syndrome (OAS)
- Superior orbital fissure syndrome (SOFS)
- Masticatory oscillopsia: this occurs in about 40% of patients, but usually settles in most
- Blindness is reported in 0.56% of cases
- Residual eyelid retraction

SURGICAL TECHNIQUE

In essence, surgery involves creating fenestrations in one or more orbital walls. Through these, orbital fat may herniate out, or (as is our preference) be removed. Various techniques in decompression have been published, varying in approach and which part of the orbit is opened. Commonly the lateral wall, medial wall and orbital floor are fenestrated. Rarely does decompression require fenestration of the orbital roof.

Lateral decompression

In this procedure, the lateral wall is fenestrated, leaving the rim intact. Variations in this technique remove the rim, either temporarily to provide access, or permanently.

Key steps

Lignocaine or bupivicaine with adrenaline is infiltrated around a suitable crow's foot, down to bone (*Figure 49.2*). An eye shield is placed.

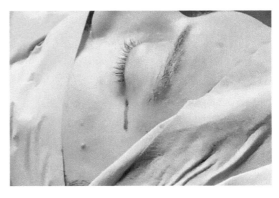

Figure 49.2 Skin marking.

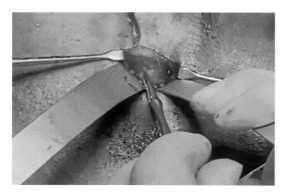

Figure 49.3 Exposure of the outer surface of the lateral rim.

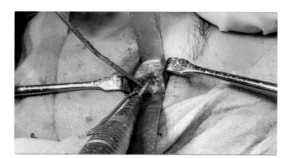

Figure 49.4 Rim reduction with bur.

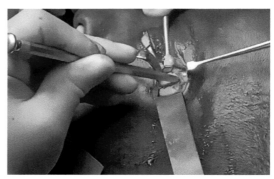

Figure 49.5 Rim reduction with osteotome.

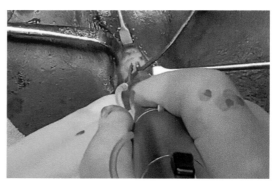

Figure 49.6 Lateral wall fenestrated with bur.

Using a scalpel/Colorado needle, the skin is incised about 2 cm, leaving the canthal region intact.

Using tenotomy scissors or fine elevator, the underlaying soft tissues are gently dissected and retracted off the periosteum of the lateral rim, from the frontozygomatic (FZ) suture above, to the zygomatic arch below. Careful dissection and retraction is necessary to avoid traction on the temporal branch of the facial nerve. The aim is to expose the entire outer surface of the lateral rim.

The periosteum is then incised along the rim and elevated off the outer bone, passing around the edge of the rim, and along the entire inner (orbital) side of the lateral wall, from orbital roof to floor (*Figure 49.3*). If the zygomaticotemporal or zygomaticofacial neurovascular bundles are encountered, these are cauterised and divided. The remaining outer periosteum is then elevated to fully expose the lateral rim.

The bony width of the outer lateral rim can vary from several mm to several cm. This bone effectively forms an overhanging ledge, obscuring access to the lateral orbital wall. On its deep surface is attached the temporalis muscle. Therefore, this bone needs to be reduced, either by removal of the entire rim, or by reducing its width, leaving 5 mm of the anterior rim *in situ* (*Figure 49.4*). The muscle can then be retracted.

Reduction of the bone can be achieved using a drill, saw or osteotomes (*Figure 49.5*). Bone is removed from the FZ suture, to the root of the zygomatic arch. As the bone is removed, the temporalis attachment will need to be gently divided.

The next step is to fenestrate the lateral wall using a small bur (*Figure 49.6*). Prior to this, a suitable retractor is placed within the orbit, lifting the inner periosteum/orbital contents away from the lateral wall. Either a malleable retractor or sheet of contoured silastic will suffice. If a retractor is manually held, it is important that the assistant does not retract or press on the orbital tissues too hard.

Once fenestrated, the hole is gradually enlarged, initially with a bur, but later using rongeurs (*Figure 49.7*). This is progressed in all directions to create a defect approximately the size of a postage stamp. Deeper bone removal in the trigone area of the greater wing of sphenoid is most effective, but requires care not to breach the dura (preoperative CTs are useful). Once the fenestration is complete, the edges are smoothed with a bur (*Figure 49.8a* and *b*).

The retractor is then removed so that the periosteum enclosing the orbital contents can be seen bulging through the fenestration. Using a sharp tip (No. 11) scalpel, this is then gently opened (*Figure 49.9*),

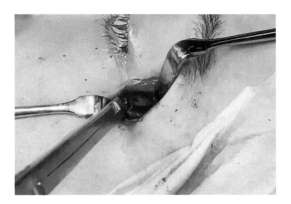

Figure 49.7 Enlargement of fenestration.

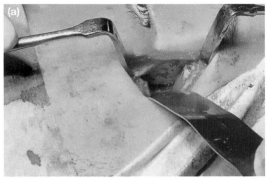

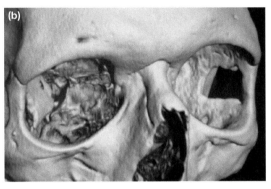

Figure 49.8 (a) Completed fenestration. (b) Lateral wall fenestration.

bearing in mind that the lateral rectus may be directly underneath (preoperative MRI scans are helpful in assessment). The opening incision can be either cruciate, unfolding each corner, or a simple rectangle approximating in size to the fenestration.

Following opening of the periosteum, the orbital fat above and below the rectus is then gently 'teased out' and removed (*Figure 49.10*). This can be augmented by having the assistant apply gentle pressure on the globe through the lids. In our experience, the quality of the fat may vary from a fibrous-fatty mass, to more satisfying locules of fat, resembling tiny lipomata (*Figure 49.11*). Fat and fibrous septae are carefully opened using fine tenotomy scissors and the herniating fat removed. Both extraconal and intraconal fat may be removed this way.

Following removal, the cutaneous wound is closed in layers. A small suction drain is recommended, although this must be carefully placed to avoid suction on the exposed orbital contents. A firm pressure dressing is then applied for 6–12 hours.

Medial wall

This may be done in isolation or as part of a two-wall procedure. Access to the medial wall is undertaken in a similar fashion to the retrocaruncular (medial transconjunctival) approach used in the repair of medial wall fractures (see *Chapter 18*). This is a much quicker exposure. Once the wall is exposed, it can be easily out-fractured into the nose, removing the fragments, with focus on the posterior-medial bulge. The periosteum is then opened and fat removed in the same way as for the lateral technique. No closure is required.

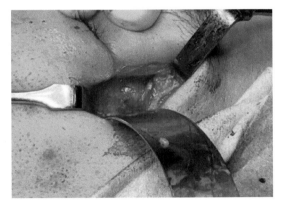

Figure 49.9 Periosteum opened. Lateral rectus can be seen.

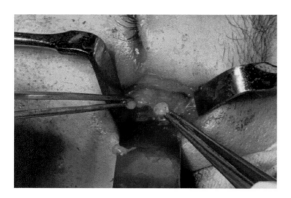

Figure 49.10 Removal of fat.

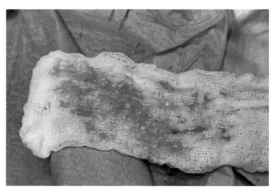

Figure 49.11 Fat is collected.

TOP TIPS AND HAZARDS

- Only electively decompress when the patient's thyroid status is stabilised.
- Blue silastic placed along the inside of the lateral orbital wall is a useful protector of contents and a good visual indicator of size of fenestration.
- Avoid over-retraction of orbital contents, which can stretch the nerves.
- The lateral approach is our preferred first choice. If the medial wall only is decompressed, the eyes can 'drift' medially.
- Acute decompression is best undertaken endoscopically to decompress the apex (usually undertaken by ENT).

FURTHER READING

Brożek-Mądry E, Jurek-Matusiak O, Krzeski A. Post-surgical complications in orbital decompression for thyroid eye disease. *B-ENT* 11 May 2022; 10.5152/B-ENT.2022.21708 [Epub Ahead of Print].

Fichter N, Guthoff RF, Schittkowski MP. Orbital decompression in thyroid eye disease. *ISRN Ophthalmol* 2012;**2012**:739236.

Gibson A, Kothapudi VN, Czyz CN. *Graves Disease Orbital Decompression*. Treasure Island (FL): StatPearls Publishing; 2023 Jan, https://www.ncbi.nlm.nih.gov/books/NBK470345/.

Lee V. A multidisciplinary (MDT) approach to Graves Orbitopathy (GO) Thyroid Eye disease (TED): the most common inflammatory disease of the orbit. Imperial College Healthcare NHS Trust; 2019.

Chapter 50

Temporomandibular Joint Arthroscopy: Diagnostic and Operative Technique

Joseph P. McCain, Briana J. Burris

INTRODUCTION

Arthroscopy of the human temporomandibular joint (TMJ) (*Figure 50.1*) was first introduced by Dr. Ohnishi in 1975 and this procedure has been further pioneered by surgeons including Drs Holmlund, Murakami, Sanders and McCain. The pioneers of TMJ arthroscopy have demonstrated the ability to successfully accomplish many surgical maneuvers that historically required open surgery. Operative maneuvers achievable during arthroscopy include diagnostic sweep, arthrocentesis, synovial biopsy, lysis of adhesions, debridement, smoothing area of frayed chondromalacia, contouring irregularities of exposed subchondral bone, lateral pterygoid myotomy, targeted deposition of medication and orthobiologics, disc mobilization, discoplasty and discopexy. Good outcomes following TMJ arthroscopy are dependent on meticulous attention to detail intra-operatively and initiation of a detailed rehabilitation regimen postoperatively. Contemporary diagnostic and operative arthroscopic techniques are presented in this chapter.

INDICATIONS

Clinical indications for TMJ arthroscopy include:

- Functional disturbances
  - Dysfunctional range of motion
    - Mandibular hypomobility
    - Mandibular hypermobility
  - Painful joint noise
- Desire to enhance or complete the diagnosis
  - High clinical suspicion of synovial membrane disease
  - Unexplained pain with negative diagnostic imaging
  - Unexplained pain with reported occlusal changes

Patients who present for consultation with symptoms related to the TMJ are first initiated on a period of non-surgical treatments, prior to surgical intervention. Non-surgical treatment should always include patient education and conservative treatment adjuncts,

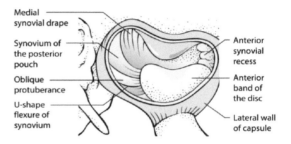

Figure 50.1 Anatomy of the temporomandibular joint (TMJ) as it relates to arthroscopy.

with the goal of reducing joint-load and inflammation. Our non-surgical treatment algorithm is based on Boering therapy and includes behavioral modification, non-clenching techniques, attempts to reduce frequency of existing parafunctional habits (i.e. dental splint, self-massage), soft diet and pharmacotherapy. Ideal pharmacotherapeutic agents reduce acute intra-articular inflammation and reduce masticatory muscle spasms. The period of non-surgical treatment is often overlooked, although holds the potential to further specify a diagnosis. We recommend utilizing this time during non-surgical treatment to concurrently obtain advanced diagnostics (i.e. advanced imaging, serology, additional consults).

After a minimum of 6–8 weeks of non-surgical management, patient symptoms are clinically re-evaluated and advanced diagnostics are reviewed. If the debilitating symptoms are refractory to non-surgical management, a discussion about minimally invasive arthroscopic treatment options is indicated.

Goals of an arthroscopic procedure include establishment of diagnosis, changing joint chemistry, smoothing surfaces, increasing joint space, mobilizing/stabilizing the articular disc and ligament contracture. Depending on a patient's medical history, symptoms, diagnostic exam findings and working-diagnosis, we select a level of arthroscopy that can accomplish the greatest number of intraoperative goals with the lowest risk of adverse outcomes.

Classification of arthroscopy from least advanced/invasive to most advanced:

- *Level I arthroscopy:* Single-puncture diagnostic arthroscopy with arthroscopic arthrocentesis
- *Level II arthroscopy:* Double-puncture operative arthroscopy with biopsy, debridement
- *Level III arthroscopy:* Multipuncture advanced operative arthroscopy with advanced debridement, discopexy or contracture for mandibular dislocation

A diagrammatic view of the relevant TMJ anatomy as it relates to arthroscopic puncture is shown in *Figures 50.2* and *50.3.*

PERIOPERATIVE CONSIDERATIONS

Diagnostic and operative arthroscopies are best performed under general anesthesia via nasal intubation. Nasal intubation allows oral cavity access for intraoperative jaw manipulation, without risk of damaging the endotracheal tube. The assistant will be asked repeatedly to translate the condyles forward into protrusion then backwards into closed mouth position.

Selection of perioperative pharmacotherapy regimens is an often-overlooked aspect of attaining optimal results with TMJ arthroscopy. Consider options for: perioperative prophylactic antibiotics and corticosteroids; intraoperative paralytics and anti-cholinergics; and a short-course of postoperative analgesics. Lastly, consider an extended course of postoperative anti-inflammatory and anti-spasmodic medications.

SURGICAL TECHNIQUES

Regardless of the level of arthroscopy planned, the procedure always begins and ends with an examination under anesthesia. The TMJs are palpated one side at a time, while the jaw is manipulated to assess rotation, translation and joint noises of each condyle.

There are two technical requirements during all TMJ arthroscopies: (1) establish appropriate arthroscopic port(s); and (2) maintain the optical cavity. Deviation from the step-by-step surgical sequence will alter the ability to accomplish those intraoperative requirements and will compromise the surgical outcome. Arthroscopy is performed within the superior joint space, with the exception of patients found to have a perforation, allowing for navigation of the scope into the inferior joint space. To allow for maximal superior joint space, the assistant will translate the patient into a protruded position during initial establishment of the arthroscopic port and when the operator is working in the posterior recess. A diagram of patient positioning in the operating room setting is shown in *Figure 50.4.*

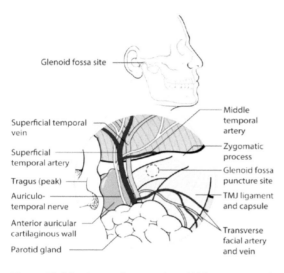

Figure 50.2 Anatomy relevant to Level I (single puncture) arthroscopy. *Abbreviation*: TMJ, temporomandibular joint.

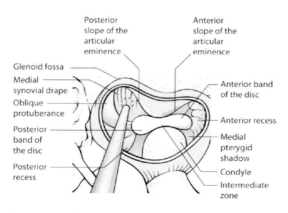

Figure 50.3 Glenoid fossa portal puncture in relation to intra-articular anatomy.

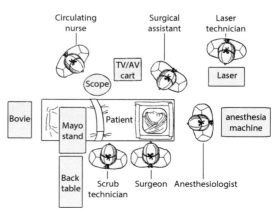

Figure 50.4 Patient positioning in the operating room.

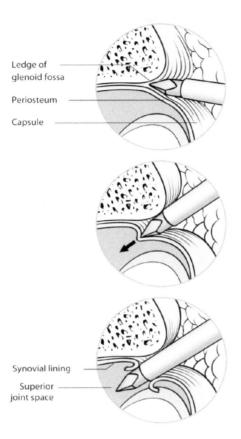

Figure 50.5 Establishing the arthroscopic portal at the superolateral aspect of the temporomandibular joint.

Level I arthroscopy

The initial surgical steps during TMJ arthroscopy result in establishment of an arthroscopic port, the fossa portal, where the arthroscope will be inserted and utilized throughout the procedure. The steps described below for establishing the fossa portal are followed, in the same way, as the initial steps for all TMJ arthroscopies, regardless of whether additional portals are eventually added (i.e. Level II and III arthroscopies). The single puncture technique, in the context of Level I arthroscopy, is described below and shown in *Figure 50.5*.

First, the thumb is used to palpate the maximum concavity of the glenoid fossa; this bony landmark is located at the inferior aspect of the zygomatic process of the temporal bone, posterior to the articular eminence and anterior to the post-glenoid process. The maximum concavity of the glenoid fossa corresponds to the soft tissue target during trocar puncture: the junction between the fossa's periosteum and the joint's superolateral synovial capsule. Using the McCain technique of joint insufflation, 3 cc of lactated ringers is injected using a 25–27 gauge needle. Insufflation is confirmed with 0.5 mm of

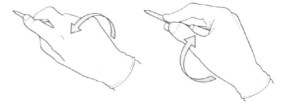

Figure 50.6 Rotational hand movement for puncturing superior joint space.

plunger rebound. Overinsufflation could lead to thinning or iatrogenic perforation of the medial synovial drape. Throughout the puncture into the superior joint space, the assistant holds the mandible in protrusion while the trocar and cannula are advanced deeper into tissues utilizing a twisting and rotational motion to prevent injury to the facial nerve and to provide better control of the sharp instrument (*Figure 50.6*). After spinning the trocar-cannula through skin, haptic feedback of reaching the bony zygomatic process should be encountered at a trocar-cannula depth of about 5 mm. The trocar is used to sound the most lateral and inferior aspect of the zygomatic process and feel the transition of the bony ledge to soft tissue of the capsule. This ledge to soft tissue junction is repeatedly scraped with the sharp trocar to develop a subperiosteal plane, at the maximum concavity of the glenoid fossa. The trocar and cannula are then redirected anteromedially to puncture the capsule and enter the superior joint space. A depth of 20–25 mm indicates a safe puncture. A depth beyond 25 mm assumes the risk of perforating through the medial synovial drape or worse, damaging the auditory ossicles. Remove the trocar while maintaining a cannula-depth of 20–25 mm. To avoid inadvertently advancing the cannula, utilize a finger rest for the hand stabilizing the cannula, while your opposite hand engages the trocar-cannula twist and lock mechanism. Connect irrigation tubing and flush out any blood clots through the open cannula. Insert the arthroscope into the cannula, with the irrigation port and light cord stacked. Small pushes of 1–2 cc lactated ringers allow for maintenance of the optical cavity. Once you confirm entry in the joint, the irrigating needle (outflow) is placed 5 mm anterior and 5 mm inferior to the arthroscopic cannula, to allow for continued maintenance of the optical cavity. It is important to insufflate with 2–3 cc of fluid prior to placing the irrigating needle to prevent collapse of the joint space (*Figures 50.6–50.8*). The 22-gauge irrigating needle should not require a depth greater than 20 mm. With the fossa portal and outflow tract established, complete your arthroscopic arthrocentesis by irrigating the joint space with a minimum of 120 cc warmed lactated ringers. After completing an arthroscopic arthrocentesis, perform a diagnostic arthroscopy. Maneuver to the seven points of interest, capturing images and noting the presence of both normal and pathological findings.

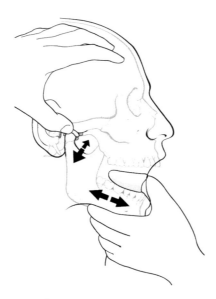

Figure 50.7 Operator and assistant collaborating to locate correct puncture location.

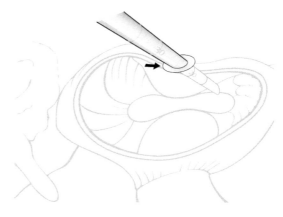

Figure 50.8 Diagrammatic representation of depth of puncture.

(a)

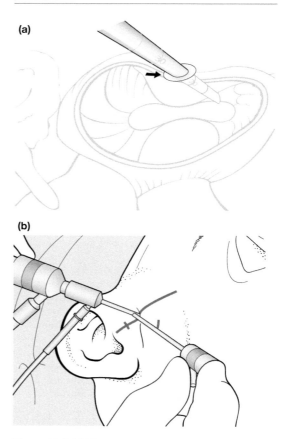

(b)

Figure 50.9 (a) Measuring depth of scope to triangulate second puncture point. (b) Measuring second puncture point.

Checklist for TMJ arthroscopy (Levels I, II and III)

- During puncture: orient trocar anterosuperior and never blindly advance cannula >25 mm.
- Ensure irrigation with a minimum of 120 cc of fluid, as <50 cc is shown to be inadequate.
- Observe oropharynx for evidence of extravasated fluid in lateral pharyngeal space, prior to extubation.
- Provide detailed post-arthroscopy rehabilitation plan that includes clear instructions on: diet consistency, medications, self-physiotherapy, wound care.

Level II arthroscopy

This procedure involves the double puncture technique. The fossa portal for the arthroscopic cannula is created as described in the Level I technique. Once the arthroscopic cannula and arthroscope are inserted, the articular eminence portal is then created by triangulation, using a second trocar-cannula to establish the working cannula. To perform this technique, the most anterior, superior and lateral aspects of the articular eminence are targeted, with the mandible in a closed-mouth position. The lavage needle is removed, irrigation is reduced to a 2 cc push while a 2.0 mm trocar and cannula is introduced into the superior joint space. The working cannula is then used to accommodate instrumentation such as holmium lasers, shavers, graspers, straight probes, hook probes and long needles for deposition of medication (*Figures 50.9–50.12*).

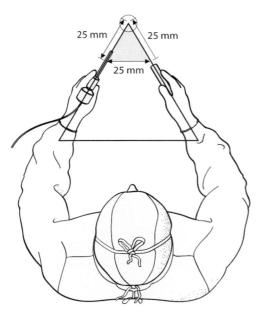

Figure 50.10 Triangulation concept.

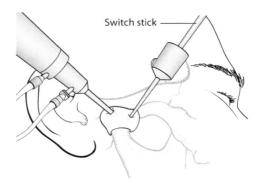

Figure 50.11 Triangulation on patient.

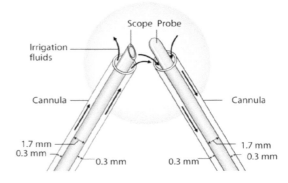

Figure 50.12 Instrumentation through both cannulas.

Level III arthroscopy

This procedure, which is the most complex, involves three to four punctures into the superior joint space. The fossa portal for the arthroscopic cannula and articular eminence portal for the working cannula are created as described in the Level I and II techniques. For semi-rigid arthroscopic discopexy (fixating the reduced disc with resorbable suture), four punctures are utilized: the arthroscopic cannula, working cannula and two fixation portals. The two fixation portals are established with 18-gauge needles in lieu of trocar-cannulas. Alternative techniques for semi-rigid discopexy and rigid discopexy are beyond the scope of this chapter.

During Level III arthroscopic discopexy, an anterior release and pterygoid myotomy is performed prior to establishing fixation portals. The anterior release is best performed through the working cannula with a holmium laser. The disc-synovial crease is delineated and scored with a hook probe, and the holmium laser on cut-mode is used to incise along the scored area, deepening the cut to simultaneously perform a ptery-goid myotomy (*Figure 50.13*), ensuring disruption of the attachment between the superior head of the lateral pterygoid and the anterior aspect of the articular disc. After adequate release is performed, the straight probe is utilized to reduce the disc posteriorly, while the mandible is in the forward position. The retrodiscal tissues, at this time, can be contracted with bipolar cautery or a holmium laser using weld-mode in an effort to tighten/shrink the retrodiscal tissue and prevent recurrent disc displacement.

Through the fixation portal, a vector is aimed at the posterolateral attachment. A straight meniscus mender is then punctured under the reduction cannula to the condylar head then superiorly through the posterior lateral portion of the disc. A second meniscus mender is then punctured through skin and is used to catch the suture. A 0-PDS suture is then passed anteriorly and a snare is used to catch it posteriorly (*Figure 50.14*). The location of the suture when it is pulled through skin is parallel and inferior to the apex of the tragal cartilage. A small skin incision is made after the suture is passed through, and a surgeon's knot is tied to the capsule and disc (*Figure 50.15*).

COMPLICATIONS

When performed using proper technique, by surgeons with arthroscopic training, TMJ arthroscopy is a safe and effective procedure. It is minimally invasive and can be performed in an outpatient setting with low incidence of complications. Complications, albeit rare, include: facial nerve injury, arthrofibrosis, infection, third-spacing of extravasated fluid into

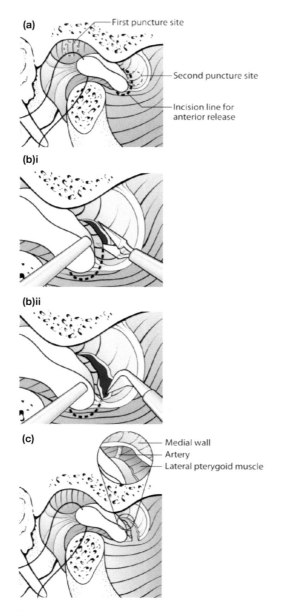

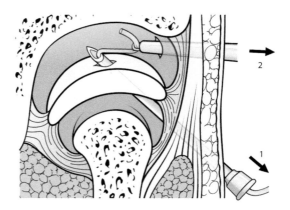

Figure 50.14 Suture discopexy. A snare is used to catch the PDS suture.

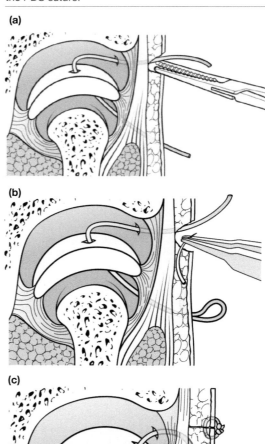

Figure 50.13 (a) Outlined location of anterior release. (b) Making anterior release. (c) Anterior release completed with associate anatomical structures.

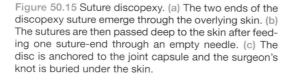

Figure 50.15 Suture discopexy. (a) The two ends of the discopexy suture emerge through the overlying skin. (b) The sutures are then passed deep to the skin after feeding one suture-end through an empty needle. (c) The disc is anchored to the joint capsule and the surgeon's knot is buried under the skin.

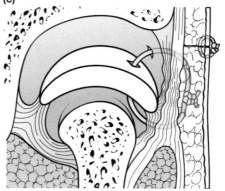

- Patient positioning is paramount. To avoid distortion of anatomy, make sure the patient's head is turned and flat on the table. Each step of arthroscopy is dependent on successful completion of the previous one. It is impossible to perform advanced procedures if this principle is not strictly adhered to.
- Always use landmarks. It is easy to become lost during a puncture. If you feel like no progress is being made, then back away, orient yourself with the known landmarks (zygomatic process of temporal bone, glenoid fossa and condylar head) and use these to make an accurate puncture. Use the vectoring measuring system for all multiple punctures.
- Make sure to gather all information. Once inside the joint, a thorough diagnostic arthroscopy is crucial to treating the condition. Make note of everything that comes into view (perforated disc, hyperemic retrodiscal tissues, amount of dislocation, etc.) and use this knowledge to come up with the best possible treatment.
- Do not rush. The temptation to rush through a part or all of this procedure will most likely lead to unfavorable results. Make sure to take extra time to explore the entire posterior pouch, the anterior recess, and if the second or third punctures are not entering the joint space in a timely fashion, be patient and do it right. It is not the job of the practitioner to make the patient worse.
- Be aware of all danger zones inside the joint space. It is important to keep the depth of fossa puncture to 25 mm or less and the vector of puncture anterior. Avoid aiming trocar-cannula too far superiorly, due to risk of glenoid fossa perforation, or too far posteriorly, due to risk of tympanic membrane or external auditory canal violation. Failure to do so may result in damage to middle ear ossicles. Never move the operative system deeper than 25 mm or redirect trocar-cannula, unless under direct arthroscopic control. Blind maneuvers risk perforation or violation of the aforementioned structures.
- Make sure to prevent extravasation. Avoid careless multiple punctures. Always maintain a patent irrigation system. Lack of a good outflow needle to drain the insufflated joint space will result in extravasation of irrigating fluid, which can be seen clinically as a swelling of the affected side of the face. Extravasation into extracapsular tissues can lead to trismus, pain, malocclusion, facial nerve paresis and increased recovery time. Extravasation into lateral pharyngeal space can lead to airway obstruction and is seen in cases when anterior release of the disc is performed. Fluid can then extravasate into the lateral pharyngeal space via the pterygomandibular space. Checking for tonsillar or uvula asymmetry and/or deviation to the contralateral side is paramount, prior to extubation. If evidence of lateral pharyngeal oedema is present, delaying extubation is recommended. Airway embarrassment is prevented by allowing time for the fluid to absorb, while the airway is protected.

lateral pharyngeal space resulting in a potential airway obstruction, perforation into the ear canal or tympanic membrane, and subdural or epidural hematoma from perforation into the middle cranial fossa.

POSTOPERATIVE REHABILITATION

The importance of establishing a complete postoperative rehabilitation plan cannot be overemphasized, as the rehabilitation phase begins prior to discharge from the facility. In the post-anesthesia recovery unit, an in-person review of the postoperative rehabilitation packets led by an OMFS team member is recommended. With the patient and their escort present, the arthroscopic images and postoperative instructions are reviewed, along with an enthusiastic demonstration of the selected physiotherapy regimen.

Postoperative rehabilitation plans should include a detailed plan, including timelines, for:

- Wound care
- Diet (staged)
- Pharmacotherapy (acute and chronic postoperative periods)
- Physiotherapy (staged)
- Physical activity (staged)

FURTHER READING

Bert J, Giannini D, Nace L. Antibiotic prophylaxis for arthroscopy of the knee: is it necessary? *Arthroscopy* 2007;**23**:4.

Kurzweil PR. Antibiotic prophylaxis for arthroscopic surgery. *Arthroscopy* 2006;**22**:452.

Ohnishi M. Arthroscopy of the temporomandibular joint. *Jap Stomatol Sot* 1975;**42**:207.

Smolka W, Iizuka T. Arthroscopic lysis and lavage in different stages of internal derangement of the temporomandibular joint: correlation of preoperative staging to arthroscopic findings and treatment outcome. *J Oral Maxillofac Surg* 2005;**63**:471–8.

Wilkes CH. Internal derangements of the temporomandibular joint: pathological variations. *Arch Otolaryngol Head Neck Surg* 1989;**115**:469.

Chapter 51

Open Surgery of the Temporomandibular Joint

Nadeem Saeed, Florencio Monje, George Dimitroulis

INTRODUCTION

The role for open surgery of the temporomandibular joint (TMJ) is diminishing. The realisation that many patients with temporomandibular disorders (TMD) improve with or without conservative therapy and the success of minimally invasive techniques for those with articular disease has led to a conceptual shift.

Early arthroscopy coupled with early TMJ replacement for end-stage disease appears to provide better patient-reported outcomes. These techniques and conditions are discussed elsewhere, and this chapter will focus on open surgery for those patients with failed conservative and closed treatment, diagnosed articular disease but not requiring formal TMJ reconstruction.

The surgical approaches to the TMJ have developed to minimise potential damage to a host of adjacent structures including the facial nerve, terminal branches of the external carotid artery (superficial temporal artery and internal maxillary artery), auriculotemporal nerve, middle cranial fossa and the middle ear.

INDICATIONS FOR OPEN TMJ SURGERY

Absolute indications

In many conditions, there is an undisputed role for surgery, but still variance in the ideal management plan. These uncommon joint disorders include:

- *Neoplasia and benign aggressive lesions (such as chondromatosis and osteochondroma)*: such lesions are rare and management is tailored to the specific tissue diagnosis and urgency for treatment
- *Ankylosis*: this can be an endpoint for a myriad of conditions and is discussed elsewhere
- *Growth and developmental disturbances (hypoplasia or condylar hyperactivity)*: such patients often benefit from a multidisciplinary approach with surgical interventions linked to growth potential and severity

Relative indications

The role of TMJ surgery in many common joint disorders remains less clear and includes:

- *Recurrent or chronic dislocation*: minimal invasive techniques are becoming more popular, but many

patients will still benefit from open surgery. The common treatment strategy of all these procedures is to promote capsular and joint scarring with resultant hypomobility

- *Arthritis*: the ideal management for patients not responding to minimally invasive techniques remains difficult. In end-stage disease, TMJ replacement is now regarded as the gold standard
- *TMJ disc derangements*: these are movement disturbances in which the articular disc plays a central role. Disc derangements and osteoarthritis are intimately related as much of their clinical course overlaps
- *Trauma*: open treatment of condylar fractures appears to offer many advantages and the treatment of soft tissue injuries is becoming a new area of interest

Open surgery is reserved only for patients with articular pain and dysfunction that is severe, disabling and refractory to non-surgical and arthroscopic management, and should be pathology based as demonstrated on arthroscopy and imaging.

PREOPERATIVE PREPARATION

Anaesthesia and positioning

Surgery is performed under general anaesthesia, ideally using a nasal endotracheal tube to permit manipulation of the mandible and hence condyle. The patient is positioned in the reverse Trendelenburg slant with the head raised above the rest of the body to reduce venous flow. The head is turned away on a 60° angle. Hypotensive anaesthesia and the use of tranexamic acid will also reduce bleeding.

Preparation of surgical site

Hair is shaved in front of the ear to the level of the superior tip of the pinna. Waterproof or barrier tape is placed horizontally and vertically above and behind the ear to cover the hair (*Figure 51.1*). A marking pen is used to outline the proposed incision line. The surgical site, adjacent ear and ear canal is liberally washed with antiseptic solution. A sterile ear pledget with Vaseline is inserted to protect the ear canal. A turban head drape is wrapped around the head which covers the anaesthetic

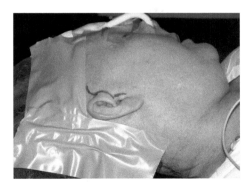

Figure 51.1 Tape used to keep hair away from surgical site.

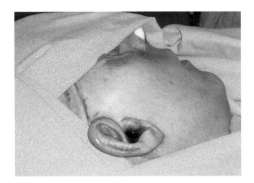

Figure 51.2 Draping of surgical site.

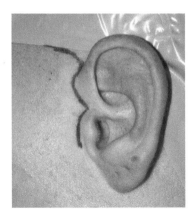

Figure 51.3 Preauricular incision with temporal extension.

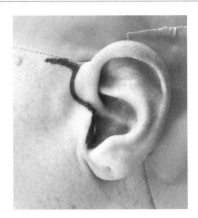

Figure 51.4 Endaural preauricular incision.

tube exiting the nose (*Figure 51.2*). Local anaesthetic of choice is infiltrated into the subcutaneous tissues along the incision line and into the joint proper.

OPERATION

Numerous surgical approaches to the TMJ are described in the literature, but the most popular are a double curved preauricular (butterfly) incision (*Figure 51.3*) or an endaural incision (*Figure 51.4*), each with or without a small temporal extension.

Incision

A 5–6-cm curvilinear 'butterfly' preauricular incision (*Figure 51.3*) is made through skin and subcutaneous tissues. The preauricular incision runs around the anterior insertion of the pinna, extending down to the insertion of the ear lobe to preauricular skin. Alternatively, the inferior incision is made over the crest of the tragus down to cartilage (*Figure 51.4*), taking care not to cut into the tragal cartilage. Superiorly, a small temporal extension of the incision is made in a forward arc about 45° relative to the zygomatic arch down to subcutaneous fat.

Skin flap development

Beginning superiorly, the temporal extension is dissected towards temporalis fascia with fine curved dissection scissors. Any superficial temporal vessels encountered are either surgically cut and tied or retracted into the anterior flap that is extended anteriorly by blunt dissection with a periosteal elevator.

Inferiorly, the flap is developed with fine curved scissors in a relatively avascular plane parallel to the base of the external auditory (tragal) cartilage (*Figure 51.5*), which runs anteromedially or along the plane of the tragal cartilage if the endaural approach is used (*Figure 51.6*).

Temporalis fascia and exposure of lateral capsule

Once the skin flap is sufficiently developed to expose the underlying temporalis fascia, the assistant manipulates the mandible while the surgeon uses their index finger to feel for the movement of the condyle under the

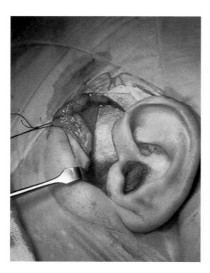

Figure 51.5 Raising full-thickness skin flap to expose temporalis fascia.

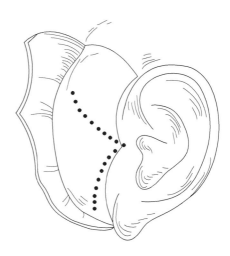

Figure 51.7 Incision of temporalis fascia.

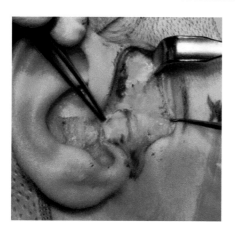

Figure 51.6 Exposed temporalis fascia.

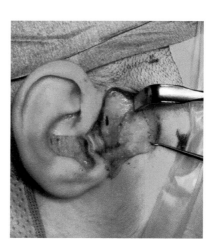

Figure 51.8 Incision of temporalis fascia.

temporalis fascia. Once the position of the condylar head is established, the root of the zygoma is identified. The temporalis fascia splits into a deep and superficial layer 2 cm above the zygomatic arch. Between these layers is loose fatty tissue and the upper trunk of the facial nerve which crosses the zygomatic arch between 8 and 35 mm in front of the most anterior portion of the bony ear canal. Dissection posterior to this allows safe forward reflection of the tissues and facial nerve. Incision of the periosteum over the root of the zygomatic arch and the temporalis fascia at 45° upwards (*Figure 51.7*) aids the tissues being swept forward by blunt dissection along the zygomatic arch using a periosteal elevator (*Figure 51.8*). Aided by a similar incision from the root of the arch downwards, the entire lateral ligament and then capsule of the TMJ can be exposed. This layer is relatively avascular, except inferiorly where branches of

the superficial temporal vessels will be encountered and may be cauterised. Access may be extended anteriorly and inferiorly depending on the degree of joint exposure required. At this point, more local anaesthetic is injected through the capsule to distend the joint space (*Figure 51.9*).

Entry through the joint capsule

Different capsule incisions (horizontal, vertical, inverted L or T shaped) are described allowing access to different areas of the joint (*Figure 51.10*). It is important to keep a cuff of capsule tissue superiorly to aid closure of the capsule. With the condyle distracted inferiorly by the surgical assistant, pointed scissors are used to bluntly enter the superior joint space and opened to reveal the superior surface of the articular disc.

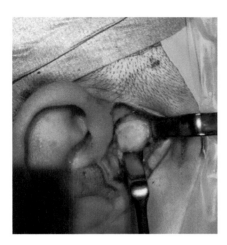

Figure 51.9 Exposed lateral joint capsule.

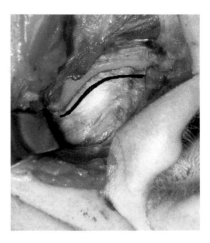

Figure 51.11 Incision into superior joint space.

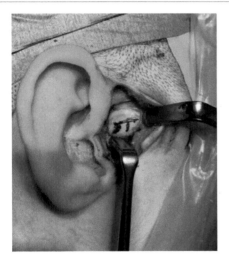

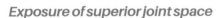

Figure 51.10 Possible incisions through capsule.

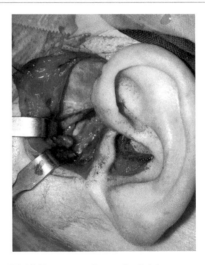

Figure 51.12 Exposure of superior joint space.

Exposure of superior joint space

With a small blade, the opening is extended anteriorly and posteriorly by cutting along the lateral aspect of the eminence and fossa (*Figure 51.11*). The capsule is reflected laterally to reveal the superior joint space (*Figures 51.12* and *51.13*). A broad periosteal elevator is then inserted into the superior joint space to help further distract the joint and expose the superior joint space as well as the glenoid fossa and eminence. The use of a Wilkes retractor can distend the upper joint space (*Figure 51.14*).

Exposure of the articular eminence

Using a periosteal elevator, the periosteum covering the lateral aspect of the articular eminence is stripped off with forward blunt dissection along the root of the zygomatic arch. Once the anterior and posterior slopes

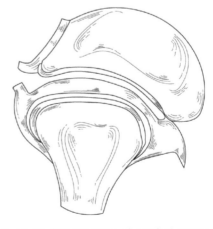

Figure 51.13 Coronal view of surgical approach to superior joint space.

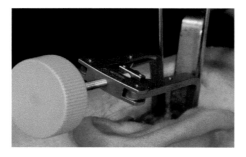

Figure 51.14 Wilkes retractor to aid visualisation.

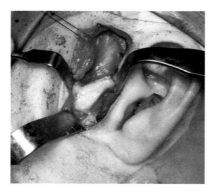

Figure 51.15 Surgical exposure of articular eminence.

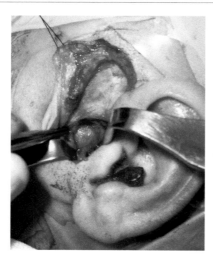

Figure 51.16 Exposure of condylar head.

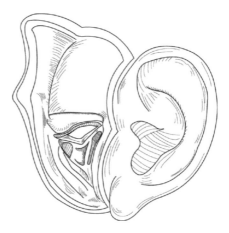

Figure 51.17 Diagram of exposed articular cartilage covering condylar head.

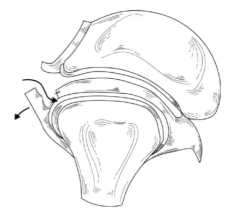

Figure 51.18 Coronal view of surgical approach to inferior joint space.

Exposure of inferior joint space

An incision is made along the lateral attachment of the disc to the condyle within the inferior recess of the capsule (*Figures 51.16–51.18*). Brisk haemorrhage may occur if the posterior attachment of the disc is cut. A fine periosteal elevator is inserted into the inferior joint space to separate the disc from the condylar head and retract the disc superiorly to expose the articular surface of the condyle.

Exposure of the condylar head

To further expose the condylar head, a vertical relieving incision is made downwards behind the condyle to produce an inverted L incision. A stay suture can be placed in the apex of this capsule incision to aid retraction and approximation at closure.

Special right-angle condylar retractors may then be inserted behind and in front of the condyle to fully expose and stabilise the condyle (*Figures 51.19*

are fully exposed, a small sharp periosteal elevator is directed medially below the greatest convexity of the articular eminence. The medial dissection through the capsule will expose the inferior aspect of the articular eminence which makes up the anterior boundary of the glenoid fossa (*Figure 51.15*).

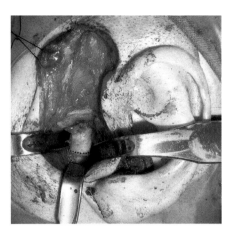

Figure 51.19 Dotted line showing osteotomy of condylar neck.

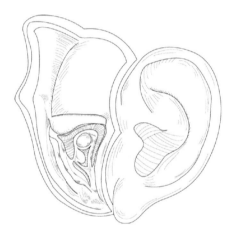

Figure 51.20 Exposure of condylar neck.

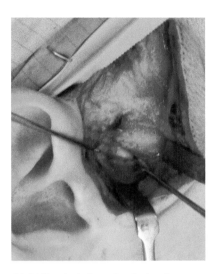

Figure 51.21 Surgical view of articular disc.

and *51.20*). Anteriorly, the condylar retractor may be inserted below the attachment of the lateral pterygoid muscle to the fovea of the condyle.

SURGICAL PROCEDURES

Articular disc

The articular disc plays a pivotal role in the complex mechanics of joint function. Any change in its physical structure, integrity or position may result in pain and joint dysfunction, referred to as internal derangement.

The two most common surgical procedures performed on the articular disc are disc repositioning and discectomy.

Disc repositioning

Upon exposing the superior joint space (*Figure 51.12*), a blunt periosteal elevator is inserted to help free up the disc anteriorly and medially. The assistant then manipulates the mandible to determine the functional position and integrity of the disc (*Figure 51.21*). At this point, further local anaesthetic is injected into the posterior disc attachment and bilaminar tissues before the disc is freed up posteriorly and the vascular retrodiscal tissues are exposed. With minor anteromedial displacements, sufficient redundant tissue within the bilaminar zone can be surgically removed and the disc repositioned posteriorly and laterally. Multiple 4-0 interrupted (non-resorbing) sutures are placed to anchor the disc to the bilaminar tissues. In situations where the disc is severely displaced, the inferior joint capsule is also exposed (*Figure 51.18*). A blunt instrument is inserted into the inferior joint space to release the disc from the condylar head and mobilise it further. Redundant tissue lateral and posterior to the posterior band of the meniscus is excised using fine scissors, leaving a rim of vascularised tissue 2 mm from the avascular posterior band of the meniscus.

Buried horizontal mattress sutures are used to fix the disc to the remaining retrodiscal tissues in its new position (*Figure 51.22*). Various anchoring devices attached to the condylar head, such as the Mitek mini anchor, have also been reported as more stable fixation points for the disc.

Discectomy

In cases where the disc is found to be unsalvageable, it is completely excised. Both upper and lower joint spaces are exposed (*Figures 51.12* and *51.18*) and a vascular clamp is placed across the retrodiscal tissues (*Figure 51.23*). As the assistant distracts the mandible (and condyle) downwards and forwards, the posterolateral part of the disc is first excised with fine pointed scissors. The remaining anteromedial part of the disc is then clamped with Allis tissue forceps to help

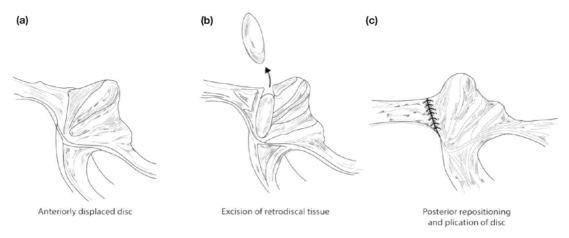

(a)   (b)   (c)

Anteriorly displaced disc   Excision of retrodiscal tissue   Posterior repositioning and plication of disc

Figure 51.22 Excision of retrodiscal tissues (a) and (b), and posterior repositioning of disc (c).

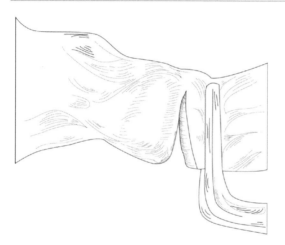

Figure 51.23 Partial excision of articular disc. A vascular clamp is placed across the retrodiscal tissues.

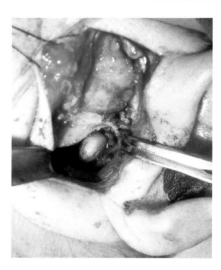

Figure 51.24 Exposed condylar head following discectomy.

retract it laterally and posteriorly to facilitate excision of the remaining part of the disc (*Figures 51.24* and *51.25*). Infiltration with local anaesthesia and judicious diathermy of bleeding points will help reduce bleeding in the resultant joint cavity. It is imperative that a complete discectomy is performed as residual anterior disc remnants will lead to persistent issues.

Many surgeons leave the space empty following discectomy with good long-term results, whilst other surgeons prefer to use free fat or free dermis-fat grafts or pedicled temporalis muscle flaps.

Articular eminence

The articular eminence is often surgically remodelled in cases of recurrent dislocation, joint replacement or in conjugation with disc procedures to facilitate free movement of the operated disc. The articular eminence may either be surgically reduced (eminoplasty) or augmented with osteotomies and/or grafts.

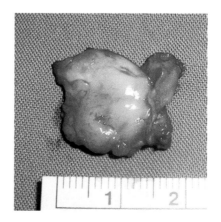

Figure 51.25 Disc specimen.

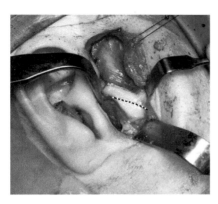

Figure 51.26 Dotted line showing osteotomy for eminoplasty.

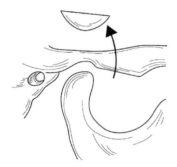

Figure 51.27 Eminoplasty.

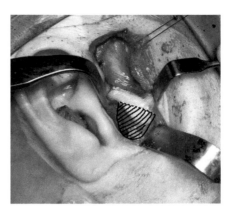

Figure 51.28 Shaded area showing bone removal required for eminence reduction.

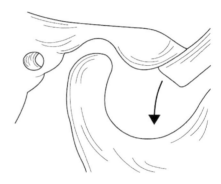

Figure 51.29 Downfracture of zygomatic arch to prevent forward translation of condyle.

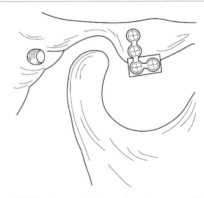

Figure 51.30 Augmentation of eminence with onlay grafts fixed with plate and screws.

Eminoplasty

This results in upper joint space scarring and so is often used to induce hypomobility in recurrent dislocation. The base of the eminence is identified by scoring the bone with a fine bur in a horizontal line joining the anterior and posterior slopes (*Figure 51.26*). The lateral part of the eminence is best removed with a fine curved chisel (*Figure 51.27*). The medial extension of the eminence is not as prominent as the lateral part and so bone files mounted on a reciprocating powered handpiece can be used to reduce the bony prominence (*Figure 51.28*) until the glenoid fossa is flush with the root of the zygomatic arch. Complete removal of the medial aspect is now felt unnecessary by some surgeons.

Eminence augmentation

Several augmentation procedures have been described to prevent forward movement of the condyle in cases of recurrent dislocation. Unfortunately, the success of the following techniques is limited, especially where the condylar head is small or atrophic and may slip medial to the augmented site:

- *Dautrey's osteotomy*: the zygomatic arch is divided just in front of the eminence and is then infractured. No fixation is used to hold the infractured arch, which is held in position by friction alone (*Figure 51.29*)
- *Onlay graft*: autogenous bone or allograft cartilage blocks are secured to the anterior slope of the eminence with miniplates and screws (*Figure 51.30*)
- *Interpositional graft*: a horizontal osteotomy is made along the base of the articular eminence. The inferior portion is downfractured and an

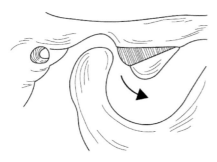

Figure 51.31 Augmentation of eminence by downfracture with interpositional grafting.

autogenous bone graft is placed as an interpositional graft, which is secured with miniplates and screws (*Figure 51.31*)

- *Alloplastic fixation:* metallic screws or plates are secured to the inferior surface of the eminence and left prominent to act as a physical barrier to the forward translation of the condyle. These may, however, damage the condylar surface due to uneven wear characteristics

Condyle

The condyle is pivotal to the development, form and function of the mandible. Trauma, disease or developmental disorders that afflict the condyle will also have a significant impact on the mandible, in particular, the occlusion. Surgery to the condylar head may range from simple smoothing of irregularities in the fibrocartilaginous articular surface, and removal of osteophytes, to complete amputation of the condyle itself in cases of severe disease or tumours. Following are descriptions of some of the surgeries.

Debridement

Upon entering the lower joint space (*Figure 51.18*), close inspection of the condylar head may reveal irregularities or defects within the fibrocartilaginous articular surface (*Figure 51.24*). With the condyle inferiorly distracted, a curette is used to gently shave the surface irregularities.

Removal of osteophytes

These bony projections are often found on the lateral and anterior pole of the condyle and should be removed with fine osteotomes rather than powered handpieces so as to minimise surgical trauma to the condyle itself.

High condylar shave

With the lateral pole of the condyle exposed, the top 5 mm layer is surgically removed with an osteotomy cut from the lateral aspect of the condylar head, which is completed medially by chisel. The remaining surface is surgically smoothed with a bone file, ensuring there are no sharp margins around the circumference of the osteotomy site.

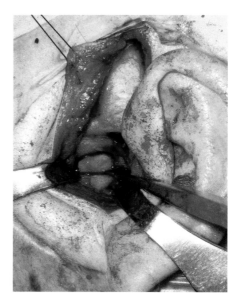

Figure 51.32 Osteotomy of condylar head.

Partial condylectomy

The lateral pole of the condyle may be excised (*Figure 51.32*) with the deep margin up to half the width of the condylar head. The aim is to preserve the medial pole of the condyle to maintain the height of the ascending mandibular ramus. A diagonal osteotomy is made from the posterior aspect of the condylar head (*Figure 51.33*), which is completed with chisels. Any sharp edges in the remaining defect are smoothly rounded with bone files.

Total condylectomy

Blunt dissection is carried inferiorly to expose the neck of the condyle to the level of the sigmoid notch (*Figures 51.19, 51.20* and *51.34*). With two condylar retractors helping to stabilise the condyle, a reciprocating saw is used to section the condylar neck. A fine chisel is used to complete the osteotomy. The amputated condylar fragment is then held with bone holding forceps while the medial attachment of the articular disc is released with sharp scissors. Anteriorly, the thick attachment of the lateral pterygoid muscle is released with dissection scissors as a traction force is placed on the condylar fragment with the bone holding forceps. Once the condylar process is extracted from its tissue bed, attention must be paid to the multiple bleeding sites.

Total joint replacement with autogenous grafts or alloplastic prosthesis should always be considered at the same time as the condylectomy to prevent severe mandibular functional and structural deformity. The alternative is to control the occlusion with intermaxillary traction until a stable occlusion can be maintained.

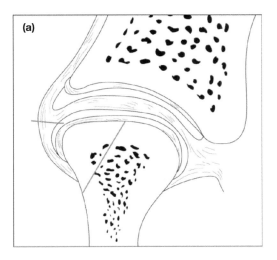

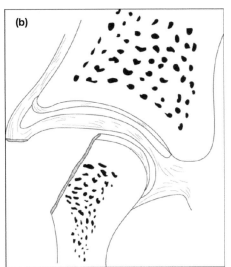

Figure 51.33 Sagittal ostectomy of lateral pole of condyle.

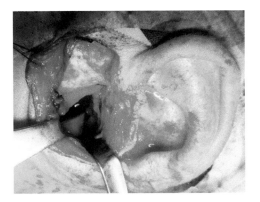

Figure 51.34 Osteotomy used for high condylectomy.

Such procedures and the management of ankylosis are discussed in *Chapters 52* and *53*.

Closure

Following careful attention to haemostasis, the surgical wound should be repaired in layers, that is, capsule, temporalis fascia, subcutaneous tissues and skin. Resorbable 4-0 sutures such as vicryl are used for the deep layers and 5-0 nylon may be used for skin either as simple interrupted or subcuticular sutures that are removed after 7 days. A mastoid-type pressure dressing is applied for 24 hours. The ear must be padded with gauze or cotton before placing the dressing. Drains are rarely indicated.

POSTOPERATIVE CARE

Physiotherapy, pharmacological and splint therapies can be employed to achieve postoperative pain control and encourage mandibular motion. Some patients, regardless of the procedure, achieve an acceptable range of motion within 7–14 days while others need to follow a strict physiotherapy regimen. Light passive opening and protrusion stretching exercises are encouraged from 5 days postoperatively. With disc repair procedures, the physiotherapy exercises should be more gradual and splint therapy can be used to maintain a stable occlusal relation in the immediate postoperative phase. Patients should be maintained on a liquid to soft diet for the first 2 postoperative weeks, but should be able to return to a normal mechanical diet with minimal dietary restrictions in due course. Joint sounds may develop or persist. After primary surgery (no previous open TMJ surgery), the hope would be to achieve a maximum interincisal opening of 35–40 mm, lateral excursive movements of 4–6 mm and protrusive excursive movements of 4–6 mm. However, patient-reported quality of life outcomes are the real measure of success with elimination of pain during function as the usual predominant concern.

COMPLICATIONS OF TMJ SURGERY (ARTHROPLASTY)

- Poor patient selection
  - Patient is an unreliable historian – secondary gain or compensation seeking
  - Patient has unrealistic expectations of surgical outcome – never tell the patient you will cure them
  - Psychiatric history
  - Significant medical history
- Inexperienced clinician
  - Poor diagnostic skills
  - Limited experience in TMJ surgery
- Poor surgical technique
  - Infection – haematoma, wound breakdown
  - Bleeding

- Facial nerve paresis
- Scarring
- Deafness – middle ear surgically breached
- Malocclusion
  - Condylar resorption
  - Overzealous arthroplasty and disc surgery
- Limited mouth opening
- Adhesions
- Fibrosis
- Ankylosis
  - Persistent symptoms
  - Failure to continue supportive non-surgical therapy
  - Poor patient compliance – cannot follow instructions
  - Misdiagnosis – chronic pain syndrome

TOP TIPS AND HAZARDS

- The operating table should be slightly inclined with the head elevated above the level of the heart to help reduce intraoperative bleeding.
- The skin/fascia flap should be developed down to the temporalis fascia, which is minimally disturbed if the temporalis is not going to be used as an interpositional flap.
- Strict dissection under the periosteum at the root of the zygomatic arch aids safe reflection of the facial nerve upwards and forwards.
- Keeping a small periosteal elevator firmly on bone, the soft tissues enveloping the condylar process can be bluntly dissected off the condyle as far inferiorly as the level of the mandibular notch.
- The role of disc repositioning surgery has diminished in light of the success of less invasive procedures such as TMJ arthroscopy and arthrocentesis.
- Bleeding is best controlled with a curved vascular clamp that is placed across the retrodiscal tissues immediately behind where the wedge excision of redundant tissue takes place.
- Autogenous fat or dermis-fat graft procured from the patient's lower abdomen can be used to fill the resultant joint cavity.
- Aggressive debridement of articular cartilage must be avoided as this will result in severe remodelling of the condyle.
- Avoid using burs to section the condyle and always use oscillating saws which do little harm to the surrounding soft tissues.

FURTHER READING

De Leeuw R, Boering G, Stegenga B, de Bont LGM. Clinical signs of TMJ osteoarthrosis and internal derangement 30 years after nonsurgical treatment. *J Orofac Pain* 1994;**54**:55–61.

Dimitroulis G. The role of surgery in the management of disorders of the temporomandibular joint: a critical review of the literature. Part 2. *Int J Oral Maxillofac Surg* 2005;**34**:231.

Gonzalez-Garcia R, Rodriguez-Campo FJ. Arthroscopic lysis and lavage versus operative arthroscopy in the outcome of temporomandibular joint internal derangement: a comparative study based on Wilkes stages. *J Oral Maxillofac Surg* 2011;**69**:2513.

Nitzan DW, Dolwick MF, Martinez GA. Temporomandibular joint arthrocentesis: a simplified treatment for severe, limited mouth opening. *J Oral Maxillofac Surg* 1991;**49**:1163–7.

Tzanidakis K, Sidebottom AJ. Outcomes of open temporomandibular joint surgery following failure to improve after arthroscopy: is there an algorithm for success? *Br J Oral Maxillofac Surg* 2013;**51**:818–21.

Chapter 52

Treatment of Temporomandibular Joint Ankylosis

Ajoy Roychoudhury, Poonam Yadav

INTRODUCTION

Temporomandibular joint (TMJ) ankylosis is a fibrous or bony fusion of the skull base with the mandibular condyle leading to trismus. Etiology can be trauma, infection, degenerative or inflammatory joint disease. Ankylosis affects chewing efficiency, speech, airway and aesthetics. The universal feature of ankylosis is restricted/no mouth opening. Other clinical features of ankylosis are varied and depend on the age of onset, involvement of unilateral or bilateral joint and duration of ankylosis. If ankylosis develops during development, then in unilateral cases limited mouth opening is associated with facial asymmetry (*Figure 52.1*). Long-standing bilateral ankylosis leads to severe retrognathia (*Figure 52.2*). Other clinical features include fullness and deepening of the antegonial notch with loss of ramus height on the ankylosed side and flatness on the non-ankylosed side. There is associated maxillary undergrowth with upwards occlusal cant, malocclusion and poor oral hygiene secondary to inability to open mouth.

PREOPERATIVE ASSESSMENT AND INVESTIGATIONS

Computed tomography (CT) imaging is the gold standard for diagnosis and treatment planning. Measurement of the ankylotic mass in all dimensions will prepare the surgeon for possible intraoperative complications such as haemorrhage from the maxillary artery. Preoperative vascular imaging and arterial embolisation may be considered in cases with recurrent and large ankylosis. History of symptoms such as disturbed night sleep, daytime somnolence and neuro-behavioural problems are suggestive of obstructive sleep apnoea. CT imaging also helps in 3D planning of safe and adequate osteoarthrectomy.

Anaesthetic consideration

Anaesthesia in TMJ ankylosis requires an experienced anaesthetic team to perform fibreoptic-assisted intubation. Fibreoptic intubation under sedation with spontaneous ventilation is the safest option. Ankylosis

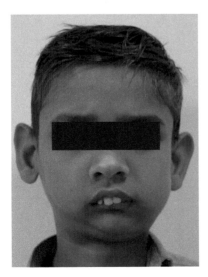

Figure 52.1 Case of left temporomandibular joint ankylosis showing facial asymmetry.

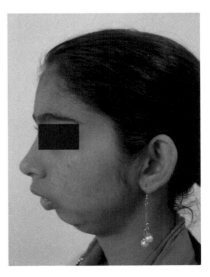

Figure 52.2 Bilateral case of temporomandibular joint ankylosis showing retrognathia/bird facies.

TABLE 52.1 Goals of treatment of temporomandibular joint ankylosis depending on age of the patient

	Goals	Treatment options
Infants and children	<ul><li>To provide mandibular range of motion</li><li>To improve airway space</li><li>To permit ongoing growth</li><li>To prevent development of facial asymmetry</li><li>To reduce chances of re-ankylosis</li><li>To improve overall quality of life</li></ul>	<ul><li>Gap arthroplasty with reconstruction of ramus-condyle unit with autogenous graft (costochondral graft – most preferred)</li><li>Distraction osteogenesis – less preferred option</li></ul>
Adults	<ul><li>To provide mandibular range of motion</li><li>To correct facial asymmetry, if any</li><li>To correct obstructive sleep apnoea, if any</li><li>To reduce chances of re-ankylosis</li><li>To improve overall quality of life</li></ul>	<ul><li>Gap arthroplasty, with reconstruction of ramus-condyle unit (alloplastic total joint prosthesis – most preferred)</li></ul>

patients have increased risk of airway obstruction and associated obstructive sleep apnoea. Mandibular retrognathia with associated pseudo-macroglossia further leads to airway narrowing. In addition, if the ankylosis is secondary to systemic inflammatory arthropathy, there may be other considerations such as fixed flexion deformity of the neck or instability of the atlantoaxial joint and restrictive pulmonary disease. Hypotensive anaesthesia should be considered as this will help to reduce intraoperative bleeding. A 30° head-up position with no neck flexion will reduce venous filling.

MANAGEMENT

Treatment modality depends on the age of the patient and to some extent on the duration and extent of ankylosis. Goals of management of TMJ ankylosis are given in *Table 52.1*.

Infancy

Ankylosis in infancy can be due to birth trauma from forceps delivery, infection and agenesis. The main aim of treatment during this period is to improve the compromised airway, provide function and to permit ongoing growth. Providing function restores functional muscle matrix and thereby allows continued growth. Early mobilisation may also permit decannulation where there is associated airway compromise requiring tracheostomy.

Childhood

Osteoarthrectomy followed by ramus-condyle unit reconstruction with an autogenous graft is the mainstay of the treatment. In bilateral ankylosis along with functional disturbances, the airway can be compromised due to retardation of mandibular growth. In these cases, improvement in airway spaces is the main goal along with restoration of mouth opening. Distraction osteogenesis to increase the corpus length of the mandible can be considered to improve airway prior to osteoarthrectomy. Autogenous grafts are currently

preferred over alloplastic prostheses for ramus-condyle unit reconstruction in paediatric/growing patients, although there is increasing consideration for alloplastic reconstruction in patients where previous reconstruction has failed. The costochondral graft is the most common graft chosen; however, unpredictable growth and re-ankylosis are the main disadvantages. Should the graft fail later in life (post-puberty), it should be converted to a total joint replacement. Other treatment modalities are gap arthroplasty, interposition arthroplasty with temporalis muscle, fat grafts, dermal grafts and free bone grafts. The growth potential is absent with these grafts and stability is limited.

Adults

Management of adult onset ankylosis aims to provide function and prevent re-ankylosis. Ramus-condyle unit reconstruction with an alloplastic prosthesis is the accepted standard of care in adults. Concomitant total joint replacement and orthognathic surgery with counter clockwise rotation of mandible (in bilateral cases) or contralateral sagittal split osteotomy with cant correction is usually done in unilateral cases. An alloplastic prosthesis allows immediate mouth-opening physiotherapy, to reduce the risk of heterotopic bone formation and re-ankylosis, and avoids additional donor site morbidity with good long-term outcomes.

Preparation of the patient before surgical procedure

The patient should be asked to rinse their oral cavity with chlorhexidine and the temporal region is shaved to provide a clean operative field. The head is placed on a headring with the nasal tube secured over the patient's forehead. Skin preparation should also include thorough cleansing of the ear canal. Separation of oral cavity, nasal cavity and ear is performed with an antimicrobial drape (*Figure 52.3*). The area supplied by the facial nerve should be free of the dressing to permit visualisation for twitching of the facial nerve during the procedure.

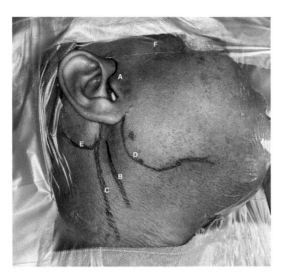

Figure 52.3 Figure showing draping and marking for endaural and retromandibular approach (A endaural incision, B retromandibular incision, C anterior border of sternocleidomastoid, D posterior border of the mandible, E mastoid process, F antimicrobial drape).

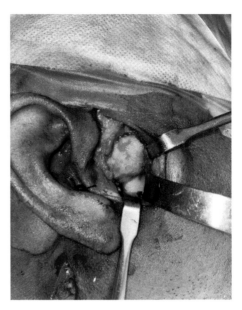

Figure 52.4 Figure showing exposure of ankylosis by endaural approach.

Incision and approach

Preauricular approach

A preauricular approach with temporal extension can be used to expose the ankylosis. The endaural approach may be preferred due to increased cosmesis (*Figure 52.4*).

The natural skin crease above the tragus is marked in front of the helix of the ear. While marking at the tragus, it should be pulled forwards. The endaural incision includes two separate areas of dissection separated by the zygomatic arch: one area below (tragal incision) and the other area above the zygomatic arch.

After marking the incision, local anaesthesia is injected into the subcutaneous plane to aid in hydrodissection and reduce haemorrhage.

The tragal incision is started from skin and subcutaneous tissue, with traction by a skin hook anteriorly. The aim is to open the avascular plane in front of the tragal cartilage. Blunt dissection is done in the avascular plane along the tragal cartilage to reach the posterior border of the condylar neck. Pre-tragal dissection is complete after reaching the condylar neck.

Moving to the portion of dissection, above the zygomatic arch, the aim is to reach the superficial layer of temporal fascia (white glistening layer). After identifying this layer, the superior dissection is connected to the pre-tragal dissection. With the root of zygoma identified, an incision can be made obliquely upwards through the temporalis fascia to expose the intervening temporal fat and zygomatic arch (if a temporalis flap is to be used, this incision should be the vertical posterior limb of the flap).

The facial nerve is superficial to periosteum on the zygomatic arch and superficial to temporalis fascia, hence the dissection should be subperiosteal on the zygomatic arch and below the temporalis fascia, above the arch. The tissue overlying the joint can be dissected bluntly off the capsule. The capsule is then opened along the posterior border of the condylar neck and head.

The dissection is completed by exposing the condylar neck posteriorly, zygomatic arch superiorly, sigmoid notch anteriorly and according to the required osteotomy inferiorly in a subperiosteal plane.

For further access, temporal extension of the superior incision can be carried out.

Retromandibular approach

A retromandibular/submandibular approach is used to expose the ramus if ramus-condyle unit reconstruction is planned with autogenous/alloplastic material. The retromandibular incision is marked parallel to the anterior border of sternocleidomastoid muscle, halfway between its anterior border and the angle of the mandible and ascending ramus.

After incising through skin and subcutaneous tissue, a skin hook is applied with superior traction. The avascular plane is opened up between the parotid fascia and anterior border of sternocleidomastoid muscle.

The tail of the parotid is retracted anteriorly to prevent violation of the parotid capsule and to allow identification of the deep cervical fascia. The posterior belly of digastric is identified, which is the limit of posterior dissection.

Next, the pterygomasseteric sling is incised and released at the inferior and posterior border of mandible and the ramus of mandible exposed in a subperiosteal plane up to the sigmoid notch to join the superior dissection using a periosteal elevator.

Damage to the marginal mandibular nerve can be avoided by nerve monitoring and careful dissection throughout the procedure. Nerve damage has not persisted in primary cases as any branches traversing the wound can be seen lying on the masseteric epimysium and retracted.

Resection of ankylotic bone

The ankylotic mass can extend a long way along the base of the skull and therefore resection may be compromised by cranial nerves emerging from the skull base, the maxillary, middle meningeal and ultimately internal jugular and carotid vessels. Preoperative evaluation of the extent of the ankylotic mass and vascular imaging will have determined the extent of dissection required and the assistance of a vascular or skull base surgeon may be required. CT data of the patient are transferred to the medical imaging software and superior and inferior osteotomy are planned. Superior osteotomy should be 5–8 mm away from the external auditory canal. A gap of approximately 1.5 cm between the superior and inferior osteotomies is planned. Cutting guides can be fabricated for exact superior and inferior osteotomy transfer from the virtual platform to the operating table. The osteotomy should be smooth and regular. The authors prefer to use a piezoelectric saw as its use results in a flat temporal surface and reduces the chances of heterotopic bone formation. An incremental technique (*Figure 52.5*) may be used for osteoarthrectomy as removing the bigger ankylotic mass *in toto* may avulse

deeper structures and haemorrhage control down a deep dark hole can prove troublesome. If using a saw or drill, attempts should be made to cut from deep to superficial to reduce the risk of inadvertent damage deep to the medial periosteum. Any residual haemorrhage from the pterygoid venous plexus can be controlled with pressure, bipolar diathermy and oxidised cellulose gauze. Maximal incisal opening should be assessed after osteoarthrectomy and if less than 30 mm, an ipsilateral coronoidectomy is performed via the same incision. Intraoral contralateral coronoidectomy is done if the opening still remains less than 30 mm.

Lining of the temporal bone

A temporalis muscle flap either full thickness or split can be elevated by extending the preauricular incision in the temporal area. The flap is rotated over the arch and sutured to the medial tissues (*Figure 52.6*). This acts as a cushion to the costochondral graft and a barrier future to bone formation between the cut ends. The authors prefer fat packing over temporalis muscle as the blood supply of the latter can get occluded when rotated over the arch and lead to dystrophic calcification and increased fibrosis. Fat grafting can be performed by mobilising the nearby buccal fat pad from the anterior portion of the wound at the anterior border of coronoid process after bluntly opening the temporalis

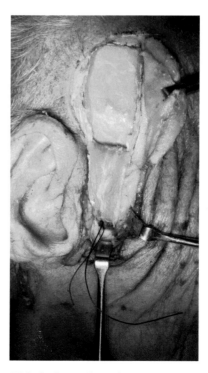

Figure 52.6 Cadaver dissection showing temporalis fascial flap interpositioning by rotation over zygomatic arch and suturing to medial tissues.

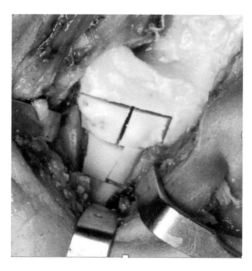

Figure 52.5 Figure showing incremental cutting of ankylotic mass.

muscle/tendon with a haemostat and simultaneous milking of the cheek towards the incision. Alternately, periumbilical abdominal fat can be harvested and grafted. A temporalis flap is not required if an allo-plastic replacement is being used (see *Chapter 53*), but fat graft packed around the prosthesis is advised to reduce heterotopic bone formation.

Costochondral graft

Costochondral graft is the most commonly used graft for TMJ reconstruction in growing patients. Costo-chondral graft can permit growth but its unpredictabil-ity can lead to overgrowth and re-ankylosis. In multiply operated cases, where re-vascularisation of the graft is limited due to fibrous tissue formation and limited capillary permeability around the operated site, take-up of costochondral graft is questionable. There is no clear consensus in the literature about whether the growth after costochondral graft is due to cartilage or activation of the functional matrix after regaining function of the mandible. Both cartilage and functional matrix may be required to work in tandem for growth.

Harvesting technique

Usually, the 5th, 6th or 7th rib is harvested. The anatomical landmarks considered are the medial axillary line, midclavicular line and the contour of the rib to be harvested. Ribs are palpated and marked (*Figure 52.7*). In females, the incision is placed in the inframammary crease. In males, the incision should follow contours of the rib.

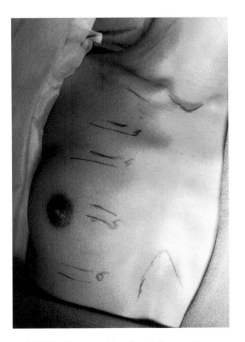

Figure 52.7 Surface marking for rib harvesting.

At all times, the surgeon's middle finger and thumb should be placed at the superior and inferior border of rib, while the index finger can palpate the rib to be harvested.

Skin and subcutaneous tissue is incised to expose the underlying muscle. With electrocautery, incision is made directly up to the bone. Dissection of periosteum should be performed with meticulous care as slippage of the instrument can lead to pleural puncture.

A Doyen rib stripper is used to separate the peri-osteum inferiorly (*Figure 52.8*). The bone end is cut with either a rib shear or by piezoelectric saw. After bone cutting, the incision should be continued towards the junction of cartilage and bone. The cartilage is cut using a blade (*Figure 52.9*).

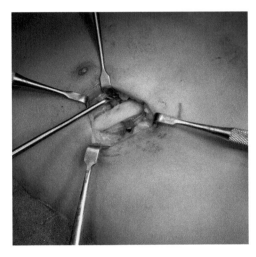

Figure 52.8 Exposure of rib and inner dissection by Doyen rib stripper to minimize the injury to pleura.

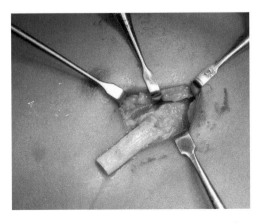

Figure 52.9 Harvesting technique from bone cutting to cartilage cutting. Note the periosteum-perichondrium sleeve to the bone–cartilage junction.

A diamond-shaped cuff of perichondrium should be maintained at the bony and cartilage junction to prevent separation (*Figure 52.10*). The authors prefer to take a 2–4 mm length of the cartilage to prevent overgrowth.

After harvest, the cavity should be filled with saline and the anaesthetist is asked to give positive pressure ventilation to check for pleural tear. A chest drain should be inserted in the usual manner if a pleural tear is detected. The periosteum of the rib should be sutured and the wound is closed in layers.

Placement of rib for joint reconstruction

The cartilaginous rib is trimmed according to the defect dimensions and contour of the condyle (*Figure 52.11*). Temporalis fascial interposition may be placed prior to rib fixation. Fat interposition (buccal fat pad/ abdominal) can be performed prior to insertion of the costochondral graft. The lateral surface of the mandible and medial surface of the rib (side facing the lateral surface of mandible) can be pre-prepared to enable direct fixation of the rib to cancellous bone permitting a more accurate fit and better chance of integration. The rib may be greenstick fractured to permit more accurate adaptation. Fixation is done with a 2 mm miniplate or washer plate with screws (*Figure 52.12*). The pediatric rib is softer than the mandible, requiring care to avoid overtightening of screws. The wound is closed in layers. The jaws are immobilised for 7–10 days for initial healing. This is followed by active mouth-opening exercises.

Transport disc distraction osteogenesis

In 2009, distraction osteogenesis was suggested for TMJ reconstruction. After osteoarthrectomy, an 'L-shaped'

osteotomy of the ramus is done, and the distractor is placed (*Figure 52.13*). The vertical limb of 'L' starts at the midpoint of the sigmoid notch and drops down to a distance slightly greater than the gap created. The horizontal limb of 'L' is then directed towards the posterior border to form an advancing disc. The distractor is then fixed and is activated at 1 mm/day. The advancing bone disc docks at the temporal bone and remodels as condyle. Temporalis fascia/muscle flap can be used as a barrier between temporal bone and the advancing neocondyle. Fat (buccal fat pad/abdominal) can also be used for similar purposes. Due to various advantages of fat interpositioning, the authors prefer to use fat as a barrier to prevent heterotopic bone formation. The distractor is removed after consolidation of the regenerate bone (3 months).

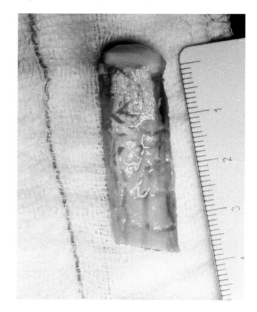

Figure 52.11 Trimming of the cartilage to mimic the condylar shape and decortication of bony part.

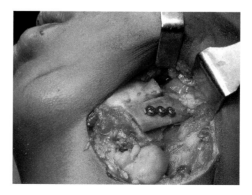

Figure 52.12 Fixation of costochondral graft with miniplate and screws with fat packing.

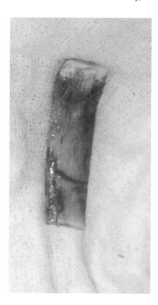

Figure 52.10 Harvested costochondral graft.

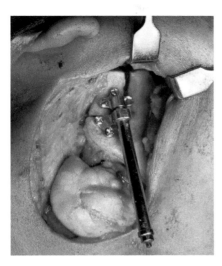

Figure 52.13 Transport disc is made using an 'L' oste-otomy and fixing the distractor.

POSTOPERATIVE CARE AND RECOVERY

Postoperative recovery is often uneventful. Active mouth-opening exercises should be started as early as possible depending on the pain threshold of the patient. Patients should be encouraged to eat food requiring active mastication. Mouth-opening exercises should be continued for at least 6 months. Any signs of reduced mouth opening in the follow-up period should be investigated for heterotopic bone formation.

POSSIBLE COMPLICATIONS AND HOW TO DEAL WITH THEM

Intraoperative haemorrhage from damage to the maxillary artery, inferior alveolar artery or pterygoid plexus of veins is often encountered. Pressure pack and isolation to clamp and cauterise the bleeding vessel usually achieves haemostasis. If uncontrolled, then the terminal branch of the external carotid is accessed and ligated after dividing the posterior belly of digastric muscle, which is already exposed in retromandibular incision. Although rare, injudicious use of chisel and mallet in bone removal can result in fracture of temporal bone and dura exposure or a cerebrospinal fluid (CSF) leak may occur. Neurosurgical support is required, and temporalis muscle is rotated into the defect with copious use of fibrin glue to manage the CSF leak.

Re-ankylosis occurs due to heterotopic bone formation. Complete removal of the ankylotic mass using a piezoelectric saw, parallel osteotomy, copious irrigation with saline to remove bone slurry and chips, fat grafting, use of a vacuum drain and aggressive physiotherapy reduces the chances of postoperative heterotopic bone formation.

TOP TIPS AND HAZARDS

- Ankylosis of the TMJ is an uncommon problem in the Western world and should be dealt with by a surgeon with experience in this area. The surgeon should have experience of the various approaches and methods of reconstruction, and access to a neurosurgeon and an anaesthetic team with expertise in fibreoptic-assisted intubation.
- Preoperative vascular imaging should be considered in patients with extensive ankylosis or several previous procedures as the vessels can lie in the ankylotic mass.
- Access to the carotid can be achieved by deepening the retromandibular wound onto digastric and anterior to the sternocleidomastoid muscles.
- These patients should always have 'group and save' samples as blood loss can be sudden and catastrophic.
- Rapid access to the joint is facilitated by the pretemporal fascial dissection approach.
- If inadequate opening is achieved intraoperatively, coronoidectomy should be considered.
- Fat packing is required in the defect to reduce heterotopic bone formation.
- Adequate mobilisation can be ensured postoperatively by regular use of the TheraBite or an equivalent physiotherapy device.

FURTHER READING

Kaban LB, Perrott DH, Fisher K. A protocol for management of temporomandibular joint ankylosis. *J Oral Maxillofac Surg* 1990;**48**:1145–51; discussion 1152.

Mercuri LG, Edibam NR, Giobbie-Hurder A. Fourteen-year follow-up of a patient-fitted total temporomandibular joint reconstruction system. *J Oral Maxillofac Surg* 2007;**65**:1140–8.

Roychoudhury A, Yadav P, Alagarsamy R, Bhutia O, Goswami D. Outcome of stock total joint replacement with fat grafting in adult temporomandibular joint ankylosis patients. *J Oral Maxillofac Surg* 2021;**79**:75–87.

Sidebottom AJ, Gruber E. One-year prospective outcome analysis and complications following total replacement of the temporomandibular joint with the TMJ Concepts system. *Br J Oral Maxillofac Surg* 2013;**51**:621–4.

Yadav P, Roychoudhury A, Bhutia O. Strategies to reduce re-ankylosis in temporomandibular joint ankylosis patients. *Br J Oral Maxillofac Surg* 2021;S0266-4356(21)00073-5.

Chapter 53

Total Prosthetic Replacement of the Temporomandibular Joint

Andrew J. Sidebottom, Nabeela Ahmed

THE EVOLUTION OF THE TMJ REPLACEMENT PROSTHESIS

Total replacement of the temporomandibular joint (TMJ) has been an option since the 19th century, but the recent prosthetic choices arose following development of the Christensen prosthesis in 1963. While initially this was cobalt chrome on acrylic, the subsequent modification to metal-on-metal led to metallosis and it was removed from the market. The current two commonly used prostheses are either a stock or custom-made variant (Stryker TMJ Concepts and Zimmer Biomet) and consist of a metal on ultrahigh molecular weight polyethylene (UHMWPE) fossa. Hemi-arthroplasty with a fossa prosthesis has also been abandoned as a result of early failure through condylar head wear.

Various other prostheses have been trialled and failed or have no long-term follow-up and the following relates to the placement of a Stryker TMJ Concepts custom-made prosthesis as this is currently the authors' first choice of prosthesis. It requires a Protomed 3D computed tomography (CT) scan to create a CAD–CAM model on which the surgical cuts are determined and the prosthesis is subsequently made. The construction technique can be seen in *Figure 53.1*. In patients with component part allergy to cobalt–chromium alloy, an all-titanium condylar component can be constructed, although the wear characteristics of a hardened titanium surface are less certain than for the cobalt–chromium alloy. The prosthetic fit is superior with a custom-made prosthesis compared with a stock prosthesis and therefore less mobility in theory should

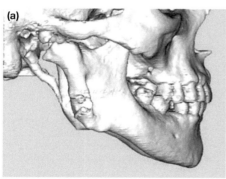
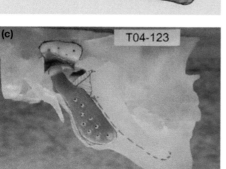
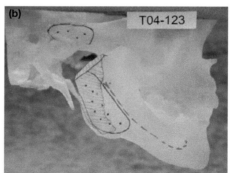
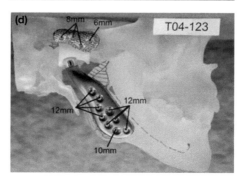

Figure 53.1 Illustration of (a) three-dimensional model, (b) resection, (c) wax up and (d) prosthesis on model using the Stryker TMJ Concepts prosthesis.

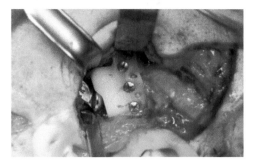

Figure 53.2 Zimmer Biomet prosthesis *in situ*.

lead to better success rates based on simple orthopaedic principles.

Zimmer Biomet (formerly Lorenz) make a stock and custom prosthesis with similar components to the Stryker TMJ Concepts system (*Figure 53.2*). The Concepts system fossa has a titanium mesh base bonded to UHMWPE, whereas the Zimmer Biomet fossa is all UHMWPE. The Zimmer Biomet stock prosthesis has five choices of ramus component and three choices of fossa size. This requires eminoplasty with a standardised drill piece or oscillating blade to permit the fit of the fossa. It also requires accurate preoperative assessment of the ramus and base of skull anatomy to determine whether the ramus component will fit against the ramus and into the fossa component, as ramus yaw and fossa lateral and sagittal angulation may not permit this to occur in some cases.

Metal-on-metal prostheses have a tendency to early metal wear and have led to the abandonment of this type of prosthesis in orthopaedic devices. Around 10% of the general population are nickel allergic with less than 1% allergic to the other alloy components, and a type 4 hypersensitivity reaction may develop in allergic individuals. An immune-mediated response to wear debris may also develop. Approximately 10% of metal-on-metal TMJ prostheses in a UK series have failed and been found to have a giant cell foreign body reaction surrounding them. For this reason, patients should be patch tested for allergy to nickel, cobalt, chromium and molybdenum individually and if necessary, consider a lymphocyte transformation test prior to recommending a cobalt–chromium alloy-based prosthesis. In allergic individuals, an all-titanium condylar head is indicated.

INDICATIONS AND CONTRAINDICATIONS

The indications and contraindications for total replacement of the TMJ were published by a UK consensus study group (*Table 53.1*). It is essential, prior to consideration of prosthetic replacement, that an appropriate trial of conservative management (including arthroscopy if possible) has been attempted and failed.

Diagnosis of condylar disease should be made with the aid of CT or magnetic resonance imaging (MRI) scan as a minimum. CT scan is required to show the bony anatomy and is acquired using a Protomed protocol (3D) if a custom-made prosthesis is to be constructed.

The clinical indicators (*Table 53.2*) give an idea of the severity of disability of the patient (similar to walking distance for total hip replacement) and also permit assessment of outcome following the procedure. Contraindications are rare (*Table 53.3*)

TABLE 53.1 Indications for total prosthetic replacement of the temporomandibular joint

Disease processes (involving condylar bone loss)
Degenerative joint disease/osteoarthrosis
Inflammatory joint disease (rheumatoid, ankylosing spondylitis, psoriatic)
Ankylosis
Post-traumatic condylar loss/damage
Post-surgical condylar loss (including neoplastic ablation)
Previous prosthetic reconstruction
Previous costochondral graft
Major congenital deformity
Multiple previous procedures

TABLE 53.2 Clinical indicators for total prosthetic replacement of the temporomandibular joint

Usually a combination of the following
Dietary score of <5/10 (liquid scores 0, full diet scores 10)
Restricted mouth opening (<35 mm)
Occlusal collapse/anterior open bite/retrusion
Excessive condylar resorption and loss of vertical ramus height
Pain score >5 out of 10 on visual analogue (in combination with any of above)
Quality of life issues other than above

TABLE 53.3 Contraindications to total prosthetic replacement of the temporomandibular joint

Contraindications
Ongoing local infective process
Severe immune compromise
Severe ASA 3 disease processes (relative)

Abbreviation: ASA, American Society of Anesthesiologists.

but include severe local infective process or radiation reaction or associated severe immune compromise. These are relative, however, as most inflammatory arthritis patients are on disease-modifying drugs, and with appropriate short-term adjustment of medication, prosthetic replacement can be safely carried out with minimal added risk. Bisphosphonate use does not seem to cause any issues.

Dental status should be checked preoperatively and any teeth restored with compromised teeth being removed. Postoperative dental infection risks prosthetic biofilm infection, which requires removal of the prosthesis. Revision surgery increases morbidity and cost (UK £10,000, US $12,000 per prosthesis). Postoperative infection should be dealt with aggressively, preferably with extraction or drainage of any abscess. Prophylactic antibiotics are recommended according to the American Association of Orthopaedics guidelines for invasive dental procedures for the 2 years following prosthetic insertion.

SURGICAL TECHNIQUE

Intravenous antibiotic prophylaxis aimed at the common skin commensals should be given on induction and continued for 24 hours postoperatively, and then oral antibiotics should be given for 5 days postoperatively. Catheterisation, if needed, will aid in fluid monitoring, but should aim to be removed at the end of the procedure. Hypotensive anaesthetic techniques and a head-up table help to reduce blood loss perioperatively.

The standard preauricular and retromandibular approaches to the TMJ are adopted. The patient is anaesthetised with a centreline tube extending over the vertex of the head. Consideration of anaesthetic technique should be borne in mind when planning surgery as fibreoptic-aided intubation or tracheostomy may be required due to restricted mouth opening. Hair is trimmed with clippers such that this does not get into the wound. *Propionibacterium acnes* is a common cause of postoperative biofilm infection, so the hair is washed and then formally prepared, including the ear canal. Towels are sutured into position to hold the hair out of the way and a Steri-Drape is placed over the operation site. Arch bars or intermaxillary fixation (IMF) screws are placed and the operating field around the mouth kept free from contaminating the operating field of the prosthetic replacement. The mouth is covered by the Steri-Drape free ends and local analgesic with adrenaline is infiltrated into the preauricular and retromandibular incision sites.

The joint is exposed from below and above (see *Chapter 51* and *Chapter 52*). It is vital to ensure that a subperiosteal approach is used with retractors holding away the medial tissues during the condylectomy, which can be performed with drill, saw or piezo saw. The required condylectomy is carried out and the soft tissues of the capsule, disc, lateral pterygoid and periosteum

are dissected gently with copious diathermy to maintain a blood-free field, while trying not to extend the dissection too far medially where the maxillary, middle meningeal and masseteric vessels and the mandibular division of the trigeminal nerve lie within a few millimetres. It is essential that all disc and capsular tissue is removed to provide sufficient space for the prosthesis. Residual disc tissue may interfere with prosthetic function and the disc can be removed most safely with the aid of diathermy and subsequent scissor freeing from the lateral pterygoid, which tends to ooze if just cut. If adequate mouth opening (>30 mm) is not achieved, an ipsilateral coronoidectomy can be completed through either the superior or inferior wound under direct vision. Contralateral coronoidectomy (transorally if the other joint does not require replacement) may also be required if the opening still does not exceed 30 mm.

Once the fossa is completely cleared of soft tissue, placement of the prosthetic fossa is attempted. The fossa is irrigated with gentamicin-containing saline and the fit of the prosthesis checked and if necessary, the fossa adjusted if there is any rocking. The different types of prosthesis require slightly different techniques at this stage and will not be further described. The following relates to the technique of placement of a custom-made Stryker TMJ Concepts prosthesis.

The fit of the fossa is confirmed by pushing it into place upwards and backwards and checking for mobility. The patient is placed in IMF to the desired occlusion and then all gowns and gloves are changed and the instruments for the intraoral procedure kept totally separate. The fossa is again trialled to ensure that adequate condyle and coronoid have been removed to enable free fitting of the fossa and rotation of the condylar component on mouth opening. There should be at least a 5-mm gap between the prosthetic fossa and the mandibular stump. The cavity is again irrigated with gentamicin solution and the fossa fitted and secured with three to four screws into the zygomatic arch.

The lower incision is then entered and the fit of the condylar component checked. It may be necessary to smooth down the lateral border of the mandible according to the preoperative planning on the CT model, with particular consideration of the gonial angle due to eversion of the bone tissues in this area at the lower attachment of masseter, most notable in long-standing ankylosis cases. Once the fit to the lateral border has been confirmed, the fit into the fossa component is confirmed. This should match that seen on the photos of the prosthesis on the model (*Figure 53.3*). Usually, it lies about 1/2 to 2/3 of the way into the fossa. If the head lies too superficial it suggests that insufficient condylar neck has been removed, which can be confirmed by direct vision, and usually the prosthesis will rock in the superoinferior plane and there will be a gap between the prosthesis and the proximal ramus.

Once the fit of the condylar prosthesis is confirmed, this is secured initially with three screws to the length

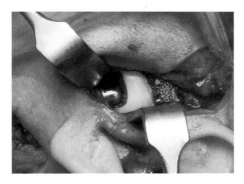

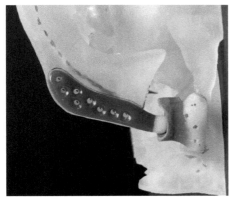

Figure 53.3 Fit of the condylar component in the fossa on the model and *in situ* should match (Stryker TMJ Concepts prosthesis).

marked on the diagrams supplied by the company. The use of three screws only does less damage to the ramus if adjustment of position is subsequently required. The IMF is removed and the occlusion is checked. If this is not correct, the position of the prosthesis requires adjustment. Once the position and occlusion are correct, a total of at least five bicortical screws should be inserted using copious irrigation with the most proximal screw being the most important as this is the point of maximum torque. The prosthesis should sit flush to the mandible along its entire length. Movement of the articulation should now be confirmed in function. If less than 30 mm movement can be achieved, either the position is incorrect or a coronoidectomy may be required. If there is dislocation, then light IMF elastics will be required postoperatively for 1 week until the vertical stability is re-established. This can occur following previous coronoidectomy or with closure of anterior open bites, where the vertical pull of the temporalis has been reduced. Once the occlusion is satisfactory, gown and gloves contaminated intraorally are changed. The fit and movement of the condyle within the fossa are checked and the wound is irrigated with gentamicin solution. If all is satisfactory, the wounds can then be closed.

The authors prefer a single 12 suction drain introduced through the upper wound extending over the prosthesis into the lower wound subperiosteally as this covers all the areas of potential wound leakage. This is secured behind the ear with black silk and is removed on the first postoperative day.

For cases which are ankylosed at this stage, an abdominal fat graft is placed if desired and packed around the articulating surfaces. The upper wound is closed with continuous resorbable sutures (Vicryl or PDS) to the temporalis fascia to cover the joint but ensuring that the drain is not inadvertently held too tightly into the wound. The subcutaneous tissues are then closed with Vicryl to bring the wound edges together and the skin with 6/0 monofilament. The lower wound is closed with continuous Vicryl to provide a watertight closure of the parotid fascia and subcutaneous tissues. This avoids involving the branches of the facial nerve in the closure and prevents sialocele. Monofilament is used to close the skin. The masseter is not directly closed as this shortening may reduce postoperative myofascial pain due to the muscle shortening achieved.

Antibiotics should be continued intravenously for 24 hours then for 5 days orally. Passive mobilisation is commenced at day 1 using a mouth-opening device and continued for at least 6 months using the minimum recommended protocol of 7 seconds maximal opening, seven times, at least seven times a day, initially aiming to improve opening by 1–2 mm per day. The opening at the start of the day will have declined compared with the night before, so the measurements should be taken at the same time every day. Most primary joint replacement patients should achieve opening of above 25 mm within 6 weeks and 30 mm by 3 months, with the pain scores diminishing rapidly towards zero. Dietary improvements take a little longer to achieve.

Postoperative stay is between 24 and 72 hours in most instances. Sutures are removed at 5–7 days.

COMPLICATIONS

Haemorrhage

This can occur from the superficial temporal vessels, the retromandibular vein behind the ramus, the masseteric vessels deep to the sigmoid notch/condylar periosteum, the pterygoid venous plexus or occasionally deeper vessels medial to the condyle such as the maxillary artery, the middle meningeal and even the internal jugular vein, which can be in close proximity either with a large ankylotic mass or following contracture due to previous surgeries. It is often difficult to control haemorrhage through the 1 cm × 1 cm wound following condylectomy hence the best method of control of haemorrhage is prevention by a careful technique. Blood samples should have been 'grouped and saved' as transfusion can occasionally be required. Occasionally, more proximal ligation of the external carotid or

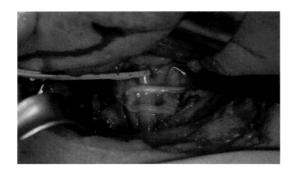

Figure 53.4 Exposure and tie of the terminal external carotid artery may be required when uncontrollable haemorrhage persists.

jugular may be required (*Figure 53.4*) and these can be accessed by a suitable extension of the retromandibular wound. Surgicel and pressure can also be used to control pterygoid oozing.

Dislocation

Dislocation of the prosthesis is rare and usually associated with previous coronoidectomy reducing vertical stability of the joint. Occasionally, closure of an open bite will cause a similar effect. It should be checked intraoperatively and the arch bars should be left *in situ* and 1 week light IMF elastic used to control inadvertent wide opening. Postoperative dislocation may also be due to joint malpositioning or dystonic contractions.

Facial nerve injury

Facial nerve palsies are common postoperatively, particularly in the temporal branch and especially following revision surgery. They are usually temporary due to stretching of the tissues to gain adequate access for placement of the prosthesis. Permanent palsies can be dealt with by brow lift and other 'cosmetic' procedures and in extreme cases cross-facial nerve grafting can be considered (*Chapter 43*).

Infection

The authors recommend prophylaxis for invasive procedures causing bacteraemia similar to those for bacterial endocarditis prevention for 2 years postoperatively according to the American Association of Orthopaedic Surgeons guidelines. Infection may present with obvious signs of redness and drainage of pus from the wounds. Usually, low-grade infection will present as increasing restriction of opening and pain. Prosthetic removal is almost inevitable and should be followed by a period of occlusal stabilisation with a gentamicin-containing acrylic spacer. Biofilm formation – whereby colonies of bacteria are covered by an almost impermeable polysaccharide membrane – may present more insidiously with ongoing pain and restriction,

but with no other clinical or haematological signs of infection. Antibiotics cannot penetrate the biofilm and prosthetic removal is indicated.

Allergy

Allergy to the prosthetic material can occur to any of the components of the prosthesis. Prevention by appropriate allergy testing preoperatively may reduce this phenomenon, although there is a suggestion that patients with failing prosthetic hip replacements develop allergy due to sensitisation and lymphocyte activation. Other factors may be involved; however, where allergy is suspected, the ongoing swelling may lead to traction facial nerve palsy and the prosthesis requires removal and ultimate revision to an all-titanium prosthesis (*Figure 53.5*).

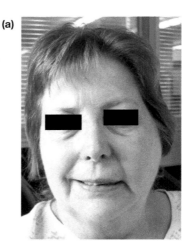

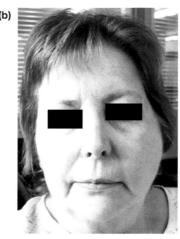

Figure 53.5 (a) Traction palsy of facial nerve due to swelling consequent upon chromium allergy. (b) This resolved following replacement of the prosthesis with all-titanium.

Myofascial pain

This occurs when opening improves around 6 weeks when postoperative mouth opening tends to exceed the preoperative level. Low-dose tricyclic medication or botulinum injections will help to control this, although this pain tends to have ceased by 1 year.

Long-term complications are rare and the majority of patients gain significant improvements within 1 year in pain scores (90%), dietary scores (90%) and mouth opening, which persist for more than 10 years.

TOP TIPS AND HAZARDS

- Consider preoperative vascular imaging in patients with extensive ankylosis or multiple previous procedures as the vessels can lie in the ankylotic mass.
- Assess all patients for metal allergy if an alloplastic prosthesis is to be used and use an all-titanium prosthesis if allergy exists.
- Rapid access to the joint is facilitated by the pretemporal fascial dissection approach.
- Access to the internal carotid artery can be achieved by deepening the retromandibular wound onto digastric and anterior to the sternocleidomastoid muscles.
- Always arrange a 'group and save' as blood loss can be sudden and catastrophic.
- If inadequate opening is achieved intraoperatively, consider coronoidectomy.
- Always check for dislocation of the prosthesis intraoperatively and place in light elastic traction for 1 week if this can be achieved.
- Ensure adequate mobilisation postoperatively by regular use of a mouth-opening device.

FURTHER READING

Gruber E, McCullough J, Sidebottom A. Medium-term outcomes and complications after total replacement of the temporomandibular joint. Prospective outcome analysis after 3 and 5 years. *Br J Oral Maxillofac Surg* 2015;**53**:412–15.

Rajkumar A, Sidebottom AJ. Prospective study of the long-term outcomes and complications after total temporomandibular joint replacement: analysis at 10 years. *Int J Oral Maxillofac Surg* 2021;**51**:665-8.

Sidebottom A. Risk factors for intraoperative dislocation of the total temporomandibular joint replacement and its management. *Br J Oral Maxillofac Surg* 2014;**52**:190–2.

Sidebottom A, Speculand B, Hensher R. Foreign body response around total prosthetic metal-on-metal replacements of the temporomandibular joint in the UK. *Br J Oral Maxillofac Surg* 2008;**46**:288–92.

Sidebottom AJ. Guidelines for the replacement of temporomandibular joints in the United Kingdom. *Br J Oral Maxillofac Surg* 2008;**46**:146–7.

Chapter

54

Orthognathic Surgery of the Mandible

Tom Aldridge, Mohammed Al-Gholmy

INTRODUCTION

Osteotomy of the mandible can be used to address prognathic, retrognathic or asymmetric discrepancies. Mandibular procedures can be used in isolation or in combination with operations to the maxilla or chin. The key to all these procedures is a stable condyle–glenoid fossa relationship that must be maintained.

Modern techniques have evolved from earlier methods to minimise relapse, iatrogenic nerve injury and complications. As with all orthognathic surgery, successful treatment relies on making the correct diagnosis to address the patient concerns and underlying aetiology. Mandibular procedures are indicated for dentofacial abnormality, correction of post-traumatic deformity, surgical treatment of obstructive sleep apnoea (OSA) and can be used in combination with temporomandibular joint (TMJ) replacement in cases of condylar resorption or degeneration.

Surgical techniques include a bilateral sagittal split osteotomy (BSSO), vertical subsigmoid osteotomy (VSSO) as well as inverted L and subapical osteotomies.

ESSENTIAL ANATOMY

The morphology of mandibles undergoing orthognathic procedures will, by definition, vary. Careful clinical and radiographic assessment must be carried out preoperatively to avoid iatrogenic nerve injury, tooth damage or unfavourable split. The use of 3D imaging and digital planning does assist visualisation of key structures and identification of interferences with osteotomy movements. The key structures and landmarks are all present but their form and relative position may vary. Class II mandibles often are hypoplastic in all three planes and with thinner rami with reduced cancellous bone which can complicate osteotomy. Class III mandibles are often hypertrophic, have an obtuse ramus:body angle and often a thinner elongated body (*Figure 54.1a, b*).

The TMJ forms the foundation of any mandibular procedure and deserves specific assessment, investigation and care to ensure long-term joint health.

PREOPERATIVE ASSESSMENT

Radiographic assessment

The inferior alveolar (or dental) nerve canal should be assessed in terms of its position and relationship to

(a)

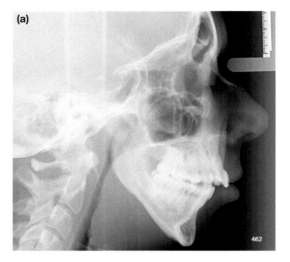

(b)

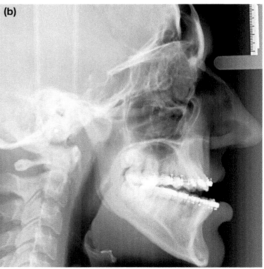

Figure 54.1 Radiographs of Class II (a) and Class III (b) mandible.

dental roots to ensure maximum protection intraoperatively. Particular attention should be paid to the canal for the Dal Pont cut and position of the mental foramen when plating.

The decision to remove lower third molars prior to a mandibular osteotomy is debatable but the authors

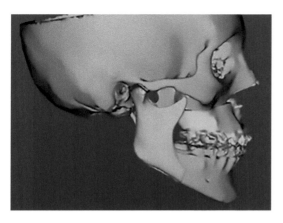

Figure 54.2 Image of digital planning.

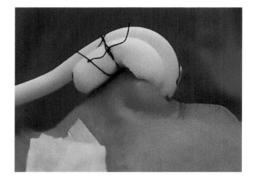

Figure 54.3 Merocel pack in place to minimise distortion of nose.

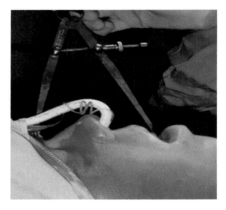

Figure 54.4 Measurement of vertical face height.

feel the teeth are best left *in situ* and removed at osteotomy time to avoid operating on abnormal bone.

Surgical planning

The required anterior, posterior and transverse movements to achieve the desired postoperative occlusion are determined in the planning phase. This can be done with choosing the final planned occlusion on study models and carrying out model surgery with the wafer produced by hand, or alternatively the movements can be determined using digital planning (*Figure 54.2*).

Digital planning, cutting guides and custom-made plates

The role of virtual planning, 3D-printed cutting guides and pre-bent plates has been shown to reduce inaccuracies and some complications compared with conventional model surgery planning. Specific to mandibular surgery there are also certain advantages. The inferior alveolar nerve (IAN) canal can be identified and hence avoided during surgery. The digitally produced plates (and/or wafers) are designed to ensure the condyle position is maintained, which is key to stability and to avoid relapse. Also, after osteotomy, bone interferences can be visualised digitally and hence reduced.

BILATERAL SAGITTAL SPLIT OSTEOTOMY: INDICATIONS AND SURGICAL TECHNIQUE

The BSSO is the workhorse of mandibular osteotomies, which has evolved to its current form from its early form in the mid-19th century.

The BSSO is versatile and allows forward and backward movements to address Class II and Class III discrepancies as well as some asymmetrical correction. Advancements up to 10 mm are stable, with excess movement being offered with distraction techniques (see *Chapter 57*).

The patient is anaesthetised with a supported passive nasal tube with minimal distortion to the nasal tissues (*Figure 54.3*). A throat pack is placed but not overpacked so as to limit mandibular setback. Induction antibiotics and steroids are administered.

The patient is prepped and draped for surgery, with some surgeons indicating mouthwash and toothbrushing to attempt to reduce postoperative infection. Local anaesthetic with adrenaline is injected by inferior alveolar block and long buccal block. At this point, standard measurements are recorded of vertical face height from a fixed point at the glabella to the fixed point on the wafer (*Figure 54.4*). The alar base measurement is recorded between two needle marks.

An extended third molar incision is made with subperiosteal dissection. If present, lower third molars are planned for removal and the incision should be designed to allow primary closure. Subperiosteal dissection is continued to the lower mandibular border below the lower first molar with extension inferiorly. Any masseter muscle fibres are stripped to allow sufficient space to facilitate the split later in the operation.

Subperiosteal dissection is extended superiorposteriorly up the leading edge of the coronoid process.

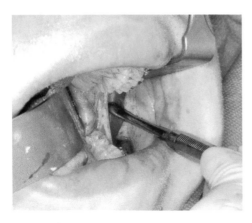

Figure 54.5 Subperiosteal dissection of buccal tissues.

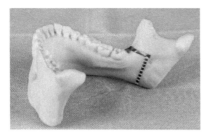

Figure 54.6 Design of the bilateral sagittal split oste-otomy (BSSO) (blue line, Hunsuck lingual cut; dashed line, propagated fracture line).

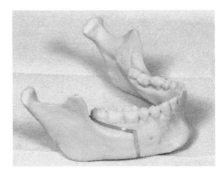

Figure 54.7 Design of the bilateral sagittal split oste-otomy (BSSO) (red line, external bone cut; orange line, Dal Pont cut).

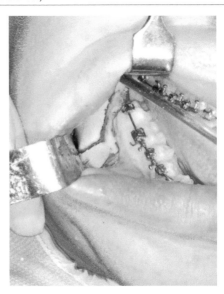

Figure 54.8 Mandible with bone cuts complete.

Temporalis muscle fibres are stripped from the bone until the crest of the coronoid process is reached (*Figure 54.5*).

Subperiosteal dissection is then continued onto the lingual side of the mandible with an elevator directed towards the sigmoid notch. The instrument can then be advanced inferiorly to allow the periosteum to be raised on a wide front to give the best chance of identifying the lingula and inferior alveolar nerve. Good light is essential and often the lingual nerve can be seen within the elevated periosteum. For a right-handed surgeon operating on the left side, this part of the operation is often best carried out from the right. Assessment of the orthopantomogram (OPG) can help locate the lingula but it is often at the level of the occlusal plane of the mandibular teeth. The mandibular foramen can vary in form from a narrow tunnel to a much wider opening.

The BSSO is part bone cut, part bone split (*Figures 54.6* and *54.7*). The first part of the osteotomy is the Hunsuck cut through the lingual cortex from the anterior edge of the ramus to the lingula or just into the mandibular foramen. Soft tissue protection on the lingual side is essential to minimise iatrogenic nerve damage. The bone cut can be made with an irrigated bur, reciprocating saw or Piezo saw at the level of the lingula with slight inferior angulation to encourage

split propagation away from the condyle. The ramus in the axial plane is dumbbell shaped, with a broader anterior and posterior band. Sometimes, reducing the lingual edge of the anterior ramus with a larger bur can facilitate visualisation of the lingula. The bone-cutting instrument is for cortical bone only and the lingual cut is then continued to the midpoint of the anterior ramus along the crest of the retromolar mandible. The idea is to be able to separate the buccal cortex from the remainder of the mandible. This may involve cutting through buried lower third molars.

This external oblique ridge cortical cut is extended to the midpoint of the lower first molar at which point the Dal Pont cut is made, once again through cortical bone and the lower border only. The correct depth is reached with the recognition of bleeding cancellous bone.

With the cortical bone cut made (*Figure 54.8*), the remainder of the operation relies on splitting the

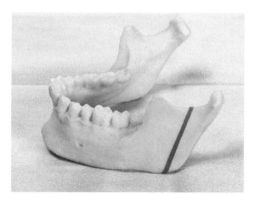 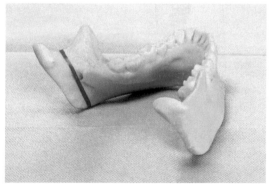

Figure 54.9 Positioning of vertical subsigmoid osteotomy (VSSO).

buccal/condylar segment from the teeth-bearing segment. The split relies on propagation of fractures created with chisels and osteotomes. A safe technique is to use a curved osteotome angled laterally away from the inferior alveolar bundle. The first applications are parallel to the Hunsuck cut, with progressive uprighting of the osteotome as anterior progress is made. Adequate depth with this instrument is often signalled with a change of tone. A lower third molar must not cause deviation of the osteotomy and may require splitting. To complete the sagittal split, the authors favour an anterior to posterior approach conceptualising 'opening a book' from front to back. It is vital to ensure the anterior lower border is free and a curved Warwick James elevator is useful to encourage this. Smith spreaders are used to control the propagation of the split with application of the tips below the IAN to separate the most inferior segment.

Successful sagittal split is confirmed with independent vertical movement of the buccal and teeth-bearing segment. Care is taken to ensure the IAN remains on the teeth-bearing segment. If present, lower third molar(s) are then removed.

For BSSO advancements, the inferior fibres of the pterygomasseteric sling are stripped from the lower border of the teeth-bearing segment. Positioning of the teeth-bearing segment is confirmed with use of the wafer and intermaxillary fixation (IMF) or custom plates. For BSSO set-back procedures, the excess buccal plate will need reducing.

The authors favour fixation with miniplates and 5-mm mini-screws, although bicortical screws can also be used. Mucosa closure is with 3/0 vicryl rapide.

VERTICAL SUBSIGMOID OSTEOTOMY: INDICATIONS AND SURGICAL TECHNIQUE

In 1968, Winstanley performed the first intraoral vertical ramus osteotomy (IVRO) to manage horizontal mandibular excess, distal segment advancement of less than 2 mm, and rotation of the mandible. Extraoral vertical ramus osteotomy (EVRO) was introduced in 1925 by Limberg to manage anterior open bite (AOB) deformity cases. In this era, BSSO and EVRO are the most commonly performed osteotomies for the correction of Class III deformities.

EVRO surgical technique

A standard submandibular incision is performed 1 cm below the lower border of the mandible close to the angle of the mandible (*Figure 54.9*). Following wide undermining, an incision is made sharply through platysma and blunt dissection undertaken. This is where the lower branches of the facial nerve are identified. Once the masseter is exposed, it is incised to expose the mandibular angle. Wide subperiosteal elevation is essential to expose the ramus of the mandible. Fibreoptic retractors are ideal as they allow easy visualisation of the sigmoid notch and the lateral aspect of the ramus.

Applied anatomy

The anti-lingula is a crucial landmark present in 44% of individuals, with 18% of patients presenting with a 3-mm deviation of the IAN either in front or behind the anti-lingula, and is a reliable identifier of the position of the lingula on the medial aspect of the mandible. Finding the anti-lingula is essential as it represents a landmark for the vertical bone cut, which extends from the sigmoid notch to the lower border of the mandible.

The osteotomy could be undertaken by a fissure bur or a piezosurgery saw/conventional air-driven saw. Careful retraction of the medial soft tissues including the IAN and vessels is undertaken.

Sufficient width of the proximal segment needs to be maintained so as to allow sufficient space for fixation and for positioning of the condylar section anatomically into the fossa to reduce the risk of relapse.

Following intraoral IMF into the desired occlusion, miniplate fixation is achieved as standard. Vertical upward force is applied to the proximal segment during fixation to prevent condylar sag.

Closure is achieved in layers with vicryl/monocryl for the deep tissues and a resorbable/non-resorbable skin suture of the surgeon's choice to maintain the aesthetics.

One of the main reasons to choose EVRO over BSSO is the reduced risk of IAN damage; however, the aesthetics of an extraoral scar need to be consented for. If a retromandibular approach is used, as has been described by many authors, the risk of a sialocele of the parotid tissues is to be considered.

In the authors' opinion, EVRO is ideal for hemifacial microsomia patients where a vertical discrepancy in the mandible requires correction. The risk of relapse is reduced with such cases due to the higher degree of control over the proximal segment during application of the fixation method of choice.

IVRO

When a VSSO is contemplated, invariably, an IVRO is performed with a vertical cut from the sigmoid notch down to the lower border of the mandible. This is known as the 'straight' IVRO. A modification has been described to undertake a horizontal osteotomy to the posterior border of the ramus at the antegonial notch. This allows preservation of the angle of the mandible for aesthetics and allows for more options of miniplate fixation. As above, the bone cuts can be performed with a bur, a saw or a piezosurgery saw.

One significant aspect of applied anatomy that requires recognition is the presence of a laterally deviated coronoid process. If this is the case and visibility is hindered, then a coronoidectomy is performed.

Fixation can be achieved either via an intraoral approach using a right-angled screwdriver, or via a transbuccal approach.

The main advantage of the IVRO is the avoidance of the extraoral scar. However, no other main advantage has been demonstrated over the years.

Advantages

- Reduced IAN injury
- Reduced horizontal relapse compared with BSSO
- Larger setbacks achievable
- More vertical correction possible

Disadvantages

- Fixation technically difficult (endoscopic technique described)
- IMF required
- Right-angled saw required
- Risk to facial nerve, cutaneous scar from extraoral approach

COMPLICATIONS

Condylar sag

Condylar sag can be defined as an immediate or late change in position of the condyle in the glenoid fossa after surgical establishment of a preplanned occlusion and rigid fixation of the bone fragments, leading to a change in the occlusion. Condylar sag is further described as central or peripheral.

Meticulous examination of the occlusion and an understanding of the occlusal changes secondary to condylar sag can reliably identify condylar sag intraoperatively. The need to position the condyle accurately in its fossa has been emphasised by the increasingly common use of rigid fixation after BSSO surgery.

Two techniques have been advocated to aid positioning of the condylar head in the glenoid fossa, either the use of intraoperative splints to try and reproduce the position of the condyles, or the use of intraoperative imaging modalities. The authors favour the former method.

Two types of condylar sag have been described:

- *Central condylar sag* is when the condyle is positioned inferiorly in the glenoid fossa and makes no contact with any part of the fossa. On release of the intraoperative IMF, the condyle moves superiorly and an AOB is seen leaning towards the affected side. If the sag is bilateral, then the AOB is more symmetrical and can extend to the posterior teeth
- *Peripheral condylar sag* occurs when the condyle is positioned inferiorly with peripheral contact with the fossa (lateral, medial, posterior or anterior). This is also known as type I condylar sag. Type II occurs when the condyle is positioned correctly in the fossa, but a disproportionate degree of force is applied to the proximal segment during fixation leading to a downward and lateral movement of that side of the mandible as the flexural stresses are released with the release of the IMF

Condylar sag should be recognisable intraoperatively as the malocclusions produced are reliably predictable as described above.

Several techniques have been described to prevent condylar sag by meticulous positioning of the proximal segment in the fossa and by removing any potential interferences that may be stopping the split mandibular segments from freely sliding against each other.

Resorption/relapse

Resorption of the condyles is closely related and almost synonymous with relapse. The mechanism of relapse is well understood, and the vectoral resorption of the condylar heads is one of the most attributable reasons for this condition.

The degree of relapse is directly related to the magnitude of the original planned movement of the mandible and that has been well established by many authors. Several aetiological factors have been described including surgical versus non-surgical causes. The most important is pre-existing condylar pathology with potential pre-existing loss of cortication of the condylar head. Small condylar heads and a high Frankfort mandibular plane angle are well-established risk factors associated with post-operating resorption of the condyles and consequent relapse.

Management involves early identification of the problem postoperatively and attempting IMF for a short period of time. If this fails, then the authors recommend removal of all orthodontic appliances and unloading the joint to allow the condylar head to heal and remodel appropriately. Invariably, this may be a progressing picture known as progressive condylar resorption (PCR), the management of which has been well described.

It is recommended to allow the disease process to burn out while the joint is unloaded with confirmational cross-sectional imaging to assess the degree of condylar pathology while assessing the state of cortication of the mandibular condyles. If loss of cortication is evident, then a further period of watchful waiting is recommended, and once remodelling and cortication has occurred, a full re-evaluation of the situation is required clinically and radiographically as if the patient was a newly referred patient with the standard preoperative records and imaging. If the resorption/relapse is minimal, re-operating is an option; however, the PCR may be so severe that TMJ replacements may be indicated along with further orthognathic surgery (bimax or mandibular surgery) depending on the type of the malocclusion and the aesthetic requirements.

Unfavourable split

There are a number of ways the mandible can split that will complicate the operation and increase the risk of IAN injury. The ultimate goal is to ensure separation of the teeth-bearing segment from the buccal plate and condyle. Incorrectly angled cuts, insufficient depth of bone cuts or misdirected force may result in fracture of the buccal plate and no condyle body separation. The osteotomy must be completed with the use of chisels and fixation has to be adapted to the fracture pattern. This may involve IMF. Failure to ensure the anterior lower border is splitting may result in a J split with difficulty achieving buccal plate alignment with plating.

Nerve injury V

The IAN is the most commonly injured nerve during BSSO surgery, with varying prevalence reported in the literature. Most UK surgeons quote close to 100% temporary altered sensation of the IAN and the prevalence of permanent numbness quoted ranges

from 20% to 33% at 2 years postoperation. The authors quote 25% based on their own results when audited.

The mechanism of injury varies with poor consensus in the literature about the cause behind the aetiology of the damaging event. The most quoted reasons include traction injuries of the IAN during retraction to protect the nerve, to direct trauma during splitting of the jaw either with rotary instruments or retractors. Combining BSSO with a genioplasty significantly increases the risk of permanent numbness of the IAN to 42%, which is not a figure with which the present authors would disagree. Malpositioned fixation techniques can damage the nerve with a more permanent injury described by most authors.

Temporary numbness is most commonly caused by a traction injury that demyelates the nerve, while permanent sensory problems arise from axonal injuries of the nerves.

There is little consensus on the difference between subjective and objective assessment of the numbness; subjectively, most patients are numb immediately postoperation, and objectively, only patients with a visible nerve injury perioperatively show signs of a sensory deficit.

The authors consent all their patients to the risk of sensory nerve damage, and they quote close to 100% temporary numbness and 25–35% permanent numbness, with a slightly increased risk if a genioplasty is recommended.

Fixation failure

The two most common current methods of fixation in BSSO surgery include miniplate monocortical fixation (semi-rigid) and rigid fixation in the form of bicortical screws and locking plate fixation.

It is essential to maintain a very close degree of adaptability between the plate and the bone to prevent excessive micromovements, which would lead to fixation failure. A well-adapted plate is able to loadshare much more efficiently than a poorly adapted plate. Adaptation to the bone is less stringently required when using locking plates. Early loading of the mandible by chewing forces will also increase the risk of plate failure as will infection leading to loosening of the screws. Wound breakdown and consequent plate infections will lead to fixation failures.

Infection

Infection is a well-recognised complication of any surgical procedure, and plate infections are reported in the literature to be as low as 10% and as high as 17%. It is common practice to prescribe intravenous antibiotics to be given at induction. There is some variation in the literature about whether postoperative oral antibiotics are of significant value. The authors recommend a shot of intravenous (IV) antibiotics at induction followed by two postoperative IV doses of antibiotics. Referral to the local microbiology guidance is essential.

Careful positioning of the mucosal incision away from the miniplates is of vital importance to prevent the risk of bacterial ingress and consequent biofilm formation and loss or failure of the fixation system due to infection.

Plate removal is the natural consequence of infection or fixation failure. The authors quote a 10–17% risk of plate removal.

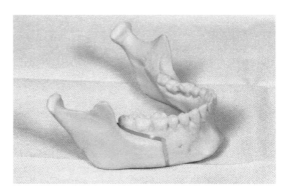

Figure 54.10 Point of maximum bone split resistance in bilateral sagittal split osteotomy (BSSO).

TOP TIPS AND HAZARDS

- Lower border stripping of pterygomasseteric sling for BSSO advancement will reduce the risk of surgical relapse.
- Condyle positioning at time of fixation is key to reduce the risk of condylar sag. Experience in positioning the condyle can be assisted with the use of digital planning with cutting guides and custom-made plates.
- Ensure all bone cuts are designed (to correct depth) to reduce compounding of factors that would result in an unfavourable split.
- When splitting the mandible, be aware of the area of bone between the IAN and the angle where there is the highest concentration of bony resistance (*Figure 54.10*).
- When completing the Dal Pont bone cut, leave a 2-mm bridge of bone at the superior end to avoid blood draining into the vertical bone cut and hindering view.

FURTHER READING

Al-Mossaissi E, Wolford L, Perez D, et al. Does orthognathic surgery cause or cure temporomandibular disorder? A systematic review and meta-analysis. *J Oral Maxillofac Surg* 2017;**75**:1835–47.

Joss C, Vassalli I. Stability after bilateral sagittal split osteotomy advancement surgery with rigid fixation: a systematic review. *J Oral Maxillofac Surg* 2009;**67**:301–13.

Naini FB, Gill DS (eds). *Orthognathic Surgery: Principles, Planning and Practice*. Wiley Blackwell; 2017.

Öhrnell Malekzadeh B, Ivanoff C-J, Westerlund A. Extraoral vertical ramus osteotomy combined with internal fixation for the treatment of mandibular deformities. *Br J Oral Maxillofac Surg* 2022;**60**:190–5.

Precious, DS. Removal of third molars with the sagittal split osteotomies: the case for. *J Oral Maxillofac Surg* 2004;**62**:1144–6.

<table>
| Chapter 55 | Orthognathic Surgery of the Maxilla |
</table>

Chapter 55
Orthognathic Surgery of the Maxilla

Ben Gurney

INTRODUCTION AND A BRIEF HISTORY OF MAXILLARY OSTEOTOMIES

Maxillary osteotomy allows independent repositioning of the maxilla in three dimensions and so can correct skeletal deformity of the midface. The history of this commonly utilised orthognathic procedure is diverse. Although initially described as an access procedure to remove maxillary polyps in the late 19th century, it was René Le Fort's experiments in the early 1900s that classified the patterns of midface fracture. This contributed to the development of maxillary osteotomy as an elective technique used to address facial deformity.

In 1927, Wassmund performed an osteotomy at the Le Fort I level to treat an anterior open bite, without pterygoid plate dysjunction, which although successful, ended with occlusal relapse. Axhausen, in 1934, described the first maxillary advance, again without full mobilisation and use of postoperative elastic traction. Further modifications followed from Schuchardt and Willmar, and in 1965 Obwegeser reported how complete maxillary mobilisation could allow passive repositioning to give a more stable postoperative result. Further understanding of the resilient maxillary blood supply was presented by Bell in 1973 and this gave confidence to the surgical community that maxillary osteotomy and repositioning could be used more routinely.

Since then, further modifications, developments in bone cutting, grafting and fixation techniques, as well as the advent of hypotensive anaesthesia and reduced surgical access have allowed the maxillary osteotomy technique to evolve, and surgical outcomes to improve. Furthermore, planning accuracy has increased with the use of digital hard and soft tissue registration, virtual surgical planning software development and 3D printing techniques.

SURGICAL ANATOMY

The paired maxillae comprises a pneumatised pyramidal body and four projections: the alveolar, palatine, zygomatic and frontal processes. Fusing at the midline intermaxillary suture, this bony structure forms the upper jaw supporting the maxillary teeth but also forms the orbit, nose and palate (*Figure 55.1*).

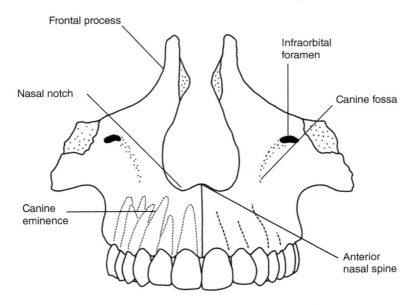

Frontal process

Infraorbital foramen

Nasal notch

Canine fossa

Canine eminence

Anterior nasal spine

Figure 55.1 Bony anatomy of maxilla. (Reproduced courtesy of Daniel R. van Gijn.)

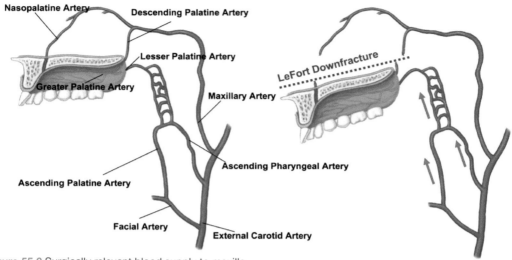

Figure 55.2 Surgically relevant blood supply to maxilla.

Maxillary blood supply is via branches of the maxillary artery, including the descending palatine artery which can be disrupted by Le Fort I osteotomy, or preserved with care. Importantly, there is additional supply from the ascending palatine branch of the facial artery and the ascending pharyngeal artery, anastomosing to supply the palatal soft tissues and gingivae, ensuring maxillary perfusion after osteotomy, providing the palatal tissues are not torn (*Figure 55.2*).

ORTHOGNATHIC TECHNIQUES FOR THE MAXILLA

Le Fort I osteotomy and variations

Le Fort I osteotomy

This is characterised by detaching the entire alveolar process of the maxilla with the centre at the inferior border of the bony nasal cavity. This creates a mobile upper jaw housing the maxillary dentition, and is the workhorse technique for orthognathic surgery. The cut extends posteriorly on a horizontal plane from the piriform aperture through the zygomatico-alveolar crest to maxillary tuberosities into the pterygopalatine fossa, separating the hard palate and alveolar process from the facial skull (*Figure 55.3*).

Operative steps

- Anaesthesia is accomplished with a nasotracheal tube, secured to the forehead
- An alternative option is submental intubation if the nose is to be better visualised throughout the procedure
- Hypotensive anaesthesia is useful, particularly at the time of down-fracture
- Local anaesthetic with adrenaline is infiltrated in the buccal vestibule

- A wire or screw placed in the superior bridge of nose provides a fixed reference marker to help measure the planned vertical maxillary change and central incisor position
- A circumvestibular access incision is made using a blade or Colorado needle. Care should be taken not to extend laterally to risk damage to the parotid papillae or exposure of the buccal fat pad
- The piriform aperture, lateral nasal walls, infra-orbital nerve and zygomatic buttresses are exposed.

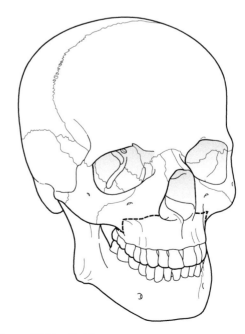

Figure 55.3 Le Fort I osteotomy.

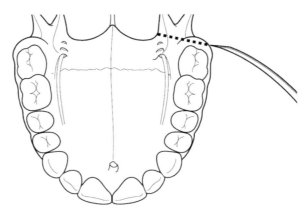

Figure 55.4 Pterygomaxillary dysjunction.

The posterior maxilla and pterygomaxillary junction are accessed with subperiosteal tunnelling laterally

- The floor of nose mucoperiosteum is dissected and protected to avoid bleeding or perforation. Placement of a Howarth periosteal elevator beneath the floor of nose, a Czerny retractor around the infraorbital nerve and a reverse Langenbeck retractor laterally will protect the soft tissues prior to osteotomy
- The hemi-Le Fort I osteotomy cut is completed with a reciprocating saw from the pterygomaxillary suture posterolaterally to the lateral nasal aperture anteriorly
- The level should be below the zygomatic buttress and 4–5 mm above the apices of the maxillary teeth. Care should be taken medially to prevent the tip of the saw damaging the nasal endotracheal tube, nasal mucosa or the descending palatine artery
- Pterygomaxillary dysjunction (*Figure 55.4*) is performed bilaterally by placing a curved chisel behind the maxillary tuberosity in an inferior and medial direction (to avoid damage to the internal maxillary artery) and controlled mallet taps until separation of the posterior maxilla and pterygoid plate can be felt
- Division of the nasal cartilaginous septum and bony septum is completed using a double-beaded septal chisel and mallet, aiming downwards and backwards. The lateral nasal side walls are carefully tapped through with a chisel
- Down-fracture of the maxilla can be encouraged by engaging spreaders at the lateral nasal side walls and applying downward pressure to the anterior maxilla. If the pterygoid plates have not been fully separated, movement of the maxilla will be markedly restricted
- Options to fully mobilise the maxilla include the use of spreaders between the pterygoid plate and

maxillary tuberosity, the use of Tessier maxillary mobilisers or Rowe disimpaction forceps. There is a degree of stretch to the descending palatine vessels, but if they tear, they should be clipped or coagulated

- Great care should be taken not to tear the palatal tissues to preserve the mobilised maxillary blood supply
- Once mobilised, the maxilla should position into the intermediate or final wafer passively and the occlusion is supported with wire or elastic intermaxillary fixation (IMF) (*Figure 55.5*)
- It is vital that all deep bony interferences are removed prior to fixation, such that the condyles are not distracted by the new position of the maxilla. These interferences may include the lateral nasal side walls, the caudal nasal septum, the pterygoid plates and the posterolateral walls of the maxillary sinus
- Maxillary impaction may additionally require reduction of the caudal septal cartilage and removal of inferior turbinates to prevent nasal airway obstruction

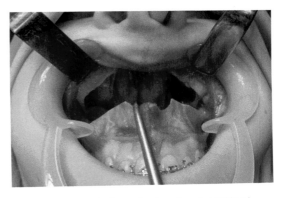

Figure 55.5 Maxilla down-fractured and mobilised.

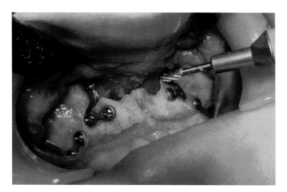

Figure 55.6 Typical fixation and piriform aperture/anterior nasal spine (ANS) sculpting.

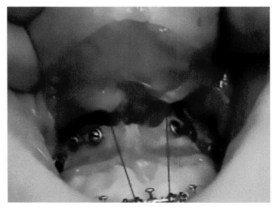

Figure 55.7 Cinch suture.

- The maxilla–mandible complex is positioned passively without any interferences to its final position using mandibular condylar rotation as a guide, ensuring the condylar heads are fully seated in the glenoid fossae
- The vertical height of the repositioned maxilla is checked against the external reference point, as well as the relationship between the anterior incisors and upper lip, ensuring there is no upward pull from the nasal tube
- Maximum bone contact in the newly fixed position will aid healing. If the maxilla has been elongated vertically, a free interpositional bone graft may be required for healing and stability purposes
- Ensure that the maxillary dental centre line is coincident with the facial midline before fixing
- Fixation is ideally achieved with two plates on each side, placed at the piriform rim area and the malar buttress region
- The maxilla should be held rigidly in the new position with no vertical, horizontal or rotational movement and the plates bent accurately so they apply passively to the bone
- Accuracy of fixation can be verified by manually maintaining the mandible in occlusion while removing the IMF wires. Observing any shift of occlusion while the teeth are slowly released is helpful in recognising a fixation error, or condylar distraction. Malocclusion secondary to inaccurate plating should be addressed at this stage (*Figure 55.6*)
- The piriform aperture corners and the anterior nasal spine can be sculpted if they are flaring the alar base
- Alar cinch suture can also help control alar flare resulting from maxillary repositioning. The lip should be everted and the fibrous tissue grasped located immediately below the alar cartilage. A suture is passed through the tissue and the pulling effect can be visualised on the alar region to ensure proper placement. This should then be repeated on the

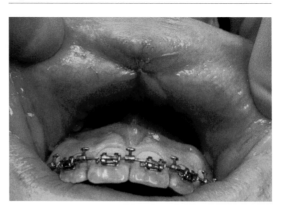

Figure 55.8 V-Y suture.

opposite side. The suture is tied to the desired tension in the midline (*Figure 55.7*)
- V-Y closure of the vestibular incision can increase the protrusion of the upper lip by enhancing its length. The rest of the maxillary incision is closed with a running 4-0 resorbable suture (*Figure 55.8*)

Postoperative care
- The patient should be placed at 45° with a cold pack or cooling mask applied to limit swelling and ease discomfort
- It is important to check for postoperative dental occlusion. Any minor interdigitation problems can be improved with light IMF elastics
- Panoramic and cephalometric radiographs are obtained to verify the planned movement and fixation

Variation: Subspinal Le Fort I osteotomy
This modification can prevent undesirable transverse soft tissue changes of the nose, reducing changes to alar width, nasal length and nasofrontal angle (*Figure 55.9*). It preserves the perinasal musculature insertions and may prevent the need for piriform sculpting or removal of the anterior nasal spine when advancing the maxilla.

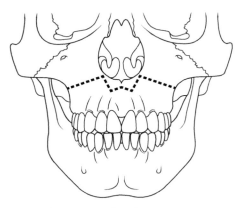
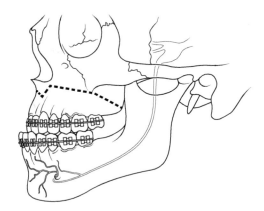

Figure 55.9 Subspinal Le Fort I osteotomy.

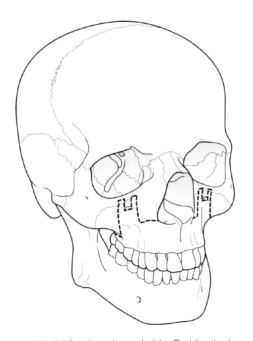

Figure 55.10 High (quadrangular) Le Fort I osteotomy.

Variation: Quadrangular Le Fort I osteotomy

If there are maxillary and zygomatic deficiencies in patients who have normal nasal projection, a high or quadrangular Le Fort I can be used (*Figure 55.10*). This cut extends higher on the anterior wall of the maxilla and body of zygoma, avoiding the infraorbital nerve.

Variation: Segmental maxillary surgery

Segmentation can be used in conjunction with Le Fort I osteotomy to move sections of the maxillary teeth independently, and several variations have been described (*Figure 55.11*). Indications include transverse discrepancy or a stepped/dual occlusal plane.

Operative technique

- If segmentation is required, interdental buccal cortical osteotomies are performed in the desired areas between roots of the teeth connecting to the horizontal Le Fort I osteotomy cut prior to maxillary down-fracture, for stability purposes
- After down-fracture, a fine bur, saw or piezoelectric cutting instrument can cut the full-thickness segmental osteotomy superiorly
- Subperiosteal dissection of the mucosal cuff, without full incisions to the attached mucosa, will give

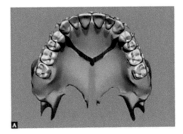
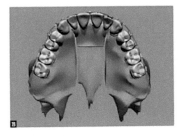
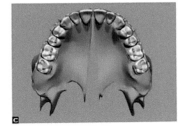

Figure 55.11 Segmental variations. (a) Three-piece segmental osteotomy. (b) Four-piece segmental osteotomy. (c) Two-piece segmental (midline) osteotomy. (Reproduced from *Dental Press J Orthod* 2016;21:Jan–Feb under the terms of the Creative Commons Attribution License. Attribution 4.0 (CC BY 4.0), https://doi.org/10.1590/2177-6709.21.1.110-125.sar.)

good access for marking and completing the segmental osteotomies with a bur or oscillating saw
- The maxillary teeth-bearing segments require arch support for healing, so an acrylic wafer is used to position the segments and aid intermaxillary fixation of the new dental occlusion; then fixation can be applied to the Le Fort I osteotomy
- A lower-profile fixation system can be used to secure the segments on the buccal surface of the bone if needed, and bone grafting can be used if there are large gaps between the maxillary segments

Postoperative considerations

The segmented maxilla should be held in the occlusal wafer wired to the maxillary teeth for 4–6 weeks for extra support.

Le Fort II osteotomy and variations

Le Fort II osteotomy

This osteotomy is pyramidal in shape, involving the alveolar process, midface and nasal bones. It is used for adult patients with nasomaxillary hypoplasia to accomplish mostly advancement and some downward movements to lengthen the face.

Operative steps

- Access is via an intraoral circumvestibular incision from molar to molar and bilateral oblique paranasal incisions or coronal flap
- The bony cuts traverse the nasofrontal suture, extend vertically downwards through lacrimal bone, keeping the canthal ligaments intact and continuing posteriorly to the lacrimal apparatus to cross the medial aspect of the infraorbital rim

- The cut is continued from the intraoral side in a downward and lateral direction to finish in the pterygomaxillary fissure
- The nasal septum is separated from the base of the skull with an osteotome starting at the level of the bridge of nose and sloping in a posterior and inferior direction. Preoperative computed tomography (CT)/cone beam computed tomography (CBCT) can help assess the midline structures and their proximity to the proposed septal osteotomy (*Figure 55.12*)
- Rowe disimpaction forceps and Tessier mobilisers are used to mobilise
- Once secured in the new position, fixation is done via miniplates and screws with bone grafting at the bridge of the nose and other areas as required (*Figure 55.13*)

Variation: Quadrangular Le Fort II osteotomy

This follows a similar outline to the quadrangular Le Fort I osteotomy with the exception of including the infraorbital rims. The infraorbital nerve tends to be overmanipulated in this osteotomy, increasing risk of permanent injury. It is used for maxillary and zygomatic deficiencies in patients displaying scleral show but normal nasal projection (*Figure 55.14*).

Le Fort III osteotomy

Le Fort III osteotomy is indicated for concurrent nasal, orbital, zygomatic and maxillary deficiencies in mostly syndromic or post-traumatic patients. Abnormalities of

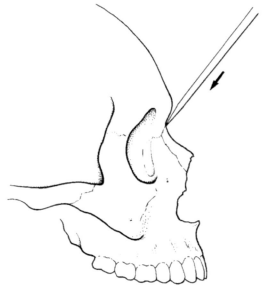

Figure 55.12 Direction of nasal septum cut at the nasal dorsal root.

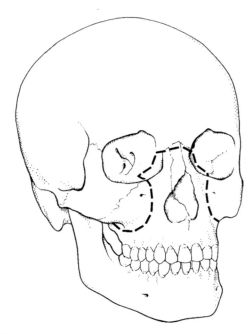

Figure 55.13 Outline of Le Fort II osteotomy cut.

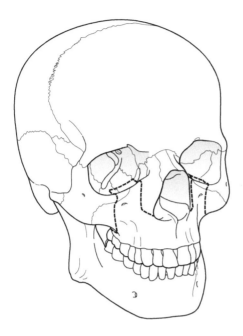

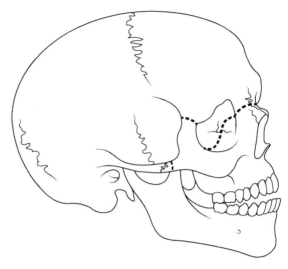

Figure 55.15 Outline of Le Fort III osteotomy cut.

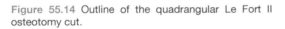

Figure 55.14 Outline of the quadrangular Le Fort II osteotomy cut.

forehead shape will affect selection between a transcranial approach and subcranial Le Fort III osteotomy.

Timing of surgery is selected on a case-by-case basis, with early intervention often influenced by severe proptosis, sleep apnoea and the need to improve the child's appearance around school age. It is important to take into account that early intervention will result in restrictive growth on the facial skeleton. Even with overcorrection, repeat surgery may be indicated once growth is completed (*Figure 55.15*).

Operative steps

- Tracheostomy may be indicated
- A coronal flap with additional access to the orbital floor requires lower cutaneous eyelid incision or a transconjunctival approach
- The bilateral bone cuts for the Le Fort III osteotomy involve the following: the zygomatic arch, frontozygomatic suture and lateral orbital wall, extending to the floor of the orbit and the infraorbital fissure
- The cut continues behind the nasolacrimal apparatus onto the medial wall of the orbit to the nasal bridge
- The nasal septum is separated from the base of skull as described for Le Fort II osteotomy. The pterygoid plates are separated from the tuberosity with an osteotome introduced from either the coronal flap approach or through a small intraoral incision in the tuberosity region

- Concurrent midfacial and supraorbital rim deficiencies require a transcranial approach whereby the supraorbital rims and the midface are advanced as a single unit 'monobloc'. The outline for this osteotomy differs from that of the Le Fort III procedure in that superior cuts run across the anterior cranial fossa to include the entire orbital rim
- Spreaders, Rowe disimpaction forceps and Tessier mobilisers can be used to mobilise, with care taken to avoid unplanned fractures which are common in the infraorbital rim and palate
- Medial canthal attachment should be preserved whenever possible
- Should there be need to detach it, appropriate canthopexy is done at the conclusion of surgery
- The face is mobilised to the planned position, with the maxillary and mandibular teeth temporarily wired together. Blocks of autogenous bone graft, calvarial, rib or iliac crest, are placed primarily in the areas of the zygomatic arch, lateral orbit wall and nasal bridge
- Miniplates and screws are used to stabilise the osteotomy and the grafted bone. Concerns of migration of metal plates and restriction of growth make a strong case for the use of resorbable plates and screws in younger children

Postoperative considerations

The decision to release intermaxillary fixation depends on the stability of the osteotomy. Dental arch discrepancies may require an additional Le Fort I osteotomy, which can be done concurrently with midface advancement, or it is often preferable to perform separately at a later date.

PLANNING TECHNIQUES SPECIFIC TO THE MIDFACE

Conventional surgical planning

Conventional surgical planning (CSP) is traditionally completed once the dental arches are decompensated, coordinated and sufficiently prepared orthodontically, so the surgical moves can be planned for the maxilla, mandible and, if necessary, the chin. However, it is possible to complete the surgical moves prior to the orthodontic decompensation, and this approach is being adopted increasingly for appropriate cases.

The key considerations with regard to the maxilla are as follows:

- *Vertical position*: the preoperative upper incisal exposure relative to the upper lip can guide planned maxillary moves in the vertical and anteroposterior dimensions. The aim is to achieve or maintain at least 2–3 mm of incisal show at rest and the whole clinical crown height ±1 mm of gingiva when smiling. This measurement depends on a normal upper lip length of 18–24 mm. If the lip is abnormally short, then plans should be made for the final upper incisor position based on the vertical proportions of the face, with the aim to achieve or maintain equal facial thirds when measured from hairline to glabella, glabella to subnasale and subnasale to soft tissue menton
- *Anteroposterior position*: anterior moves in the maxilla are usually aesthetically favourable as they enhance facial projection, but if there are concerns with respect to nasal changes, the corrective move may be minimised in Class III cases by concurrently setting the mandible back with a bimaxillary procedure. The paranasal areas, the support of the upper lip and the midpoint of the labial surface of the clinical crown of the central incisor as it relates to the forehead in profile should be observed while smiling (*Figure 55.16*). In a well-balanced face, this point does not project beyond the glabella. This relationship is universal and is consistent across age, gender and racial groups
- *Midline position*: this is demonstrated by the centreline between the maxillary central incisors and should relate to the philtrum, nose and forehead midline, as well as the lower central incisors and chin. The planned maxillary midline move may be bodily or rotational
- *Maxillary cant*: best measured preoperatively with calipers from a fixed point such as the medial canthus to the tip of the canine incisal edge. Cant correction can be addressed by impacting the elongated side or down-grafting the shortened side, or a combination of both. The 'fulcrum' position of the maxillary tilt should also be considered
- *Occlusal plane inclination*: the occlusal plane can be rotated 'clockwise or anticlockwise' (assessed from the right lateral profile of the facial skeleton).

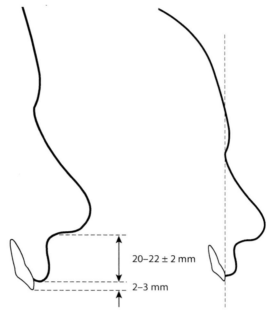

Figure 55.16 Maxillary positioning: vertical, upper lip length/incisal show; anteroposterior, upper incisor relationship to forehead.

Maxillary clockwise rotation will protrude the piriform apertures, potentially widening the alar base, and with corresponding lower jaw osteotomy and clockwise rotation may tuck the lower jaw and chin in, reducing the chin/throat distance and closing the posterior airways, so should generally be avoided from a functional and aesthetic point of view. Anticlockwise maxillary rotation may require posterior bone grafting and can reduce nasal changes and favour incisal upper lip support, but will require significant advancement and anticlockwise rotation of the mandible. Soft tissues will be better supported by a projected and vertically proportioned facial skeleton and this will be an aesthetic advantage as the patient ages

Virtual surgical planning

Virtual surgical planning (VSP) is believed to reduce inaccuracies in maxillary positioning compared with CSP due to elimination of face-bow transfer and laboratory model surgery steps. Three dimensional (3D) reconstructed data are obtained from CBCT of the facial skeleton and are merged with the patient's dental anatomy from an intraoral digital scan, or scan of poured dental casts. There are increasing planning software options that allow import of these data. Additionally, 2D or 3D photography can be superimposed to represent the soft tissues. The software can then orientate, clean up, merge and segmentalise the data so that prescribed movements of the segments can be performed virtually.

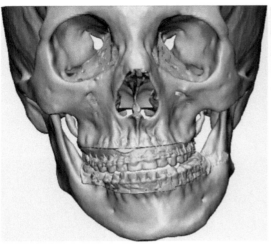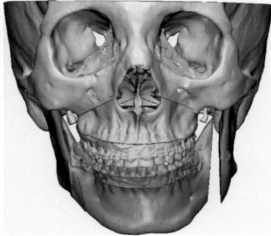

Figure 55.17 Before and after VSP images.

The huge advantage of this approach is the ability to test virtual maxillary positions and predict discrepancy between the upper and lower jaws, with relation to the facial skeleton, at the intermediate stage of bimaxillary surgery, and whether there are likely to be interferences. It can additionally control and check the maxillary midline, cant and inclination of occlusal plane. It is particularly relevant in analysing and correcting yaw deformities of the maxilla in the axial plane. Although prediction of soft tissue change is not yet entirely accurate, bony and dental relationships are precise, meaning that surgical wafers can be 3D printed once the plan is confirmed.

Meta-analyses of VSP compared with CSP have demonstrated reduced time for splint production and overall preoperative processing time, but not necessarily reduced clinical planning time. VSP is a largely office-based workflow, as opposed to a lab-based approach. Apart from the initial financial investment of software and hardware, the total cost of the VSP technique per patient is currently similar to that of CSP.

Although both techniques have demonstrated significantly better surgical accuracy for maxillary than mandibular osteotomies, VSP shows greater accuracy in the sagittal plane, and is significantly more accurate in certain reference areas, especially the anterior area of the maxilla (*Figure 55.17*).

COMPLICATIONS

A lengthy list of complications has been associated with maxillary osteotomy. This includes maxillary sinusitis, loss of tooth vitality, sensory nerve morbidity, aseptic necrosis, vascular complications, nasal septum deviation, unfavourable fractures of the skull base and pterygoid plates, cranial nerve palsy, ophthalmic complications, canthal drift, lacrimal drainage issues, malpositioning, dental malocclusion, asymmetry, non-union, maxilla instability and relapse. The reality is that complications are rare for Le Fort I maxillary osteotomy performed by well-trained surgeons, but do increase for the higher-level maxillary osteotomies, or in patients with major anatomical irregularities, such as cleft lip and palate.

TOP TIPS AND HAZARDS

- Hypotensive anaesthesia and positioning the patient with head up can dramatically control intraoperative bleeding.
- A lower or subspinal osteotomy design can significantly reduce nasal flaring and unwanted soft tissue changes.
- A well-mobilised maxilla will be more stable, but continue to check colour and capillary refill of attached gingiva when mobilising to ensure good blood supply is maintained.
- Check and double-check the maxillary dental midline with the facial midline before, during and after fixation.
- Check that upper lip/incisal show with soft tissue pull of nasal tube is neutralised before fixing.
- Ensure paranasal plates are low profile and do not extend too superiorly or a thin patient will be aware of them.

FURTHER READING

Chen Z, Mo S, Fan X, et al. A meta-analysis and systematic review comparing the effectiveness of traditional and virtual surgical planning for orthognathic surgery: based on randomized clinical trials. *J Oral Maxillofac Surg* 2021;**79**:471.e1–471.e19.

Heufelder M, Wilde F, Pietzka S, et al. Clinical accuracy of waferless maxillary positioning using customized surgical guides and patient specific osteosynthesis in bimaxillary orthognathic surgery. *J Craniomaxillofac Surg* 2017;**45**:1578–85.

Naini FB, Gill DS. *Orthognathic Surgery: Principles, Planning and Practice*, First Edition. John Wiley & Sons Ltd; 2016.

Peiró-Guijarro MA, Guijarro-Martínez R, Hernández-Alfaro F. Surgery first in orthognathic surgery: a systematic review of the literature. *Am J Orthod Dentofacial Orthop* 2016;**149**:448–62.

Posnick JC. *Orthognathic Surgery, Principles & Practice*, Second Edition. Elsevier; 2022.

Bailey & Love's Essential Operations Bailey & Love's Essential Operations
Bailey & Love's Essential Operations Bailey & Love's Essential Operations
Bailey & Love's Essential Operations Bailey & Love's Essential Operations

PART 8 | Orthognathic and craniofacial surgery

Chapter

56

Genioplasty

James Sloane

INTRODUCTION

The chin is a cornerstone of facial composition and any imbalance of proportion or symmetry can have a negative impact on facial harmony. Genioplasty is routinely performed to redress this either in isolation or in conjunction with orthognathic surgery. While alloplastic techniques are described, this chapter will focus on the osseous genioplasty which has far greater versatility of application. The horizontal sliding genioplasty, first described via an extraoral approach by Hofer in 1942, was later modified by Trauner and Obwegeser in 1957 to access the osseous chin via an intraoral approach. It allows for corrections of chin deformities in all three planes of movement to balance the chin with overall facial proportions. Since these original descriptions using wire fixation, modern genioplasty typically employs miniplates, including a variety of preformed designs and sizes giving predictable, stable outcomes with minimal morbidity.

ANATOMY OF THE CHIN

The chin can be defined by the labiomental crease superiorly, the oral commissures laterally and the submental-cervical crease inferiorly. Anteriorly, paired mentalis muscles originate from the incisive fossa and attach into the labiomental sulcus to elevate, evert and protrude the lip and dimple the chin. The mental protuberance has a triangular shape with slight concavity centrally but rises laterally to form the mental tubercles (*Figure 56.1*). Other muscles that attach anteriorly to the chin region include the depressor anguli oris and depressor labii inferioris. The inferior alveolar nerve exits the mandible through the mental foramen and becomes the mental nerve, supplying innervation to the lower lip and chin. Of clinical significance in genioplasty is the path of the nerve within the mandible prior to exiting, which can lie anterior and inferior to the foramen. This becomes relevant when planning osteotomy cuts and so 5-mm clearance should be given around the foramen, which lies inferior to the roots of the first and second premolar teeth.

Lingually, the genial tubercles are the site of attachment for paired geniohyoid and genioglossus muscles, while the digastric fossa provides attachment for the anterior belly of the digastric muscle (*Figure 56.2*).

PREOPERATIVE ANALYSIS OF THE CHIN

Evaluation of the chin and lower third of the face should be assessed in relation to the middle and upper thirds, with teeth in occlusion, relaxed lips and natural head posture. Consideration of lip position, labiomental fold, chin/neck angle, chin projection, contour and symmetry are important. Both frontal and profile view

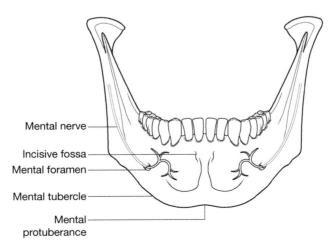

Mental nerve
Incisive fossa
Mental foramen
Mental tubercle
Mental protuberance

Figure 56.1 Anterior view of mandible showing key anatomical points relevant to genioplasty.

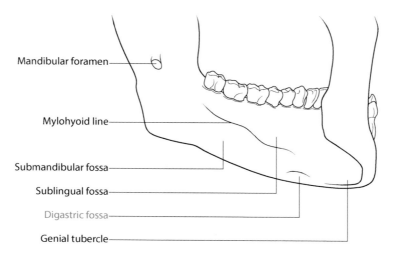

Figure 56.2 Posterior view of anterior mandible.

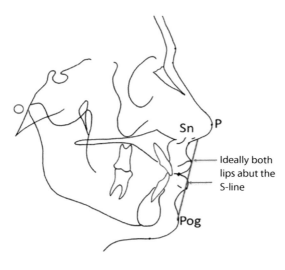

Figure 56.3 Analysis using the S-line (Steiner line) for assessing chin proportion in profile view. (Modified from *Oral Maxillofac Surg Clin* 2021; https://doi.org/10.1007/978-981-15-1346-6_66. Published under CC BY 4.0.)

assessment are vital clinically and radiographically, with either lateral cephalogram and orthopantomogram (OPG) or, increasingly, cone beam computed tomography (CBCT).

A wide variety of cephalometric and soft tissue assessment tools exist such as the Steiner or 'S-line'. This connects the midpoint of subnasale and nasal tip with soft tissue pogonion, and gives an indication of the chin point relative to the lower face landmarks such as the lips (*Figure 56.3*). These will have variation based on racial and gender norms and should be viewed as an adjunct to help planning rather than being prescriptive. Frequently, patient concerns with chin position may be associated with underlying dental malocclusions. It is important, therefore, that the patient is comprehensively assessed in relation to both soft and hard tissues to ensure appropriate treatment is planned as orthognathic surgery may well be indicated. The effects of genioplasty in altering facial balance can be measured clinically but also have an element of subjectivity, so it is vital to ensure the patient's primary concerns have been fully elicited and that there is concordance of patient expectation and surgical plan in advance of surgery.

ROLE FOR 3D PLANNING USING CBCT AND CUTTING GUIDES

Orthognathic surgery is increasingly planned virtually based on merged CBCT of the facial skeleton and intraoral occlusal scans for sufficient resolution of the dentition. This software is also used to segmentalise the chin and visualise genioplasty movements, which is particularly valuable in asymmetry cases and provides excellent accuracy when measuring the hard-tissue changes in three dimensions. Soft tissue movement does not follow in a 1:1 ratio with bony changes and, although software algorithms are improving, should be interpreted with caution on most current platforms. Patient-specific preformed plates can also be used, providing further levels of precision, although this additional hardware comes at increased cost. It is likely computer-aided planning will soon become the standard of care as technology develops further (*Figures 56.4* and *56.5*).

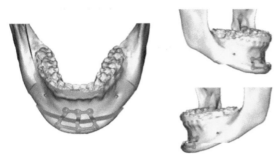

Figure 56.4 Three-dimensional planning using cone beam computed tomography to virtually plan osteotomy cut and surgical movements. (Courtesy of DePuy-Synthes/Materialise.)

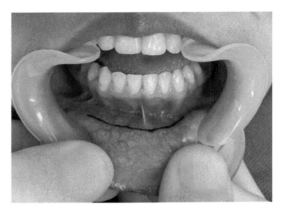

Figure 56.6 Access incision marking on labial mucosa from canine to canine.

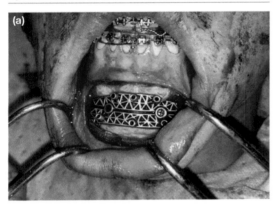

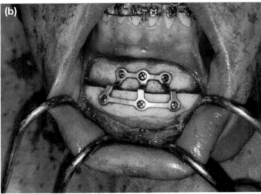

Figure 56.5 (a) Custom cutting guide for genioplasty. (b) Patient-specific preformed plate.

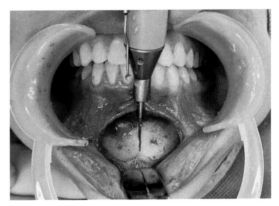

Figure 56.7 Marking of the midline with fine fissure bur.

SURGICAL TECHNIQUE

Incision and access

- Lidocaine/adrenaline (1:80 000, 2.2 mL) is infiltrated into the labial soft tissues and allowed to dissipate
- *Mucosal incision:* with an assistant holding out the lip, the labial mucosa is incised parallel to the teeth, leaving a 5–10-mm cuff from the labial sulcus (*Figure 56.6*). This incision is approximately 3–4 cm in length from canine to canine. Care must be taken to identify and protect branches of the mental nerve which may be visible superficially
- *Muscular incision:* the scalpel is then angled perpendicular to the mandible and mentalis transected down to bone
- *Periosteal stripping:* careful stripping using an Obwegeser periosteal elevator should enable direct visualisation of the mental nerve bilaterally and access extends posteroinferiorly to the lower border, preserving much of the periosteal attachment of genial segment anteriorly to ensure more predictable soft tissue changes

Reference marks

- A fine fissure bur is used to mark the midline vertically and two further optional vertical references may be placed approximately 7–10 mm on either side of the midline (*Figure 56.7*). These provide a landmark for accurate repositioning and should

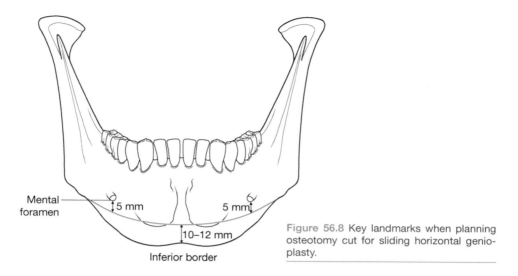

Mental foramen

5 mm   5 mm

10–12 mm

Inferior border

Figure 56.8 Key landmarks when planning osteotomy cut for sliding horizontal genioplasty.

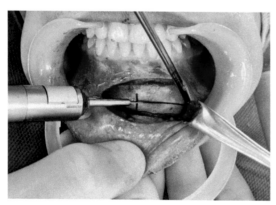

Figure 56.9 Sliding horizontal genioplasty cut.

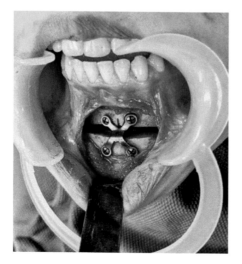

Figure 56.10 Genioplasty fixation with pre-bent miniplate fixation.

extend both superiorly and inferiorly of the subsequent osteotomy line. It is best to undertake these markings standing at the top of the table looking downwards to achieve accurate orientation. A small horizontal mark may also be placed in the midline to identify the planned position of the osteotomy cut in the vertical dimension. This should be at least 10–12 mm above the lower border and 5 mm below the root apices and mental foramen to prevent sensorineural damage (*Figure 56.8*)

Osteotomy

- An Aufricht retractor is used to allow visualisation of the lower border and protect the mental nerve while a reciprocating or potentially piezoelectric saw passes from posterior to anterior to produce the osteotomy (*Figure 56.9*) and is then repeated on the opposite side to complete the osteotomy. It is important to include both cortices of the mandible, particularly at the lower border while avoiding injury to the deeper soft tissues and maintain the same saw blade angulation on both sides
- An osteotome can be used to gently complete the osteotomy if required. For a sliding horizontal advancement osteotomy, the lower border cut usually extends back to the first molar region to avoid excessive notching

Positioning

- Depending on whether the chin is being advanced, set back, impacted or down-grafted, the inferior segment can be controlled with a Kocher or temporary positioning screw

Fixation

- Usually, low-profile preformed plates are used to fix the chin in the new desired position (*Figure 56.10*),

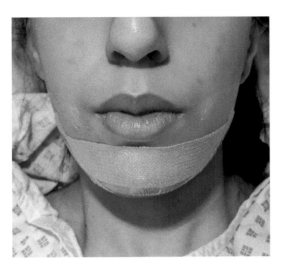

Figure 56.11 Genioplasty postop dressing.

or miniplate fixation bilaterally. Bicortical screw techniques are also described
- It is important to check the lower border is smooth at this point and ensure no winging or significant palpable steps and that there is good bony contact posteriorly. If a setback has taken place, any palpable spurs will require careful reduction with a bur

Closure

- Two-layer closure is achieved using 4.0 monocryl, first reattaching mentalis muscle bilaterally preventing subsequent ptosis of the chin and then the labial mucosa is closed as a continuous suture

- Elastoplast tape and clear Tegaderm are used to support the chin anteriorly and inferiorly to reduce swelling and risk of haematoma formation. This is kept in place for 1 week postoperatively (*Figure 56.11*)

Variations of genioplasty cut

The horizontal sliding genioplasty to advance or set back the mandible can also be used to make vertical changes altering the angle of the osteotomy cut. The steeper this angle becomes, the greater the vertical change with anteroposterior (AP) movement, for example setting back the chin will result in increased vertical height and vice versa (*Figure 56.12*).

Bone grafting for increased vertical change

If the desired vertical increase does not correspond to the associated sliding AP change, for example advancement and increased vertical height, an open book approach can be used. Autologous or xenograft can be used to increase stability for larger moves (*Figure 56.13*).

Similarly, a bony segment can be removed for vertical reduction. Changing the thickness of this segment into a wedge shape can allow additional control over the AP change in either direction (*Figure 56.14*).

Asymmetry correction

Depending on the desired vertical changes, the genial segment can either be bodily moved to align the chin point with the facial midline or an intermediary segment of chin can be removed and reversed to correct significant asymmetry (*Figure 56.15*).

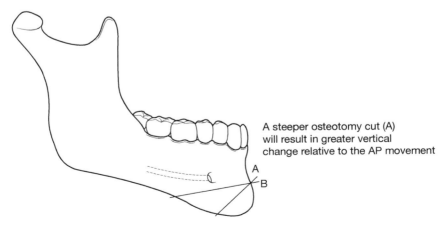

A steeper osteotomy cut (A) will result in greater vertical change relative to the AP movement

Figure 56.12 The impact of altering steepness of osteotomy cut on vertical movement.

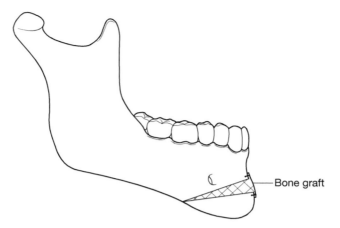

Figure 56.13 Genioplasty advancement and vertical increase with interpositional bone graft.

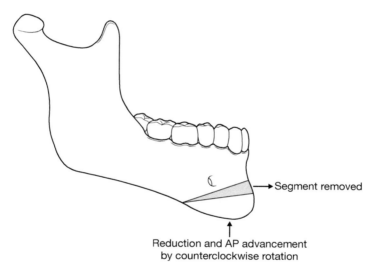

Figure 56.14 Vertical reduction genioplasty by removing a segment of bone with counterclockwise rotation of the chin point.

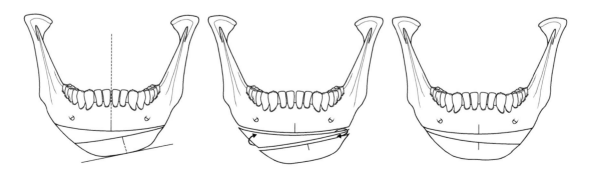

Figure 56.15 Correction of mandibular asymmetry by rotating the wedge segment 180°.

TOP TIPS AND HAZARDS

- Ensure osteotomy cuts are at least 5 mm below the mental foramen nerve to avoid potential nerve injury.
- Complete the osteotomy through both cortices, specifically checking at the lower border to avoid unfavourable propagation.
- Resuspend mentalis muscle carefully to avoid ptosis of the lower lip/chin and support with pressure dressing in the early postoperative period.
- Maintain maximal periosteal attachment over the genial segment to optimise soft tissue changes following osteotomy.
- Feel for the lower border bilaterally before closing to ensure no bony spurs, notching or asymmetry, which could be easily addressed at this stage.

FURTHER READING

Ferretti C, Reyneke JP. Genioplasty. *Atlas Oral Maxillofac Surg Clin North Am* 2016;**24**:79–85.

Lee N, Komath D, Lloyd T. Genioplasty. In: Farhadieh R, Bulstrode N, Cugno S (eds). *Plastic and Reconstructive Surgery: Approaches and Techniques*. Wiley-Blackwell; 2015:1047–62.

Moragas JSM, Büttner OM, Mommaerts MY. A systematic review on soft-to-hard tissue ratios in orthognathic surgery part II: Chin procedures. *J Craniomaxillofac Surg* 2015;**43**:1530–40.

Sati S, Havlik R. An evidence-based approach to genioplasty. *Plast Reconstr Surg* 2011;**127**:898–904.

Trauner R, Obwegeser H. The surgical correction of mandibular prognathism and retrognathia with consideration of genioplasty. I. Surgical procedures to correct mandibular prognathism and reshaping of the chin. *Oral Surg Oral Med Oral Path* 1957;**10**:677–89.

Bailey & Love's Essential Operations Bailey & Love's Essential Operations
Bailey & Love's Essential Operations Bailey & Love's Essential Operations
Bailey & Love's Essential Operations Bailey & Love's Essential Operations

PART 8 | Orthognathic and craniofacial surgery

Chapter 57

Mandibular and Maxillary Distraction Osteogenesis

Will Rodgers, Caroline Mills

INTRODUCTION

Distraction osteogenesis (DO) is a technique to create new bone by gradually separating the segments following an osteotomy. It was first described by Codivilla in 1905 and later refined by Ilizarov in the long bones and McCarthy for the craniofacial skeleton. The technique is employed in the craniofacial skeleton when large movements are required. Indications for distraction are multiple (*Table 57.1*), and can include soft tissue only distraction, which may be undertaken in the management of scarred or deficient tissue prior to temporomandibular joint reconstruction.

There are three stages of distraction. The latency stage is that period following the corticotomy/osteotomy and before active separation (distraction) begins. This period may vary according to the age of the patient though is typically around 5 days, but may be less than 24 hours in an infant. The distraction stage then commences and the bony segments are distracted. The rate of distraction is typically quoted as 0.5 mm twice per day, although this will vary according to patient factors and may be as high as 2–3 mm/day in infants, divided into multiple increments. The final stage is consolidation, that period following distraction and before the removal of the distraction device to allow for ossification of the callus and is usually 3–6 months.

DO can be achieved with either an internal or external device. Increasingly, semi-buried internal devices are preferred (*Figure 57.1*), having fewer complications and being better tolerated and less bulky than external devices. The advantages of external devices include vector control throughout the distraction process in three planes. Advantages and disadvantages of each are listed in *Tables 57.2–57.5*.

TABLE 57.1 Indications for distraction osteogenesis

Severe mandibular/maxillary retrognathia or micrognathia

Syndromic deformity: e.g. cleft lip and palate, craniofacial microsomia, Treacher Collins, Nager, Apert, Crouzon

Post-traumatic deficient mandibular growth and temporomandibular joint ankylosis

Retrognathia with obstructive sleep apnoea/tracheostomy-dependent

Late reconstruction of defects following oncological ablation

To address bony advancements with concurrent tight soft tissue envelope

PREOPERATIVE WORK-UP

Patients should be seen in a multidisciplinary setting to include speech and language therapists, psychologists, orthodontists, and relevant surgical and medical specialties to decide appropriate timing and aims of intervention. Many patients undergoing maxillary and mandibular DO have severe retrognathia with significantly compromised airway for whom preoperative polysomnography and respiratory physician review should be considered. Cleft patients should be seen by their cleft team to assess the risk of postoperative velopharyngeal insufficiency.

Standard preoperative medical work-up and anaesthetic consultation are essential. Patients may require

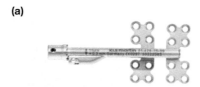

(a)

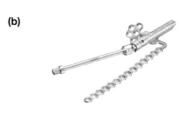

(b)

Figure 57.1 (a) Internal mandibular distractor. (b) Internal maxillary distractor. (Courtesy of KLS Martin.)

TABLE 57.2 Advantages of internal distraction devices

Single exit point for distraction arm

Allows longer consolidation times

Generally better tolerated

In some devices the actuator arm can be removed in clinic at the end of the distraction phase thus reducing the risk of infection

TABLE 57.3 Disadvantages of internal distraction devices

Requires additional preoperative work-up and is technique-sensitive

Requires patient compliance, increased postoperative care and monitoring

TABLE 57.4 Advantages of external distraction devices

External devices may result in less disruption to periosteum and blood supply

Able to distract greater distances than internal devices

Potential for three-dimensional vector adjustments after device placement

TABLE 57.5 Disadvantages of external distraction devices

External skin scars

Distraction pin loosening

Pin tract infections

awake fibreoptic nasoendotracheal intubation, submental intubation or a covering tracheostomy, and discussion with an anaesthetic colleague with an interest in difficult airways should be had at an early stage.

Pre-surgical planning is crucial to a successful outcome in DO. Imaging should be appropriate to the relevant case, although will commonly include an orthopantomogram, fine-cut CT with 3D reconstructions and scanned or physical study models. Consideration must be given to the location and angulation of the osteotomy with respect to key anatomy and with regard to the vector of distraction. When bilateral distractors are used, the combined vector of distraction should be respected to avoid interference and device failure. Although distractors can be placed freehand,

results may be unpredictable. Virtual planning allows for the production of cutting and drilling guides to ensure accurate placement of the device in sound bone while avoiding relevant anatomy.

OPERATIVE TECHNIQUE

Mandibular internal distraction device placement via an intraoral approach

- This approach is used for anteroposterior distraction with an osteotomy just posterior to the dentition
- Under general anaesthetic with an appropriate airway, and nasoendotracheal intubation, the patient is placed in a supine position with head support and is prepped and draped in the normal fashion
- An incision is made over the external oblique ridge; the length is judged on the site of osteotomy and surgical access required (*Figure 57.2*)
- Subperiosteal dissection is undertaken to allow sufficient space for placement of the distraction device. Care is taken to protect the inferior alveolar nerve, mental nerve and, if necessary, the lingual nerve with reference to preoperative diagnostic imaging
- If using a patient-specific device and virtual surgical planning, cutting guides should be placed and the drill holes may be pre-drilled prior to making the osteotomy
- The planned osteotomy may be made with a fissure bur, reciprocating saw or piezoelectric saw according to preference. The entirety of the osteotomy site must be visualised with good retraction, using for example a forked-ramus retractor to the coronoid and an Awty retractor for the lower border. The mandible is brought to the occlusal plane to improve access for the inferior border osteotomy, ensuring the whole of the lower cortex is osteotomised. The superior aspect of the osteotomy cut is not completed at this time (see *Mandibular Internal Device Placement*). Care is taken to only cut the buccal plate in the region of the inferior dental nerve to prevent damage to the nerve

Mandibular internal distraction device placement via an extraoral approach

- This approach is commonly used for vertical ramus distraction with a horizontal ramus osteotomy above the lingula, although is also appropriate for anteroposterior distraction depending on patient factors
- The patient is placed in a supine position, a bolster underneath the shoulders with neck extension improves access to the submandibular region, and is prepped and draped in the normal fashion
- Several approaches may be used including the classic Risdon and periangular approaches; the

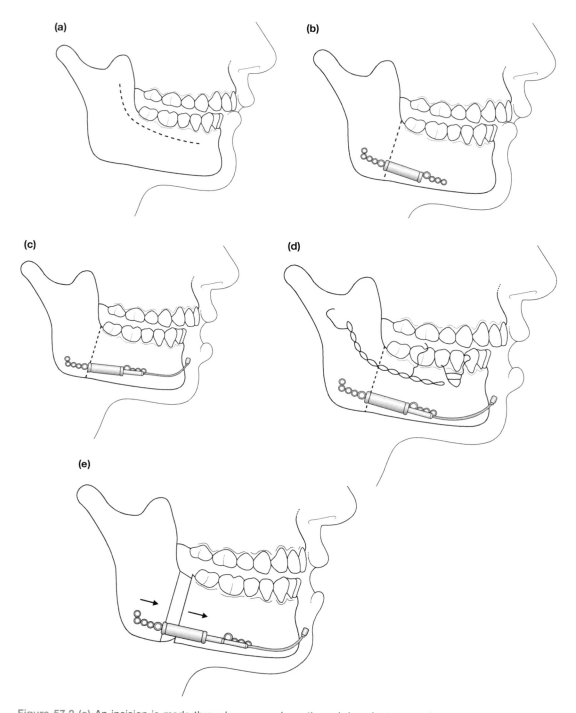

Figure 57.2 (a) An incision is made through mucosa down through buccinator muscle over the external oblique ridge. The distance is 2–3 cm based on planned surgical access and distraction device size. (b) The mandibular distractor is contoured and secured on the lateral aspect of the mandible after partial completion of the osteotomy at the body ramus junction. (c) The mandibular distractor has been secured with monocortical and bicortical screws and the osteotomy is completed. (d) The activation arm can be placed so that it emerges transmucosally or percutaneously depending on the size of the mandible and surgical access. (e) The distraction device is activated to ensure complete movement of both segments of the mandible and the inspection of the inferior alveolar neurovascular bundle.

authors prefer the periangular incision. The skin and subcutaneous tissues are incised and the platysma muscle is divided, with care being taken to ensure preservation of the marginal mandibular branch of the facial nerve. Dissection is continued to the inferior border of the mandible and angle region. To provide adequate surgical access, the facial artery and vein frequently require dissection and ligation

- Subperiosteal dissection is carried out, stripping off masseter anteriorly and superiorly to visualise the site of device placement
- If using a patient-specific device and virtual surgical planning, cutting guides should be placed and the drill holes may be pre-drilled prior to making the osteotomy
- The planned osteotomy may be made with a fissure bur, reciprocating saw or piezoelectric saw according to preference. The entirety of the osteotomy site must be visualised with good retraction. A Howarth's to the coronoid notch, malleable to the posterior border of the mandible and careful exposure and retraction anteriorly, taking care not to breach intraorally, allows for excellent visualisation. The posterior aspect of the osteotomy cut is not completed at this time (see *Mandibular Internal Device Placement*)

Mandibular internal device placement

- Before placing the distraction device (see *Figure 57.1a*), it is important to open and close the device to ensure all components are functional. If using cutting guides, these may now be removed and the device placement can be checked against virtual plans to ensure fitting to the pre-drilled holes. Otherwise, the appropriate device should be selected, contoured with plate-bending forceps to lie passively on the lateral aspect of the mandible and placed *in situ* ensuring the correct vector for distraction in three planes of space (*Figure 57.2*). For vertical ramus distraction, the device is placed towards the posterior border of the mandible for mechanical stability. For anteroposterior distraction the device is placed towards the lower border below the nerve and tooth roots/buds
- Screw holes are drilled, one anteriorly and one posteriorly, and screws (preferably 2.0 mm) are utilised to secure the device. If access is difficult posteriorly, a 5-mm percutaneous stab incision can be utilised for introduction of a trocar through which drilling and screw placement can occur. When device positioning is confirmed, it is then removed to allow completion of the osteotomy. Free movement of the segments should be confirmed
- The device can now be placed; it is advisable to place at least three screws per bony segment a minimum of 5 mm away from the edge of the osteotomy. The length of screws are dependent

on local anatomy, including the inferior alveolar neurovascular bundle, teeth roots and tooth buds. The device should now be checked to ensure proper function. Bony interferences may need adjustment

- The distraction activation arm is placed prior to closure. Given the variety of options available, it is important to be familiar with the system being used, including arm extensions and unidirectional locks. The activation arm can emerge transmucosally or percutaneously depending on access and patient factors. If it is elected to have the activation arm exit percutaneously, a small incision is made and an artery clip can be tunnelled to deliver the arm ensuring no soft tissue drag. Typically, the arm is sited posteroinferior to the ear or transmucosally for anteroposterior distraction, although it may also exit in submental area; however, scarring can be an issue.. For vertical distraction, the arm exits in the submandibular area, either retroauricular or superior to the root of the helix. The authors' preference is for percutaneous exit of the distractor arm, which is better tolerated by patients
- If concurrent contralateral distraction is required, the second device should also be placed and function should be confirmed in tandem prior to closure
- Irrigation is carried out after haemostasis is achieved. Intraorally, the mucosa is closed with 3/0 or 4/0 vicryl. Extraorally, the tissues are closed in layers, platysma 3/0 vicryl, subcutaneous tissue 4/0 vicryl and skin with 5/0 monofilament nylon or vicryl rapide

Mandibular external distraction device placement via a combined intra-/extraoral approach

- The intraoral approach is performed and the planned osteotomy is partially completed as previously described
- Percutaneous stab incisions are made according to the planned osteotomy site. Pin sites relate to the initial vector of distraction and should be placed according to preoperative diagnostic studies. Note that the skin and soft tissue is pinched between the two pairs of pins to reduce the length of resulting scar, therefore skin incisions should be positioned more eccentrically to the bony site
- On bone, the pins are usually placed 5 mm from the osteotomy site and more than 4 mm apart depending on the distraction device (*Figure 57.3*), with at least two pins on each segment. Pins (50 mm) are inserted through a trocar through the external incisions and drilled into bone with care to ensure correct angulation to allow placement of the distraction device, which can now be attached in the zero position

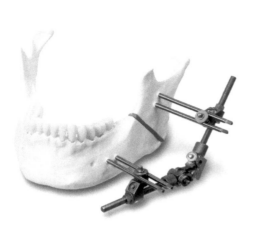

Figure 57.3 External mandibular distractor. Device can control distraction in three planes. (Courtesy of KLS Martin.)

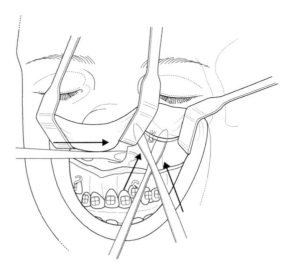

Figure 57.4 The subperiosteal dissection is carried out exposing the piriform rim, the infraorbital nerve and the zygoma, and a subperiosteal tunnel is carried out posteriorly back to the pterygomaxillary junction.

- The osteotomy may now be completed as previously described and the device actioned (see *Figure 57.2e*) to ensure good function before returning to the zero position
- Closure as previously described

Maxillary internal distraction

- The Le Fort I osteotomy described in *Chapter 55* is generally used, with some important modifications. Osteotomies at Le Fort II/III/Monobloc may also be used
- The vestibular incision should be made with consideration to the placement of the distractor arms and, particularly in the case of cleft, kept as minimal as possible
- Subperiosteal dissection should expose the piriform rim, infraorbital nerve and zygoma, and a subperiosteal tunnel is carried out posteriorly back to the pterygomaxillary junction (*Figure 57.4*)
- Osteotomy location and angulation must respect local bone quality to ensure stable application of the device and avoidance of key anatomy, and respect the distraction vector to avoid interference according to the pre-surgical plan (*Figures 57.5* and *57.6*). If virtual surgical planning has been used, cutting guides can be placed and holes pre-drilled. The osteotomy then proceeds as described in *Chapter 55* (*Figure 57.6*); however, prior to down-fracture, the left and right distraction devices are contoured and their position confirmed with two screws above and below the osteotomy. The device may now be removed and the osteotomy completed

- Following down-fracture, bony prominences that may interfere at any point in distraction should be removed
- The distraction devices (see *Figure 57.1b*) are now placed as described above and activated to ensure good function before being reset to their starting position (*Figure 57.7*). The distraction arm is attached and exits transmucosally through the incision, which is closed with 3/0 or 4/0 vicryl

Maxillary external distraction

- The approach is as described above; however, external maxillary distraction with a rigid external halo frame may be tooth-borne (*Figure 57.8*) or, more often, use bone plates attached with stainless steel wire to the external vertical bar (*Figures 57.9* and *57.10*)
- As with the internal device, plate placement respects local bone quality and desired distraction vector according to preoperative planning
- It is important to familiarise yourself with the construction and function of the external distractor and to ensure all relevant equipment is available. The halo frame is oriented parallel to the Frankfort plane and sized to fit the patient's head. Screws fix the device to the cranium and should penetrate the scalp to the outer cortex only. Four screws per side are placed 2–4 cm above the helix of the ear
- Plates are placed at the pyriform rim and wires can be looped beneath and passed percutaneously to be attached to the frame

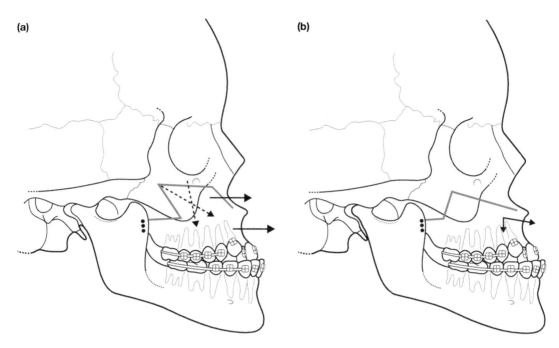

Figure 57.5 (a) The angle of the osteotomy is in the horizontal plane with a step at the zygoma for bone-borne distraction device. (b) The angle of the osteotomy will also control the vector of distraction and this is placed in a superior-to-inferior position allowing vertical lengthening of the maxilla during distraction, depending on available bone stock.

Device removal

In some internal distraction systems, the distraction arm can be removed at the end of the distraction stage. Adequate ossification in the distraction gap should be visualised on radiographs, CT scan or ultrasound before removal. The device is removed under general anaesthetic following the consolidation stage via the same approach as inset. In the case of non-union of incomplete bony infill, internal fixation may be required on device removal. This may require load-bearing plates with bone graft and should be anticipated following preoperative imaging.

POSTOPERATIVE CARE AND RECOVERY

Level of care for recovery and in-patient stay should be agreed with anaesthetic colleagues preoperatively and may include admission to the intensive care unit or respiratory ward depending on patient requirements. Early application of ice packs or a Hilotherm temperature-controlled cooling device helps to limit postoperative pain and swelling. Antibiotic prophylaxis is given per local protocol and should be used judiciously. Excellent wound care is essential to a good outcome and is started on the first postoperative day. Prior to

discharge, the patient should have adequate pain control and oral intake. A soft diet is recommended for 6 weeks. Distraction commences following the latency stage, as discussed above.

COMPLICATIONS

Intraoperative complications include injury to neuro-vascular structures, tooth buds, incomplete corticotomy and difficulty with planned distractor placement position. These can be mitigated with good pre-surgical planning. Complications following this procedure are seen in 20–35% of cases, the majority of which relate to relapse (65%), infection (9.5%), pain (9%) and inappropriate vector distraction (8.8%). Relapse can be mitigated to an extent by ensuring an adequate length for the consolidation stage. Pin site infections are common. Good wound hygiene and careful use of antibiotics are usually sufficient to prevent/treat infection; however, device removal may rarely be required. Vector modification is possible with external devices. With internal devices the options are to accept the vector with late revision or to replace the device. Late complications include growth disturbance and temporomandibular joint ankylosis. Early consolidation can be seen in younger age groups and may require adjustment to rate and frequency of distraction.

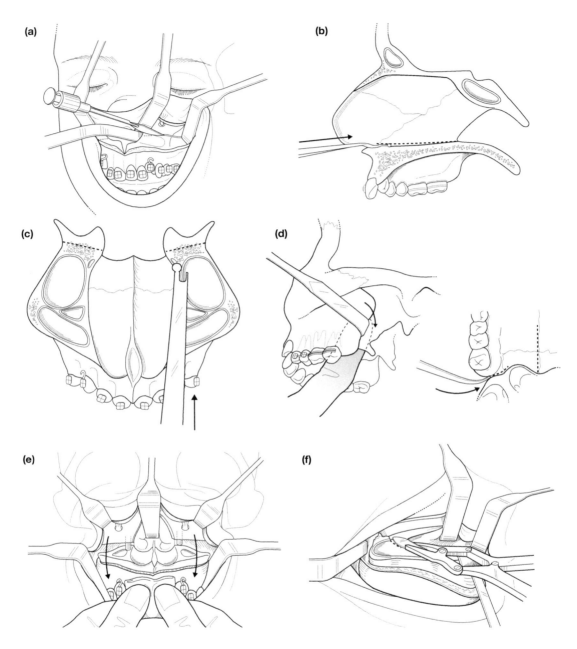

Figure 57.6 (a) A periosteal retractor is placed along the lateral nasal wall to prevent tearing of the tissues. An osteotomy is made with the reciprocating saw from the zygoma to the piriform rim at the appropriate level. With the Langenbeck toe-out retractor placed to the pterygomaxillary junction, the osteotomy is carried out posteriorly and inferiorly back to the pterygomaxillary junction. (b) With adequate tissue retraction and a finger placed at the posterior nasal spine (oral side), the nasal septal osteotome is tapped with a mallet separating cartilaginous septum and vomer from the maxilla. (c) With a periosteal elevator in place protecting lateral nasal mucosa, a spatula osteotome is gently tapped along the lateral nasal wall until an increase in resistance is felt, ensuring the descending palatine neurovascular bundle is not transacted. (d) It is important to place the osteotome near the inferior aspect of the pterygomaxillary junction and angled inferiorly to avoid the internal maxillary artery and have a finger palpating the pterygomaxillary junction from the oral side. (e) The maxilla is digitally down-fractured with pressure on the anterior maxilla and midface. Extensive mobilisation is not required, just enough to free up the maxilla. (f) It is advisable to remove the sinus mucosa from the inferior aspect of the maxillary sinus and to remove any bony irregularities along the Le Fort I cut that may impede distraction movement.

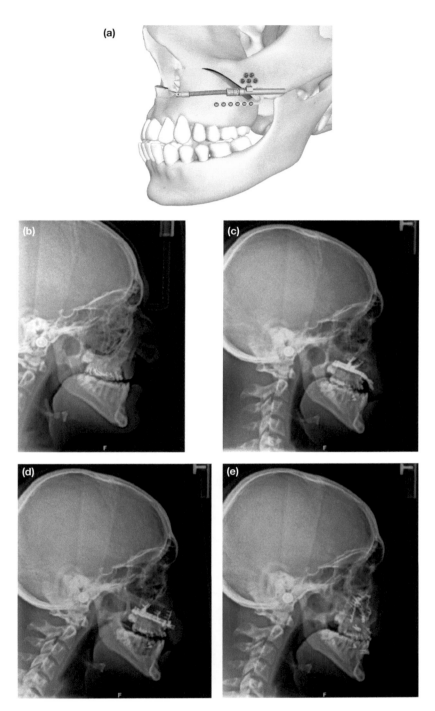

Figure 57.7 Bone-borne distractor after osteotomy and placement. (Courtesy of KLS Martin.) (a) Bone-borne maxillary distractor. (b) Preoperative showing severe maxillary hypoplasia in keeping with cleft diagnosis. (c) At the start of distraction. (d) At the end of distraction. (e) Following removal of distractors and definitive fixation.

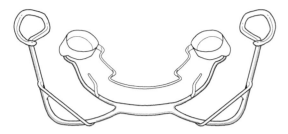

Figure 57.8 Orthodontic device to be cemented onto molars with external arms to be connected to external distraction.

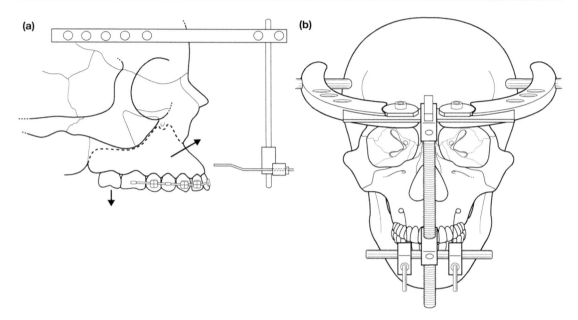

Figure 57.9 Rigid external distractor (RED) device with attachment. (a) Lateral view. (b) Front view. (Courtesy of KLS Martin.)

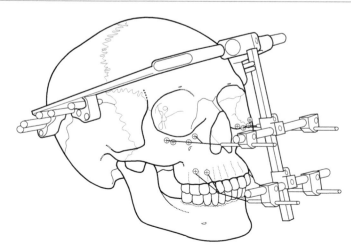

Figure 57.10 Halo frame external distractor with bone plate attachments on the maxilla and midface. (Courtesy of KLS Martin.)

TOP TIPS AND HAZARDS

- When using external distraction, scarring of the tissue can be limited by gathering the soft tissues towards the osteotomy site to reduce tension during distraction.

- Beware that if planning virtually, the condyles can be inadequately imaged on cone beam CT and medical CT may be preferred.

- Special attention must be paid to the cleft cohort, including knowledge of relevant surgical history, such as a pharyngeal flap which may change airway plan, and thorough preoperative speech assessment with lateral videofluoroscopy and/or fibreoptic nasopharyngoscopy as preferred.

- Ensure screw placement is more than 5 mm from the osteotomy site with correct angulation to avoid trespassing the osteotomy.

- When using cutting guides, ensure passive placement without distortion prior to pre-drilling holes and making the osteotomy. Additional time spent confirming placement will not be wasted.

- Following contouring of an internal distraction device, it is important to confirm that the device is still able to traverse the full length of distraction. Excessive contouring of the device can lead to device failure.

- Following consolidation and removal of maxillary distractors, it is important to confirm stability of the maxilla and, if any concern, to secure with plates and consider the use of bone grafts.

- Familiarise yourself with the devices preoperatively and ensure all relevant equipment is available.

- Review the CT imaging preoperatively to ensure sound bone placement for internal and external devices and particularly with respect to the calvarium for placement of the rigid external distractor device.

FURTHER READING

Davidson EH, Brown D, Shetye PR, et al. The evolution of mandibular distraction: device selection. *Plast Reconstr Surg* 2010;**126**:2061–70.

Guerrero CA, Arnaud E. Osteodistraction: the present and the future. In: Brennan PA, Schliephake H, Ghali GE, Cascarini L. *Maxillofacial Surgery* 3rd Edition. Elsevier; 2016.

Ilizarov GA. The tension-stress effect on the genesis and growth of tissues. Part II. *Clin Orthop Relat Res* 1989;**239**:263–85.

Master DL, Hanson PR, Gosain AK. Complications of mandibular distraction osteogenesis. *J Craniofac Surg* 2010;**21**:1565–70.

McCarthy JG. *Craniofacial Distraction*. Springer; 2017.

Chapter

58

Surgical Management of Craniosynostosis

Martin Evans

INTRODUCTION

Craniosynostosis, the premature fusion of sutures of the cranial vault or skull base *in utero*, is a rare condition affecting approximately 1:2000–1:2500 live births in the UK and Europe. Cranial sutures, located between calvarial bone plates, are important sites of rapid calvarial growth in the first 2 years of life (*Figure 58.1*). This sutural bone formation and consequent calvarial growth occurs due to brain expansion which induces growth at the sutural interface. In patients with poor 'brain drive', such as in cases of microcephaly or over-shunted hydrocephalic infants and children, calvarial expansion is reduced or absent.

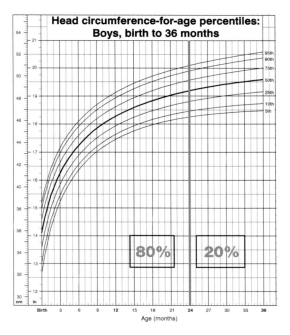

Figure 58.1 Growth chart – 'head circumference', showing rapid increase in head circumference hence calvarial growth in the first 2 years of life. (Modified from the National Center for Health Statistics in collaboration with the National Center for Chronic Disease Prevention and Health Promotion [2000].)

Following the early years of life, sutural bony expansion becomes less important, and further calvarial growth is more dependent on appositional bone deposition and internal resorption.

Premature fusion of the bones of the skull (craniosynostosis) can impede calvarial growth and cause distortion of the normal shape of the skull in infancy and beyond.

Craniosynostosis can be broadly subdivided into non-syndromic, single-suture types or more complex multisuture/syndromic types. The syndromic craniosynostoses will have other manifestations specific to the condition in many cases. There are known to be at least 150 genetic conditions that have craniosynostotic phenotypes, and the coronal cranial sutures are most commonly fused in these cases, with other cranial sutures being less frequently involved.

The rare nature of non-syndromic craniosynostosis, with a prevalence of approximately 1:2000 live births, and of the syndromic craniosynostosis conditions, such as Crouzon syndrome (1:25000 live births) or Apert syndrome (1:100000 live births), mandates that management of the cases should be dealt with in craniofacial centres that offer the full multidisciplinary team of surgeons – neurosurgery/plastics/maxillofacial surgeons plus ophthalmic surgeons/otolaryngologists, skilled anaesthetists and allied health professionals such as speech and language therapists, clinical nurse specialists and psychologists.

CLINICAL MANIFESTATIONS OF CRANIOSYNOSTOSIS

The clinical manifestations of craniosynostosis include:

● Raised intracranial pressure (ICP)
● Airway issues
● Ocular issues
● Neurodevelopmental limitations
● Psychosocial difficulties (including aesthetic compromise)

Figure 58.2 illustrates the effect on calvarial bone of raised ICP in a child with Crouzon syndrome. Bony lacunae and bony perforations are evident.

Adverse sequelae as listed above are more prevalent in syndromic craniosynostosis, although non-syndromic

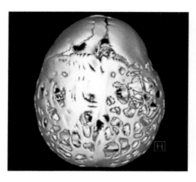
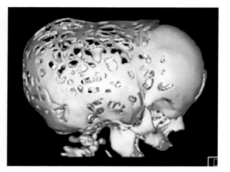

Figure 58.2 Effect on calvarial bone of raised intracranial pressure in a child with Crouzon syndrome.

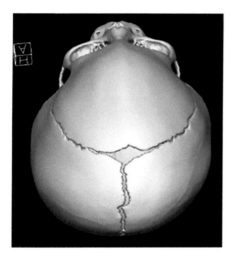

Figure 58.3 Trigonocephaly with fusion of the metopic suture visible in an infant aged 6 months. There is bilateral supraorbital recession in addition to the wedging of the forehead and biparietal widening.

craniosynostosis can give rise to raised ICP, and also have aesthetic challenges for the patient and parents, if untreated.

The goals of surgical management of craniosynostosis should therefore be to reduce the impact or to remove the potential sequelae listed above. It follows that this should be undertaken at the time of maximal calvarial growth, in the early years of life, to achieve optimal results.

The following will be a discussion on the types of surgical management for both syndromic and non-syndromic craniosynostosis, noting that there is some overlap in the procedures undertaken.

SURGICAL MANAGEMENT OF NON-SYNDROMIC CRANIOSYNOSTOSIS

Virchow's law describes how perpendicular calvarial bone growth to a prematurely fused suture is absent, and this leads to consequential 'overgrowth' of other calvarial bones and distortion of shape. This results in the classical abnormal calvarial morphologies seen in the various single-suture synostoses (*Figures 58.3–58.5*).

The surgical management of single-suture synostosis is usually undertaken with only one procedure necessary, up to the age of 12–15 months in most UK centres. Sagittal synostosis is managed earlier if possible. However, age of referral and craniofacial unit protocol are important in determining the exact time of surgery. Other factors that might be considered are that there is a noted increase in revision surgery in some patients who undergo early surgery and also there are known to be concerns regarding the impact of general anaesthetic on infants under 12 months. Resilience for a prolonged surgical procedure is also better tolerated at a slightly older age in these patients.

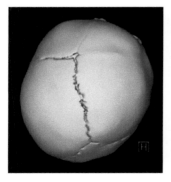
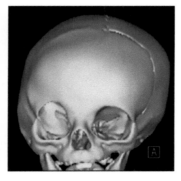

Figure 58.4 Right anterior plagiocephaly as a result of unicoronal synostosis including right orbital changes. There is also concurrent (but unrelated) posterior right plagiocephaly due to 'moulding' in this case.

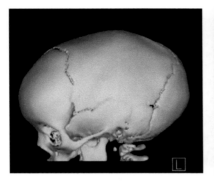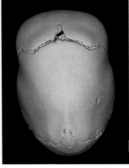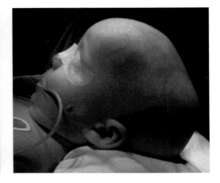

Figure 58.5 Scaphocephaly as a result of sagittal synostosis in infant aged 6 months. There is a saddle deformity, occipital bullet, frontal bossing and temporal pinching consistent with this type of craniosynostosis.

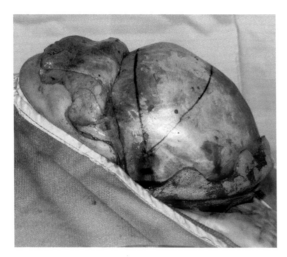

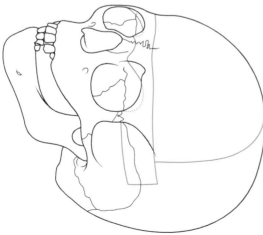

Figure 58.6 Marking of bone cuts of frontal bone and frontal bandeau for a fronto-orbital advancement with remodelling (FOAR) procedure. In this case, the patient has bicoronal synostosis. Note that the pericranial flap has been raised as a separate layer in the bicoronal flap access.

Surgical management of metopic and unicoronal/bicoronal suture synostosis

For metopic suture synostosis and coronal suture synostosis, removal of the fused suture, the distorted frontal bandeau and frontal bone, and replacement with a reshaped 'bony construct', constitutes the classical fronto-orbital advancement with calvarial remodelling (FOAR) procedure (*Figures 58.6–58.8*).

Surgical management of sagittal synostosis

There are various options for management of sagittal synostosis, dependent on the preference of the surgical team and also the age of presentation. In essence, the purpose of operative intervention is to remove the fused suture and address the anteroposterior growth excess. Procedures for managing this condition can be classified as active or passive. For example, calvarial remodelling procedure (passive), spring-mediated cranioplasty (active) or endoscopic/open suturectomy plus postoperative helmet (active).

The conventional procedure to correct a scaphocephalic calvarium due to sagittal synostosis is a calvarial remodelling procedure (*Figure 58.9*), whereby the fused suture is removed and the distorted shape of the calvarium is disassembled and reconstructed into a more conventional shape (*Figure 58.10*).

Gaining more acceptance in the craniofacial worldwide community, following the pioneering work of Lauritzen et al., is the use of preformed metallic springs (spring-mediated cranioplasty) to open up and expand the calvarium following surgical removal of a fused suture (*Figure 58.11*). The advantage of this type of procedure is it is less morbid and more time-efficient, and hence postoperative recovery of the infant is more rapid. In addition, multiple springs can be applied to multiple sites in the calvarium offering a more uniform expansion, if desired.

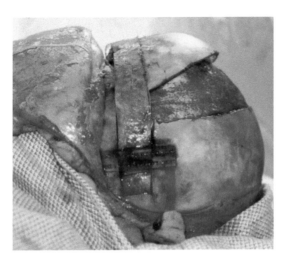

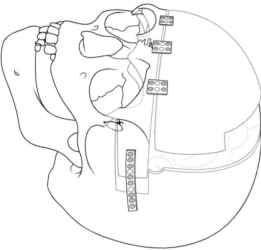

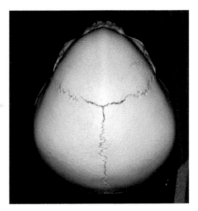

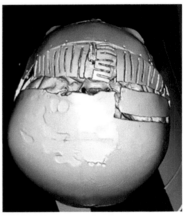

Figure 58.8 Three-dimensional reconstructed computed tomography scans showing trigonocephaly. Postoperative fronto-orbital advancement with remodelling (FOAR) and the shape, position and fixation of the bony construct in the same patient.

Figure 58.7 Advancement (fronto-orbital advancement with remodelling, FOAR) of the bony construct to the desired position addressing anteroposterior concerns, and expanding the anterior cranial fossa. Fixation with resorbable plates and screws is shown.

The disadvantage of spring-mediated cranioplasty is that this process requires a second procedure under general anaesthetic to remove the springs once the expansion has occurred. There is increasing research in the worldwide literature comparing this procedure favourably with conventional calvarial remodelling procedures. Spring-mediated cranioplasty procedures are usually undertaken at an earlier age than calvarial remodelling, offering another potential advantage.

A further option for management which is gaining acceptance in the UK, but used more frequently worldwide, over 20 years in some units, to manage sagittal and other forms of unisutural synostosis is endoscopic suturectomy. This process, where the fused suture is excised through minimal incisions, relies on the use of a helmet to 'mould' the deformed calvarium in the postoperative period. Again, this procedure has the advantage of being undertaken at a younger age, and also due to the limited access wounds and minimal cranial bone excision, it is less morbid than the more comprehensive calvarial remodelling procedures described above. The disadvantage of this procedure is the need for continuous wear of a 'moulding helmet' in the 12–18 months post surgery.

SURGICAL MANAGEMENT OF SYNDROMIC CRANIOSYNOSTOSIS

In contrast to the (usually) single-staged procedure for non-syndromic craniosynostosis, the management of syndromic craniosynostosis is more prolonged and complex and involves multiple procedures in many cases. Multidisciplinary care of craniofacial patients in the UK is 'from the cradle to the grave' and

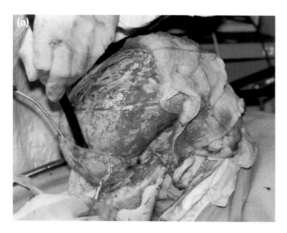

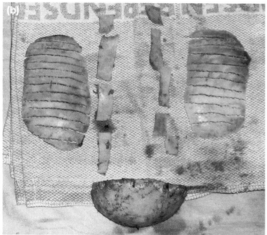

Figure 58.9 Sequence of a calvarial remodelling procedure. (a) The patient is supine with removal of the 'occipital bullet' in progress. (b) Disassembled calvarial bones shown prior to reassembly.

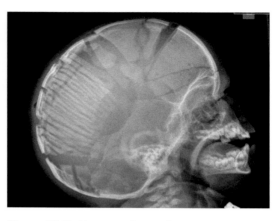

Figure 58.10 Postoperative radiograph demonstrating calvarial remodelling, showing repositioned and reshaped frontal bone (to correct frontal bossing) plus reduction of occipital 'bullet' as well as lateral (temporoparietal) panels and sagittal strip removal and remodelling.

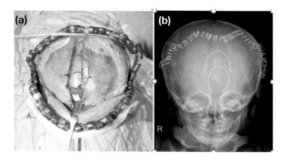

Figure 58.11 (a) Springs inserted into an infant with metopic synostosis and (b) postoperative radiograph. A strip craniectomy is performed and the springs inserted into the bony space to allow active expansion. (Images courtesy of Mr P. Subash, craniofacial surgeon, Kochi, India.)

Supraregional Craniofacial Centre funding facilitates this. In practice, however, most treatment of even the most severely affected syndromic patients is completed by early adult life.

The goals of management are geared toward facilitating optimal brain development and consequently the child overall, and this includes both functional and aesthetic sequelae. The treatment 'protocols' will vary among craniofacial centres, but all clinicians will appreciate that syndromic craniosynostotic infants and children may require emergent procedures to manage acute problems and will also require more frequent review to manage evolving clinical sequelae, as the child grows. Therefore, treatment protocols are only loosely employed, as the phenotypic variation of craniosynostotic patients, even within the same syndrome, ensures

that treatment decisions are tailored to the individual child's needs.

The functional impact of syndromic craniosynostosis centres, in the main, around the effect that the condition may have on the development of the child. Surgery is therefore designed to reduce or alleviate the effects on the developing brain – in essence providing symptom relief and prevention of related sequelae. Repeat surgery is often required in this group, as early procedures rarely address the inherent abnormal calvarial and facial growth pattern completely. Procedures undertaken may have manifold effects on the developing child's brain, for example a decompressive craniectomy or calvarial remodelling procedure may reduce raised ICP, but may also improve central sleep apnoea and improve the appearance of the growing calvarium.

Raised intracranial pressure in syndromic craniosynostosis

Raised ICP is well documented (*Figure 58.12a*) and can affect up to 67% of complex craniosynostoses. It is complex in pathogenesis, and incompletely understood, but is thought to be an interaction between cranio-cephalic mismatch, a restrictive growth pattern and an expanding brain demanding more space, venous hypertension as a result of reduction in the diameter of skull base foraminae and cerebrospinal fluid (CSF) flow-dynamic disorders.

Surgery to manage raised ICP/intracranial hypertension might include one or more of:

- *Decompressive calvariectomy*: removal of bone to allow brain expansion (*Figure 58.12b*)
- *Posterior calvarial expansion (posterior calvarial vault release - PCVR, or posterior calvarial distraction - PCVD)*: to increase both infratentorial and supratentorial volume (*Figure 58.13*)
- *Endoscopic third ventriculostomy (ETV) or an extra ventricular shunting procedure*: to improve CSF flow dynamics

Obstructive sleep apnoea/ airway obstruction in syndromic craniosynostosis

Obstructive pathology of the upper airways is present in up to 68% of syndromic craniosynostosis patients.

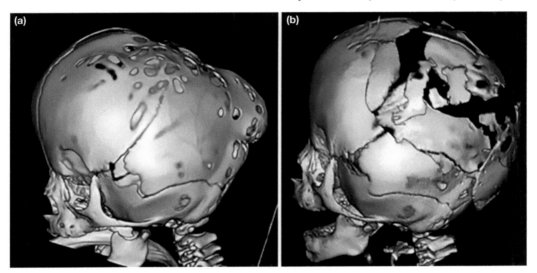

Figure 58.12 (a) Pansynostotic calvarium (3D CT scan) with signs of raised intracranial pressure (bony perforations). (b) The same patient having undergone subtotal calvariectomy – a decompressive procedure to allow expansion of the brain and reduce overall intracranial pressure. This procedure may require to be repeated in some cases.

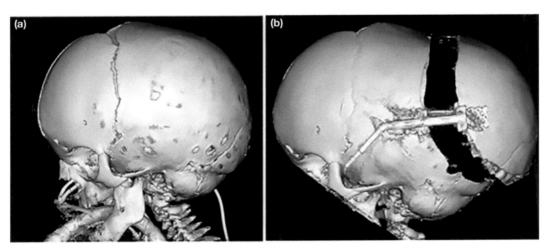

Figure 58.13 (a) Syndromic craniosynostosis patient undergoing (b) posterior calvarial vault distraction (PCVD).

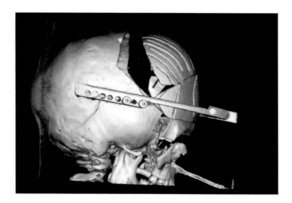

Figure 58.14 Apert child (age 5 years) undergoing Le Fort III maxillary advancement plus concomitant fixed fronto-orbital advancement with external rigid distractor frame *in situ*. This was undertaken to manage peripheral sleep apnoea plus exorbitism.

This is mainly due to midfacial hypoplasia reducing the nasopharyngeal and oropharyngeal spaces. A relationship has been identified between obstructive breathing during sleep and ICP, and consequently cerebral perfusion pressure (CPP). This chronic reduction in CPP is not autoregulated, and therefore has a detrimental effect on the developing brain.

Management strategies aim to minimise this chronic insult to the brain from obstructive airways, and can include:

- Surgery to relieve choanal atresia or stenosis
- Adeno-tonsillectomy
- Soft palate surgery
- Continuous positive airways pressure via mask (CPAP)
- Tracheostomy
- Midface advancement (Le Fort III or frontofacial advancement) (*Figure 58.14*)
- Mandibular advancement to correct retrognathia

Ocular disorders in syndromic craniosynostosis

The eyes are commonly affected in syndromic craniosynostosis. A common feature seen in Apert and Crouzon syndromes, for example, is a proptosis (exorbitism). In Crouzon syndrome, this is due to the deficient anteroposterior (AP) length of the orbital floor. This can lead to problems with corneal dessication and in some cases to globe subluxation. For this reason, surgery to manage the orbital anatomic deficiencies is often required. Refractive errors are common in these patients, as are eye movement and coordination issues, some of which is explained by the aberrant osteology of the syndromic orbits. Apert syndrome infants are usually hyperteloric, and may have asymmetrically positioned orbits (dystopia).

Management of orbital structural anomalies may require bony surgery to restore normal anatomy. Orbital surgery might include Le Fort III maxillary osteotomy, to address the infraorbital and lateral aspect of the orbit or a combined frontofacial (monobloc) advancement, to address the supraorbital and infraorbital bony deficiency. If these procedures are undertaken in early years, then they are likely to need to be repeated as the child matures, and as clinical needs dictate.

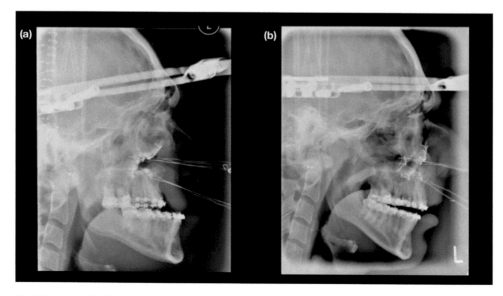

Figure 58.15 Le Fort III advancement of the maxilla by distraction osteogenesis in a Crouzon adult patient. (a) Pre-distraction and (b) post-distraction plain radiograph views. Note orthodontic appliances and external distractor frame *in situ*.

Figure 58.15 shows Le Fort III advancement surgery in a syndromic adult, compared with frontofacial advancement in the child (*Figure 58.14*). It is important to note that if the patient does not require midfacial advancement surgery as an emergent procedure in infancy/childhood, then the craniofacial growth deficiencies related to syndromic craniosynostosis will determine that facial advancement at Le Fort II/III level plus mandibular surgery will be required to optimise and normalise the midface/lower face in late teens/adulthood.

ANAESTHETIC CONSIDERATIONS IN PAEDIATRIC CRANIOFACIAL SURGERY

The infant listed for surgery usually undergoes gaseous induction and once a cuffed, reinforced and well-fitting ET tube is inserted, and secured very securely with copious adhesive tape, attention is given to obtaining intravenous access. Multiple peripheral cannulae can be secured, along with an arterial line (usually via the radial artery) and a central line (usually the internal jugular vein).

Infants/children in this age group have a circulating blood volume of 80 mL/kg, and therefore blood loss intraoperatively, due to the low volume, will pose the greatest threat to a safe procedure. To prevent blood loss, the infant can be given a tranexamic acid infusion intraoperatively. Blood loss should be anticipated during elective cases at specific points, such as when the bone cuts are commenced by the surgeon. Cell salvage (autotransfusion) is used routinely, but this does have limitations in some cases, in terms of acquiring enough volume to 'process' through the autotransfusion cycle in a timely fashion without causing undue delay in transfusion and harm as a result. A low threshold to transfuse intraoperatively is employed at the author's unit, to ensure safe continuation of surgery. Blood coagulation products for replacement of clotting factors are typically used only when more than 100% total blood volume is lost during the procedure.

At the author's unit, the majority of non-syndromic and syndromic cases are nursed postoperatively on a neurosurgical high dependency unit.

TOP TIPS AND HAZARDS

- Craniosynostosis management should be undertaken in designated craniofacial units.
- Syndromic or multisuture craniosynostosis management should be tailored to the individual patient's needs.
- The use of resorbable fixation for fronto-orbital advancement surgery prevents the need for procedures for fixation removal.

FURTHER READING

Jimenez DF, Barone CM, Cartwright CC, et al. Early management of craniosynostosis using endoscopic-assisted strip craniectomies and cranial orthotic molding therapy. *Pediatrics* 2002;**110**:97–104.

Lauritzen C, Sugawara Y, Kocabalkan O, Olsson R. Spring mediated dynamic craniofacial reshaping. Case report. *Scand J Plast Reconstr Surg Hand Surg* 1998; **32**:331-8.

Mathijssen IM. Guideline for care of patients with the diagnoses of craniosynostosis: Working Group on Craniosynostosis. *J Craniofac Surg* 2015;**26**:1735–807.

Tamburrini G, Caldarelli M, Massimi L, et al. Complex craniosynostoses: a review of the prominent clinical features and the related management strategies. *Childs Nerv Syst* 2012;**28**:1511–23.

Chapter 59

Surgical Management of Obstructive Sleep Apnoea

Tom Aldridge, Ashraf Messiha, Sirisha Ponduri

INTRODUCTION

Obstructive sleep apnoea (OSA) is caused by airway collapse due to anatomical and pathophysiological muscular changes in nasal aperture and nasopharyngeal and pharyngeal structures. The narrower the airway, the more likely complete collapse is to occur. Complete airway collapse leads to increased respiratory effort with relative hypercarbia and hypoxaemia. The increased respiratory effort also causes arousal and increased sympathetic activity with resultant tachycardia and hypertension and risk of arrhythmia. Global estimates of OSA prevalence vary but a conservative estimate is between 5% and 7%, with certain groups at higher risk. Symptoms from OSA vary in severity (*Table 59.1*) and are associated with health risks (*Table 59.2*). Apnoea is result of complete occlusion for more than 10 seconds and hypopnea is 50% occlusion for more than 10 seconds. The Apnoea Hypopnea Index (AHI) grades the number of events per hour as mild (at least 5 per hour, but fewer than 15), moderate (at least 15 per hour, but fewer than 30) or severe (at least 30 per hour).

OSA is diagnosed by clinical symptoms, questionnaires (Epworth Sleepiness Scale or STOP-Bang) and by polysomnography. These will exclude central sleep apnoea or other sleep disordered breathing conditions. The mainstay treatment for OSA is continuous positive airway pressure (CPAP) but it is important to address reversible risk factors such as raised body mass index (BMI), poor sleep hygiene, excess alcohol intake and sedative medications. For patients unable to tolerate CPAP, there are surgical and non-surgical treatments that may be beneficial.

Risk factors include raised BMI (>30 kg/m^2), menopause, male and increasing age but there are specific morphological patterns common to OSA patients.

PATIENT ASSESSMENT

The surgical management of OSA patients must be a multidisciplinary team (MDT) exercise and involve oral and maxillofacial surgeons; ear, nose and throat surgeons; orthodontists; sleep physicians; and, when required, specialist anaesthetists. Patient selection, diagnosis and correct operation choice is essential and this is only possible after thorough head and neck examination, polysomnography and upper airway assessment. It is important to consider the upper airway in three dimensions and appreciate lateral and posterior collapse.

Assessment will include:

- Skeletal/soft tissue assessment
- *Nasal assessment, external*: nostril patency, turbinate size
- *Nasal assessment, internal*: septal alignment, polyps, internal nasal valve
- *Oral examination*: incisal relationship, tongue size, tonsil and adenoid assessment and Mallampati scoring
- *Nasendoscopy*: to assess functional and anatomical loss of patency
- Muller's manoeuvre

TABLE 59.1 Symptoms of obstructive sleep apnoea (OSA)

OSA symptoms when asleep	OSA symptoms when awake
Snoring	Waking sleepy and unrefreshed
Apnoea/struggling to breath	Headache
Sensation of choking	Difficulty concentrating, poor memory
Myotonic jerks, restless sleep	Depression, irritable
Need to use toilet	Poor coordination, reduced libido

TABLE 59.2 Risks associated with obstructive sleep apnoea (OSA)

Increased risk of Type II diabetes
Increased risk of cerebral vascular accident
Hypertension
Increased risk of myocardial infarction
Reduced cognitive function

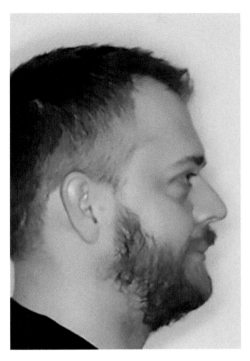

Figure 59.1 Clinical assessment. 1: short chin-neck <36 mm; 2: chin-throat angle >110°; 3: increased neck circumference >38 cm; 4: retrognathic mandible; 5: hypoplastic maxilla; 6: high mandibular plane angle.

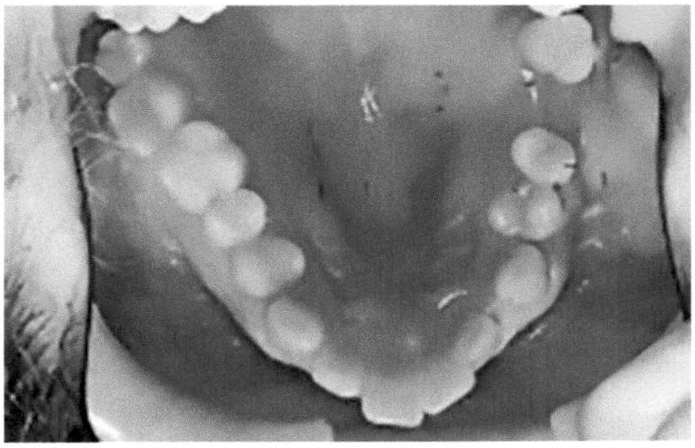

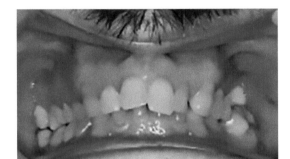

Figure 59.2 Narrow maxillary arch with high palate vault.

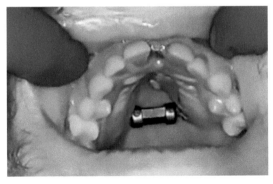

Figure 59.3 Narrow maxillary arch.

Anatomical features related to potential airway compromise (*Figure 59.1*) include:

- Retruded mandible
- Retruded maxilla
- Posterior vertical maxillary deficiency
- Repositioned tongue
- High occlusal plane
- High mandibular plane angle
- Short chin-neck line

In addition to these, there is a characteristic morphology of the palate and nasal floor in patients with OSA. These are often the findings in patients with normal **BMI** or normal neck circumference. The palate may be narrow with a high vault with the posterior teeth in crossbite with subsequent narrowing of the nasal airway and posterior nasal aperture. In such cases, surgically assisted rapid palatal expansion (SARPE) will benefit the nasal airway volume prior to maxillary advancement (*Figures 59.2–59.5*).

Volumetric assessment

Manipulation of computed tomography (CT) or magnetic resonance imaging (MRI) images can isolate

Figure 59.4 SARPE in active phase.

and recreate a 3D representation of the airway to visualise the points and aetiology of airway compromise (*Figure 59.6*). By dividing the airway into superior to inferior thirds, the point of airway collapse can be identified and hence addressed. Upper third collapse requires maxillary advancement, middle third requires mandibular advancement and lower third requires genioplasty or hyoid advancement. In reality, all three are often advanced.

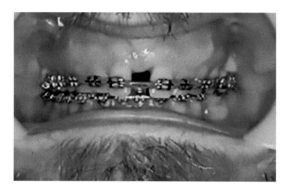

Figure 59.5 Widened maxillary arch at end of pre-surgical orthodontic phase.

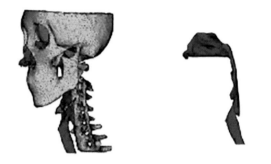

Figure 59.6 Reconstruction of airway.

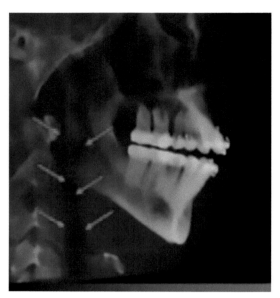

Figure 59.7 Lateral cephalogram showing airway dimensions.

be recorded. Orthopantomogram (OPG) and lateral cephalomatic assessment (*Figure 59.7*) can help to diagnose a dentofacial deformity. The anterior-posterior distance from the tongue base pharyngeal wall can also be assessed.

The goal of these assessments is to identify the point of airway compromise and hence find the simplest intervention to correct it. Recreating the airway collapse in an awake supine patient can be difficult and further investigation may be required. Drug-induced sleep nasendoscopy can be helpful, especially to identify patients with multilevel collapse.

Historically, a systematic approach advising a conservative Phase 1 with uvulopalatopharyngoplasty and/or mandibular osteotomy with genioglossus advancement-hyoid myotomy and suspension has been successful for a substantial number of patients. However, if Phase 1 was unsuccessful, Phase 2 involved maxillary mandibular advancement (MMA) osteotomy. Some of these techniques have been superseded but the need to diagnose and individualise treatment modality remains paramount.

Investigations

In addition to a thorough clinical examination and nasendoscopy, there is a need for more targeted investigations. A full set of facial clinical photographs with full face-frontal, profile and 45°, worm's-eye view, and a record of chin and neck form are required both in terms of diagnosis and for records. The patient's BMI, neck circumference and chin-neck length should

ROLE OF ORTHODONTICS

Mandibular advancement appliances (MAA) provide a valuable and viable alternative non-surgical option in the management of sleep apnoea in patients who are unable to tolerate CPAP. MAA offer the additional advantage of being able to be easily transported with the patient when travelling and for areas where electrical power supply may not be available. Within the authors' department, an integrated approach has been developed to ensure each patient receives a comprehensive assessment from various specialties. Referrals are almost exclusively from respiratory physicians integrated with an ENT assessment where considered appropriate. Following a diagnosis of sleep apnoea and exploration of CPAP as a gold standard treatment option, patients are referred to the maxillofacial team to explore a mandibular advancement device as an alternative approach. *Figure 59.8* illustrates the OSA patient pathway developed within the authors' department.

PREOPERATIVE CONSIDERATIONS

Part of the preoperative assessment must be to ensure the airway compromise is not due to reversible conditions such as nasal polyps or enlarged tonsils. An

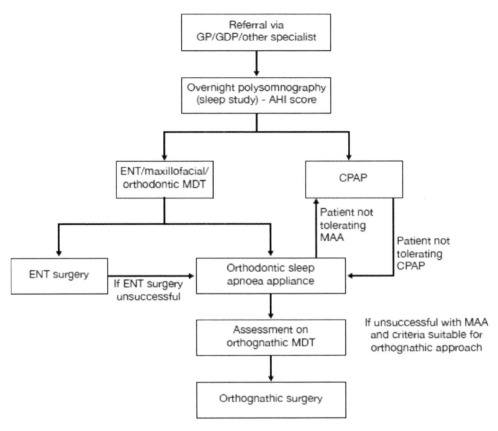

Figure 59.8 Obstructive sleep apnoea patient pathway. *Abbreviations*: AHI, Apnoea Hypopnea Index; CPAP, continuous positive airway pressure; ENT, ear, nose and throat; GDP, general dental practitioner; GP, general practitioner; MAA, mandibular advancement appliances; MDT, multidisciplinary team.

anaesthetic assessment is often warranted as there may be comorbidities related to the OSA or a potentially difficult airway to intubate. An experienced anaesthetist is essential to look after specific risks associated with OSA patients, as well as to ensure hypotension at the time of maxillary down fracture and to ensure a controlled extubation to avoid the need for airway adjuncts or forceful jaw thrust that may disturb the plated mandible.

SURGICAL MANAGEMENT AND TECHNIQUE

Intranasal surgery

Reduced nasal airflow and subsequent mouth breathing has marked effects on sleep quality. Increased nasal airflow resistance results in oropharynx and hypopharynx collapse as well as posterior tongue displacement. Although nasal surgery alone has little effect on AHI, there will be benefits for sleep quality and it may contribute to treatment of OSA when combined with other airway treatments. Findings of septal deviation,

turbinate hypertrophy and valve dysfunction can be addressed with septoplasty, turbinoplasty or valve reconstruction.

Oropharynx surgery

Soft palate collapse remains the main focus for many clinicians treating OSA with uvulopalatopharyngoplasty (UPPP) being the most commonly used operation for OSA worldwide. Multiple variations of the original non-ablative technique have evolved to address the individual patterns of airway collapse.

Tongue base surgery

In cases with large lingual tonsils, the use of transoral robotic surgery (TORS) to remove the excess tissue with laser or cutting diathermy has been shown to be beneficial in 75% of non-obese and 50% of obese patients. In the authors' experience, the procedure has significant morbidity with postoperative pain.

An alternative approach to achieve tongue base level airway improvement is to advance the genioglossus muscle with osteotomy of the genial tubercle.

This is rarely in isolation but with MMA to maximise hypopharynx enlargement and to improve postoperative facial profile.

Maxillary mandibular advancement

MMA is becoming the mainstay of surgical management of OSA with a counterclockwise rotation to maximise airway expansion and to minimise negative aesthetic changes. The surgical steps in MMA surgery are similar in many ways to conventional orthognathic surgery for dentofacial deformity. The movement will usually be greater and based around the position of the lower central incisors as opposed to the uppers as in conventional orthognathic surgery. A mean mandibular movement of 12 mm is required for successful correction. This requires particular attention to limit any potential causes of postoperative relapse. Results of outcomes can be similar to those from CPAP.

As with conventional orthognathic surgery, a passively seated nasal tube is required with intravenous antibiotic and steroid use as per protocol. The patient must be positioned and draped to ensure the head is naturally aligned on the shoulders and the full face and enough neck is exposed to assess the profile and chin–throat angle. Standard measurements of vertical face height and alar base must be recorded.

Mandible

The bilateral sagittal splint osteotomy is the most reliable and versatile for mandibular advancement. The surgical technique is very similar to that for standard orthognathic surgery and is explained in more detail in *Chapter 54*. The adaption for OSA patients involves directing the Dal Pont cut (lateral corticotomy) more anteriorly along the body of the mandible to allow some bone overlap after the split.

Advancements up to 12–15 mm are required and can be planned with a counterclockwise rotation to achieve a more balanced profile and more aesthetic nasal complex. Thorough lower border stripping is essential to fully release the pterygomasseteric sling to allow advancement and reduce relapse risk. Due to excess stretch to the lip, fixation may require a transbuccal approach to ensure good screw angulation.

Maxilla

The Le Fort I osteotomy as described in *Chapter 55* is well suited to allow maxillary movement to follow any mandibular advancement. Particular attention to widening the nasal aperture and to vomer reduction after down-fracture is essential to ensure nasal airflow with no septal deviation is achieved.

Chin

Inclusion of an advancement genioplasty to project the tongue base forward and suspend the hyoid is beneficial in terms of aesthetics and also to augment any mandibular movement to maximise airway expansion. By bringing forward the genial tubercle and inferior mental spine, the genioglossus and geniohyoid muscles are elevated and advanced. Various techniques have been suggested including a box genioplasty and tunnelled genial tubercle advancement. The authors favour a horizontal sliding genioplasty (*Chapter 56*) but with absolute care to ensure the muscle attachment remains on the posterior cortex.

The sequencing of the MMA can be customised to each patient. This is to ensure the point of airway collapse identified on the 3D volumetric study is prioritised. If the primary point of collapse is the tongue base, the authors suggest completing the BSSO first to ensure condyle position is maintained and any resorption is

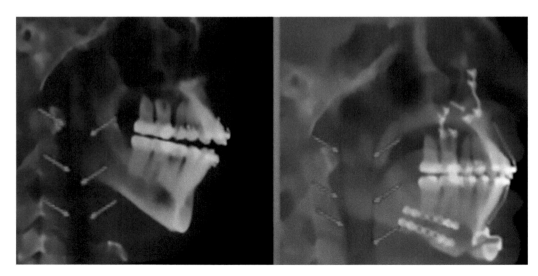

Figure 59.9 Preoperative and postoperative lateral cephalograms showing airway expansion.

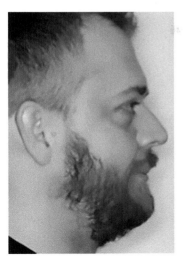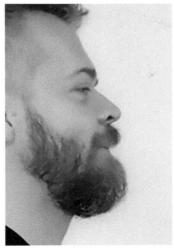

Figure 59.10 Preoperative and post-operative photographs showing soft tissue changes.

minimised. This will require preoperative consideration to ensure the correct wafers are constructed.

POSTOPERATIVE CARE AND RECOVERY

The postoperative care for OSA osteotomy patients is very similar to that for deformity osteotomy patients. The authors recommend administration of two postoperative intravenous (IV) antibiotics and steroids, and the use of a cooling mask such as Hilotherm. An OPG is taken to assess condyle position and a lateral cephalogram is taken to assess bone and soft tissue advancement (*Figure 59.9*). After surgical recovery, a repeat sleep study and Epworth questionnaire are carried out to assess outcome.

POSSIBLE COMPLICATIONS

As well as the risks of standard orthognathic surgery and general anaesthetic risks, there are specific complications related to OSA MMA. The risk of relapse of movement is higher due to the larger changes but also the risk of symptom relapse is increased due to the multifactorial nature of the condition. For example, there are changes in brown fat deposition with advancing age.

Hypernasal speech/velopharyngeal incompetence has been reported post MMA and UPPP with nasal regurgitation of fluids, but most patients seem to recover.

There is a perception that bimaxillary advancement for OSA patients will have a negative effect on facial aesthetics concerns. As some patients will have a Class II appearance, there will be improvement postoperatively with more jaw projection and widening of the chin neck angle. For Class I patients, however,

advancing the midface will upset the facial profile. By using a counterclockwise rotation as opposed to a straight advancement, this can be minimised. Patients should be warned about the potential for facial changes and this must be balanced against the health benefits of treating OSA. Most patients are satisfied, however, with their postoperative appearance (*Figure 59.10*).

TOP TIPS AND HAZARDS

- Manage OSA patients in an MDT setting.
- Maximise non-surgical options before considering surgery.
- With large mandibular advancements, lower border stripping is essential to minimise muscle drag as a source of relapse.
- Plan to sequence any operation to focus on main cause of airway collapse.

FURTHER READING

Camacho M, Certal V, Capasso R. Comprehensive review of surgeries for obstructive sleep apnea syndrome. *Braz J Otorhonolaryngol* 2013;**79**:780–8.

Ishman S, Ishii L, Gourin C. Temporal trends in sleep apnea surgery: 1993–2010. *Laryngoscope* 2014;**124**:1251–8.

Liu S, Yi H, Yin S, et al. Primary maxillomandibular advancement with concomitant revised uvulopalatopharyngoplasty with uvula preservation for severe obstructive sleep apnea-hypopnea syndrome. *J Craniofac Surg* 2021;**23**:1649–52.

Messiha A, Gurney B, Haers P. Obstructive sleep apnoea syndrome. In: Naini FB, Gill DS (eds), *Orthognathic Surgery – Principles, Planning and Practice*. Wiley-Blackwell; 2017.

Chapter 60

Primary Closure of the Unilateral Cleft Lip

Serryth Colbert, David Drake

INTRODUCTION

Clefts of the lip and/or palate are the most common craniofacial birth anomalies and are among the most common of all birth anomalies, with birth prevalence ranging from 1 in 500 to 1 in 2 000 depending on the population. Successful management of patients born with cleft lip and/or palate requires multidisciplinary, highly specialised team management from birth to adulthood. Our technique of repairing a unilateral cleft lip is outlined.

OBJECTIVES OF CLEFT LIP REPAIR

The essential objectives of cleft lip repair are the restoration of normal function and appearance of the lip and nose. This is achieved by re-establishing normal insertions of the nasolabial muscles and correct anatomical position of the soft tissues, including the mucocutaneous elements. This will re-establish the anatomic and functional balance between the soft tissues and the skeleton.

Skin: The skin of the lip is corrected in both vertical and horizontal orientation. To restore normal height of both sides of the cleft relative to the non-cleft side, it is necessary to restore the normal length of the skin on the cleft side using various techniques, such as the rotation advancement design (Delaire and Millard), undulating wavy flaps (Pfeifer), straight-line design (Rose–Thompson), lower lip Z-plasties/triangular flaps (Tennison–Randall, Skoog, Trauner or Malek), the quadrangular flap (Le Mesurier) or a combination of different techniques and principles (Fisher and Afroze). The skin of the lip on the medial element is short as a consequence of the change in normal muscular insertion and actions. Careful reconstruction of the nasolabial muscles allows the overlying skin to lengthen to the correct lip height.

Muscle: The fundamental goal of surgery is to achieve anatomic muscular reconstruction, particularly with respect to anchorage of the complex nasolabial muscles of the cleft side to the anterior nasal spine, the nasal septum and muscles on the non-cleft side (*Figure 60.1*). It is necessary to reconstruct the nasolabial muscles of the cleft such that the skin margins are not under tension during skin closure. If the primary nasolabial muscle reconstruction is good, anatomy,

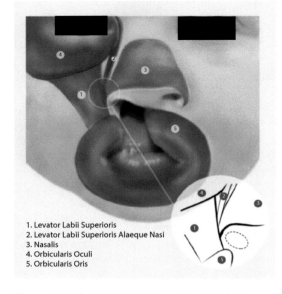

1. Levator Labii Superioris
2. Levator Labii Superioris Alaeque Nasi
3. Nasalis
4. Orbicularis Oculi
5. Orbicularis Oris

Figure 60.1 Muscle anatomy in unilateral cleft lip.

function, skeletal growth and total facial aesthetics can be excellent.

Nose: The nasal septum is deviated in unilateral cleft lip. There are two reasons:

- *Position of the anterior nasal spine (ANS)*: it is positioned towards the non-cleft side and the septum which is attached to it is deviated towards the non-cleft side
- *Muscle attachments of the medial side*: the most nasal and deep bundles of orbicularis muscle insert into the mucoperichondrium and anterior nasal spine and therefore they pull the caudal part of the septum towards the medial side

Septal deviation causes the upper lateral cartilage to buckle, depressing the radix, and also causes the lower lateral cartilagenous framework to shift and thereby collapse the dome on the lateral side (*Figure 60.2*).

Septoplasty at the time of lip repair produces a straighter nasal septum positioned in the facial midline and restores the patency and natural width of the

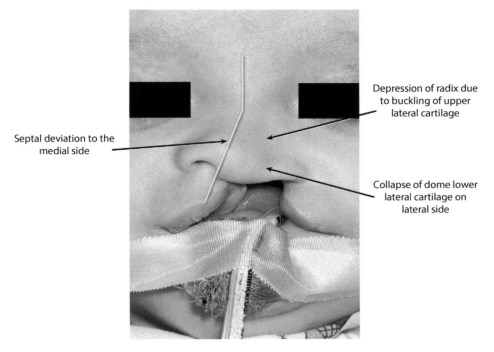

Figure 60.2 Deviation of nasal septum to non-cleft side.

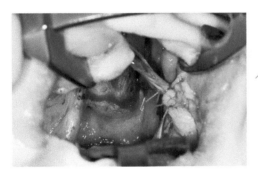

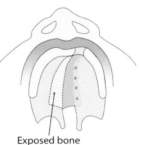

Figure 60.3 Insetting a vomer flap into the anterior hard palate.

nostril. To achieve the proper midline position and atti-tude of the nasal septum, the surgeon must perform a wide subperichondrial dissection on both sides of the septum. Once the deviated nasal septum is reposi-tioned, nostril patency is restored on the cleft side.

The nasal floor is also reconstructed to eliminate the vestibular oral nasal communication if the palate is involved. A vomer flap is used when possible to repair the anterior hard palate in continuity with the floor of nose. There is no evidence to support the hypothesis that use of vomer flaps causes restriction in maxillary growth.

Alveolar cleft segments: the distance between the greater and lesser segments is proportional to the width of the cleft lip. The segments will be approxi-mated from pressure exerted on them by the repaired cleft lip moulding the anterior element of the greater segment into its correct position.

Anterior hard palate: a vomer flap is raised and inset into the lateral cleft margin to close the ante-rior hard palate at the time of repair of the cleft lip to establish continuity of nasal floor closure (*Figure 60.3*). There may be some narrowing of the width of the pos-terior cleft palate following vomer flap closure.

OUR TECHNIQUE FOR CLEFT LIP REPAIR: ADVANCEMENT/ROTATION LIP REPAIR WITH AN INFERIOR TRIANGULAR FLAP

The authors close the cleft lip at 3 months of age and the repair involves the following key steps:

- An advancement/rotation repair of the cleft lip incorporating an inferior triangular flap addressing the medial shortening and lateral displacement while restoring normal anatomy, lip length and symmetry. The scar is positioned in the line of the normal philtral ridge
- Achieving a functional muscular repair by restoring the displaced muscles to their correct anatomical position and recreating the muscular rings of mid and lower face
- Using a vomer flap to repair the anterior hard palate in continuity with the repair of the floor of nose
- Performing a McComb's nasal dissection if required to release the lower lateral cartilage allowing it to sit in a correct anatomical position
- Straightening of the caudal aspect of the nasal septum if significantly deviated to place the septum in its correct central anatomical position

The key surgical steps in the authors' surgical protocol are as follows:

- *Left complete cleft lip*: identification of key surgical landmarks (*Figure 60.4*)
- *Skin markings*: these include:
  - *Cupid's Bow markings*: non-cleft-side peak, trough and peak on the cleft side (a point on the cleft side equidistant from the trough of the Cupid's Bow)
  - *First change in the appearance of the white roll on the lateral element*: the point of first change of the white roll and where the white roll and vermilion start to converge
  - *Base of columella*: this is rotated
  - *Alar base*: the inferior medial point
- *Medial element incision*: a curved incision is made along the short medial element. The aim is to place the scar in the line of the natural philtral ridge. The medial side of the philtrum must be lengthened to match the non-cleft length. The incision does not extend onto the base of columella at its superior aspect. The incision extends from the base of columella on the cleft side to the cleft side peak of the Cupid's Bow curving parallel to, and just above, the white line. It is curved medially and turns across the vermilion through 90° at the Cupid's Bow peak and extends just past the wet–dry mucosal junction. A back cut tangential to the inferior curve 1–2 mm above the white roll is made as the medial element of the inferior triangular flap (see below)
- *Lateral element incision*: the incision on the lateral side extends from the alar base along the junction of the nasal and lip skin to meet the mucosa at 90°.

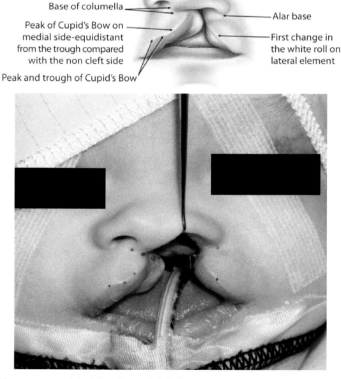

Base of columella

Peak of Cupid's Bow on medial side-equidistant from the trough compared with the non cleft side

Peak and trough of Cupid's Bow

Alar base

First change in the white roll on lateral element

Figure 60.4 Skin markings on complete left unilateral cleft lip.

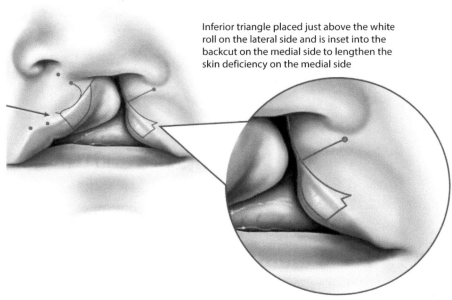

Inferior triangle placed just above the white roll on the lateral side and is inset into the backcut on the medial side to lengthen the skin deficiency on the medial side

Figure 60.5 Inferior triangle and backcut.

The incision then extends from this point along the white roll parallel to the skin/mucosal junction to meet the upper point of the lateral triangular flap

- *Inferior triangle incision*: an inferior triangular flap is incorporated along the incision in the lateral element and is inset into a backcut in the medial element to lengthen the deficient medial element (*Figure 60.5*). The triangle and the backcut must be the same height above the white roll. The addition of an inferior triangle to the advancement/rotation repair of a cleft lip allows full restoration of length without the overextension of the medial incision under the base of the columella. The lip length must not be shorter than the non-cleft columella height side at the end of the surgery
- *Advancement/rotation*: advancement of the lateral side to align with the rotated medial element (*Figure 60.6*)
- *Intranasal incision*:
  - The incision on the medial element extends at a tangent to the curved incision extending into the floor of the nose along the nasal/oral mucosal junction. It will connect to the vomer flap and the flap raised will form the medial floor of the nose
  - The incision on the lateral element is a continuation of the lateral element incision into the nose parallel to the junction of the skin–mucosal junction. This incision extends to the alveolus and sits just inferior to the inferior turbinate

Advancement of the lateral element to upper landmark to base of columella mark on the medial segment

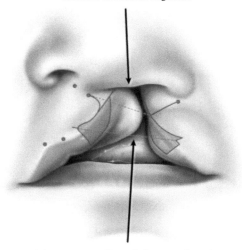

Advancement of lateral element triangular flap to the back cut on the medial segment

Figure 60.6 Advancement and rotation.

- *Sterile mucosa incision*: the incisions are extended across the white roll medially and laterally at 90° to the white roll. They extend through the wet–dry junction and then up into the nose. The mucosa outlined is the sterile mucosa

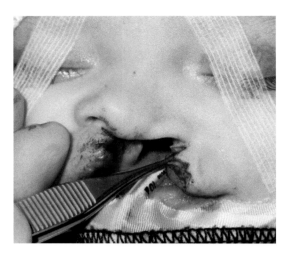

Figure 60.7 Dissection of muscle on the lateral side.

- *Advancement/rotation*: advancement rotation skin markings with an inferior triangle. The vermilion border is tattooed with temporary ink – these points act as landmarks to allow accurate reconstruction of the white roll. Local anaesthetic is infiltrated and the marking incised. The sterile mucosa is excised and the muscle edges are identified along both sides of the cleft margin
- *Muscle dissection*: the muscle is dissected on both sides of the cleft to separate the muscle from the mucosa and dermal layers
    - On the medial side, dissection of the muscle is carried out to relieve the abnormal attachments from the anterior nasal spine and the columella base allowing lengthening and rotation of the skin of the medial element
    - On the lateral side, muscle dissection is done to identify and mobilise the head of the transverse nasalis and the length of orbicularis (*Figure 60.7*)

- *Subperiosteal dissection*: this is performed if the transverse nasalis muscle will not reach the anterior nasal spine. After the muscle dissection is completed, an incision is made in the buccal sulcus up to the nasal alveolar margin of the cleft. A wide subperiosteal dissection is made from the vestibule on the cleft side over the piriform rim, nasal bone, infraorbital and malar regions to lift the facial mask, taking care to protect the infraorbital nerve (*Figure 60.8*)
- *McComb's nasal dissection*: this is required if the lower lateral cartilage buckles and will not sit in the correct position when the nasal muscle is approximated. Access is gained to the lower lateral cartilages through a medial approach allowing blunt dissection of the cartilage from the overlying skin/nasal mucosa. The plane of dissection is subdermal and submucosal. The lower lateral cartilage can also be approached from the lateral aspect if required, but this is not commonly performed (*Figure 60.9*). The McComb's dissection reduces the buckling effect of the lateral crus of the lower lateral cartilage, allowing it to sit in a more natural position
- *Septoplasty*: correction of the caudal aspect to the deviated nasal septum provides stability and exact positioning of the previously lifted alar crus of the cleft side and nasal tip. This allows the nose to grow in a balanced way with equal muscular force being exerted on both sides. The caudal aspect of the nasal septum is then carefully isolated and freed through the same cleft incision by splitting and raising the perichondrium on both sides
- The septum is detached from its attachment to the nasal spine and maxillary crest, straightened and repositioned centrally (*Figure 60.10*)
- *Nasal floor reconstruction*: the nasal floor is reconstructed by suturing the hair-bearing nasal mucosa on both sides, posteriorly closing the lateral nasal floor to the vomer flap (*Figure 60.11*)

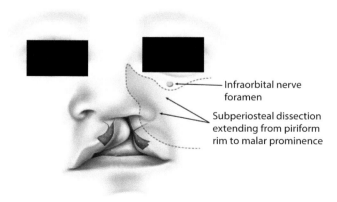

Infraorbital nerve foramen

Subperiosteal dissection extending from piriform rim to malar prominence

Figure 60.8 Subperiosteal dissection on lateral side.

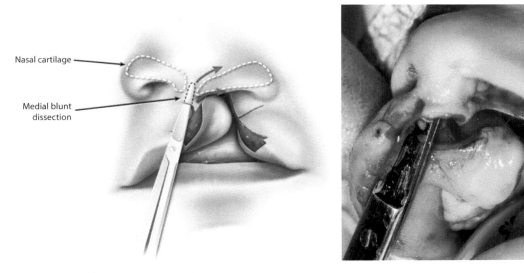

Nasal cartilage

Medial blunt
dissection

Figure 60.9 McComb's nasal dissection.

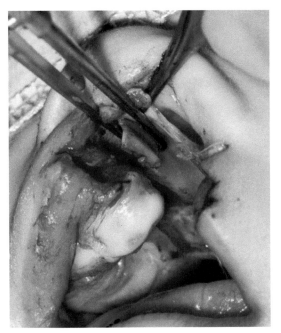

Figure 60.10 Detachment and straightening of caudal
aspect of nasal septum.

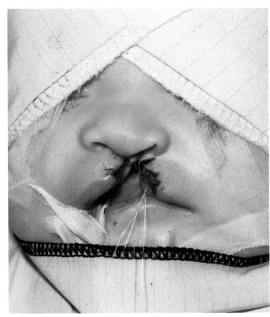

Figure 60.11 Reconstruction of nasal floor.

- *Suturing of transverse nasalis to ANS/septum*: this is to secure the position of the base of the septum (*Figure 60.12*)
- *Natural approximation of orbicularis oris*: the orbicularis is approximated and sutured to a natural position, maintaining the muscle length (*Figure 60.13*)

- *Skin closure*: tension-free skin closure is performed (*Figure 60.14*). This is made possible by the subperiosteal dissection, radical mobilisation and suturing of the transverse nasalis and orbicularis muscles

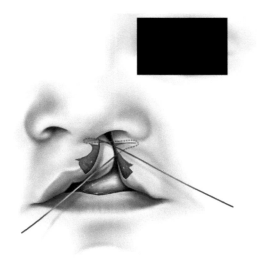

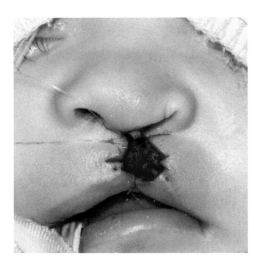

Figure 60.13 Functional repair of orbicularis oris.

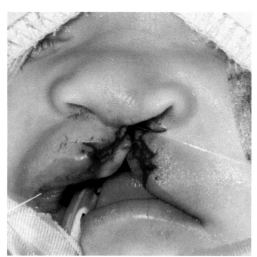

Figure 60.12 Suturing of transverse nasalis to anterior nasal spine (ANS)/septum.

COMMON TECHNIQUES OF CLEFT LIP REPAIR

Millard cleft lip repair

Flap design

The Millard repair is based on a rotation flap on the medial cleft side coupled with an advancement flap on the cleft lateral side. The incision is then bowed in a curvilinear fashion near the base of the columella crossing the philtrum towards the far lateral extent of the columellar base. In one form or another, it is the most widely practiced method today.

The rotation advancement technique relies on a 'cut as you go' strategy that allows continuous modifications during the design and execution of the repair. It does not adhere to strict geometrical principles or

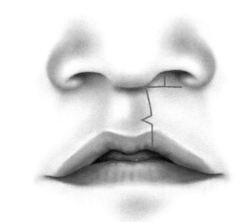

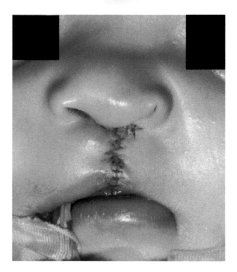

Figure 60.14 Tension-free closure of skin.

measurements. However, it may leave a scar crossing the midline at the base of the columella and cause shortening of the lip on the cleft side with resultant vermilion notching and whistle deformity.

Delaire cleft lip repair

Delaire's cleft lip technique incorporates a curvilinear incision that extends up and parallels the medial cleft margin but stops near the medial edge of the base of the columella. The lateral lip element advancement incision curves outward and then medially as it extends superiorly before it again extends to the alar base.

Delaire does not incorporate an inferior triangle into his cleft lip repair, which limits the extra length that can be gained. A Delaire repair does not include a vomer flap.

Pfeifer cleft lip repair

Flap design

Pfeifer described a wavy-line repair that allowed downward rotation as the curves were approximated into a straight line. The two curves are brought together such that the highest and lowest points of one curve are approximated with the corresponding highest and lowest points of the other, thus creating a straight line.

The Pfeifer repair achieves good vertical-length soft tissue reconstruction, but in some cases this can be at the expense of soft tissue reconstruction in the horizontal dimension.

Afroze cleft lip repair

Flap design

The Afroze incision is a combination of two incisions: the Millard incision on the medial cleft side and the Pfeifer incision on the cleft side. The flap is designed so that the Millard flap on the cleft side rotates downwards and the peak of the distal curve on the Pfeifer flap is positioned in the triangular defect formed by the downward movement of the Millard flap.

The lip scar does not lie along the philtrum – this is the only disadvantage of this technique. However, the scar heals exceptionally well as the wound is closed under no tension whatsoever.

Tennison cleft lip repair

Flap design

The triangular flap repair was initially described in 1952 by Tennison. Tennison's technique made use of an inferior backcut that begins not far above the cleft-side peak of the Cupid's Bow of the medial lip element and is angled superolaterally. Precisely measured

triangle flaps allow vertical lengthening of the medial lip element while enabling lengthening of what is often an otherwise short transverse lateral lip element without compromising the ideal basal position of the philtral column incision.

The main disadvantage of the triangular flap repair technique is that the philtrum on the cleft side is violated by the triangular flap. Some authors believe this leaves a more noticeable scar. Another potential disadvantage is the difficulty in modifying the repair or performing secondary revision at a later stage due to the zigzag scars.

Fisher cleft lip repair

Flap design

The repair allows for a repair line that ascends the lip at the seams of anatomical subunits. Applying the principle of anatomic subunits to cleft lip repair, the 'ideal line of repair' should be one that ascends the lip from the cleft-side peak of Cupid's Bow to the base of the nose along a line exactly mirroring the non-cleft-side philtral column. These manoeuvres help to preserve natural subunit boundaries allowing for rotation and medial lip lengthening at the expense of narrowing the philtrum to a degree.

Fisher often adds a small inferior triangle just above the cutaneous roll for additional rotation and feels that this accentuates the pout of the lip. While this technique is included in the category of rotation/advancement repairs, it is clearly a hybrid of multiple principles, including triangle-flap techniques and use of geometric and curvilinear incisions to approach a vertically oriented closure.

REPAIR OF THE INCOMPLETE CLEFT LIP

The repair of the incomplete cleft lip follows the same principles as outlined for the repair of the complete cleft lip. The incision is modified to divide the nasal skin from the lip skin in a line along the base of the nasal sill (*Figure 60.15*). The texture of the nasal skin is different to the texture of the skin of the lip and the incision line is placed between the junction of both skin types. The texture of the skin that is excised is abnormal due to the lack of underlying muscle insertion. A small wedge excision into the nasal sill may be used to prevent a prominence of scar tissue from developing in this area. The authors do not include this extension into the nasal sill as it may lead to nostril narrowing and flattening of the nasal sill.

The postoperative result for an incomplete cleft lip repair is illustrated in *Figure 60.16*.

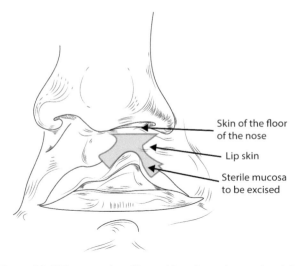
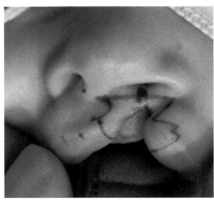

Skin of the floor of the nose

Lip skin

Sterile mucosa to be excised

Figure 60.15 Preoperative skin markings for an incomplete left side cleft lip repair.

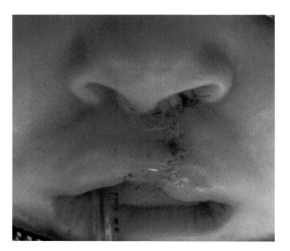

Figure 60.16 Postoperative result for the repair of an incomplete left side cleft lip.

TOP TIPS AND HAZARDS

- Careful identification of anatomical landmarks and respect for anatomical boundaries between the nose and lip.
- Wide subperiosteal undermining of the anterior maxilla to allow tension-free muscle repair.
- Identification of the anterior border of the septum, subperichondrial undermining of the nasal septum and release of alar cartilage from the vestibular skin.
- Identification and dissection of the nasalis and orbicularis muscle.
- Reconstruction of the upper and middle muscle rings with fixation of the nasalis muscle to the periosteum, just below the ANS, and fixation of the oblique part of orbicularis to the ANS and septum.
- Correct alignment of the alar base, anterior septum and columella.
- Careful reconstruction of the horizontal fibres of orbicularis.

ACKNOWLEDGEMENTS

Illustrations by Steve Atherton and Heather Goodrum, additional graphics by Amy Shorter and additional photography by Belinda Colton of Medical Illustration, Abertawe Bro Morgannwg University Health Board, Heol Maes Eglwys, Morriston, Swansea, Wales.

FURTHER READING

Fisher DM. Unilateral cleft lip repair: an anatomical subunit approximation technique. *Plast Reconstr Surg* 2005;**116**:61–71.

Markus AF, Delaire J. Functional primary closure of the cleft lip. *Br J Oral Maxillofac Surg* 1993;**31**:281–91.

McComb H. Treatment of the unilateral cleft nose. *Plast Reconstr Surg* 1975;**55**:591–601.

Millard RD, Jr. Refinements in rotation advancement cleft lip technique. *Plast Reconstr Surg* 1964;**33**:26–38.

Randall P. A triangular flap operation for the primary repair of unilateral clefts of the lip. *Plast Reconstr Surg* 1959;**23**:331–47.

Chapter 61

Primary Closure of Bilateral Cleft Lip

Krishna Shama Rao

ANATOMY

- The prolabium located centrally is devoid of muscle and consists of skin, vermilion and oral mucosa
- There is no definitive line of demarcation between the columella and prolabium
- The premaxilla, containing the tooth buds for future permanent incisors, may be situated centrally or asymmetrically to the right or left, anteriorly, superiorly or inferiorly or a combination thereof
- Sometimes permanent lateral incisors are missing/hypoplastic
- On the lateral segments, the lip vermilion is turned upwards to join the alar base. This is because both the extrinsic muscles (levator alaeque nasi, levator labii superioris, nasalis) as well as the intrinsic upper lip muscles (orbicularis marginalis and peripheralis) are oriented upwards and inserted into the alar base and maxilla along the pyriform ring (*Figure 61.1*)
- The lower lateral cartilages are pulled laterally, resulting in a flattened appearance of the nose
- The septum and premaxilla are attached to the vomer as a thin stalk

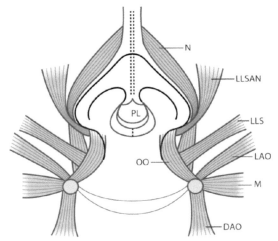

Figure 61.1 Anatomy. *Abbreviations*: PL, prolabium; N, nasalis; LLSAN, levator labii superioris alaeque nasi; LLS, levator labii superioris; LAO, levator anguli oris; M, modiolus; DAO, depressor anguli oris; OO, orbicularis oris.

CLINICAL EVALUATION/RECORD KEEPING

- Photographs, both extraoral and intraoral
- Study models
- Orthopantomogram after 5 years of age
- Check premaxilla for mobility and fracture

TIMING OF SURGERY

- The ideal age for lip repair is 3 months
- In less-informed societies, patients may present at any age
- Protocols for primary repair of bilateral cleft lip presenting at any age is as follows:
  - *3 months to 2 years*: lip repair
  - *2–7 years*: palatoplasty first and then lip repair
  - *7 years to adulthood*: palatoplasty first and then lip repair with alveolar bone grafting

When the patient presents for surgery after the age of 7 years, the premaxilla may be severely displaced and may occasionally require surgical repositioning.

HOW TO HANDLE THE PREMAXILLA

In minimally displaced premaxilla in the newborn or when the child presents early (at less than 3 months of age), strapping of prolabium with dynaplast or elastics is helpful.

In the more displaced premaxilla, nasoalveolar moulding with specially developed plates with nasal prongs to guide premaxilla and lateral segments into position can be fitted. This requires repeated visits to the clinic to adjust the plates (*Figures 61.2–61.4*).

Lip adhesion

This is a surgical procedure which allows mobilisation of the nasal layer and closure of the lateral segment margins with the prolabium without mobilisation and anastomosis of the orbicularis oris muscle. This allows repositioning of the premaxilla and definitive repair at the second stage some 3 months after the lip adhesion (*Figure 61.4*).

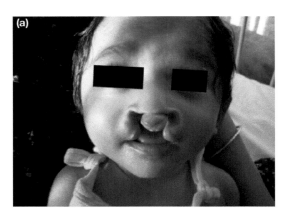
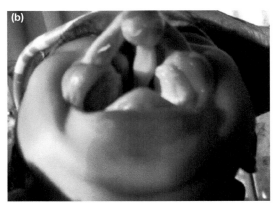

Figure 61.2 (a) Premaxilla at the tip of the nose, absence of columella and deficient prolabial tissue; (b) protruded premaxilla and deviated nasal septum.

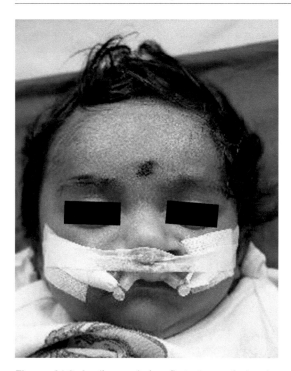

Figure 61.3 Appliance during first stage of alveolar moulding.

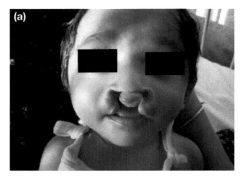
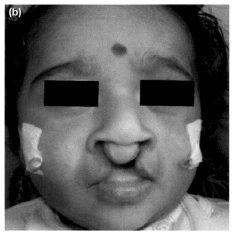

Figure 61.4 Treatment progression using an appliance and strapping to guide the premaxilla.

Premaxillary osteotomy

Indication

Premaxillary osteotomy is indicated when:

- Patient is aged about 7 years
- Premaxilla is more than 1 cm protruded and/or deviated
- When other conservative techniques are not appropriate

Primary premaxillary osteotomy is performed using a longitudinal mucosal incision, use of cutting instruments to perform a predetermined oblique ostectomy, separation of the nasal septum from the vomer and retropositioning the premaxilla and stabilisation with

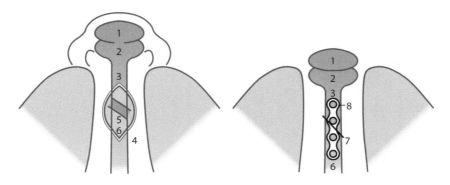

Figure 61.5 Premaxillary osteotomy. 1, prolabium; 2, premaxilla; 3, vomerine stalk; 4, vomerine mucosa; 5, osteotomy site; 6, vomer exposed; 7, osteotomy site after reduction; 8, resorbable bone plates.

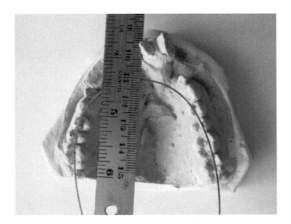

Figure 61.6 Model analysis prior to premaxillary osteotomy.

resorbable bone plates. After 3 months, primary repair of lip can be undertaken (*Figure 61.5*).

Preoperative assessment and postoperative view are shown in *Figures 61.6* and *61.7*.

DEFINITIVE PRIMARY REPAIR OF BILATERAL CLEFT LIP

Anaesthesia

Surgery is carried out under general anaesthesia, using an oral endotracheal, reinforced tube.

Position

Patients are positioned with the neck extended and a mouth gag applied.

Procedure

After the mouth gag is applied, marginal incisions are made along the medial aspects of the palatal shelves up to the end of the hard palate. On the premaxilla,

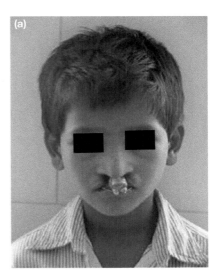

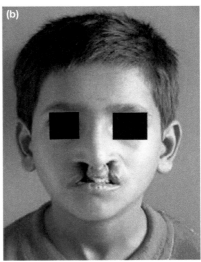

Figure 61.7 (a) Preoperative and (b) postoperative photographs.

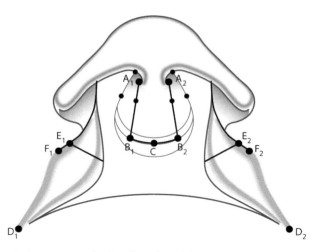

$A_1 A_2$ – junction of columella with prolabium.
$B_1 B_2$ – highest point of Cupid's bow. C – lowest point of Cupid's bow.
$D_1 D_2$ – commisure of lip. $E_1 E_2$ – white roll fades.
$F_1 F_2$ – back cut along white roll such that $E_1 F_1 = E_2 F_2 = B_1 C = B_2 C$.

Figure 61.8 Anatomic points for lip marking.

a Y-shaped incision is made with the two short limbs encircling the premaxilla and the long limb along the vomerine mucoperiosteum. The nasal layers are elevated using Mitchell's trimmer or a plastic instrument. A single-layer mucosal closure of the nasal lining is achieved from the lip to the hard palate using interrupted resorbable vicryl 4/0 sutures with the knots inverted into the nasal cavity. The mouth gag and neck extension are then removed.

Next, lip marking should be planned. The key points to mark on the prolabium are the apparent junction between columella and prolabium. A1 and A2 are marked at the corner of the base of the columella on either side. Two divergent lines are drawn down to the white roll to end at B1 and B2 (*Figure 61.8*), B1 and B2 being slightly wider than A1 and A2. Point C is the midpoint between B1 and B2, and it is the lowest point of the Cupid's Bow. On the cleft side's right and left points, D1 and D2 are marked to represent the commissure of the lips. Points E1 and E2 are marked at the spot where the white roll just begins to fade. Thus, D1–E1 is equal to D2–E2. At E1 and E2, a perpendicular line is drawn towards the free margin of the lip. Points F1 and F2 are marked such that E1–F1 is equal to E2–F2 is equal to B1–C is equal to B2–C. F1–E1 continues along the white roll into the internal aspect of the nostril on either side. The incision is made using a no. 15 blade starting from A1 to B1 and then again on the other side from A2 to B2. The two are joined together across C. The incision goes through the skin and incorporates a little of the underlying tissue. On the cleft sides, that is the lateral sides, incisions are started at E1 and continued along the white roll into the nostril and extended laterally to the point F1. At E1, the incision is also taken perpendicular to the white roll to the free margin of the

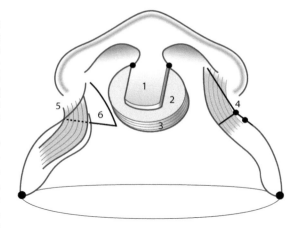

Figure 61.9 Muscle dissection. 1, prolabial skin flap; 2, excess skin and mucosa; 3, premaxilla, 4, unoperated side showing orbicularis muscle bundle under intact skin/mucosa; 5, exposed orbicularis oris muscle; 6, mucosa elevated.

mucosa and a mucosal flap is elevated on right side. A similar flap is elevated on the left side.

Once the incisions are completed, the orbicularis oris muscle is dissected free from its abnormal attachments on either side of the base of the ala and maxilla. The muscle is freed from its attachments to the skin, mucosa and vermilion using a no. 15 blade up to a distance of about 5 mm (*Figure 61.9*). Superiorly, where the abnormal insertion of the muscle into the ala is seen, the muscle is freed using a combination of sharp and blunt dissection to free the entire corpus of orbicularis oris muscle along with the bundles of the nasalis and the other associated muscles. To mobilise the lip completely, the muscles are also freed from the underlying maxillary bone in a subperiosteal manner. The orbicularis and nasalis muscles are freed as far as the base of the alar margin and a sulcular incision is made into the depth of the sulcus from the free margin of the lip up to the pre-molar area. The subperiosteal dissection is carried out to elevate the entire lip complex along with its under-lying and associated muscles away from the maxilla. The tissues are freed along the pyriform margin and also extended into the lateral aspects of the ala of the nose on either side. The incision along the white roll towards the nostril is carried on until it reaches the inferior aspect of the inferior turbinate mucosa. The mucosal flaps are raised to coincide with the nasal layer of the anterior aspect of the palatal mucosa. On the prolabial side, the incision B1–A1 is carried further backwards along the nasal mucosa over the vomer bone, such that the nasal flaps can be elevated on either side. This helps in having a continuous nasal lining from the palate forwards into the lip. As soon as the mobilisation is complete, it will be seen that the lateral segments of the lip now assume a very comfortable horizontal position and they can be brought together with minimal or no tension at all. The excess lip mucosa which is medial to points E1 and E2 is used to form the sulcus of the future upper lip.

Mobilisation of nasal cartilages

Blunt dissection of the lateral crura of the lower lateral cartilages on either side is performed using curved blunt-tipped tenotomy scissors. The scissors are placed through the lateral incision and blunt dissection proceeds along the superior and inferior and the outer and inner aspects of the lower lateral cartilage up to the dome (intermediate crura). The medial crura of the lower lateral cartilage is approached from the prolabial side and also freed on all aspects. This mobilises the lower cartilage completely and allows it to attain its natural form during closure of the lip.

Closure

Closure is performed in three layers (*Figure 61.10*). First, the nasal layer is closed in continuity with the closure of the premaxillary nasal mucosa which was performed earlier. Once the nasal layer closure is complete, the mucosa on the inner aspect of the upper lip on either side is sutured to the prolabial mucosa to form the sulcus of the oral cavity. Closure is obtained using 4/0 vicryl sutures (5/8 of a circle cutting needle).

The next layer of the closure is the muscle. The nasalis is identified on either side by pulling it medially and seeing the inwards movements of lower lateral cartilage and the base of ala on either side. The orbicularis oris muscles are also identified and three sutures are placed using 4/0 vicryl to bring together the orbicularis and nasalis muscles comfortably in the midline over the prolabial mucosa. Along its length, skin hooks are posi-tioned actively, giving a slight downward traction to

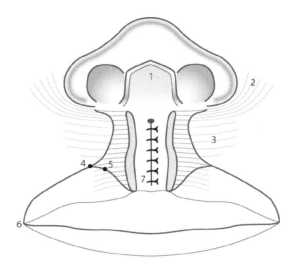

Figure 61.10 Closure of nasal layer and apposition of the muscles. 1, elevated prolabium; 2, nasalis muscle; 3, orbicularis oris muscle; 4, point F1; 5, point E1; 6, commissure point D; 7, mucosa sutured with 4.0 vicryl.

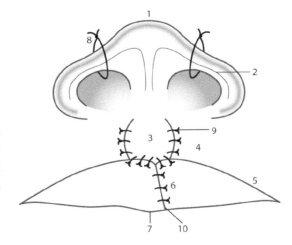

Figure 61.11 Skin closure. 1, dome; 2, lower lateral cartilage; 3, prolabial skin; 4, lateral element skin; 5, Cupid's Bow; 6, vermilion; 7, central tubercle; 8, bolster stitch with 3.0 Prolene; 9, skin closure with 5.0 Prolene; 10, mucosal closure with 4.0 vicryl.

the lip, to ensure that the entire nasalis and orbicularis muscles have been brought together.

Skin closure

The prolabial skin is allowed to fall gently upon the closed orbicularis muscles, and the two lateral segments are then gently pulled across and held together with two skin hooks held in parallel along the long axis of the body of the patient (*Figure 61.11*). Any excess skin in the lateral segments resulting from the closure of the

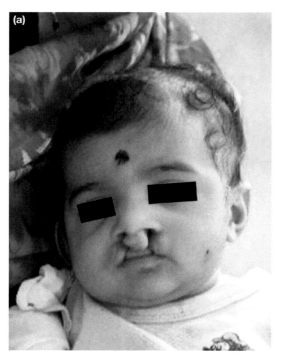 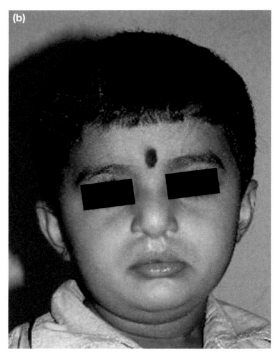

Figure 61.12 Primary closure of bilateral cleft lip surgery: (a) preoperative and (b) postoperative.

muscles can be incised to accommodate the prolabial skin in the midline and the wound is closed using 5/0 Prolene sutures. The vermilion and the oral mucosa are closed using 4/0 vicryl. Care is taken to achieve a central tubercle in the midline of the lip, thus giving the upper lip a pleasant and natural appearance. Bolster sutures are placed through the dome (intermediate crura) of the lower lateral cartilages to hold them up in a new position allowing the skin and the mucosa to adapt and heal in the new relaxed positions of the cartilages. The skin sutures and bolster sutures are removed after 7 days.

Postoperative care

Steri-Strips are placed immediately after the suturing and they are removed after 2–3 days to inspect and clean the wound. The wound is meticulously cleaned with normal saline and hydrogen peroxide and beta-dine and Steri-Strips are replaced. On the seventh day, the sutures are removed under sedation, the wound is cleaned again and new Steri-Strips are placed.

Results

The results of primary closure of bilateral cleft lip surgery are shown in a series of different patients in *Figures 61.12* and *61.13*.

COMPLICATIONS

Intraoperative

Fracture of the premaxilla

The premaxilla is continuous with the vomer along a very thin stalk and may sometimes be traumatised, especially if it is protuberant either prior to the surgery or during the procedure.

Avulsion of the premaxilla

This is a rare, but unacceptable, iatrogenic complication.

Postoperative

Early

- *Infection*: the wound may get infected, especially in chronically malnourished children in developing countries due to decreased immunity. Use of anti-biotics and local wound management should sal-vage the surgical procedure
- *Dehiscence of the wound*: as a sequela to either wound infection or tension during closure, partial break-down of the surgical repair may occur. Conserva-tive management is followed by secondary correc-tion after 6 months

Late

- *Oronasal fistula*: partial breakdown of the nasal layer may lead to small oronasal communications in the

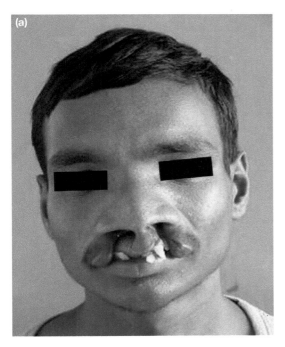
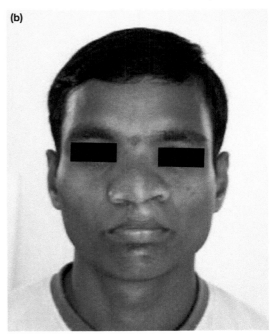

Figure 61.13 Primary closure of bilateral cleft lip surgery: **(a)** preoperative and **(b)** postoperative.

region of the premaxilla and lateral segments. Definitive repair of the fistula in two layers is taken up as a secondary procedure after 6 months

- *Cupid's Bow deformity*: mismatch of the white roll during suturing or wound contracture may lead to a deformed Cupid's Bow, which is corrected with Z-plasties or scar revision
- *Whistling deformity*: generally, this is a severe deformity due to inadequate mobilisation of nasalis and orbicularis oris muscles or dehiscence of these muscles due to closure with tension. Secondary repair is carried out in the form of a complete revision cheiloplasty
- *Hypertrophic scar*: hypertrophic scar is a common sequela due to excessive tension in skin closure and is all the more apparent in pigmented skin (types IV–VI). Hypertrophic scars can be managed initially conservatively using vitamin E cream, massage, Contratubex ointment, etc. Minimally hypertrophic scars can be resurfaced with erbium YAG lasers. Severely hypertrophic scars would need excision and resuturing in a tension-free environment

MOBILISATION: OPEN TECHNIQUE

The incisions of the lip which extend into the nasal cavity along the inferior margin of the lower lateral cartilage are continued to meet the prolabial incision at the medial crura. This allows a complete reflection of prolabial and columellar skin to expose the dorsal aspect of the right and left lower lateral cartilages completed up to its attachments laterally to the pyriform rim.

Next, the nasal mucosa is freed from the inner aspect of the lower lateral cartilages from lateral to medial to mobilise the lateral crura completely. The superior end of the lower lateral cartilage is freed from its fibrous overlapping attachment with the upper lateral cartilage.

The lateral crura is now free-floating while the medial crura continues to be attached to the columellar mucosa.

An interdomal stitch is taken after medialisation of the two lateral crura such that a new better projected nasal tip is achieved.

Closure is then achieved by redrawing the columella–prolabial skin, and suturing the infracartilaginous incision.

The rest of the lip–nose correction is exactly as before.

The nasal septum is generally addressed at the same time and it is excess mobilised and trimmed along the axillary crest.

This allows the septum to swing freely and reposition itself in the midline as balance is restored between two sides of facial and lip muscles.

There was a hypothetical concept that nasal and facial growth might be affected if an open lip–nose correction were to be performed. However, this is not the case as can be seen in 10-year follow-up of patients.

The results of mobilisation – open techniques are shown in *Figure 61.14*.

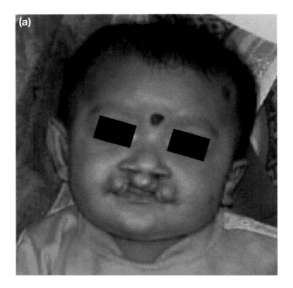

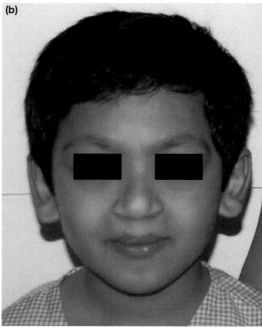

Figure 61.14 (a) Preoperative and (b) postoperative photographs of a patient treated with the 'open' technique.

TOP TIPS AND HAZARDS

- The prolabium is devoid of muscle.
- The premaxilla may be situated centrally or asymmetrically in three dimensions.
- The ideal age of repair of the bilateral cleft lip is 3 months, but patients may present at any age in less-informed societies.
- There are several techniques to manage the premaxilla, which include simple strapping, nasoalveolar moulding, lip adhesion and premaxillary osteotomy (very occasionally).
- In the definitive repair of the bilateral cleft lip, it is important to first repair the nasal floor.
- Further important steps include careful marking of the incisions and meticulous mobilisation of the muscles.
- The lip–nose complex is treated simultaneously and hence careful closed dissection and mobilisation of the lower lateral cartilages are performed.
- During mucosal closure, care is taken to achieve a good sulcus and, on the labial side of the alveolus, a gingivo-alveolar periosteoplasty is achieved.
- Skin closure achieves symmetry of the lip and nose, and pleasing Cupid's Bow, philtral ridges and central tubercle.

FURTHER READING

Bardach J. *Salyer & Bardach's Atlas of Craniofacial and Cleft Surgery: Cleft Lip and Palate Surgery*, vol. 2. Philadelphia, PA: Lippincott; 1999.

Delaire J, Precious D, Gordeef A. The advantage of wide subperiosteal exposure in primary surgical correction of labial maxillary cleft. *Scand J Plast Reconstr Surg Hand Surg* 1988;**22**:147–51.

Jackson IT, Yavuzer R, Kelly C, et al. The central lip flap and nasal mucosal rotation advancement: Important aspects of composite correction of the bilateral cleft lip nose deformity. *J Craniofac Surg* 2005;**16**:255–61.

Markus AF, Delaire J. Functional primary closure of cleft lip. *Br J Oral Maxillofac Surg* 1993;**31**:281–91.

Mulliken JB, Wu JK, Padwa BL. Repair of bilateral cleft lip: review, revisions, and reflections. *J Craniofac Surg* 2003;**14**:609–20.

Chapter

62

Primary Repair of Cleft Palate

Simon van Eeden

INTRODUCTION

The palate separates the nose from the oral cavity and is made up of the bony hard palate anteriorly and the muscular soft palate posteriorly. The palate facilitates simultaneous breathing and eating and is important in feeding, swallowing, speech and hearing. Coordinated movement of the soft palate during feeding and swallowing prevents food and fluid regurgitation into the nose and encourages caudal propulsion of the food bolus. During speech, the soft palate must remain open for some sounds and must close for others meaning that it must be of sufficient length with adequately functioning muscles to be able to effect these changes rapidly and efficiently.

Babies born with a cleft of the palate are unable to adequately breastfeed, and early diagnosis and management is therefore imperative to prevent a failure to thrive and, in extreme circumstances, death. The diagnosis of a cleft palate should be made at the initial baby check after birth following the guidelines published by the Royal College of Paediatrics and Child Health. Once feeding has been established and the baby is thriving, attention can then be focussed on their specific treatment.

The aims of cleft palate repair are to create a mechanical barrier between the oral cavity and the nasal cavity and to provide a functioning soft palate to facilitate feeding, swallowing, speech and hearing.

Clefts involving the palate may occur in combination with clefts of the lip, which may be either unilateral or bilateral, or they may occur as isolated clefts of the palate. The aim is to repair the palate by 1 year of age as there is evidence to suggest that repair of the palate before 13 months of age results in better speech. In an isolated cleft palate (iCP), repair is usually undertaken in one surgical procedure whether the cleft involves the soft palate only or whether it involves both the hard and soft palate. In clefts involving both the lip and palate, consideration must be given to the sequencing of the lip and palatal repair. For unilateral clefts of the lip and palate (UCLP), there are many different protocols and sequences described to do this and although practitioners of each sequence point to advantages of their preferred choice, a recent randomised trial comparing three different sequences did not show benefit of one sequence over another when looking at speech outcomes at 5 years of age. Many follow the Oslo protocol, repairing the lip and hard palate at the first operation followed by repair of the soft palate at the second operation.

There are also many sequences and protocols described for the repair of bilateral clefts of the lip and palate (BCLP) and in many units a BCLP will be repaired in three operations: repair of the lip or lip adhesion and one side of the hard palate at the first operation followed by repair of the contralateral hard palate if a definitive lip repair was done at the first operation or definitive lip repair with contralateral hard palate repair if a lip adhesion was done at the first operation, followed by repair of the soft palate.

This chapter will therefore describe repair of the hard palate using a superiorly pedicled single layered vomerine flap in clefts of the lip and palate; repair of the hard palate in an isolated cleft palate (iCP), and repair of the soft palate, which is common to all these cleft types.

REPAIR OF THE HARD PALATE IN A UNILATERAL CLEFT OF THE LIP AND PALATE

In a UCLP, the vomer is inserted into the major segment of the palate and the junction of the vomerine mucosa with the palatal mucosa is easily discerned as the vomerine mucosa is pseudo-ciliated mucosa and appears red, whereas the hard palate mucosa is keratinised squamous mucosa and has a coral pink appearance.

The vomerine incision

The incisions are marked and local anaesthetic (2% lignocaine in 1:80 000 adrenaline) is given. Starting posteriorly, the incision made through the muco-perichondrium begins anterior to the adenoidal pad and is brought forward at the junction of the hard palate mucosa and the vomerine mucosa, and is advanced below and beyond the alveolus anteriorly on the medial aspect of the cleft to become continuous with the lip incision at the junction of the attached mucosa of the alveolus inferiorly and septal mucosa superiorly.

If there is tension on the vomerine flap, a backcut running from the posterior limit of the vomerine incision laterally can be made to relieve the tension and ensure a tension-free closure.

Once the mucoperichondrial flap is raised, a marginal incision is made on the lesser segment at the junction of the hard palate mucosa and the nasal mucosa and runs anteriorly from the junction of the hard and soft palate below the alveolus to become continuous with the lateral lip incision. A mucoperiosteal flap is then raised on the minor segment.

The vomerine flap is turned over to be inserted below the flap raised on the minor segment so that the raw surface of the vomerine flap is in continuity with the raw surface of the hard palate mucosa.

The flap is sutured in position with horizontal double breasting mattress sutures using 5/0 vicryl on a compound curved needle. The small gap left between the mucosal edges on the minor segment and the vomerine flap is closed with two or three 6/0 PDS sutures on a round needle.

This completes the superiorly pedicled single-layered vomerine flap repair of the hard palate in a UCLP.

REPAIR OF THE HARD PALATE IN A BILATERAL CLEFT OF THE LIP AND PALATE

In a BCLP, the vomer and nasal septum occupy a midline position and the clefts run lateral to the septum/vomer from the lip through the alveolus to the hard and soft palate.

Hard palate repair using vomer flaps in BCLPs is usually done on two separate operations at least 6 weeks apart to ensure the blood supply to the premaxilla. The blood supply to the premaxilla and prolabium in a BCLP is mainly through the posterior septal artery and partially through the lateral nasal and terminal branches of the anterior ethmoidal vessels passing through the columella. There is no continuity of the superior labial vessels across the cleft nor is there an incisive papilla meaning that once the philtral incisions have been made in the prolabium and the skin raised, the blood supply from the vessels passing through the columella to the premaxilla is disrupted. This means that the premaxilla is reliant on the posterior septal arteries. It is therefore important to keep one side of the vomerine mucosa undisturbed to maintain this blood supply, meaning that only one side of the hard palate will be repaired at the time of the lip repair.

The incisions are marked and local anaesthetic (2% lignocaine in 1:80 000 adrenaline) is given. A midline incision is made in the vomer starting posteriorly just anterior to the adenoidal pad.

This is brought forward onto the premaxilla and is then taken below the alveolus on one side at the junction of the septal mucosa and attached alveolar mucosa forward to become continuous with the lip incision.

A full mucoperichondrial vomerine flap is then raised taking care not to perforate the flap, especially where it is tightly bound down just anterior to the pre-vomerine suture. A marginal incision is made at the junction of the hard palate mucosa and the nasal mucosa on the ipsilateral segment that runs from the junction of the hard and soft palate anteriorly below the alveolus to become continuous with the lateral lip incision. A muco-periosteal flap is then raised on the lateral segment.

The steps that follow are the same as for the UCLP hard palate repair described above.

If a formal lip repair has been performed at the first operation, the patient will return to theatre at least 6 weeks following this for repair of the contralateral hard palate using a vomerine flap raised contralaterally; the steps in the procedure are the same as described above. It is, however, sometimes difficult to access the alveolar cleft once the lip has been formally repaired; if this is the case then the vomerine flap will only be taken forward to a point that is technically feasible and a small oronasal communication will be accepted at the alveolus and closed at the bone grafting stage later. If, however, a lip adhesion was performed at the first procedure, then the patient will return for a formal lip repair and contralateral vomerine flap along the whole length of the cleft (as described above) at least 6 weeks later. This completes repair of the hard palate in BCLPs.

Repair of the soft palate using an operating microscope will follow approximately 3 months after hard palate closure in UCLPs and BCLPs and the technique, a Sommerlad radical palatoplasty, described below for repair of an iCP will be followed.

REPAIR OF ISOLATED CLEFTS OF THE PALATE

When repairing an iCP, the hard palate is repaired at the same time as the soft palate. The repair is carried out using an operative microscope and a Sommerlad gag is used to gain access (*Figure 62.1*). In those cases where the extent and width of the hard palate cleft precludes tension-free closure of the nasal layer, a bilateral superiorly pedicled vomer flap is used to effect this.

The incisions are marked (*Figure 62.2*) and local anaesthetic (2% lignocaine in 1:80 000 adrenaline) is given. A central incision is made on the hard palate down to bone (if the cleft does not involve the whole of the hard palate) to the anterior aspect of the cleft and continued as marginal incisions bilaterally at the junction of the nasal and oral layers to the tip of the uvula.

Full mucoperiosteal nasal and oral flaps (*Figure 62.3*) are then raised from the hard palate followed by the soft palate dissection as described by Sommerlad, on each side of the cleft.

The oral submucoperiosteal dissection is taken laterally to the junction of the hard palate and the alveolus along the extent of the hard palate.

The greater and lesser palatine neurovascular bundles are identified as they exit from the palatine bone;

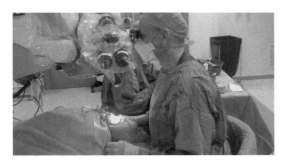

Figure 62.1 Operative microscope and Sommerlad gag.

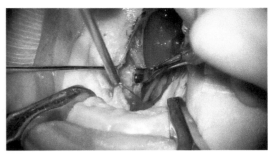

Figure 62.3 Oro-mucoperiosteal flaps and nasal muco-periosteal flaps raised from hard palate.

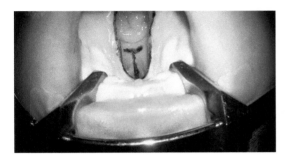

Figure 62.2 Operative marking of marginal incisions for isolated cleft palate repair and vomer flap.

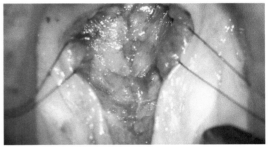

Figure 62.4 Repaired nasal layer with muscles attached.

careful dissection continues around them making sure that their tight mucoperiosteal envelope are relieved, facilitating advancement of the oral hard palate flaps towards the midline while ensuring the integrity of the neurovascular bundles.

The oral subperiosteal dissection is taken posteriorly to the junction of the hard and soft palate; at this point the minor salivary glands are firmly bound to the tensor veli palatini laterally and the palatopharyngeus medially.

The tensor veli palatini in a cleft palate, instead of forming the anterior aponeurosis of the soft palate with the contralateral muscle, is inserted into the posterior margin of the hard palate laterally.

Similarly, the palatopharyngeus, which normally forms a sling with the contralateral muscle, is inserted into the posterior margin of the hard palate medially and the margin of the cleft.

To prevent perforation of the oral flap where the salivary glands are tightly bound to the muscles described above at the junction of the hard and soft palate, it is imperative that the dissection is carried out above the minor salivary glands. This will also ensure that the rest of the soft palate dissection to separate the oral mucosa and minor salivary glands from the nasal layer and the attached palatal muscles is carried out in the correct plane.

The dissection to separate the oral mucosa and attached minor salivary glands from the nasal layer

and the attached palatal muscles is then continued posteriorly into the glandular uvula and laterally to the superior constrictor.

The nasal layer with attached palatal muscles is then repaired with 5/0 monocryl starting with the uvula posteriorly and continuing forward; it is important to evert the nasal layer by taking small bites of the mucosa and larger bites of the muscle. This ensures a convex nasal surface soft palate contact with the posterior pharyngeal wall during speech and swallowing (*Figure 62.4*).

If there is excess tension in the nasal mucosal repair, then the vomer can be utilised to complete closure of the nasal layer:

- Two mucoperichondrial vomer flaps are raised by making a midline incision along the vomer from just anterior to the adenoidal pad to the anterior margin of the cleft
- Bilateral incisions are made from the posterior limit of the vomer incision laterally just anterior to the adenoidal pad

If the vomerine flaps do not easily reach the nasal mucosal flaps raised on the lateral margins of the cleft, backcuts can be made posterolaterally to increase the reach.

The vomerine flaps are sewn to the nasal mucosa in an edge-to-edge fashion using 5/0 vicryl interrupted sutures on a compound curved needle (unlike the technique used for repair of the hard palate in unilateral

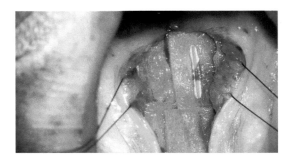

Figure 62.5 Adrenaline patties on repaired nasal layer and 4/0 Ethilon sutures retracting the oral layer.

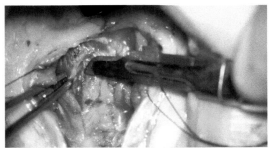

Figure 62.6 Paramedian incision through muscle to the nasal mucosa.

and bilateral clefts of the lip and palate described above). This completes closure of the nasal layer of the soft and hard palatal cleft.

4/0 Ethilon stay sutures are then used to retract the oral layer of the soft palate improving access to the lateral aspect of the soft palate as far lateral as the hamulus and the superior constrictor.

Adrenaline (1:1 000) soaked brain patties are then placed onto the nasal layer and muscles for 2–5 minutes (*Figure 62.5*). This improves haemostasis and the operative field.

Paramedian incisions taken along the medial aspect of the palatopharyngeus down to nasal mucosa are then made from the uvula to the posterior aspect of the hard palate taking care not to incise the nasal layer sutures bilaterally (*Figure 62.6*).

The dissection is then advanced from medial to lateral along the full extent of the paramedian incisions taking care to separate all muscle from the nasal layer while maintaining the integrity of the nasal layer.

When it is no longer possible to advance laterally safely, the anterior aspect of the paramedian incisions are then continued laterally at the junction of the hard palate and the soft palate, and in so doing the medial hard palate attachment of the palatopharyngeus and the lateral hard palate attachment of the tensor veli palatini are separated from the hard palate.

At the lateral extent of the hard palate this incision is continued posteriorly, medial to the hamulus, and the tensor veli palatini released from the hamulus bilaterally.

The dissection continues posteriorly in a plane just medial to the superior constrictor. This part of the dissection is then joined with the initial muscle dissection described above and advanced posteriorly and laterally so that the muscles can be moved posteriorly within the soft palate without anterior tension.

The muscle bundles from each side, made up of the levator veli palatini, palatopharyngeus and tensor veli palatini, are joined to each other in the midline with 4/0 Ethilon or 4/0 PDS (depending on surgeon preference) and in so doing the palatal muscular slings

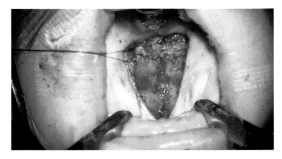

Figure 62.7 Palatal muscle sling, including levator veli palatini, palatopharyngeus and tensor veli palatini repaired in the midline.

are reconstructed (*Figure 62.7*). Adding part of the tensor veli palatini to the repair adds strength to the reconstruction. The palatoglossus remains attached to the oral layer and is reconstituted when the oral layer is repaired.

The oral layer is then repaired with:

- interrupted 5/0 monocryl sutures for the uvula
- Sommerlad looped mattress 4/0 monocryl or 4/0 vicryl sutures for the remainder of the oral layer; the first of these sutures is placed just anterior to the muscle bundle, and passes through the nasal layer closing the dead space between the oral and nasal layers and prevents forward migration of the muscular sling

If there is excess tension on the repair in the midline, Von Langenbeck relieving incisions, made in the hard palate at the junction of the palatal mucosa and the alveolar mucosa, are made bilaterally, extending posteriorly into the soft palate if necessary. The gaps left in the hard palate mucosa as a result of these incisions are filled with buccal fat pad bilaterally (*Figure 62.8*).

When complete, the throat pack is removed and bilateral palatal blocks or suprazygomatic maxillary nerve blocks are given using 0.25% or 0.5% chirocaine.

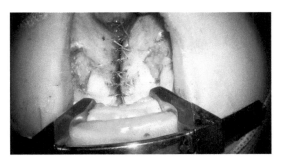

Figure 62.8 Repaired oral layer with lateral relieving incisions and buccal fat pad bilaterally.

POSTOPERATIVE CARE AND RECOVERY

- Patients are nursed routinely on the ward
- Pain is managed with routine analgesia that includes iv paracetamol, oral ibuprofen and morphine
- Babies can feed immediately following surgery; parents are encouraged to adopt a trial-and-error approach as babies often prefer solids to bottlefeeding following soft palate repair
- Discharge is usually the day following surgery if comfortable and feeding adequately

POSSIBLE COMPLICATIONS AND HOW TO DEAL WITH THEM

Immediate complications

- *Airway compromise*: this usually presents on extubation and may be caused by palatal swelling with direct contact of the soft palate with the adenoidal pad, or due to tongue swelling. This manifests with nasal flaring, tracheal tug, sternal recession, the use of accessory respiratory muscles and an inability to maintain an oxygen saturation above 96%. Management in the first instance is with a nasopharyngeal airway. In rare instances if this does not alleviate the obstruction, a second nasopharyngeal airway can be placed and if this does not overcome the obstruction, a tracheostomy may be indicated (very rarely)
- *Bleeding*: local measures (e.g. local pressure with tranexamic swabs). If local measures fail, the baby should be returned to theatre for management under general anaesthetic
- *Infection*: manage with appropriate antibiotics

Later complications

- *Fistulae*: adopt a wait and watch approach. Only repair later if influencing speech or quality of life
- *Palatal dehiscence*: carry out a re-repair 6–12 months later
- *Velopharyngeal incompetence*: speech surgery when identified

TOP TIPS AND HAZARDS

- Include the possibility of the need for a nasopharyngeal airway postoperatively when consenting for palate repair.
- Use a microscope to repair the palate.
- Protect the lip commissures in soft palate and isolated cleft palate repair using Steri-Strips.
- Ensure that the vomerine flap dissection is carried out in the subperichondral plane.
- Failure to dissect in the subperichondral plane when raising the vomer flap might result in mucosal perforation and probable oronasal fistula formation.
- Ensure initial subperiosteal hard palate dissection to prevent oral mucosa perforation at the hard and soft palate junction when repairing the soft palate.
- Failure to dissect in the subperiosteal plane when raising the oral layer of the soft palate might result in mucosal perforation at the hard and soft palate junction resulting in probable oronasal fistula formation.
- Ensure the soft palate dissection is carried out in the plane between the nasal mucosal layer and the muscles.
- Failure to dissect in the plane between the palatal muscles and the nasal mucosal layer might result in failure to raise the levator veli palatini muscle and include it in reconstruction of the muscular sling.
- Have a low threshold for carrying out Von Langenbeck relieving incisions to relieve tension on the palate repair.
- Closure of the palate under tension increases the likelihood of oronasal fistula.
- Release the mouth gag for at least 5 minutes after 2 hours of operating. Failure to release the mouth gag after prolonged operating is likely to result in significant tongue swelling with associated airway compromise.

FURTHER READING

Åbyholm FE, Borchgrevink HC, Eskeland G. Cleft lip and palate in Norway: III. Surgical treatment of CLP patients in Oslo 1954-75. *Scand J Plast Reconstr Surg* 1981;**15**:15–28.

Lohmander A, Persson C, Willadsen E, et al. Scandcleft randomised trials of primary surgery for unilateral cleft lip and palate: 4. Speech outcomes in 5 year olds – velopharyngeal competency and hypernasality. *J Plast Surg Hand Surg* 2017;**51**:27–37.

Royal College of Paediatrics and Child Health. Palate examination: identification of cleft palate in the newborn - best practice guide. 2015. https://www.rcpch.ac.uk/resources/palate-examination-identification-cleft-palate-newborn-best-practice-guide.

Shaw WC, Semb G, Nelson P, et al. The Eurocleft Project 1996-2000: overview. *J Craniomaxillofac Surg* 2001;**29**:131–40.

Sommerlad BC. A technique for palate repair. *Plast Reconstr Surg* 2003;**112**:1542–8.

Bailey & Love's Essential Operations Bailey & Love's Essential Operations
Bailey & Love's Essential Operations Bailey & Love's Essential Operations
Bailey & Love's Essential Operations Bailey & Love's Essential Operations

PART 9 | Cleft lip and palate

Chapter

63

Alveolar Bone Grafting

Alistair Smyth

INTRODUCTION

Repair of the alveolar cleft with bone is an important procedure for children with congenital clefts of the embryological primary palate (complete cleft lip and palate and isolated cleft lip and alveolus). The technique was developed and popularised in the 1970s and remains an essential component of the treatment pathway. The aim is to provide normal anatomical bony continuity with the following benefits:

- Facilitate eruption of permanent teeth into the previously grafted site (canine or lateral incisor)
- Bone support for adjacent erupted teeth (central incisor)
- Enable future orthodontic tooth alignment within cleft site
- Closure of possible oronasal fistula
- Maxillary consolidation in cleft lip and palate
- Improve nasal alar base support

In brief, the operation grafts free bone into the alveolar defect within a well-vascularised soft tissue envelope. Subsequent bony consolidation and reorganisation provides normal anatomical structure.

ESSENTIAL SURGICAL ANATOMY AND EMBRYOLOGY

Alveolar cleft

The maxillary cleft results from an embryological failure of union between the premaxilla of the primary palate and the lateral bony segment of the secondary palate. As this embryological fusion line is between the incisors and the canine tooth region, the cleft is typically paramedian and may be complete, incomplete, unilateral or less frequently bilateral. As embryological fusion progresses radially from the incisive foramen at the junction of the primary and secondary palate, incomplete clefts of the alveolus can present with an intact nasal floor and a variable degree of bone formation within the superior aspect. Consequently, congenital cleft of the alveolus without cleft lip does not occur.

The alveolar cleft can be considered as an inverted four-sided pyramid with labiobuccal, medial, distal, palatal and nasal floor aspects. While the medial and distal margins of the defect are provided by the alveolar segments, the labiobuccal, palatal and superior margins

are often incomplete or discontinuous and require soft tissue repair. To facilitate future tooth eruption, the alveolar soft tissue is repaired preferably with keratinised mucosa.

PREOPERATIVE CONSIDERATIONS

Timing

Secondary alveolar bone grafting is usually carried out before eruption of the ipsilateral permanent canine tooth. Patient age range is usually 9–11 years; however, timing is dependent on dental development and ideally when permanent canine root development is between 2/3 and 3/4 complete on radiograph. Earlier bone grafting may be considered if a viable unerupted lateral incisor is present. If the permanent canine tooth has already erupted, then there is often still significant advantage to bone grafting; however, prognostic outcomes are reduced.

Access

Good or adequate surgical access to the bony cleft is essential. Prior orthodontic preparation is often required to expand the maxillary segments anteriorly, improve tooth position adjacent to the cleft site or procline upper incisors over the bite in bilateral cleft lip and palate. Orthodontic appliances should be either removable (arch wires or quad-helix) or positioned away from the operative site (transpalatal appliance). In bilateral cases, postoperative stabilisation of the mobile premaxilla by orthodontic arch wire is necessary. In some cases, such as isolated cleft lip and alveolus or if dental arch alignment is already acceptable, then pre-surgical orthodontic appliance treatment may not be required.

Teeth

Teeth planned for removal (erupted or unerupted) can often be undertaken at the time of bone grafting; however, ectopic erupted teeth (particularly if palatally positioned) are often better removed or aligned well in advance to improve palatal flap quality. Teeth should not be retained if they prevent adequate access to the cleft alveolus and would compromise bone graft healing from bacterial contamination or tooth mobility within the early healing period.

Vomer flap

If at the time of primary cleft surgery, vomer flap closure of the anterior palate was combined with lip repair, then the nasal floor within the alveolus can be intact with no oronasal communication. This assists secondary alveolar bone grafting with no requirement for nasal floor closure at the time of graft placement. Although this nasal soft tissue border is epithelialised on both surfaces, this does not impair good outcomes.

Bilateral alveolar clefts

Bilateral simultaneous bone grafting is the norm; however, if preoperative assessment identifies a small rudimentary premaxilla then consideration should be given to a staged approach to reduce risks of premaxillary ischaemia or necrosis.

In some bilateral cases with considerable malalignment of the premaxilla (severe pro- or retroclination), simultaneous osteotomy and repositioning of the premaxilla can be considered to improve alignment and appearance. Premaxillary osteotomy also provides superior access for nasal floor repair.

Cleft lip revision

If required, cleft lip revision can be combined with alveolar bone grafting in unilateral cases. However, extensive bilateral cleft lip revision should not be combined with bilateral bone grafting as vascularity of the premaxilla can be compromised.

OPERATIVE TECHNIQUE

Autogenous cancellous bone is the gold-standard graft material. The anterior iliac crest is the preferred harvest site, providing a good volume of graft with minimal morbidity. Simultaneous two-surgeon operating reduces operating time and allows timely transfer of the harvested cellularised graft to the recipient site. A throat pack is recommended and best inserted (and subsequently removed) by the operating surgeon once the patient is prepped and draped.

Operative steps in unilateral alveolar bone graft (general anaesthesia)

- Local anaesthetic infiltration (2% lignocaine and 1:80 000 adrenaline) provides vasoconstriction
- Removal and storage of any orthodontic intraoral appliance if impeding access
- While ink marking of the outline of the labiobuccal and palatal flaps and 'fistula' is not essential, this can assist operative planning and highlight areas of potential difficulty. The labial aspect of the alveolar cleft or fistula is outlined (*Figure 63.1*). The buccal advancement mucogingival flap from the 'lesser' maxillary segment includes an oblique backcut in the first molar region (*Figure 63.2*). Marking of the

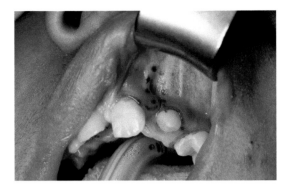

Figure 63.1 Operative marking of labial 'fistula' and labiobuccal mucoperiosteal flaps.

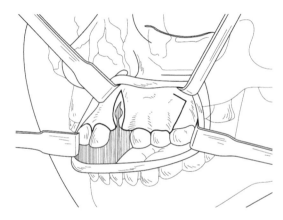

Figure 63.2 Diagram of labiobuccal incisions and flap outline.

gingival margin incision around the central incisor tooth on the 'greater' segment is often extended just beyond the midline to assist subsequent elevation of this mucoperiosteal tissue; starting in the midline. If the anterior palatal mucosa is intact and does not invaginate into the cleft alveolus, then elevation of anterior palatal flaps may not be required. However, the palatal tissue often does invaginate the cleft and therefore bilateral palatal flaps are required

- The labial soft tissue cleft or fistula is placed under tension with cheek retractors and incised around the fistula as an inverted flask-shape. While inferiorly the incision reaches the bony margins of the cleft; superiorly, the incision does not encounter bone and inadvertent fenestration of nasal floor should be avoided. The gingival margin incisions are completed along with the posterior backcut of the buccal advancement flap on the lesser segment
- The buccal and anterior labial mucogingival flaps are carefully elevated in the subperiosteal plane

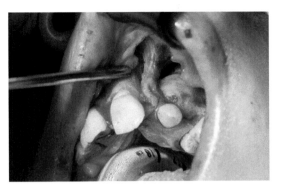

Figure 63.3 Elevation of labiobuccal flaps and nasal floor mucosa.

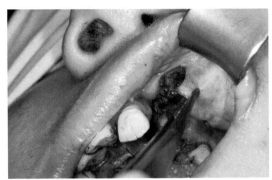

Figure 63.4 Adequate advancement of buccal flap following backcut, wide elevation and periosteal release.

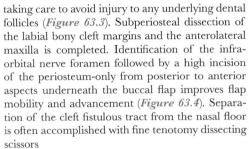

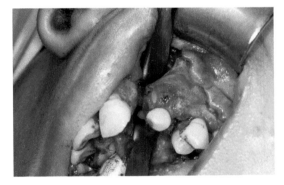

Figure 63.5 Nasal floor dissection and anterior palatal flaps.

taking care to avoid injury to any underlying dental follicles (*Figure 63.3*). Subperiosteal dissection of the labial bony cleft margins and the anterolateral maxilla is completed. Identification of the infra-orbital nerve foramen followed by a high incision of the periosteum-only from posterior to anterior aspects underneath the buccal flap improves flap mobility and advancement (*Figure 63.4*). Separation of the cleft fistulous tract from the nasal floor is often accomplished with fine tenotomy dissecting scissors

- In most cases, unless there is uninterrupted continuity of the palatal fibromucosa within the anterior palate, it is necessary to raise anterior palatal flaps (*Figure 63.5*). Following palatal gingival margin incisions, access is gained into the subperiosteal plane of the palate, often better starting some distance from the cleft alveolus. Separation of the palatal mucosa from the margin of the bony cleft with Aufricht scissors to create anterior palatal flaps is often better accomplished when the palatal tissues have been elevated up to and into the alveolar cleft. It is important to ensure that these cuts on either side of the palatal cleft margin within the anterior palate converge to an apex within the vault of the palate and do not diverge superiorly; otherwise, subsequent palatal flap closure high in the palate will be compromised
- Subperiosteal dissection within the cleft alveolus is completed up to the margins of the nasal floor and pyriform fossa of the nose. Further dissection along the nasal floor laterally is often impeded by the inferior turbinate and medially by the nasal septum. If the nasal floor mucosa is intact with no oronasal communication, then the integrity of the nasal floor is maintained. In clefts of the lip and palate, some degree of separation of the nasal and palatal tissues high in the palate at the posterior border of the cleft alveolus is required. Again, this is often better accomplished with sharp-pointed Aufricht scissors, avoiding fenestration of the nasal floor as suture placement within this area is difficult. All margins

of the alveolar cleft are now fully defined. There is no requirement to extend the dissection further into the palatal tissues unless a palatal fistula is present and planned for simultaneous closure. Redundant excess mucosa within the cleft alveolus is resected avoiding fenestration of the nasal floor. When an oronasal fistula or communication is present, then judicious resection of the excess mucosa is required to ensure that sufficient mucosa is retained to allow subsequent tension-free suture closure within the nasal floor

- Any communication in the nasal floor mucosa is closed using a resorbable suture material and a round-bodied needle with the knots positioned nasally. Occasionally, a compound curved or J-shaped needle can help suture placement. The palatal flaps are approximated and closed behind the bone defect (*Figure 63.6*). Haemostasis is checked and the defect is now ready to receive the harvested cancellous bone (*Figure 63.7*). Most of the cancellous bone is morselised into smaller more-compactable pieces, while larger pieces can be retained for placement along the nasal floor and onlay over the anterior maxilla/canine fossa region

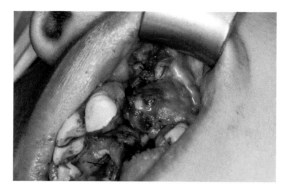

Figure 63.6 Nasal floor and anterior palatal closure.

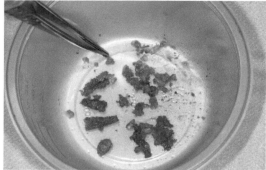

Figure 63.7 Harvested cancellous bone graft.

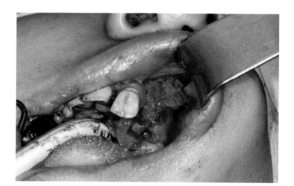

Figure 63.8 Bone graft packed into alveolar cleft and over anterior maxilla.

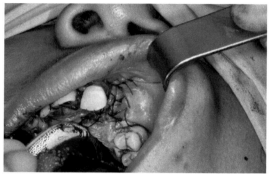

Figure 63.9 Buccal flap advancement and wound closure.

- The alveolar bone defect is filled with the small-particulate autogenous cancellous bone, starting from the extremities of the defect such as the nasal floor, pyriform rim and deep aspects. The bone is frequently compressed and moulded into the defect. The defect should be over-filled and bone also placed over the anterior maxilla lateral to the pyriform rim area to improve alar base support (*Figure 63.8*)
- The buccal flap is advanced with tension-free closure over the labial aspect of the grafted alveolus with suture placement starting from the gingival margin and extending superiorly towards the buccal sulcus. Further suture placement between the labial and palatal tissues across the alveolar crest within the cleft site, followed by interdental sutures between the palatal and labiobuccal soft tissue flaps, provide a virtual 'watertight' closure (*Figure 63.9*)
- The gingival soft tissue secondary defect within the first molar region following buccal flap advancement is left to heal by secondary intention (*Figure 63.10*)
- Any orthodontic appliance is now replaced, checking that the appliance does not compress or traumatise the repair; as otherwise it may

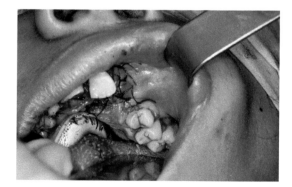

Figure 63.10 Secondary gingival defect in first molar region.

be preferable to not replace the appliance. The throat-pack is carefully removed under direct vision followed by oropharyngeal suction

POSTOPERATIVE CARE

- Early mobilisation (first postoperative day)
- Perioperative systemic antibiotics and simple analgesia

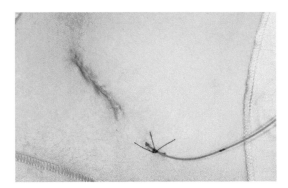

Figure 63.11 Closure of anterior iliac crest donor site with in-dwelling wound cannula infusion of local anaesthetic.

- Iliac crest donor site 'pain buster' analgesia with local anaesthetic infusion – 0.5% plain bupivacaine (*Figure 63.11*)
- Soft diet for 4–6 weeks
- Oral hygiene regime with 0.2% chlorhexidene digluconate and toothbrushing

POSSIBLE COMPLICATIONS

- *Partial wound dehiscence with graft exposure and contamination*: often associated with excessive flap tension and/or inadequate oral hygiene. Treatment is conservative with local wound hygiene measures and consideration of a systemic antibiotic such as metronidazole
- *Bone sequestration*: bony sequestra may become visible within the graft site within the first few weeks. They are usually best left to separate spontaneously with subsequent healing. Good local hygiene is important
- *Granuloma*: may occasionally occur and present as an enlarging gingival epulis. Often related to persistent local inflammation from a bone sequestrum, wound suture and poor hygiene. Most resolve spontaneously with local hygiene measures. Persistent lesions may require excision
- *Graft resorption*: bone loss may be partial or rarely complete. Early bone loss is often associated with inadequate soft tissue closure or subsequent dehiscence. Late bone resorption may occur when there is a lack of dental loading of the graft site, particularly if the permanent canine tooth is already erupted at the time of surgery. In such cases, early postoperative medial movement of the canine into the grafted site by the orthodontist would provide beneficial dental loading and inhibit late bone resorption

TOP TIPS AND HAZARDS

- Clarify treatment plan with the orthodontist, in particular which teeth are to be removed from the cleft site and which are to be retained.
- Palatally erupted teeth (supernumerary or diminutive lateral incisors) are preferably extracted at least 6 weeks before grafting to improve flap quality.
- Beware of possible dental changes between clinic visit and admission for surgery. Previously unerupted teeth may have erupted and previous erupted teeth may have exfoliated. Consider updating radiographs if doubt exists.
- Ensure any orthodontic appliance can be removed or does not obstruct access.
- Raise full gingivo-mucoperiosteal flaps and avoid attempts to preserve a periodontal gingival 'collar'.
- Nasal floor soft tissue continuity is essential and repair can be difficult. Vomerine flap repair of the anterior palate at the time of primary lip repair is advantageous.
- Keep the time period of stored cancellous bone graft to a minimum. Avoid use of cortical bone.
- Use a bone rongeur to break the bone into small fragments which compact well and improve perfusion surface area. Avoid desiccation with an overlaid damp saline swab prior to insertion at the recipient site.
- Avoid use of non-autogenous materials such as bone substitutes, biomembranes or fibrin glue within the alveolar site. If possible, reduce routine use of haemostatic materials and bone wax.
- Plan for soft tissue closure with keratinised mucosa (gingival tissue) and not non-keratinised buccal mucosal tissue. Teeth will not erupt through non-keratinised mucosa.
- For clefts of the primary palate only (cleft lip and alveolus), the bone margins of the alveolar cleft palatally are fully defined up to the intact bony hard palate posteriorly.
- In bilateral cases, ensure continued attachment of the labial soft tissue pedicle to the premaxilla. If the premaxilla is excessively malaligned vertically, horizontally or both, consider simultaneous premaxillary osteotomy and repositioning. Premaxillary stabilisation by orthodontic fixed labial arch-wire is required.

FURTHER READING

Åbyholm FE, Bergland O, Semb G. Secondary bone grafting of alveolar clefts: a surgical/orthodontic treatment enabling a non-prosthodontic rehabilitation in cleft lip and palate patients. *Scand J Plast Reconstr Surg* 1981;**15**:127–40.

Boyne PJ, Sands NR. Secondary bone grafting of residual alveolar and palatal clefts. *J Oral Surg* 1972;**30**:87–92.

Lundberg J, Jäghagen EL, Sjöström M. Outcomes after secondary alveolar bone grafting among patients with cleft lip and palate at 16 years of age: a retrospective study. *Oral Surg Oral Med Oral Pathol Oral Radiol* 2021;**132**:281–7.

Revington PJ, McNamara C, Mukarram S, et al. Alveolar bone grafting: results of a national outcome study. *Ann R Coll Surg Engl* 2010;**92**:643–6.

Scott R, Scott J, Stagnell S, et al. Outcomes of 44 consecutive complete bilateral cleft lip and palate patients treated with secondary alveolar bone grafting and premaxillary osteotomy. *Cleft Palate Craniofac J* 2017;**54**:249–55.

Bailey & Love's Essential Operations Bailey & Love's Essential Operations
Bailey & Love's Essential Operations Bailey & Love's Essential Operations
Bailey & Love's Essential Operations Bailey & Love's Essential Operations

PART 9 | Cleft lip and palate

Chapter
64

Cleft Rhinoplasty

Clare Rivers, Mark Devlin, Craig Russell

INTRODUCTION

Despite multiple descriptions of techniques for primary cleft lip/nose repair in the literature, consensus on optimal management among experienced cleft surgeons remains elusive. Within the literature, three main philosophies of approach to the primary cleft nasal deformity could be described:

- *Minimal nasal intervention within the primary surgical pathway*: this approach recognises challenges in obtaining permanent correction of the nasal deformity that will not require secondary intervention
- *Intermediate nasal intervention within the primary surgical pathway*: there is recognition of a dynamic component to the cleft nasal deformity throughout growth that may necessitate early secondary surgery
- *Extensive nasal intervention within the primary surgical pathway*: this approach aims to correct all functional and aesthetic nasal deformity at the time of primary lip/nose repair, expecting that the patient will not require secondary intervention

Whichever of the philosophies the treating surgeon considers most appropriate, recognition that no one philosophy reigns supreme throughout the cleft community is important. In the era of informed consent, surgeons treating the cleft deformity should fully discuss the challenges and limitations of cleft nasal management (and the controversies therein).

This chapter focuses on technical aspects of an intermediate surgical philosophy and highlights aspects of the alternate philosophies where relevant.

FEATURES OF THE CLEFT NOSE DEFORMITY

In the unilateral cleft lip, neither side of the nose is normal (*Figure 64.1*). The underlying bone is deformed and deficient with hypoplasia and displacement of the lesser maxillary segment and a wide piriform aperture on the cleft side. The nasal ala is flattened with the base displaced posteriorly, inferiorly and laterally due to tethering to the underlying bone. The anterior nasal spine and caudal septum are deviated to the non-cleft side while the body of the septum deviates to the cleft side causing posterior nasal obstruction. The nasal bones are widened with nasal bridge deviation. The upper lateral cartilage (ULC) is deviated to the

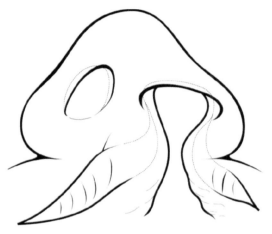

Figure 64.1 Unilateral cleft nose primary deformity.

non-cleft side and partially dislocated from the lower lateral cartilage (LLC). The lateral crus is drawn into an S-shape as the LLC is significantly deformed and rotated. The nasal tip is flattened and deviated with bifidity due to fibrofatty tissue between the two domes. Due to the displacement of the LLC in the dorsoventral plane, the columella is short and appears deficient. However, the columella 'is in the nose' as the splayed medial crus and associated soft tissue is drawn into the alar rim.

The bilateral cleft lip nasal deformity has a broad flattened nasal tip, short columella and lateral and inferior displacement of the alar bases. The maxilla is deficient bilaterally with variation in the position of the premaxilla. There is disturbed caudoventral growth of the septum with inferior displacement resulting in a lack of projection and subsequent flattening of the osseocartilaginous vault of the dorsum. The skeletal imbalances and short columella contribute to the broad nasal tip. The LLCs are deformed with downward displacement of the lateral crura bilaterally. The nostrils are therefore wide and horizontally rotated.

RHINOPLASTY PROCEDURES AT THE TIME OF THE PRIMARY CLEFT LIP SURGERY

Various methods and approaches have been described for primary rhinoplasty performed at the time of lip

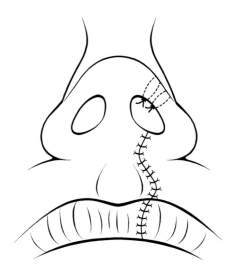

Figure 64.2 Alar transfixation to the skin at the alar crease.

repair. However, there is a growing consensus that primary rhinoplasty should and can be performed without additional scarring or incisions beyond those required for concurrent repair of the cleft lip.

Unilateral cleft lip and nose

The well-established modified McComb's technique involves closed dissection of the alar cartilages from the attached skin through the buccal sulcus and columellar incisions using sharp-pointed scissors (iris or tenotomy scissors). Through the buccal sulcus incision, dissection continues over the cleft half of the nose to the nasal bones. Using the columellar incision, dissection can be performed to release the skin from the medial crus and dome of the alar cartilage. The alar cartilage is dissected free from the nostril rim, the nasal tip and up to the nasion. This allows the alar cartilage, attached to nostril lining, to be lifted and held with one or two mattress sutures (e.g. clear 4-0 PDS) passed from the nasal vestibule, through the intercrural angle and lateral crus to the nasion. These can be passed over bolsters or buried by reintroducing the needle back through the same point in the skin (*Figure 64.2*). Further mattress sutures can address the lateral vestibule webbing as well as obliterate any dead space. There is no need for additional incisions to be made in the nasal lining. Using a non-permanent suture removes the need for suture removal unless a bolster is used.

Bilateral cleft lip and nose

The aim is to preserve and elongate the columella by repositioning the LLCs with correction of the columellar height and nasal width. A McComb's dissection can

be used; however, there is no landmark to position the alar lift. The ULCs should normally be at the same height as the LLC. Therefore, the aim of lifting is to the height of the ULC and to reduce the nostril size equally. To address the lack of columella height, forked flaps from the prolabium and nasal sill advancement flaps have been used. However, the resulting unsightly scars have meant these have fallen out of favour. The modern practice is to retrieve the columella from the nasal tip with reshaping and redraping of the nasal cartilages. The alar cartilages can be accessed medially from the prolabium under the columella without extra incisions. Subperichondrial septal dissection allows repositioning of the medial crura with support provided by interdomal suturing (*Figure 64.3*). Access can be obtained with an extended prolabial incision through the membranous septum. By going posterior to the medial crura, they can be repositioned superiorly to support the lengthened columella. To allow apposition of the medial crura, the fibroadipose tissue between the domes should be dissected. Other techniques that involve intranasal incisions and open approaches are not recommended due to concerns about long-term growth and secondary procedures.

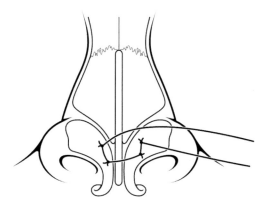

Figure 64.3 Horizontal mattress interdomal suture.

INTERMEDIARY SEPTORHINOPLASTY: FROM PRIMARY REPAIR TO END OF GROWTH

Ongoing nasal asymmetry is common in children with cleft lip and palate (particularly unilateral). The reasons for the asymmetry are well recognised and could be considered as a combination of skeletal, cartilaginous and soft tissue.

We can consider the effects of each of these factors in relation to the various extents of unilateral cleft involvement.

Unilateral cleft lip with no alveolar involvement

- *Skeletal*: there may be minimal overt skeletal asymmetry. There is likely to be an underlying maxillary hypoplasia which, though often subtle, will cause some degree of asymmetry
- *Cartilaginous*: asymmetry in the cartilaginous structures is found at two points. The LLC on the cleft side will often be hypoplastic, flattened and laterally displaced. This affects symmetry of the nasal dome and tip. Secondly, the nasal septum is often anteriorly displaced/dislocated from the maxillary crest and anterior nasal spine leading to nasal tip asymmetry
- *Soft tissue*: the healing process with scar contraction can lead to asymmetry. Overly aggressive resection of skin may cause nostril stenosis. Lateral webbing within the nostril also causes asymmetry

Unilateral cleft lip with associated alveolar cleft

- *Skeletal*: the alveolar cleft will lead to asymmetric support for the lip, nostril sill and alar base. Hypoplasia of the maxilla will have a more overt impact than in unilateral cleft lip with no alveolar involvement
- *Cartilaginous*: the degree of asymmetry of the LLC and nasal septum is greater than where no alveolar cleft is present
- *Soft tissue*: as above. In addition, the soft tissues as they heal intraorally can be drawn upwards into the alveolar cleft, which can affect both lip and nose symmetry

Unilateral cleft lip and palate (complete)

- *Skeletal*: as above but with a likely greater width of cleft and greater overall effect
- *Cartilaginous*: as above but with greater overall effect
- *Soft tissue*: as above but with greater overall effect

In relation to each of the situations above, the impact of facial growth is unpredictable. The variations in how an individual child might grow represents one of the reasons for surgical caution. Surgical intervention exposes the child to another variable, independent factor that may affect further facial growth.

Once initial healing has occurred, the surgeon's role is to provide input as requested. The likelihood of nasal asymmetry existing following cleft lip ± palate repair is significant. Parents are counselled on this. Nevertheless, parental anxiety regarding asymmetry may lead to a discussion regarding further surgery. It is important that, during this period of growth, surgical intervention is minimal. The simplest interventions are those that address the soft tissues only. Surgery confined to the lip or nasal tip is less likely to cause a negative impact

of facial and nasal growth than procedures involving the nasal septum. The decision to intervene should only be taken following discussion with the parents, patient (where appropriate) and the Cleft Clinical Psychology Team. Aesthetic outcome is important in cleft care and therefore a legitimate reason for intervention when likely to improve matters with limited risk of complication.

The role of medical management in nasal obstruction should be first considered as this may achieve a reduction in symptoms. Liaison with the patient's family doctor to ensure optimal medical management is vital.

When undertaking rhinoplasty in this age group, interventions should be combined with a planned procedure, for example alveolar bone grafting (ABG), where possible to minimise anaesthetic exposure and educational disruption.

Unilateral

A widened nostril sill width can be addressed with a wedge excision or as part of cleft lip revision with alar base re-dissection and repositioning. Addressing nasal tip asymmetry, tip-plasty can be performed through a mid-columella incision which is continued infracartilaginously. The LLC and ULCs are exposed (*Figure 64.4*). The fibrous attachment of the LLC to the ULC and the rim of the maxilla are freed by sharp dissection. The interdomal attachments between both lower lateral crura are also freed. This should allow the LLC to be free and mobile, enabling it to be evaluated for lateral mucosal tethering. The deficiency of the cleft side mucosa is evaluated by placing a hook in the intermediate crural margin and advancing the

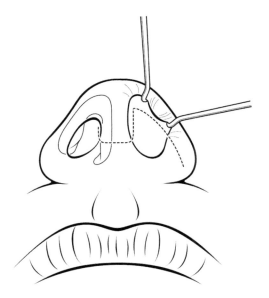

Figure 64.4 A mid-columella incision with bilateral infracartilaginous incisions.

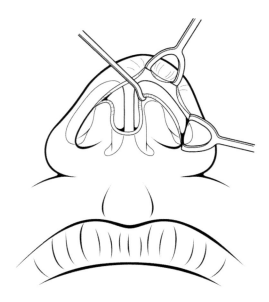

Figure 64.5 The required mobilisation on the cleft side is assessed by placing a skin hook.

freed LLC with attached mucosa to match the height of the non-cleft side (*Figure 64.5*). If there is tethering of the LLC, it should be ensured that only the mucosal attachment remains (*Figure 64.6*). If the mucosa is still tight and limits elevation of the LLC, a V-Y incision can be made to release the lateral web and rotate the LLC.

After release of the LLC and correction of the mucosal deficiency, the chondromucosal unit is advanced into its correct position. Several suturing techniques can be employed to hold the cartilages in their new position (*Figure 64.7*).

The skin is redraped and sutured. Additional support can be provided with one to three alar transfixation

sutures to the skin at the alar crease to reconstitute the alar crease, support nasal tip projection and reduce vestibular webbing.

A variety of splinting techniques are described and utilised according to surgeon preference.

Bilateral

The same approach and manoeuvres can be used in the bilateral cleft nose; however, addressing lack of tip projection is more challenging due to the shortened columella. It can be tempting to place cartilage grafts such as columella strut grafts and shield grafts to address this, but this may compromise future surgical endeavours.

DEFINITIVE CLEFT RHINOPLASTY ONCE GROWTH HAS STOPPED

Unilateral cleft lip rhinoplasty

The unilateral cleft lip nose is considered more difficult to treat than the bilateral cleft lip nose due to asymmetry. Challenges in the unilateral cleft/lip nose include:

- Nasal tip asymmetry with the dome at the cleft side lower than the non-cleft side
- The cleft side lower lateral crura is crimped, deformed or hypoplastic
- The nasal tip is often underprojected and over-rotated
- Widened nasal tip due to the LLCs spaced further apart
- Asymmetry at the naso-alar groove, with depression at the cleft side

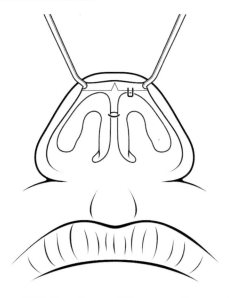

Figure 64.7 Superior medial crus mattress suture and a suture from the lateral crura to the upper lateral cartilage.

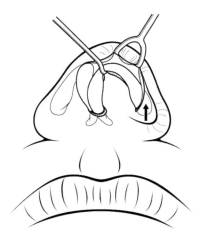

Figure 64.6 If elevation of the released LLC is limited by the mucosa, a V-Y releasing incision can be made.

- Horizontal or wider nostril at the cleft side
- Lower alar rim on the cleft side
- The septum and its bony associations are deviated in a cranial caudal and anteroposterior direction causing aesthetic and functional concerns
- Soft tissue deficiency at the cleft side with depressed nasal bony floor at the previous ABG site

Reconstructing the bony defect at the cleft side

The skeletal framework should be treated first in any craniofacial deformity before cleft rhinoplasty is performed. Patients who require maxillary advancement due to maxillary hypoplasia should ideally have this before rhinoplasty. Alternatively, the cleft lip rhinoplasty can be done simultaneously with the osteotomy but is not advocated by the authors. Bony deficiency at the piriform rim can be augmented with alloplastic material or autogenous bone. A block of contoured corticocancellous bone can be harvested from the mandible, calvarium or iliac crest and secured to the pyriform rim defect as an onlay graft via an intraoral circumvestibular incision. Two fixation screws are used to secure the bone to the underlying bony base. If a non-resorbable material is preferred, Medpore (porous polyethylene implants) can be custom-made or fashioned on table. The method of surgical access and means of securing the implant is the same as for bone grafts. Peri-implant infection is of low incidence and practice involves a standardised systemic antibiotic protocol.

Incision and exposure

Open rhinoplasty is preferred as it allows unparalleled access to the underlying asymmetric nasal tip anatomy and dorsum (*Figure 64.8*). An inverted V-transcolumellar incision can be used with bilateral infracartilaginous incisions. The nasal tip is carefully degloved and

skeletonised. The difference in size and morphology between the LLC at the cleft side and the non-cleft side can be appreciated. Dissection should continue over the ULCs and continue in the subperiosteal plane along the nasal bones.

Septal cartilage graft harvesting

The septum can be reached via a tip split technique. The fibrous attachment between the bilateral LLCs is dissected to access the septum. Following subperichondrial dissection, septal cartilage graft is dissected out leaving at least 10–12 mm of caudal and dorsal strut. Where functional internal nasal valve issues exist, a dorsal approach is favoured as, in addition to allowing access to harvest graft, it creates space for spreader grafts.

Dorsal hump

These can be removed as in standard rhinoplasty. A cartilaginous hump can be excised with a blade while the bony hump is osteotomised and removed with a Rubin osteotome. The remaining rough edges can be smoothed out by rasping or by using a diamond rasp.

Nasal bone management

Detailed preoperative assessment will guide endonasal or percutaneous osteotomies to close the open roof defect and realign any nasal deviation. For the deviated nose in the unilateral cleft lip deformity, comprehensive clinical and radiological assessment is advocated allowing preoperative planning of the management of the cartilaginous septum, vomerine crest, caudal ethmoidal plate and turbinates. This should only be undertaken by an appropriately trained and experienced surgeon.

Nasal tip surgery

There are numerous tip-grafting techniques useful in cleft lip rhinoplasty. They are as follows:

- Extended septal graft (*Figure 64.9*)
- Columellar strut (*Figure 64.9*)
- Onlay graft (*Figure 64.10*)
- Alar batten graft (*Figure 64.11*)

To acquire additional nasal projection, the extended septal graft technique is useful. The septal cartilage graft is sutured to the caudal end of the septum, projecting in a caudal direction beyond the nasal septum. This allows correction of the nasolabial angle from an obtuse angle to 90°.

For increased strength and height, the nasal tip is further supported with a columellar strut. The columellar strut can be sutured to the extended septal graft. The dome at the cleft side can be lifted to the same height as the dome of the non-cleft side and sutured to the extended septal graft and columellar strut. Onlay grafts can be secured on top of this to increase the nasal tip height, masking some of the nasal tip asymmetry. Residual asymmetry due to the hypoplastic nature of

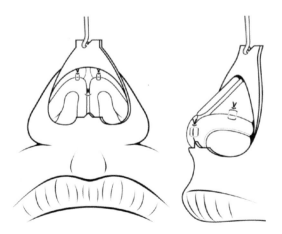

Figure 64.8 Open rhinoplasty technique with columellar stepped incision.

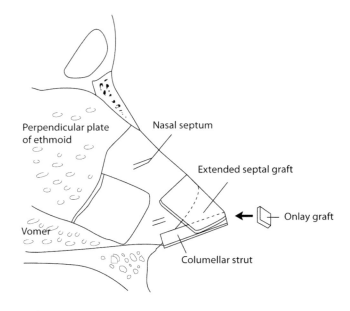

Figure 64.9 Extended septal graft is fashioned from the harvested septal graft. It is sutured to the caudal end of the septum. It can be further reinforced by a columellar strut.

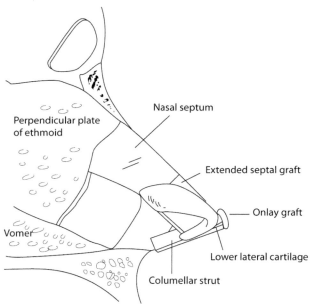

Figure 64.10 The nasal projection is directed in a caudal, anterior direction by the extended septal graft and columellar strut. Placement of an onlay graft at the nasal tip will further increase nasal projection, mask some asymmetry of the nasal tip and form a more defined nasal tip.

the LLC at the cleft side can be camouflaged with alar batten graft. The best sources of grafts are septal or conchal cartilages. Rib cartilage grafts can be useful when a large dorsal strut is required and for extended septal grafts and columellar struts. The fifth, sixth or seventh rib is harvested via an inframammary incision. The rib graft can be fashioned to a dorsal graft of the appropriate height and length. This can be placed in the subperichondrial and subperiosteal pocket. Various suturing techniques are employed to improve the nasal tip definition and refinement, including transdomal, interdomal and intercolumellar sutures.

Alar base

Alar base reduction can be achieved with appropriately sized nasal sill resection.

Bilateral cleft lip rhinoplasty

The concerns for bilateral cleft lip nose include:

- Broad nasal bridge
- Depressed nasal tip with decreased nasal projection
- Short, retracted columella
- Wide amorphous nasal tip
- Wide alar base

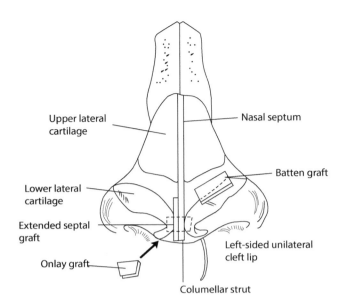

Upper lateral
cartilage

Nasal septum

Lower lateral
cartilage

Batten graft

Extended septal
graft

Left-sided unilateral
cleft lip

Onlay graft

Columellar strut

Figure 64.11 Extended septal graft sutured to the caudal end of the septum, columellar strut, left-sided batten graft and an onlay graft.

The aim of the surgery is to increase nasal tip projection, refine the nasal tip and reduce alar base width. Incision and exposure techniques are the same as that for the unilateral cleft lip nasal deformity.

Narrowing of the nasal bridge

Although hump reduction is rare, fracture of the nasal bone can narrow the nasal bridge. This can be performed with medial and lateral nasal osteotomies resulting in sharper nasofacial angles. Augmentation of the dorsum with alloplastic implants or rib grafts helps in two ways – augmenting the dorsum of the shallow bridge and creating the illusion of a narrow nasal bridge.

Nasal tip surgery

Nasal tip projection can be increased with a columellar strut, and this can be further reinforced with extended septal graft. Instead of conchal and septal grafts, rib grafts or alloplastic implants may be needed to form the strong underlying architecture. The wide nasal tip can be narrowed with transdomal and interdomal sutures. Further definition and projection of the nasal tip can be achieved with onlay grafts.

Alar base

Alar base width reduction can be performed with judicious nasal sill excision, suturing both muscle and skin to reconstruct the foundations.

TOP TIPS AND HAZARDS

- Nasal intervention at the time of lip repair should be tailored to the philosophy of whole care pathway (be it minimal with understanding of need for significant surgery later in life or a more aggressive primary rhinoplasty to avoid further surgery).
- Secondary rhinoplasty should be undertaken following psychological, functional, radiological and aesthetic assessment.
- Be cautious of undertaking multiple rhinoplasty procedures chasing perfection.

FURTHER READING

Devlin MF, Ray A, Raine P, et al. Facial symmetry in unilateral cleft lip and palate following alar base augmentation with bone graft: a three-dimensional assessment. *Cleft Palate Craniofac J* 2007;**44**:391–5.

Massie JP, Runyan CM, Stern MJ, et al. Nasal septal anatomy in skeletally mature patients with cleft lip and palate. *JAMA Facial Plast Surg* 2016;**18**:347–53.

McComb H. Primary correction of unilateral cleft lip nasal deformity: a 10-year review. *Plast Reconstr Surg* 1985;**75**:791–9.

Talmant JC, Talmant JC. Rhinoplastie de fente primaire et secondaire [Cleft rhinoplasty, from primary to secondary surgery]. *Ann Chir Plast Esthet* 2014;**59**: 555–84.

Tse RW, Mercan E, Fisher DM, et al. Unilateral cleft lip nasal deformity: foundation-based approach to primary rhinoplasty. *Plast Reconstr Surg* 2019;**144**: 1138–49.

Chapter 65

Face, Neck and Brow Lift Surgery

Dominic Bray

INTRODUCTION

There are several techniques described in relation to aesthetic surgery of the face and the neck. The author's technique detailed in this chapter involves entering the deep plane to release the deep retaining ligaments of the face before restoring proportion and reducing deep volume in the neck in the quest to create exceptional and long-lasting results.

Frank A. Clark, an American politician, wrote "If you find a path without obstacles, it probably doesn't lead anywhere". This is apt in rejuvenation of the ageing face. The dense collection of retaining ligaments in the face, necessary for retaining volume, lift and beauty in youth, become anchors of soft tissue as we age. Any technique that ignores these anchors cannot adequately elevate facial soft tissues with any longevity.

The evolution of the face and neck lift technique has progressively addressed deeper layers throughout the last 50 years; from early skin-only lifting, to a myriad of methods to tighten the underlying superficial musculoaponeurotic system (SMAS) originally described by Swedish surgeon Tord Skoog in the 1970s. SMAS lift led to acceptable results for the time, it produced a predictably tighter jawline and some short-lived neck improvement but did little for the descended midface, which often needed concomitant volume with autologous fat transfer and/or midface lifting. It regularly created deformity of tension (atrophic migrated scarring) and vector (lateral sweep) deformity over time leaving tell-tale signs of surgery caused by lifting against several immobile ligamentous anchors (*Figure 65.1*).

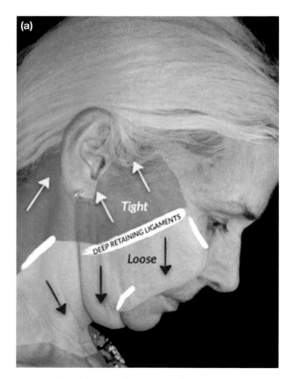
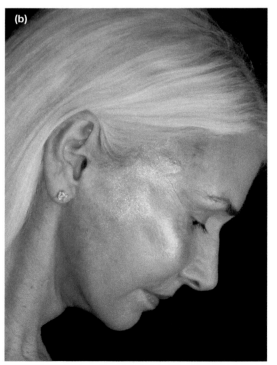

Figure 65.1 (a) Lateral sweep deformity following previous superficial musculoaponeurotic system facelift with inadequate release of the deep retaining ligaments of the face. This causes preauricular tension and central fifth laxity. (b) Three months following secondary deep plane facelift.

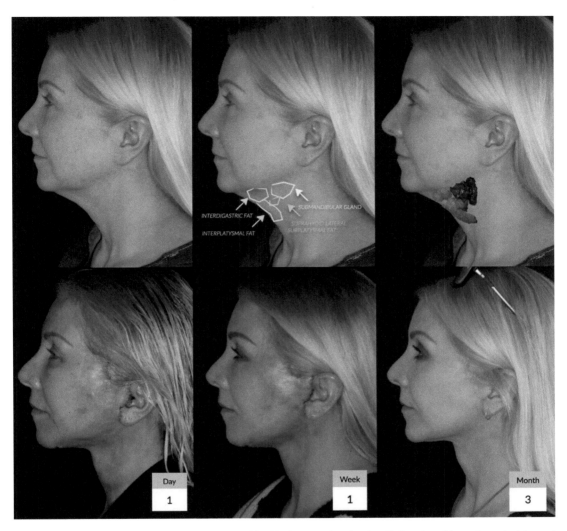

Figure 65.2 Combined deep plane face and neck lift with deep neck reduction. Failure to address the subplatysmal structures cannot create an acute neck–chin angle in patients with hypertrophied or descended submandibular glands, deep neck fat or digastric muscles.

Subcutaneous neck liposuction was used to improve profile contour but longer-term outcomes show that not only do we need superficial fat for a soft neck contour, for skin health and to mask the dynamic contraction of the underlying platysma muscle but blunting of the neck–chin angle with age is often due to subplatysmal deep fat, hypertrophic anterior digastric muscles and/or submandibular glandular hypertrophy or ptosis in addition to platysma and skin redundancy (*Figure 65.2*).

This chapter outlines the surgical technique for extended composite deep plane face and neck surgery, and browlift surgery. It assumes basic facial anatomical knowledge.

FACE AND NECK SURGERY

Surgical procedure

Positioning, preparation and anaesthesia

The procedure can be performed under local anaesthesia alone or with conscious sedation. The latter is preferred due to the duration of surgery. In a semi-recumbent position with gel head donut support, the face and neck are prepared with chlorhexidine and draped in sterile fashion. Oxygen nasal specs are positioned with CO_2 monitoring. Incision lines are injected with 1% lidocaine and tumescent fluid anaesthesia achieved with a solution of dilute lidocaine, bupivacaine, adrenaline, sodium bicarbonate and tranexamic acid. Conscious sedation is achieved with midazolam or propofol.

Deep neck reduction

A 2-cm submental incision is made in the natural submental crease with the patient's neck extended. The skin is elevated caudally with McIndoe scissors, taking care to maintain a thin layer of subcutaneous fat and an intact dermis, and extended superolaterally to divide the mandibular cutaneous retaining ligaments. A central strip of interplatysmal fat is excised and the deep neck is entered by elevating large subplatysmal muscle flaps 4 cm laterally via their central dehiscence, 2 cm below the hyoid and to the mandible superiorly superficial to the anterior belly of digastric muscle. The suprahyoid deep neck is exposed with Aufricht retractors and assessed with good retraction, headlighting and 2× loupe magnification. The deep neck contents can be variable and reduction is planned preoperatively with palpation against the patient's own tongue-based palatal pressure, 3D Vectra analysis (Canfield Scientific) and on-table examination and palpation. The subplatysmal suprahyoid fat is distinctly separated into one central and two lateral compartments. Commonly,

interdigastric fat is removed and the anterior belly of digastric muscles plicated with 2/0 vicryl. If the digastric muscles are hypertrophied, they are linear reduced by 30–60% with monopolar needle point cautery. After reduction of the suprahyoid lateral fat compartment, the inferior pole of the submandibular gland is assessed. If mildly ptotic, a lateral platysma muscular sling suffices. If significantly ptotic or hypertrophied below the level of the mandibular line, the capsule is entered for reduction. This is difficult access and dissection but is aided by good retraction of the skin flap caudally, the subplatysmal flap anteriorly and with good toothed forcep central countertraction on the suprahyoid lateral fat inferiorly.

The gland is vascular and reduced meticulously with combination bipolar and monopolar cautery. Occasionally, the facial vessels require ligation. After reduction, the capsule is oversewn and closed with interrupted 2/0 vicryl. Careful haemostasis of the newly sculpted deep neck is achieved with bipolar diathermy and tested by asking the patient to perform a Valsalva manoeuvre. A 2/0 vicryl neck defining stitch is placed anchoring the platysma on each side to the hyoid periosteum. The platysma is closed from 2 cm infrahyoid using a 2/0 vicryl horizontal mattress corset technique

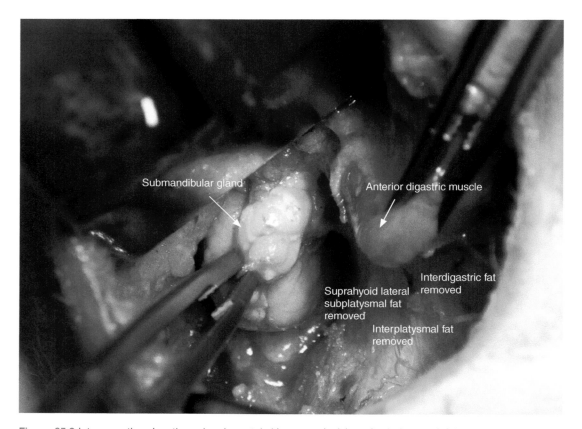

Figure 65.3 Intraoperative view through submental skin crease incision of subplatysmal right deep neck contents after removal of interdigastric fat.

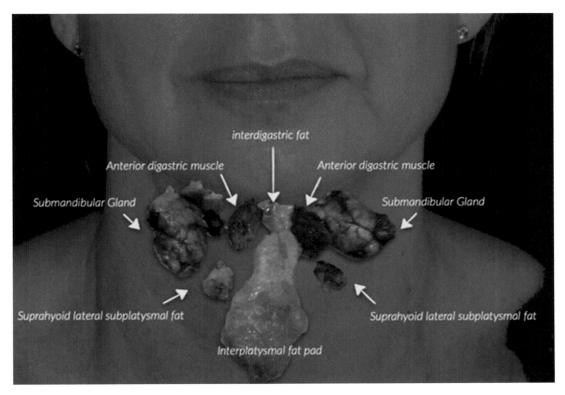

Figure 65.4 Subplatysmal structures removed in deep neck reduction surgery.

to the level of the mentum, then double-breasted back to the infrahyoid fixation point. Meticulous closure in layers redefines the deep neck visibly on the operating table. At this stage no 'lifting' has been performed, just deep volume reduction, re-sculpting and reconstruction of the anterior neck (*Figures 65.3* and *65.4*).

Composite deep plane face and neck lift

Trichophytic temporal hairline incisions are made following the helical crus, passing paratragal then 4 mm anteriorly at the incisura, down and around the earlobe and back up 2 mm anterior to the postauricular sulcus before turning posteriorly at the level of the inferior crura of the antihelix and tricophytically hugging the postauricular hairline. A back-lit skin flap is elevated to 2 cm past Pitanguy's line, which is the surface landmark of the temporal branch of the facial nerve, at which point the deep plane is entered. Using strong magnification, headlighting, superior retraction and counter-traction, the deep plane is entered with needle point monopolar cautery. Dissection progresses using scissor spreading and blunt dissection developing a composite skin/SMAS flap with the roof as the orbicularis oculi superiorly, the SMAS centrally and the platysma inferiorly following the zygomaticus major, parotid capsule and masseter inferiorly on the floor. The zygomatic cutaneous ligament (McGregor's patch), masseteric ligaments and preauricular parotid cutaneous ligaments are sharply divided and the lateral platysma is detached from its attachments to the sternocleidomastoid muscle, access having been eased with prior division of the temporoparotid fascia (Lore's fascia).

Once all ligaments have been freed, there is complete en bloc mobility of the neck, jowl, nasolabial fold, malar fat pad and midface (*Figure 65.5*). In cases of significant midface ptosis or previous lower blepharoplasty ectropion, the superior dissection of the SMAS composite flap is extended to include lateral orbicularis oculi and divide the lateral orbicularis retaining ligament. The buccal fat pad can be reduced between the visible buccal facial nerve branches and divided masseteric ligaments. The gonial angle, jawline and submandibular gland contour are assessed and if necessary, the platysma can be back cut horizontally from its lateral border deep in the neck to create a tight platysma sling, which elevates the gland back up behind the mandible when secured laterally to the mastoid fascia or to the anterior mastoid after incising the parotid capsule depending on gonial angle definition desired. At this stage, the patient is positioned in a more upright position to gauge aesthetically the ideal vector of composite deep plane orbicularic–SMAS–platysma flap lift by placing Pitanguy flap clamps on the composite cuff and mimicking the rejuvenating vector (*Figure 65.6*).

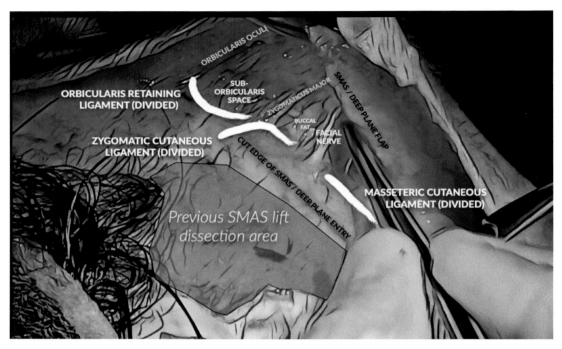

Figure 65.5 Deep plane entry anterior to Pitanguy's line. Demonstrating position of divided deep retaining ligaments, zygomaticus major and facial nerve branches.

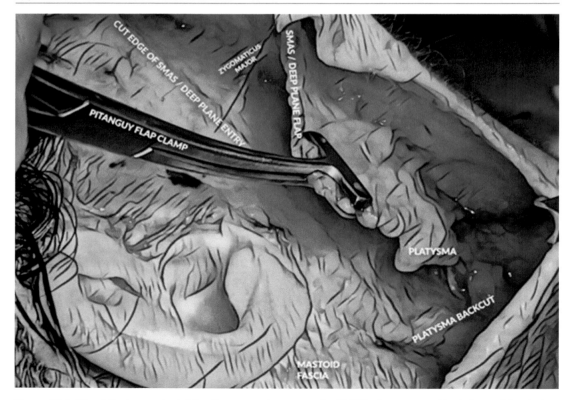

Figure 65.6 After full release of retaining ligaments, the composite SMAS–platysma ± orbicularis oculi flap is fully mobile in the glide plane.

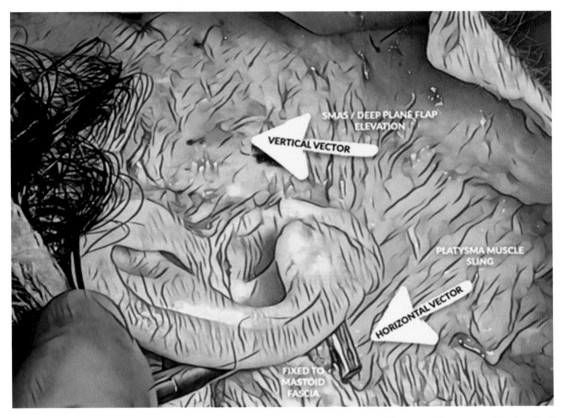

Figure 65.7 Bivector advancement of composite flap enabling posterior vector platysma advancement and vertical vector facial advancement.

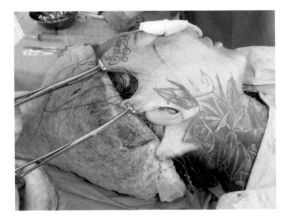

Figure 65.8 Intraoperative skin excess created with full ligamentous release in the deep plane. Note no tension is placed on the skin.

Most commonly, this is approximately 70° and follows the direction of the zygomaticus major muscle.

The flap is then fixed under no tension with vertical mattress 2/0 vicryl to the lateral immobile SMAS in the

midface, the superficial temporal fascia at the level of the brow and the mastoid and investing layer of deep cervical fascia in the neck (*Figure 65.7*). The redundant SMAS cuff is excised and if there is any lower facial third or neck subcutaneous fat contour irregularity, this can be sparingly sculpted with Kaye facelift scissors under direct vision.

The near vertical vector of this lift creates abundant skin lateral to the orbit in the lateral facial fifths, a phenomenon not seen with the backwards vector pull SMAS only lifts. The creation of this skin excess is reassuring that the lift has been performed in an appropriate vector as the frontalis elevator is deficient laterally leading to descent of the lateral brow tail with age. This skin is elevated subcutaneously over the orbital rim to the level of the arch of the eyebrow and excised by superiorly extending the trichophytic temporal incision.

The exact same procedure is performed on the other side before the skin is trimmed. This enables balance to be achieved between sides in the deep layers prior to meticulous tailoring of the more superficial skin flap under absolutely no tension (*Figure 65.8*). Delaying skin closure until both sides are completed allows time for retracted deep perforating vessels to bleed enabling

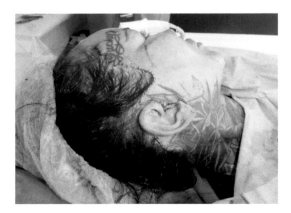

Figure 65.9 After redundant skin excision, skin flap approximates under no tension. Note trichophytic incision and limited use of straight lines.

better haemostasis. Keypoint 5/0 monocryl sutures are placed at the helix, incisura and mastoid to hold position, not forcibly appose the skin. Any hair-bearing skin is closed with a 5/0 Prolene everting interrupted vertical mattress and the ear incisions are closed with tension-free continuous 5/0 Prolene (*Figure 65.9*). A 12fr grenade suction drain is placed on each side in the neck and a head bandage applied.

Postoperative care

The patient should be nursed with the head elevated to reduce dependent swelling. Careful blood pressure monitoring and intervention if necessary reduces the risk of haematoma. Combination analgesia with paracetamol and codeine is sufficient, although the best analgesic is constant icing. Skin sutures are removed a week after surgery. In most cases, return to social and professional visibility is achieved 2 weeks after surgery and strenuous exercise at 4 weeks. Facial and neck tissues can be indurated up to 12 weeks postoperatively and patients should be counselled of this. Manual lymphatic drainage, ultrasound and/or hyperbaric oxygen therapy are good adjunctive interventions to hasten soft tissue recovery.

Complications
Haematoma/seroma

Haematoma occurs in 1% of patients, commonly in patients with hypertension, males and those of Celtic origin. Immediate closed or open evacuation, compression and ice is curative. Occasionally, reopening the wound, irrigation and cautery or ligation of SMAS perforators is required. Haematoma can lead to seroma, which is managed with serial aspiration and/or drain placement until dry.

Neuropraxia

Temporary paresis of the temporal, buccal or most commonly marginal mandibular branch of the facial nerve occurs in 1% of patients. Treatment is reassurance and time. Most neuropraxias resolve completely in 3 months. Contralateral botulinum toxin injection can mask the visible disfigurement in the interim.

Skin induration and swelling

Swelling and hard skin induration will to some degree occur in all patients. This is managed expectantly. Combination intervention with lymphatic drainage, ultrasound and dilute steroid/5FU injections are helpful in remittent cases.

> ### TOP TIPS AND HAZARDS
>
> - Patient selection is key to a successful facelift practice; meticulous assessment of extrinsic facial ageing and a candid discussion of the causes of dissatisfaction with appearance including structural volume loss and existing asymmetry are important.
> - Good retraction, countertraction and a broad field access in the subplatysmal deep neck is essential to access the submandibular glands.
> - The deep plane is most easily entered over the masseter above the mandible and below the zygomatic ligament. Once access to the glide plane is established, the dissection can be progressed inferiorly subplatysma and superiorly into the midface with blunt dissection.
> - A stepwise approach allows time for any retracted SMAS perforating vessels to bleed, allowing meticulous haemostasis at skin closure.

BROWLIFT SURGERY

The brow–upper eyelid position is an important consideration in pan-facial rejuvenation. Brow position and shape relays expression and affect more than any other facial feature. The brow and upper eyelid complex are intrinsically linked; surgical rejuvenation of the latter is discussed elsewhere (*Chapter 66*). Multiple techniques have been described to surgically restore a youthful brow position. The author predominantly uses two techniques depending on the subunit(s) requiring correction.

Positioning, preparation and anaesthesia

The patient positioning, skin preparation and the choice of anaesthesia is similar to that described under face and neck lift surgery. In addition, a supraorbital block is injected bilaterally.

Surgical procedure

Lateral browlift

A 1–2-cm trichophytic follicle-sparing incision is made parallel, and 1 cm posterior to the temple hairline above the desired brow peak to the deep temporal fascia. Blunt blind dissection with a sweeping motion of this plane is performed with a Ramirez 2 endoforehead fronto-temporal dissector inferiorly to 1 cm above the superior orbital rim. The dissection then transitions deep into the subperiosteal plane where complete release of the arcus marginalis and temporal crest (conjoint tendon) is necessary for lateral brow superior advancement. Attention is turned to blunt parietal dissection to allow forehead flap advancement. Release is confirmed with a passively repositioned brow under no tension. Various fixation techniques have been described such as Endotine devices, bone tunnels, screws and plates but lateral brow 2/0 vicryl suture fixation of the temporo-parietal fascia to the deep temporal fascia is adequate in most cases. The skin is closed with staples.

Endoscopic (or non-endoscopic) browlift

Where medial brow release is desired, the surface landmark of the supraorbital nerve is marked on the skin. The supraorbital nerve exits the supraorbital foramen of the frontal bone and can be palpated as a notch on its orbital part. The medial iris serves as the most reliable topographical landmark for the course of the supraorbital nerve at the supraorbital rim.

The steps above for lateral browlift are followed, with or without endoscopic assistance but the blunt dissection is extended medially towards but avoiding the supraorbital nerve. An additional follicle-sparing trichophytic hairline 1–2-cm incision is made in the midline. Subperiosteal blunt dissection of the forehead proceeds with release of the arcus marginalis medial to the supraorbital nerve on both sides. It is imperative that periosteal attachment over the nasal part of the frontal bone remains intact to prevent over-medial browlift, which leads to an unnatural surprised appearance.

The lateral and medial pockets are communicated with blunt dissection and a Ramirez 3 frontoparietal dissector is used to release the scalp from the parietal bone as far as necessary to allow tension-free scalp and forehead advancement. Fixation is with sutures, with or without bone tunnels, or fixation devices, and can be tailored with tension to the desired brow position and the skin closed with staples. A light head bandage is applied for the first 24 hours.

Postoperative care

Immediate postoperative care addresses swelling and bruising. The patient is nursed head upright and encouraged to ice. Headache is common and easily managed with non-opioid analgesia. Staples are removed at 1 week and exercise avoided for 4 weeks.

Complications

Temporary forehead and brow paresthesia is common and self-limiting. Haematoma and infection are rare. Temporary neuropraxia of the frontal branch might occur due to traction and resolves at 6–12 weeks. The most common complication is under- or over-correction and the patient must be counselled of this prior.

> **TOP TIPS AND HAZARDS**
>
> - Careful patient evaluation is essential to determine the segments of the brow and/or upper eyelid complex that require rejuvenation.
> - Blunt dissection laterally at the level of the deep temporal fascia avoids inadvertent damage to the frontal branch of the temporal nerve.
> - Full release of the arcus marginalis and conjoint tendon allows for passive tension-free brow repositioning.
> - Leaving uninterrupted periosteum over the nasal bone avoids over-elevation of the medial brow.

Chapter 66

Aesthetic Blepharoplasty

Velupillai Ilankovan, Tian Ee Seah

INTRODUCTION

Artists and sculptors have described eyes as the "windows to the soul". Ancient literature of the East and West compares the aesthetics and function of the eye and periorbital region to the shape of a fish, rates the eyebrow to the beauty of the young timid deer, the nasal bridge and medial canthi to the shape of the bow and denotes the existence of philosophical strength and the natural beauty.

Aesthetic blepharoplasty in essence is a surgical exercise that can improve aesthetics as well as touch the soul to enhance one's wellbeing. Restoring the shape of the eyebrow is also considered as an adjuvant exercise to support blepharoplasty.

SURGICAL ANATOMY

The topographical and anthropometric anatomy of the eyelid and eyebrow varies from ethnicity to ageing. When we looked into the shape of the eyebrow and eyelids of young patients of varied ethnicity, there was statistically significant evidence of variability and also perception of aesthetics was recognised as not universal. The shape of the eyebrow has a standard presentation but preferred aesthetics varies according to influence from the outside environment, with preferences for a flat shape, high arch or even 'S' shape. In a balanced face, the shape of the eyebrow is lower medially and higher laterally. The eyelid aesthetic, however, is standard.

The function should follow aesthetic enhancement. Any untoward surgical or non-surgical outcome can compromise the function.

The main surgical procedure to enhance eyelid aesthetics is the blepharoplasty. The other adjuvant procedures that contribute to providing a complete package are implants to enhance bony resorption, volumisation to correct deficiencies and cutaneous enhancement to remove rhytids. The indications for aesthetic blepharoplasty are related to correcting the ageing process as well as other inherent deformities and facial presentations.

The supratarsal crease of the upper eyelid is a fixed anatomical position which is formed as a result of fibrous extension from the levator aponeurosis to provide dermal insertion. An upper blepharoplasty needs to create this as a mandatory exercise. The eye shadow space is a convex contour between the crease and the eyebrow. The palpebral fissure is the opening between the eyelid margins which is lower medially and higher laterally similar to the shape of the eyebrow. The corresponding surface anatomy to the supratarsal crease in the lower lid is the lower lid crease (*Figure 66.1*).

In ageing of the upper lid, there is descent of the eyebrow particularly the lateral brow followed by upper lid hooding and to some degree medial orbital fat atrophy. In the lower lid, however, there is lower lid bulge, malar festoon, tear trough deformity, malar palpebral groove and, to some degree, deepening of the naso-jugular groove (*Figure 66.2*).

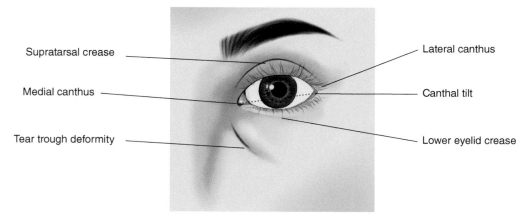

Figure 66.1 Illustration of a patient with youthful eyelids.

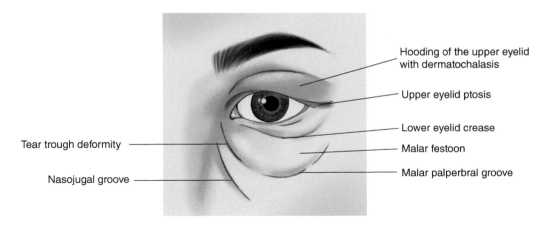

Figure 66.2 Illustration of a patient with ageing of the eyelids.

Hooding of the upper eyelid with dermatochalasis

Upper eyelid ptosis

Lower eyelid crease

Malar festoon

Malar palperbral groove

Tear trough deformity

Nasojugal groove

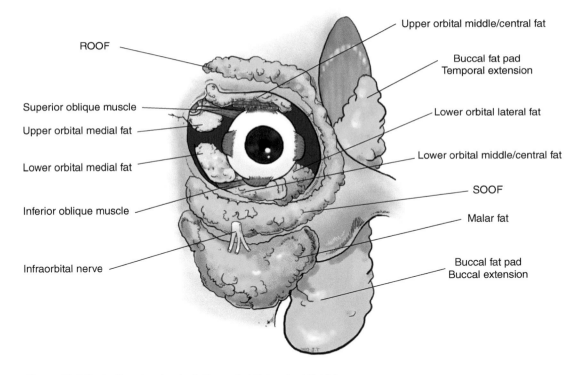

Figure 66.3 Illustration showing both the periorbital and orbital fats.

ROOF

Superior oblique muscle

Upper orbital medial fat

Lower orbital medial fat

Inferior oblique muscle

Infraorbital nerve

Upper orbital middle/central fat

Buccal fat pad Temporal extension

Lower orbital lateral fat

Lower orbital middle/central fat

SOOF

Malar fat

Buccal fat pad Buccal extension

The retro-orbicularis oculi fat (ROOF) and sub-orbicularis oculi fat (SOOF) will interfere with the aesthetic outcome unless they are addressed during standard blepharoplasty exercise (*Figure 66.3*).

The lower eyelid crease in youth is approximately 3–4 mm from the eyelashes. With ageing, it moves temporally downwards, more compared to medially. Two surface anatomical structures are important to the aesthetic surgeon: the tear trough and the malar palpebral groove in the lower lid. The former has dense fibrous dermal attachment to the maxilla. The latter is made more prominent with varying amounts of fat prolapse. This is usually a sausage shape in appearance.

The fat herniation can be described as medial, middle and lateral. Structurally the lower eyelid is made up of three layers. The external coverage of skin and orbicularis oculi is termed the anterior lamella. The middle lamella is a support layer of the eyelid which includes the tarsal plate, septum and the tarsoligamental sling. The posterior lamella is the palpebral conjunctiva. The

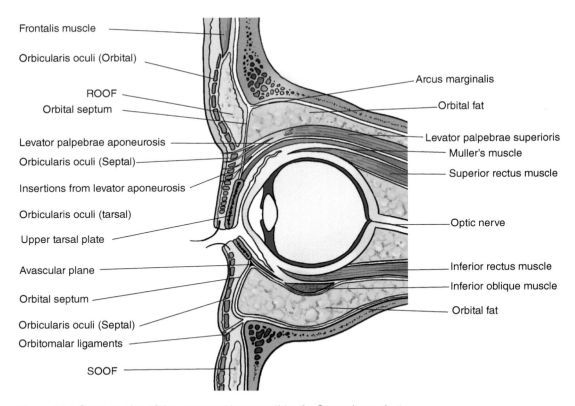

Figure 66.4 Cross-section of the upper and lower eyelids of a Caucasian patient.

orbicularis oculi is divided into pretarsal, preseptal and orbital components (*Figure 66.4*). The main function is in tear transport and eye protection.

The tarsal plates are fibrous plates of connective tissue with horizontal dimensions of approximately 30 mm in the upper lid and 25–28 mm in the lower lid, and vertical dimensions of 10 mm and 4 mm in the upper and lower lids, respectively.

The orbital septum is akin to periosteum and in the upper eyelid, is fused to the levator aponeurosis which acts as a boundary between anterior and deep orbit. In the lower lid, the septum is inherently joined with the capsulopalpebral fascia, which is the ligamental sling to the lower lid.

The levator aponeurosis, Whitnall's ligament and the ligament of Lockwood are the retractors of the upper and lower lids and knowledge of them is important in managing post-blepharoplasty complications such as ptosis and ectropion (*Figure 66.5*).

The fusion of the levator aponeuroses and the orbital septum creates the supratarsal crease which is strengthened by the dermal fibres from the levator aponeuroses and passes through the orbicularis oculi muscle to the skin. Location of this arrangement is anterior to the superior tarsus, hence orbital fat migration is prevented beyond the supratarsal crease. However, the upper eyelid anatomy is somewhat different in

East Asian people as 50% are born with no upper lid crease (*Figure 66.6*). For those who have a lid crease, this is called a double eyelid. Electron microscopy and cadaver studies in patients with lid creases have demonstrated that dermal fibres from the levator aponeuroses pass the orbicularis to subdermal attachment. This arrangement is linear in a thread-like form to create the crease. In patients with no eyelid crease, there is no such linear arrangement but rather the fibres are in coarse stratified bundles. Thus, in the upper eyelid of an East Asian person, the levator aponeuroses fibres not having subdermal attachment would explain no upper lid crease (*Figure 66.7*).

The capsular palpebral fascia is a similar structure to the levator aponeuroses which originates from the inferior rectus fascia and attaches to the ligament of Lockwood. This functions as a voluntary retractor of the lower lid.

The ROOF is a distinct anatomical adipose tissue situated between the superior lateral orbicularis and the septum. This may require contouring to improve the eyelid concave aesthetics. Similarly, it will require plication superiorly while correcting malar festoon.

There are two distinct fat pads in the upper eyelid and three in the lower lid. These are sited above the levator aponeurosis and capsulopalpebral fascia, respectively. In the upper lid, the lacrimal gland is

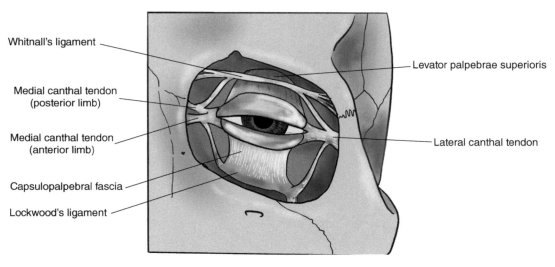

Figure 66.5 Ligaments of the upper and lower eyelids.

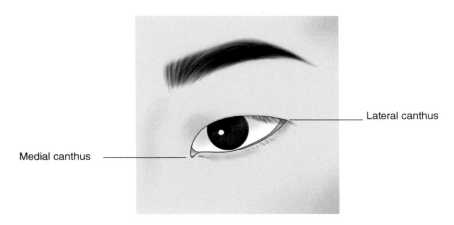

Figure 66.6 Eyelid of an Asian patient.

close to the middle fat and care must be taken to avoid resection with orbital fat during upper blepharoplasty. Similarly, in the lower lid, the inferior oblique muscle separates the middle and medial fat compartments, and in procedures such as septal reset the sutures might pull the muscle down and can cause diplopia as a postoperative complication.

Internal and external carotid artery systems provide blood supply to the eyelid. An inadvertent use of filler injections can result in retrograde flow into the ophthalmic artery and can cause central retinal artery embolism (*Figure 66.8*).

The orbitomalar ligament is an osteocutaneous structure that plays a major part in formation of the tear trough and in unmasking SOOF and orbital fat, and shows the malar festoon. Division of this osteocutaneous ligament with zygomatic cutaneous ligament will aid in treating malar descent.

In the lower lid the orbital septum and the capsulopalpebral fascia join below the tarsal plate and form an important potential space which is extremely useful in transconjunctival approach. Hence, we do not support the use of the terms 'preseptal' and 'postseptal' in an anatomical description of the approach.

CLINICAL EVALUATION

The aim of a blepharoplasty is to produce a natural, 'un-operated' outcome rather than attempting to provide accurate symmetry and measurements. Any measurements are a guide rather than determinant factors.

The eyelids should be examined for redundant skin. This is probably more important in the upper than the lower. In the upper, concomitant lateral brow ptosis

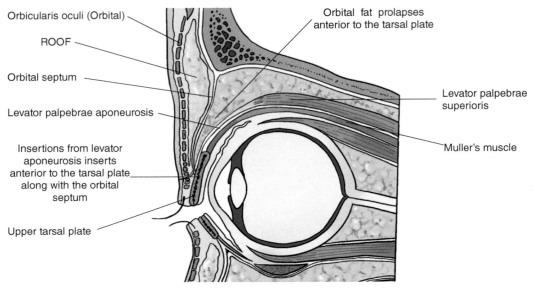

Orbicularis oculi (Orbital)

ROOF

Orbital septum

Levator palpebrae aponeurosis

Insertions from levator aponeurosis inserts anterior to the tarsal plate along with the orbital septum

Upper tarsal plate

Orbital fat prolapses anterior to the tarsal plate

Levator palpebrae superioris

Muller's muscle

Figure 66.7 Cross-section of the Asian upper eyelid anatomy.

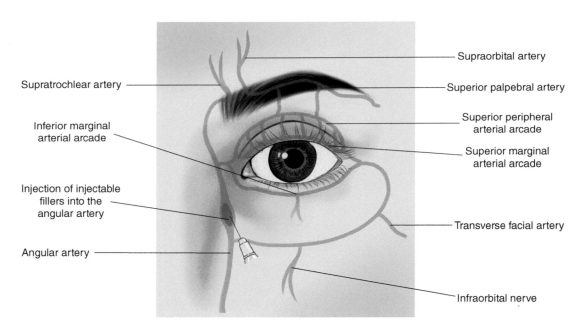

Supratrochlear artery

Inferior marginal arterial arcade

Injection of injectable fillers into the angular artery

Angular artery

Supraorbital artery

Superior palpebral artery

Superior peripheral arterial arcade

Superior marginal arterial arcade

Transverse facial artery

Infraorbital nerve

Figure 66.8 Injection of injectable fillers into the angular artery can have devastating consequences including blindness.

must be checked as it can cause apparent skin excess (*Figure 66.9*).

Evaluation of the supratarsal crease and creation of a well-defined one are the most important requirements of upper blepharoplasty. In correction of the eyelid of an East Asian person, the position of the supratarsal crease should match the patient's face as opposed to creating a number 8–10 mm from the tarsal margin.

Fat herniation is more noticeable in the lower lid than the upper. However, excess excision of the central fat can result in a cadaveric look. In the upper lid, contouring of the fat will aid in creating a well-defined crease; however, care is essential in fat excision along the middle and medial compartments. In the lower lid again, the aim is to create a natural-looking lower lid crease without sausage-shaped lower lid bulge, malar

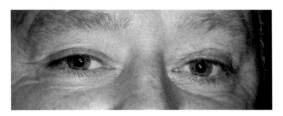

Figure 66.9 Clinical photo showing ptosis and derma-tochalasis of the upper eyelids in a Caucasian patient.

festoon, tear trough, malar palpebral groove and the deepening of the nasojugal groove. The eyelid/cheek junction must be a natural contour to a younger-looking face. The management of fat therefore is either very careful resection or careful septal reset.

Laxity of the lower lid should be evaluated correctly to provide a convex contour.

In summary, after evaluation, a good upper blepharoplasty will result in removal of sufficient redundant skin and creation of a natural supratarsal crease. In the lower lid, careful skin excision, some form of fat management and a lid-tightening procedure can be performed if necessary.

OPERATING TECHNIQUE

The aim in upper blepharoplasty is to create a contoured supratarsal crease with no fat herniation. In the lower lid, the aim is to create a concave full elevated lid with smooth contours and no tear trough or malar palpebral groove.

Preoperative preparation

Detailed informed consent, patient escort and home support should be planned in advance. The patient should be instructed to remove all eye and facial make-up before coming into the hospital.

Skin marking

This is carried out preoperatively when the patient is sitting up. A non-toothed Adson forceps is useful to assess the excess upper skin in the upper eyelids. Overcorrection can result in the patient being unable to close the eye comfortably, particularly in a patient with comorbidities and previous dry eyes. A fine-tipped

marking pen should be used (*Figure 66.10*). The shape of skin excision varies from patient to patient. In the lower lid, subtarsal marking with crow foot extension is a useful approach. If a skin-only blepharoplasty is planned, the amount of skin excision also should be marked in the lower lid in advance, keeping the superior skin marking along the subciliary line.

Anaesthesia

Most blepharoplasty procedures can be carried out under local anaesthetic. However, intravenous sedation or general anaesthesia are optional and the preparation would be carried out by the anaesthetist.

Once the patient is antiseptically prepared and draped, 2% lidocaine and 1 in 80 000 adrenaline is infiltrated in a turgid technique to minimise inadvertent haematoma formation into the orbicularis oculi muscle, which would make the muscle excision difficult. This is more important in surgery of the upper eyelid. The approximate volume of local anaesthetic agent required for the upper eyelid is 2–3 mL per lid and in the lower lid 4–5 mL of the same concentration.

Upper blepharoplasty

The inferior incision is the most important as it provides the new supratarsal crease. Extreme care should be given to the medial extension as it extends into the naso-orbital valley. Improper excision will give a postoperative epicanthal fold. Laterally the incision should not go beyond the lateral orbital rim. The superior excision is only the wrinkled eyelid skin. The lateral brow ptosis can be somewhat corrected by a skin excision making an asymmetric trapezoidal incision (*Figure 66.11*). Haematosis is obtained prior to the next step of excision of 2–3 mm of orbicularis oculi muscle. This excision should be around the supratarsal crease (*Figure 66.12*), and will expose the septum. In blepharoplasty of an East Asian patient, some of the superior portion of the pretarsal orbicularis oculi muscle may

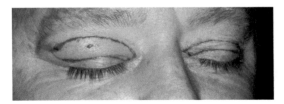

Figure 66.10 Markings for the blepharoplasty are made with a fine-tipped sterilised pen.

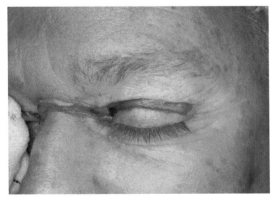

Figure 66.11 Skin is first excised with careful haemostasis.

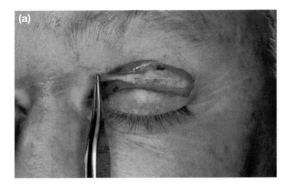

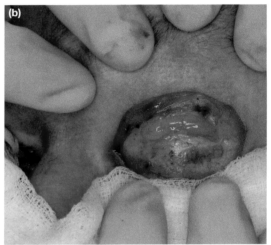

Figure 66.12 (a) A strip of orbicularis oculi is resected. (b) Pressure on the lower eyelid will make the septum more pronounced, the image shows upper central fat prolapse after incision of the orbital septum.

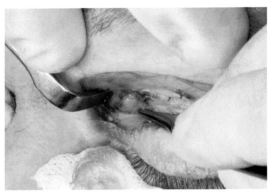

Figure 66.13 Prolapse of the upper medial fat pad, which is often lighter in appearance.

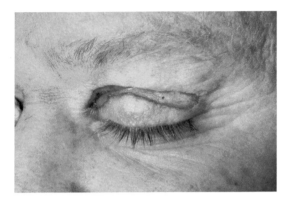

Figure 66.14 Placement of a deep 5/0 vicryl suture unites the lower orbicularis oculi to the levator aponeurosis.

be resected to prevent a bulky pretarsal flap. This may be up to 70% but varies between individuals. Pressure along the lower lid will make the septal bulge more prominent. The septum is opened to the entire length, which we call an 'open sky' approach. This exposes the pre-aponeurotic fat and facilitates access to the medial fat (*Figure 66.13*). The medial fat is lighter in colour. If the volume is small, cauterisation on its own to reduce the prominence is adequate. The central fat excision starts from the lateral end with careful cauterisation.

Fat excision should be conservative and the aim is in contouring. Achieving haemostasis is critical. Then, attention should be given to the ROOF. This gives fullness along the lateral orbital rims. Careful resection will give a better lateral definition. This fat is situated deep to the orbicularis oculi muscle and superficial to the septum.

Once the haemostasis is achieved, the repair can begin. The first suture will provide the basis for the new supratarsal crease. Different techniques are reported,

but we have been successful over the years with one deep suture placed in the middle using a 5/0 vicryl suture. This suture will unite the inferior orbicularis oculi muscle to the fascia along the Whitnall's ligament (*Figure 66.14*), and raise the upper eyelid to the open position. In the East Asian patient, the dermis or orbicularis oculi is plicated to this underlying fascia (*Figure 66.15*) The patient should be warned of this exercise if it is carried out under a local anaesthetic. Subsequently, the sutures are only placed to the skin using a 6/0 Prolene interrupted suture technique (*Figure 66.16*). A cold pack is applied for approximately 2 hours (*Figures 66.17–66.20*).

Lower blepharoplasty

The incision is placed subciliary approximately 2 mm below the ciliary margin. The lateral extension is a natural crease along the crow's foot area of approximately 5–7 mm. The skin flap is raised with care. We use

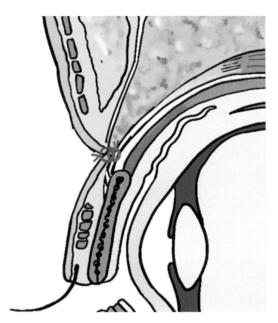

Figure 66.15 The red suture indicates the deep vicryl suture plicating the dermis to the levator aponeurosis. The blue suture indicates the nylon skin suture.

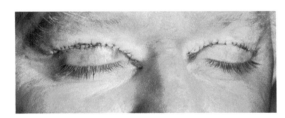

Figure 66.16 Closure using 6/0 Prolene sutures.

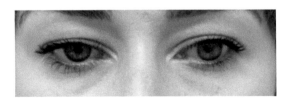

Figure 66.17 Preoperative photo of the upper eyelid showing hooding of the upper eyelids.

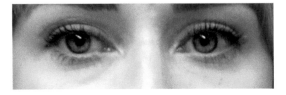

Figure 66.18 Postoperative photo showing the newly created supratarsal folds.

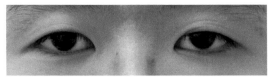

Figure 66.19 Preoperative photo showing a lack of supratarsal crease.

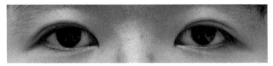

Figure 66.20 Postoperative photo showing medially tapered supratarsal folds.

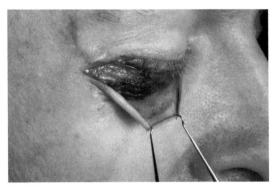

Figure 66.21 Skin-only flap is developed with careful dissection.

either a knife or monopolar cautery. Note that extreme care is essential when using the electrocautery to avoid any buttonholes (*Figure 66.21*). The elevation of the skin flap to the inferior orbital rim margin is completed. After obtaining haemostasis, a blunt dissection of the orbicularis muscle is carried out at the midline. The blunt end of the retractor is introduced and the incision of the rest of the muscle is carried out along the same line using the electrocautery. This exposes the fat enveloped in the septal capsule. Mobilisation is carried out all along the inferior orbital rim by exposing the arcus marginalis (*Figure 66.22*).

We carry out a septal reset where the mobilised fat within the septal capsule is laid along the rim and sutured to the arcus using two to four 6/0 vicryl sutures (*Figures 66.23* and *66.24*). It is important not to drag the inferior oblique muscle during this manoeuvre.

In some circumstances, rather than septal reset, careful resection of the fat is performed; however, excess removal can cause a hollow appearance at a later date. Following the fat management, the split orbicularis oculi muscle is 'spot welded' using monopolar cautery.

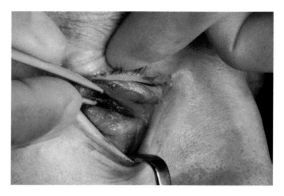

Figure 66.22 Incision along the inferior orbital rim and raising the arcus marginalis and periosteum exposes the orbital fat.

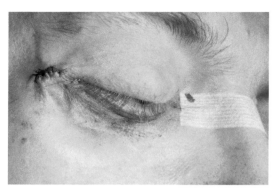

Figure 66.25 Closure is done with interrupted sutures at the lateral canthal region and subcuticular at the subciliary region with 6/0 Prolene sutures.

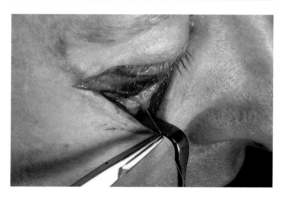

Figure 66.23 The septum is developed for septal reset.

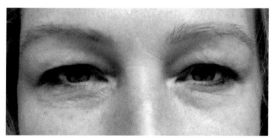

Figure 66.26 Preoperative photo showing hooding of the upper eyelids and tear trough and lower eyebags.

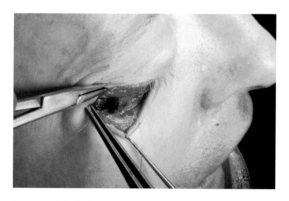

Figure 66.24 Inferior suture to the arcus marginalis and periosteum with 6/0 vicryl sutures.

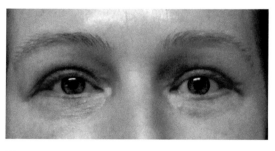

Figure 66.27 Postoperative photo showing newly created supratarsal folds from upper blepharoplasty and correction of the eyebags at the lower eyelids with lower blepharoplasty.

Laterally, the pretarsal and preseptal orbicularis muscles are incised and mobilised, a supralateral retraction is carried out and the orbicularis oculi plication is completed using a 5/0 vicryl suture to the lateral rim periosteum. Excess muscle is again trimmed. When SOOF needs support and tightening, this is suspended under the orbicularis muscle to the lateral periosteum before completing the orbicularis plication. Then the skin is draped over and a limited amount is excised, noting that overexcision will result in ectropion. The lateral sutures are placed first using 5/0 Prolene sutures. The subtarsal incision is closed using subcuticular 6/0 Prolene sutures (*Figures 66.25–66.27*).

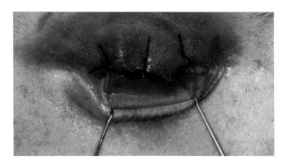

Figure 66.28 Black sutures are placed on the lower conjunctiva to the upper eyelid to allow tension during dissection via transconjunctival approach.

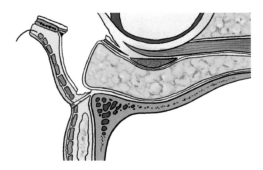

Figure 66.30 The transconjunctival approach. The incision is made on the conjunctiva approximately 4mm below the tarsus. Blunt dissection along the intraseptal plane to the arcus marginalis is then carried out.

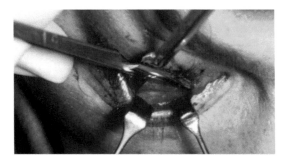

Figure 66.29 Tenotomy scissors allow blunt dissection without disrupting the orbital septum. An intraseptal approach is preferred.

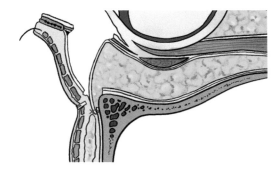

Figure 66.31 Septal reset is then performed. The septum and fat are sutured to the arcus marginalis or periosteum.

Transconjunctival blepharoplasty

Over the years, different surgical techniques have been reported. Since our publication in 1991, we have performed a transconjunctival approach as described below with good success. After the usual preparation, three 5/0 sutures are placed along the tarsal plate of the lower lid to retract (*Figure 66.28*). An incision approximately 4 mm below the tarsal plate is made starting below the lower lacrimal punctum to the extent of the whole of the lower lid. The palpebral conjunctiva is mobilised using a fine tenotomy scissor (*Figure 66.29*). The mobilised conjunctiva is sutured to the upper lid using 5/0 sutures.

It is important to recap the anatomy of the lower lid again. The capsular palpebral fascia, the lower lid retractor system arises from the fascia of the inferior rectus muscle. This joins with the orbital septum about 3–4 mm inferior to the tarsal plate, just below where the palpebral conjunctival incision is made. This united attachment joins the arcus marginalis along the infra-orbital rim. This anatomical structure is an 'intraseptal potential space'. Hence, there is no place to use the terms 'preseptal' and 'postseptal'. It is intraseptal. If

travelled along this space, one should not visualise the orbital fat unless there is preset orbital trauma and damage to the septal lining (*Figure 66.30*).

Once the arcus marginalis is mobilised, the fat with the septal cover is also mobilised and is ready for septal reset procedure, to correct the tear trough and malar palpebral groove (*Figure 66.31*). If necessary, we also place fat droplets harvested from the upper lid along the medial aspect to correct the deep nasojugal groove. If septal reset is not carried out and one wants to excise the fat, excision and cauterisation could be done after an incision along the septal cover.

All the suspension sutures are removed and checked for haemostasis, correction of tear tough, nasojugal groove and malar palpebral groove. The conjunctiva is sutured using a 6/0 vicryl rapid suture ensuring no sutures are visible at the ends to prevent conjunctival irritation.

It is important to understand preoperatively that the transconjunctival approach is only correcting the middle lamella and not the anterior lamella problem. However, a pinch blepharoplasty could also be carried out if this excess skin needs removal. It is more suitable for younger patients.

Modifications: Skin-only blepharoplasty

This is also termed a 'pinch' blepharoplasty. Only the excess skin is removed. In the upper lid, the excess skin is marked in the normal way. Maintaining a supratarsal crease is essential. The planned skin is excised. After haemostasis, the skin is repaired with 6/0 Prolene sutures.

Along the lower lid, the pinch blepharoplasty is carried out by placing a subciliary incision. The skin is raised and the planned amount is excised. After haemostasis this is repaired using 6/0 Prolene via a subcutaneous approach.

ADJUVANT PROCEDURES

Perioral laser resurfacing

This is a mechanism to remove the superficial epidermal layers with minimal dermal injury. Erbium laser produces minimal dermal damage, shortened post-treatment hyperaemia and hypopigmentation compared with CO_2 lasers.

Autologous fat volumisation

Upper lid

The fat grafting is only to the medial part of the supraorbital rim and to some degree to the infrabrow region at the position just above the periosteum. About 0.5–2.5 mL suffices.

Lower lid

Fat grafting over the infraorbital rim will enhance the bony defect. Grafting the malar area in a supraperiosteal plane will enhance periorbital aesthetics. Selective microfat grafting to tear trough and nasojugal groove are optional techniques.

COMPLICATIONS

Like any surgical procedure, complications do occur after aesthetic blepharoplasty. We group them as pre-, peri- and postoperative causes.

Patient selection and careful pharmaceutical history in planning and preparation of the patient will minimise any complications.

Inadvertent local anaesthetic infiltration into the blood vessels can cause rapid haematoma. The turgid technique of infiltrating local anaesthetic solution particularly along the upper lid will minimise trauma to the arcuate blood vessels. Local anaesthetic infiltration should be between the skin and muscle. Possible injury to the globe if the needle is placed in the deep layer is a rare complication. Every care should be taken to avoid corneal trauma during surgery. We use protective eye ointment rather than a corneal shield as the majority of our procedures are carried out under a local

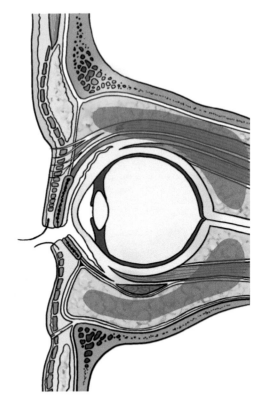

Figure 66.32 Retrobulbar haemorrhage is a rare but devastating complication. Meticulous haemostasis must be ensured during the entire surgery. Care must be given particularly to the orbital fat during manipulation and resection.

anaesthetic and the patient's tolerance would be poorer for eyeshields.

Retrobulbar haemorrhage is a very rare complication (*Figure 66.32*). This should be recognised immediately to save the eyesight. Central retinal artery occlusion is a rare occurrence. Intravascular displacement of a filler or fat from a peripheral arteriole to the ophthalmic arterial system is a known pathway (*Figure 66.8*).

During surgery, and at the completion, achievement of complete haematosis is a must. Damage to trochlea and as a result superior oblique muscle palsy is a possible complication in upper blepharoplasty. Excessive cauterisation of the superior medial palpebral artery which is inferomedial to the medial fat pad can cause damage to the trochlea. In the lower lid, the inferior oblique muscle can be traumatised during orbital fat resection as this muscle is in close proximity in between the medial and central fat pads (*Figure 66.33*). During a septal reset procedure, inadvertent suturing can also result in postoperative diplopia.

Further complications post surgery are dryer eyes, upper lid malposition (mainly ptosis), lower lid

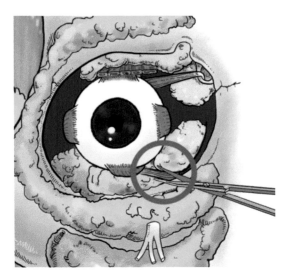

Figure 66.33 The inferior oblique muscle lies between the medial and central fat pad and care must be taken during incision with scissors or electrocautery around this area.

malposition with inferior scleral show to ectropion, eyelid crease abnormalities, hypertrophic scarring, pigmentation, loss of eyelashes and entropion, to name but a few.

In summary, aesthetic blepharoplasty with adjuvant procedures can correct intrinsic and extrinsic problems. We have summarised the problems and solutions (*Figures 66.34* and *66.35*). A holistic mindset will result in a natural-looking 'window to the soul'.

TOP TIPS AND HAZARDS

- The aim of a blepharoplasty is to produce a natural, un-operated looking outcome.
- Evaluation of the supratarsal crease and creation of a well-defined one are the most important requirements of upper blepharoplasty.
- The inferior incision of the upper blepharoplasty is the most important as it provides the new supratarsal crease.
- In upper blepharoplasty, a deep suture is placed in the middle to unite the inferior orbicularis oculi muscle to the fascia along the Whitnall's ligament to raise the upper eyelid to the open position.
- In lower blepharoplasty, septal reset or careful fat resection can be done to improve the eyebags. In both instances, care must be given to avoid pulling or traumatising the inferior oblique muscle.
- In the lower eyelid, the orbital septum and the capsulopalpebral fascia joins below the tarsal plate and forms an important potential space which is extremely useful in transconjunctival approach. We do not support use of the terms 'preseptal' and 'postseptal' in the anatomical description of the approach.
- During surgery, and at completion, achievement of complete haematosis is paramount.
- Retrobulbar haemorrhage is a very rare complication and should be recognised immediately to save the eyesight.

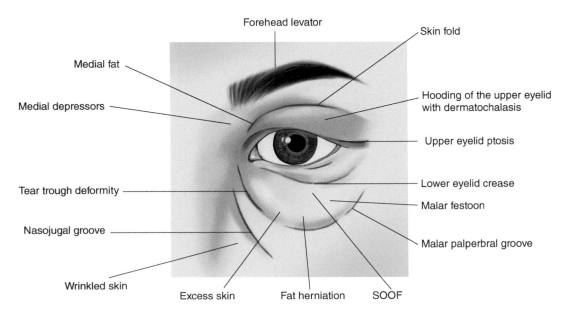

Figure 66.34 Problems of the ageing eyelid.

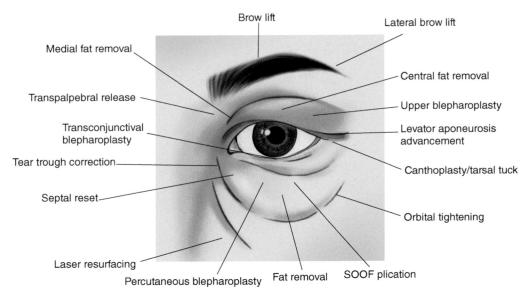

Brow lift

Lateral brow lift

Medial fat removal

Central fat removal

Transpalpebral release

Upper blepharoplasty

Transconjunctival
blepharoplasty

Levator aponeurosis
advancement

Tear trough correction

Canthoplasty/tarsal tuck

Septal reset

Orbital tightening

Laser resurfacing

Percutaneous blepharoplasty   Fat removal   SOOF plication

Figure 66.35 Solutions for the ageing eyelid.

FURTHER READING

Ilankovan V. Transconjunctival approach to the infraorbital region: a cadaveric and clinical study. *Br J Oral Maxillofac Surg* 1991;**29**:169–72.

Ilankovan V. Aesthetic blepharoplasty. *Br J Oral Maxillofac Surg* 2010;**48**:493–7.

Kunur J, Sabesan T, Ilankovan V. Anthropometric analysis of eyebrows and eyelids: an inter-racial study. *Br J Oral Maxillofac Surg* 2006;**44**:89–93.

Chapter 67

Otoplasty

Ahmed S. Mazeed, Neil W. Bulstrode

INTRODUCTION

Prominent ear is the most common congenital deformity of the auricle, with reported incidence of as high as 5% in some studies. It is commonly bilateral but can be unilateral in some cases.

Prominent ear has many psychosocial sequelae in children from bullying by other children. Otoplasty is an effective procedure in alleviating psychosocial distress in the majority of patients who undergo correction.

ANATOMICAL CONSIDERATIONS

Ear prominence occurs as a result of one or more of the following anatomical abnormalities:

- Inadequate formation of antihelical fold
- Increased conchal depth with increased angle between concha and mastoid
- Earlobe protrusion

The antihelix bifurcates inferiorly into two cartilaginous structures; the antitragus medially and a smaller less obvious structure laterally which is continuous with the tail of helix (cauda helicis), with the antitragal-helicine fissure or groove in between. The tail of helix (cauda helicis) is the lowermost part of the helical cartilage. It lies just above the lobule and is a key structure to correct lobule prominence (*Figure 67.1*).

The traditional method of passing a needle with blue dye to mark points on the posterior surface of the auricle to guide placement of the antihelical sutures is not necessary. The cartilage architecture when adequately exposed and inspected from the posterior surface can serve as a better guide to the surgeon simply because every convexity or elevation on the front of the ear (antihelix, superior crus and inferior crus) will be visualised as concavity or depression on the back of the ear (*Figure 67.2*). Likewise, any concavity or depression on the front of the ear (concha, scapha and triangular fossa) will be visualised as convexity or elevation on the back of the ear. If there is any doubt, gentle pressure medially along the helix will reveal the correct position of the antihelix.

In normal ears, the conchal floor is almost in direct contact with the mastoid. In prominent ears, the concha usually appears excessive from the frontal view giving an illusion of large conchal bowl or large ear. However, the concha is usually of normal size and the increased conchal depth is secondary to protrusion of the concha away from the mastoid. True conchal hypertrophy is very rare and can only be confirmed after the protrusion of the concha has been corrected by concha-mastoid (Furnas) sutures. The lack of the antihelical fold also contributes to increased conchal depth.

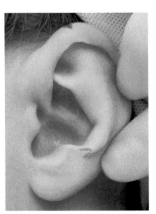
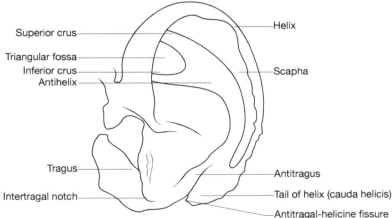

Labels: Superior crus, Triangular fossa, Inferior crus, Antihelix, Tragus, Intertragal notch, Helix, Scapha, Antitragus, Tail of helix (cauda helicis), Antitragal-helicine fissure

Figure 67.1 The V-shaped inferior bifurcation of the antihelix.

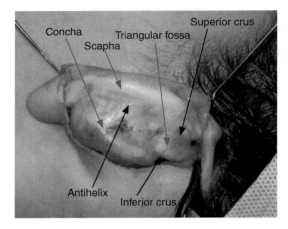

Figure 67.2 Cartilage architecture from the posterior surface. Purple arrows point to convexities or elevations. Black arrows point to concavities or depressions.

TIMING OF CORRECTION

The optimal timing should be a balance between a number of factors including auricular growth, cartilage strength and psychological impact on the patient. Age 6–7 years is a reasonable age to perform otoplasty because:

- The ear is nearly fully developed by this age
- The cartilage is strong enough to hold the sutures
- Good patient compliance can be expected in the postoperative phase

Younger patients might be operated on if the deformity is extremely severe necessitating earlier intervention due to psychosocial reasons and are advised that there may be a higher chance of recurrence or relapse.

OPERATIVE TECHNIQUES

Adequate knowledge of otoplasty techniques as well as appropriate training and experience are keys to performance of otoplasty surgery with good outcome. The goals of prominent ear correction are creating the antihelical fold, reducing conchal depth and reducing lobule protrusion.

Overall, cartilage reshaping in otoplasty can be classified as cartilage-sparing techniques (suturing only) and cartilage-cutting techniques (scoring, breaking or excision).

Cartilage suturing to define the antihelix was first described by Mustardé (1963) and forms the basis for most otoplasty techniques currently. Concha-mastoid sutures to reduce the conchal depth were popularised by Owens and Delgado (1965) and Furnas (1968).

Cartilage anterior scoring to define the antihelical fold was popularised by Chongchet (1963) and Stenstrom (1963) and is based on the principle of Gibson and Davis that cartilage tends to bend away from the

abraded perichondrium toward the side of intact perichondrium.

Various techniques have been described to correct lobule protrusion such as suturing the tail of helix to the concha, skin excision from the back of the lobule and suturing of lobule tissues to the concha, mastoid or scalp periosteum.

The author's preferred technique is based on a combined modified Mustardé and Furnas technique. It is an exclusively cartilage-suturing technique (cartilage-sparing) without performing any cartilage scoring, breaking or excision. This technique is applicable to almost all prominent ear cases whatever the patient age. It provides natural appearance, consistent results, with low-risk profile avoiding unnecessary scars and complications.

Combining both cartilage-suturing and scoring carries the combined risk of the two methods. Potential risks of anterior-scoring are anterior haematoma, anterior skin necrosis and chondritis with irreparable cartilage deformities.

STEPWISE OPERATIVE TECHNIQUE

Infiltration

The posterior surface of the auricle and the retroauricular sulcus are infiltrated with a local anaesthetic with adrenaline to help haemostasis and provide analgesia.

Positioning

The patient is placed in a comfortable supine position with shoulder support and a head roll to stabilise the head. The head is prepped and draped allowing access to both ears.

Approach

The auricle is gently pressed medially to fold it along the antihelix to reveal a V-shaped inferior bifurcation of the antihelix. This is marked and reflected to the posterior surface of the auricle. Another point is marked on the upper end of the auricle opposite to the superior crus and a point is marked on the posterior surface of the auricle 1 cm inferior to this point (*Figure 67.3a*).

A small amount of skin is excised as a double ellipse ensuring that the scar does not sit in the retroauricular sulcus or on the mastoid skin (*Figure 67.3b*).

Exposure

Skin and soft tissues are dissected sharply off the cartilage medially towards the sulcus to separate the cartilage of the conchal bowl from the mastoid soft tissue and postauricular muscles (*Figure 67.4a*), and laterally till reaching the edge of helical rim (*Figure 67.4b*, arrow). Dissection should extend inferiorly to expose the cartilage of the tail of helix (*Figure 67.4b*, the forceps).

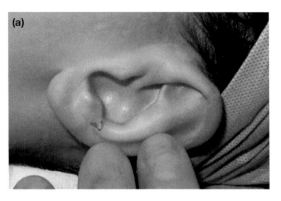
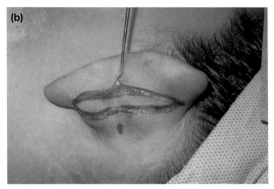

Figure 67.3 (a) Marking of the lower limit of dissection opposite to the V-shaped bifurcation of the antihelix. (b) Double ellipse.

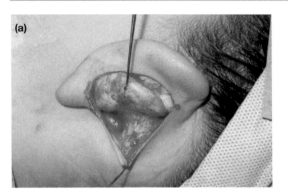
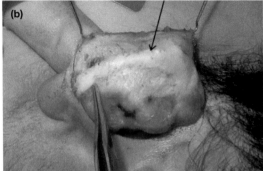

Figure 67.4 (a) Medial dissection. (b) Lateral dissection.

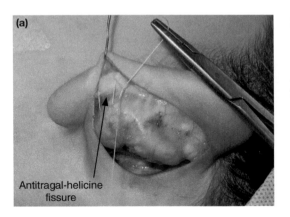
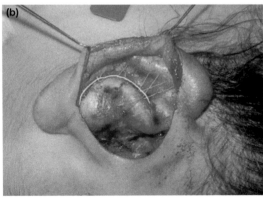

Antitragal-helicine fissure

Figure 67.5 (a) The first conchoscaphal suture. (b) The cascade of conchoscaphal sutures

Creating the antihelical fold and reducing lobule protrusion

Mustardé-type sutures are placed between the concha and scapha to define the antihelix. Suture placement is carried out in caudocephalad direction. The first Mustardé suture is placed as a double mattress suture

taking parallel passes from the posterior aspect of the tail of helix to the conchal bowl and is tied tightly. The antitragal-helicine fissure lies in between (*Figure 67.5a*, arrow). Each suture serves as a guide for correct placement of the subsequent suture in a stepwise manner moving superiorly. The second Mustardé-type suture is also tied tightly. The third, fourth and, if necessary, the

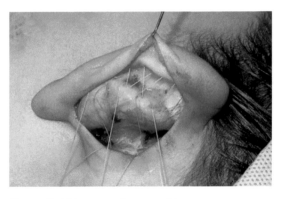

Figure 67.6 Three concha-mastoid sutures.

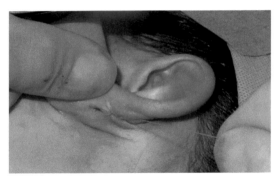

Figure 67.7 The lower 5–8 mm of the wound is left unsutured to allow drainage and prevent haematoma.

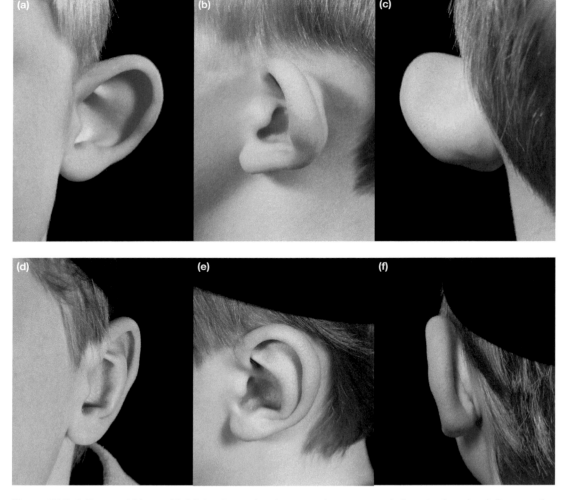

Figure 66.8 A 6-year-old boy with bilateral prominent ears and severe conchal protrusion. (a–c) Preoperative appearance. (d–f) Six months postoperative appearance without performing any conchal excision.

fifth sutures are not fully tightened. Instead, they are made bridging or spanning the conchal and scaphal cartilages. The cascade of conchoscaphal sutures should be parallel to a curvilinear line centred on the desired antihelix, not in a straight line, to reproduce its natural contour (*Figure 67.5b*).

Reducing conchal depth

Three Furnas-type concha-mastoid sutures are placed between the posterior conchal wall (just medial to the row of Mustardé sutures) and a deep bite of the mastoid soft tissues/fascia to set back the concha (*Figure 67.6*). The suture ends are left long. The upper and lower sutures are tightened first, followed by the middle one which is tightened lastly as needed. This helps to avoid telephone ear deformity, which results from excessive setback of the middle part of the auricle.

Wound closure

Once haemostasis is ensured, the wound is closed in a single layer by running rapidly absorbable sutures, e.g. 5/0 vicryl rapide. The lower 5–8 mm of the wound can be left unsutured to allow drainage and prevent haematoma formation. If at the initial dressing removal there is a collection, it can be easily evacuated by downward milking of the posterior aspect of the ear without the need to remove any stitches. The skin edges of this small open part are always well-coapted and its healing is not adversely affected (*Figure 67.7*).

Dressing

A non-adherent Vaseline gauze is applied behind the ear. Then cotton wool padding and head bandage are applied.

POSTOPERATIVE CARE

- The patient is discharged that day with the head bandage
- The dressing is removed after 2–4 days
- The patient is instructed to wear a night-time head band for 3 months
- The patient is advised to avoid swimming for 1 month
- The patient is advised to avoid contact sports for 3 months
- The patient is reviewed in the clinic after 3 months and again after 1 year (*Figure 67.8*)

COMPLICATIONS

Early complications

Haematoma

Meticulous haemostasis of any bleeding point is important before skin closure. Leaving the lower 5–8 mm of the wound unsutured allows drainage and reduces haematoma formation. This, together with the absence of any cartilage scoring, reduces the haematoma rate significantly.

Skin necrosis

The chance of developing a haematoma is higher using an anterior-scoring technique, due to the more extensive degloving and dissection of the fine cartilage and use of a more compressive postoperative dressing which can lead to severe consequences such as pressure necrosis of skin and may be followed by chondritis with irreparable cartilage deformities.

Infection

This is a rare complication that needs antibiotic cover and there is a low threshold for surgical washout to try to avoid chondritis that leads to permanent cartilage deformities.

Late complications

Suture extrusion

This is the most common complication and can be managed easily by removing the extruded suture, usually in the outpatient setting.

Recurrence or relapse

This mostly occurs due to disruption of antihelical fold sutures. Using absorbable sutures, e.g. polydioxanone, also results in higher relapse rate necessitating reoperation. Patients with relapse due to exposed sutures can undergo revisional surgery once there is no sign of ongoing infection.

We agree with a previous study which showed that high-caseload surgeons are significantly less likely to have recurrence of ear prominence compared with surgeons with low caseload and that there is association between the surgical volume or caseload and the incidence of relapse.

TOP TIPS AND HAZARDS

- The first (lowermost) Mustardé suture pulls on the tail of helix and is effective in correction of lobule prominence as it brings the lobule backwards similar to pulling on the tiller of the rudder of a boat. If this suture is accurately placed, no further procedure is needed to correct the lobule protrusion. No skin excision from the back of the lobule is needed nor suture fixation of the lobular tissues to the concha, mastoid or scalp.

- Concha-mastoid (Furnas) sutures correct conchal protrusion and cause forward and inward rotation of concha. Therefore, they should be carried out with caution to avoid narrowing of the external auditory canal.

- Mustardé sutures also help in correction of the excessively deep concha by rolling the posterior conchal wall to be incorporated into the antihelical fold.

- There is no consensus on the material of choice for cartilage suturing, but most surgeons use non-absorbable sutures such as polypropylene, nylon and Ethibond. Non-absorbable braided 4-0 sutures (e.g., Ethibond) have soft knots, and are less palpable and sharp than monofilament sutures (e.g., polypropylene), possibly resulting in lower rate of suture extrusion.

FURTHER READING

Bulstrode NW, Mazeed AS. Prominent ears. In: Bulstrode NW, Mazeed AS, ed. *Great Ormond Street Handbook of Congenital Ear Deformities: An Illustrated Surgical Guide*. CRC Press; 2022. pp. 99–115.

Cugno S, Bulstrode NW. Congenital ear anomalies. In: Ross D, Bulstrode NW, Cugno S, ed. *Plastic and Reconstructive Surgery: Approaches and Techniques* 1st ed. John Wiley & Sons, Ltd; 2015. pp. 238–54.

Firmin F. Prominent ears. In: Firmin F, Dusseldrop J, Marchac A, ed. *Auricular Reconstruction*. Thieme; 2017. pp. 321–34.

Stewart KJ, Lancerotto L. Surgical otoplasty: an evidence-based approach to prominent ears correction. *Facial Plast Surg Clin North Am* 2018;**26**:9–18.

Webster GV. The tail of the helix as a key to otoplasty. *Plast Reconstr Surg* 1969;**44**:455–61.

Bailey & Love's Essential Operations Bailey & Love's Essential Operations
Bailey & Love's Essential Operations Bailey & Love's Essential Operations
Bailey & Love's Essential Operations Bailey & Love's Essential Operations

PART 10 | Facial aesthetic surgery

Chapter 68 — Septorhinoplasty and Nasal Reconstruction

Hesham A. Saleh, Annakan V. Navaratnam

INTRODUCTION AND OVERVIEW

Rhinoplasty and septorhinoplasty are the most common facial plastic procedures. They are undertaken to augment and refine the nasal bony-cartilaginous skeleton and overlying skin to enhance the aesthetics and function of the nose. There are several approaches and a multitude of techniques that can be utilised, and these must be tailored according to the surgeon's preference, the patient's anatomy and most importantly the objectives of the operation based on shared decision making.

ESSENTIAL SURGICAL ANATOMY

The surgical anatomy of the nose relevant to septorhinoplasty surgery can be divided into thirds: the bony pyramid (upper third), the cartilaginous vault (middle third) and the tip (lower third) (*Figures 68.1–68.3*). Although a detailed description of this anatomy is beyond the scope of this chapter, a thorough understanding of these nasal structures as well as the overlying superficial musculoaponeurotic system (SMAS) and the skin–soft tissue envelope is essential when undertaking septorhinoplasty surgery.

(a)

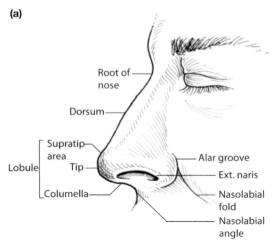

(b)

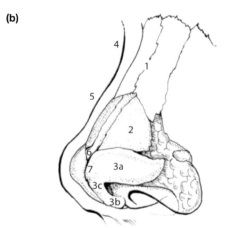

(c)

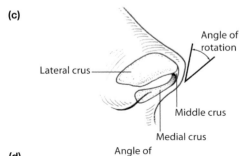

(d)

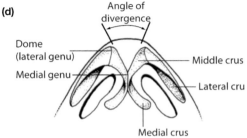

Figure 68.1 Surgical anatomy of the nose. (a) Soft tissues. (b) Osseocartilaginous structures: (1) nasal bone, (2) upper lateral cartilage (ULC), (3) lower lateral cartilage (LLC): 3a lateral crus, 3b medial crus, 3c intermediate crus, (4) nasion, (5) rhinion, (6) anterior septal angle (ASA), (7) dome. (c) Lower lateral cartilages and tip rotation. (d) Lower lateral cartilages and tip shape.

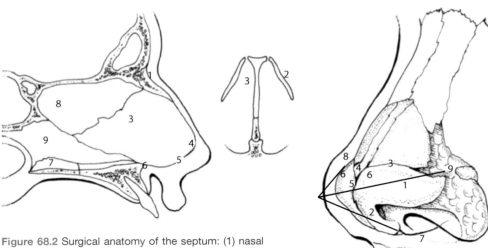

Figure 68.2 Surgical anatomy of the septum: (1) nasal bone, (2) upper lateral cartilage, (3) quadrangular septal cartilage, (4) anterior septal angle (ASA), (5) middle septal angle, (6) posterior septal angle – anterior nasal spine, (7) maxillary crest, (8) perpendicular ethmoid plate, (9) vomer.

OPERATIVE TECHNIQUE

Approach

The choice of approach is dependent on the anatomical deformity, the aims of the surgery and the preference of the operating surgeon.

Closed approach

The closed (endonasal) approach has the benefit of no external skin incisions and allows for preservation of many of the anatomical tip support mechanisms depending on the techniques employed. It provides less visualisation of nasal cartilage and therefore makes grafting techniques more difficult to utilise. However, depending on the experience of the surgeon, many of the manoeuvres employed in the open approach can be utilised endonasally.

The three main incisions used by the authors, which can be in various combinations, are the intercartilaginous incision (*Figure 68.4a*), the marginal incision (*Figure 68.4b*) and the full transfixion incision (*Figure 68.4c*).

Intercartilaginous incision
- Incision made through the nasal mucosa between the upper lateral and lower lateral cartilages
- Using an alar retractor to expose this region, bilateral incisions are made obliquely along the length of the intercartilaginous region with a No. 15 blade and the nasal skin can then be degloved to the radix with either a scalpel blade or dissecting scissors
- This incision can be joined with either hemitransfixion or full transfixion incisions depending on which closed approach is being used

Figure 68.3 Tip support mechanisms. **Major:** (1) Size, shape, strength and resilience of medial and lateral crura; (2) Attachment of medial crura foot plate to the caudal border of quadrangular cartilage; (3) Attachment of upper lateral cartilages (caudal border) to alar cartilages (cephalic border). **Minor:** (4) Dorsal portion of cartilaginous nasal septum; (5) Ligamentous sling spanning the domes of lower lateral cartilage; (6) Attachment of lower lateral cartilage to the overlying skin and musculature; (7) Nasal spine; (8) Membranous nasal septum; (9) Sesamoid complex extending the support of lateral crura to the pyriform aperture.

- If no or little manipulation of the lower lateral cartilages is required, this can be combined with a hemitransfixion incision to perform the septoplasty component
- If manipulation of the lower lateral cartilages is required, the intercartilaginous incisions are extended to a full transfixion incision and additional marginal incisions are used to perform the 'delivery technique'

Marginal incision
- This incision is made on the caudal edge of the lower lateral cartilages (lateral crura extending to medial crura)
- The caudal edge of the lower lateral cartilage can be palpated and can also be visualised laterally where the vestibular hair finishes
- This can be visualised more easily with the use of an alar retractor and pushing onto the skin overlying the lower lateral cartilage with the middle finger

Full transfixion incision
- This is a vertical incision through the entire membranous septum at the caudal end of the

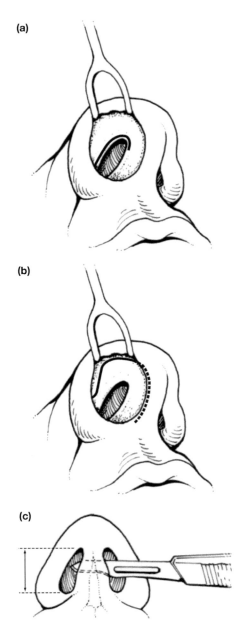

(a)

(b)

(c)

Figure 68.4 Intercartilaginous access or delivery technique. (a) Intercartilaginous, (b) marginal incisions and (c) transfixion incision (TI): the partial TI stops short of the anterior nasal spine (ANS). The complete TI divides the septo-crural ligaments with potential loss of tip projection (TP).

quadrilateral cartilage which separates the medial crural attachments from the nasal septum

Delivery of lower lateral cartilages

- This technique combines intercartilaginous, full transfixion and marginal incisions to expose the

lower lateral cartilages without requiring external skin incisions
- The lower lateral cartilages are dissected by degloving the lateral crura using curved Iris scissors through the marginal incisions extending under the nasal skin to the intercartilaginous incisions
- The incisions either side of the nasal columella are joined under the columellar skin through blunt dissection with Iris scissors
- The ligaments between the medial crura are then divided to free the medial aspect of the medial crura
- Careful dissection over the domes is required to avoid laceration to the soft triangle
- Once all attachments medially and laterally are released from the lower lateral cartilages, a closed artery clip can be passed through the nasal passage on each side into the intercartilaginous incisions and brought forward caudal to the alar rim to expose the entire lower lateral cartilages. Each lower lateral cartilage can be modified (e.g. cephalic trim, transdomal sutures)
- The two lower lateral cartilages can also be delivered through one nostril to perform interdomal sutures

Hemitransfixion incision

- This is a vertical incision in the vestibular skin of one side of the caudal border of the nasal septum
- Through one nostril, the skin is retracted using a short thin-bladed self-retaining speculum, e.g. Cottle, Killian's. The incision extends from the anterior septal angle to the nasal spine
- This incision allows elevation of the mucoperichondrial flaps either side of the nasal septum to perform the septoplasty component of the operation if require

Open approach

The open (external) approach has the advantages of excellent visualisation of the cartilages, allowing for better diagnosis of structural pathology, and the greater exposure that this approach provides enables the surgeon to utilise grafts more easily and precisely. However, the disadvantages of using this approach include increased scarring by dissection of the skin from the cartilages and potential trauma to the tip and dorsal skin by manipulation and retraction. It is usually used for severe post-traumatic deformities, secondary and revision rhinoplasties and noses with complex abnormal anatomy such as cleft noses. This approach combines transcolumellar and bilateral marginal incisions (*Figure 68.5*).

Transcolumellar incision

- A horizontal inverted 'V' incision across the mid-columella, usually at the narrowest point of the columella

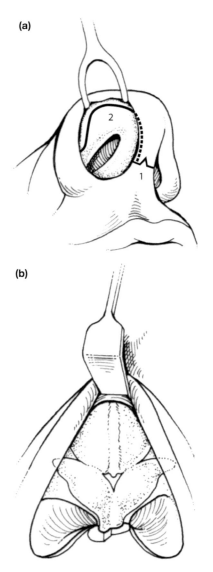

Figure 68.5 The open/external approach: (a) (1) inverted 'V' transcolumellar, (2) bilateral vertical columellar and marginal incision. (b) Elevation of the skin and soft tissue envelope (SSTE) offering a direct view on the tip and middle third.

- The incision connects the medial ends of the bilateral marginal incisions
- Care must be taken to ensure that the incision is sufficiently superficial to avoid injury to the medial crura of the lower lateral cartilages

Columellar flap

- Once the transcolumellar and marginal incisions are made, the columellar skin flap is then dissected off the caudal edge of the medial crura using a narrow double hook retractor to lift the flap up

and a mixture of sharp and blunt dissection using dissecting scissors (the authors use Iris scissors)
- As the domes are encountered, the angle of dissection needs to change to follow the contour of each lower lateral cartilage. An angled Walter scissors is useful to aid dissection at this stage
- Two single skin hooks are used to provide tension – one skin hook placed in the lateral alar rim with an assistant retracting laterally and one skin hook in the nasal side of the lower lateral cartilage dome with an assistant retracting inferiorly and anteriorly
- The marginal incision can be extended laterally by cutting down with scissors: one blade outside and one blade inside the flap under direct vision

Dorsal skin flap

- To expose osseocartilaginous dorsum, a dorsal skin flap needs to be raised using a mixture of sharp and blunt dissection in a subperiosteal place to ensure the SMAS layer is intact
- A wide double hook retractor in the nasal side of both lower domes can be used to retract the lower lateral cartilage (LLC) anteriorly and inferiorly
- A narrow double hook retractor initially can be used to retract the dorsal skin flap up and facilitate dissection initially
- As progress is made in degloving the nose, an Aufricht retractor can be used to retract the dorsal skin flap which enables further dissection to the radix
- Usually, a broad dissection across the dorsum is required to enable manipulation of the nasal bones and to provide adequate access to the middle third of the dorsum

SEPTOPLASTY AND HARVESTING OF SEPTAL CARTILAGE GRAFTS

Septal surgery is performed to correct septal deviations that are causing airway obstruction or aesthetic problems due to anterior deflections, as well as to harvest osseous or cartilaginous grafts. Resection and harvesting of quadrangular cartilage should be tailored according to the patient's anatomy and the requirement of the surgery. A minimum of 1 cm of dorsal and caudal septal structure should be preserved to prevent dorsal saddling, tip drooping and columellar retraction.

Grafts can also be utilised from autologous auricular or rib cartilage as well any irradiated allografts, xenografts and synthetic material. The extensive topic of graft materials is outside the remit of the chapter but surgeons undertaking complex and revision septorhinoplasty procedures should be aware of the potential sources of graft materials especially when undertaking cases where nasal septal cartilage may be insufficient.

Septoplasty can be approached via either closed or open approaches.

Closed approach

- Most septoplasties for nasal obstruction are performed using this approach
- The mucoperichondrial flaps, which can be unilateral or bilateral, can be raised through a hemitransfixion incision

Open approach

- This is mostly done as a part of an open septo-rhinoplasty procedure or in cases where there are complex septal deformities
- After the columellar and dorsal skin flaps have been raised, a skin hook is placed into the nasal side of the LLC domes to retract the domes laterally
- Sharp dissection of the intercrural ligaments is undertaken between the medial crura using Iris scissors
- Adson forceps can be used to palpate and grasp the caudal edge of the nasal septum to ensure dissection is in the right plane to avoid a tear in the mucoperichondrial flap
- Once the caudal edge of the nasal septum is encountered, sharp dissection using a 15 blade or closed Iris scissors should be undertaken to raise the mucoperichondrial flap on one side of the nasal septum
- Once the adhesions at the caudal edge of the nasal septum are dissected and an adequate subperichondrial plane is identified, the rest of the flap can be raised with a Freer elevator and a thin blade self-retainer such as a Cottle's speculum

Septoplasty (general)

- Elevation of the mucoperichondrial flap should proceed posteriorly to include the perpendicular plate of the ethmoid either unilaterally or bilaterally
- The osseocartilaginous junction should be dislocated, usually by a Freer dissector, from the perpen-

dicular plate of ethmoid and vomer but leaving the attachment under the nasal bones (keystone area) of at least 1.5 cm (*Figure 68.6*)
- To free the quadrangular cartilage from the osseo-cartilaginous junction fully, resection of a portion of the perpendicular plate of ethmoid and vomer is required
- This can be undertaken en bloc using superior and inferior cuts through the perpendicular plate made with turbinectomy or Caplan scissors and posterior detachment with a Freers if an osseous graft is required or via piecemeal resection with Tilley Henckel forceps

Anterior septoplasty

Anterior septal deviations can be difficult to successfully correct. The cause for the septal deviation must be carefully assessed and the correct technique employed to correct the deviation.

Augmentation of the caudal/anterior septum

- Deviation of the caudal septum is usually due to the caudal septum being too long and/or displaced to one side of the anterior nasal spine
- To correct this, the caudal septum must be detached from the anterior nasal spine by sliding a Freer elevator from the subperichondrial space medial to one mucoperichondrial flap to the other (*Figure 68.7*)
- The caudal septum can then be shortened to the correct height by resecting inferiorly segmentally, and reattached to the anterior nasal spine centrally

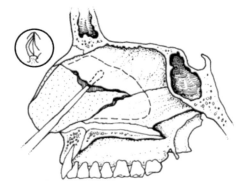

Figure 68.6 Disarticulation of the cartilaginous septum from the perpendicular plate of ethmoid.

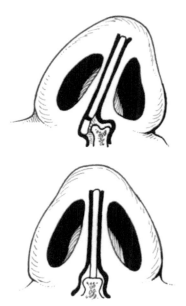

Figure 68.7 Anterior septal correction: resection of caudal septum and repositioning onto anterior nasal spine.

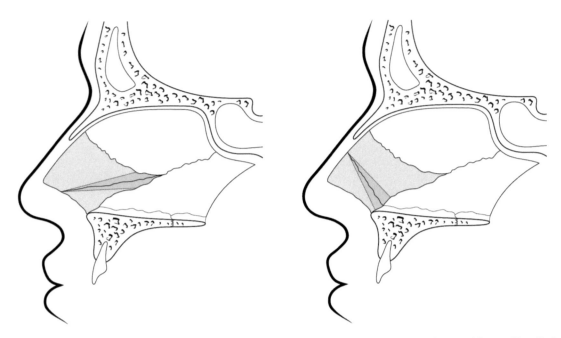

Figure 68.8 Excision of septal angulation at old fracture sites. This cartilage can also be used for grafting if of sufficient size and shape.

- The caudal septum is reattached to the anterior nasal spine with 4.0 PDS

Correction of posterior septal deviation and cartilage harvesting

- Deviations of the mid and posterior cartilaginous septum can be addressed through resection of the deviated segment of quadrangular cartilage with preservation of the dorsal strut of at least 1 cm (*Figure 68.8*)
- Cartilage here can also be harvested for use for cartilage grafts. Ensure that cartilage harvested is of adequate size for use in grafts especially if larger grafts such as septal extension grafts are required

RECONSTRUCTION

Dorsal nasal surgery

With nasal skin degloved from the upper lateral cartilages and nasal bones, the nasal dorsum can be manipulated through a range of techniques.

Hump reduction

- Hump resection can be performed with a scalpel for the cartilage to excise a unit: upper lateral cartilage (ULC) and septum, and with a Rubin-guided osteotome, introduced in the 'fish mouth' created, for the bony hump. This is known as en bloc hump resection (*Figure 68.9*)

- An alternative method, split hump technique, that can be used in an open technique and especially for large cartilaginous dorsal humps, is to detach the upper lateral cartilages at the level of the septum and resect the cartilaginous septum with Fomon scissors. It enables reconstruction of the middle third with either auto spreader grafts using upper lateral cartilages, spreader grafts or simply reattachment of the upper lateral cartilages to the nasal septum
- Bony irregularities are corrected with upwards rasping
- An 'open roof deformity' results after hump resection, which can be corrected with lateral osteotomies
- Over-resection of the bony hump and under-resection of the cartilaginous hump can lead to a 'pollybeak'

Lateral osteotomies

Lateral osteotomies are performed to narrow the nose after a dehump or to manipulate deviated nasal bones. If the indication is the latter when no dehump if performed, lateral osteotomies can be used in combination with faded medial osteotomies. Lateral osteotomies can be performed transcutaneously or endonasally. It is the authors' preference to use a transcutaneous approach to achieve better control and the stab incisions used for this technique nearly always heal without a scar.

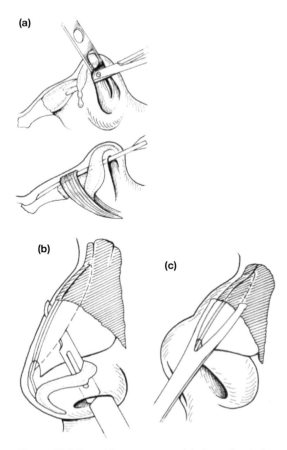

Figure 68.9 Dorsal hump surgery: **(a)** dissection below the SMAS and exactly on the perichondrium and ideally below the periosteum at the bridge leaving the lateral side of the nasal bones attached to the SSTE; **(b)** hump resection initiated with scalpel on cartilaginous portions of hump; **(c)** hump resection completed with rounded edges osteotome (Rubin) on the bony portions of hump.

- Bilateral stab incisions 2 mm long are made with a new size 15 blade at the level of the medial canthus in the direction of the relaxed skin tension lines just above the angular vein. Two other incisions should be made midway between the medial canthus and the pyriform aperture posteriorly on the side of the nose at its base
- Osteotomies are transcutaneously performed with a 2-mm micro-osteotome. The lateral osteotomy runs low in the nasofacial groove to below the medial canthus, where it is angled towards the midline (*Figure 68.10*)

Medial osteotomies

- The osteotome is engaged at the junction between the nasal bones and the upper lateral cartilages and tapped gradually, with its leading edge controlled by palpation and advancing parallel to the osseous nasal septum
- Just prior to the intercanthal line, the direction of the osteotomy should be angled laterally and not extend beyond the intercanthal line. Extension superior to this can lead to skull base injury

Manipulation of nasal bones

Following osteotomies, manipulation of nasal bones is undertaken to close the open roof deformity following a dehump or to realign the nasal bones. If the nasal bones do not mobilise easily, then the osteotomies can be performed again. Crushed cartilage camouflage grafts can be used for any irregularities that result from osteotomies.

Reconstruction of the middle third

The middle third of the nose (middle vault) can be compromised due to internal nasal valve collapse/stenosis causing airway obstruction or due to saddling post trauma or as a complication of previous rhinoplasty. Therefore, surgical management of the middle third of the nose requires consideration of both functional and aesthetic aspects.

Spreader grafts

Spreader grafts are usually used in open septorhinoplasty to reconstruct the middle third of the nose. They

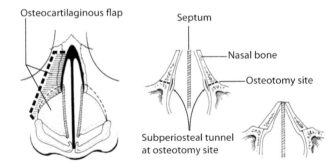

Figure 68.10 Lateral osteotomies. The 'open roof' is corrected by lateral osteotomies to mobilise the pedicled osteocartilaginous flap.

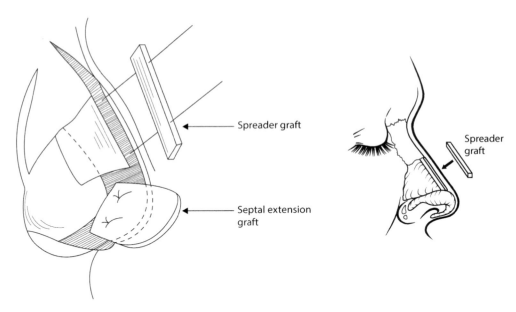

Figure 68.11 Support grafts: spreader graft and septal extension graft.

can also be used in closed approaches with a submucosal pocket, although the outcomes are more difficult to predict (*Figure 68.11*).

- This thin rectangular cartilage graft is placed between the nasal septum and the detached ULC and can be unilateral or bilateral depending on the patient's symptoms and appearance
- The graft is initially placed and held in place with a narrow bore needle before being sutured with 5.0 PDS to both the nasal septum and upper lateral cartilage
- The graft opens the nasal valve angle by moving the ULC away from the septum and decreases the resistance to nasal breathing. It can also be used to provide fullness in the middle third or to camouflage a deviated appearance of the middle third
- Typically, these grafts extend from the rhinion to the caudal medial end of the ULC. However, they can be extended caudally beyond the length of the ULC to correct a deviation of the lower nasal septum or be placed only at the lower caudal half of the ULC if the focus is to widen the internal nasal valve only
- Spreader grafts may broaden the nasal dorsum or cause irregularities in this region. This can be addressed with sculpting the ULC/spreader graft/septum complex with a scalpel or onlay grafts

Dorsal onlay grafts

A variety of dorsal onlay grafts can be used to augment the nasal dorsum and especially the middle third in cases of saddle deformity (*Figure 68.12*). Cartilage onlay grafts (crushed and intact) can be placed under the nasal skin and attached to the upper lateral cartilage with 5.0 PDS. The authors also use diced cartilage grafts wrapped in fascia or xenografts which are held in place using percutaneous sutures taped to the skin.

Nasal tip surgery

Nasal tip support

If the tip support mechanisms have been disrupted during a septorhinoplasty, it is essential that the tip is reconstructed to maintain tip support and prevent tip ptosis or columellar retraction in the future. Any reconstruction of the nasal tip can affect projection and rotation.

A multitude of augmentation, suture and grafting techniques can be employed to support the lower lateral

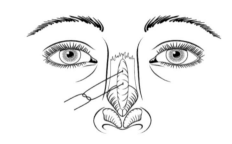

Figure 68.12 Dorsal onlay graft held with percutaneous sutures.

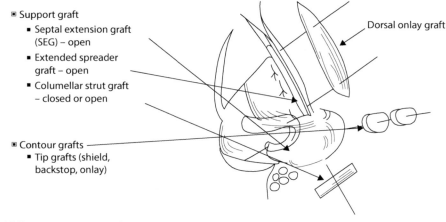

- Support graft
  - Septal extension graft (SEG) – open
  - Extended spreader graft – open
  - Columellar strut graft – closed or open
- Contour grafts
  - Tip grafts (shield, backstop, onlay)

Dorsal onlay graft

Figure 68.13 Common support grafts.

cartilages and nasal tip which are beyond the scope of this chapter. We will describe three techniques that reliably provide support to the nasal tip in septorhinoplasty surgery.

Septal extension graft

In open septorhinoplasty procedures, this wide rectangular graft can be used to project and support the nasal tip as well as correct any deviation of the lower third of the nose. As it provides significant tip support, a thick cartilaginous graft is required. It can be attached to the nasal septum side to side with 5.0 PDS or end to end with the support of bilateral spreader grafts. We describe the side-to-side technique below.

- The septal extension graft (SEG) is placed on one side of the nasal septum. If the caudal septum is attached to the anterior nasal spine, the SEG can be attached to the caudal septum alone (5.0 PDS). If, however, the caudal septum is not reliably attached to the anterior spine (e.g. if too short), then the SEG should be attached to the anterior nasal spine as well (4.0 PDS)
- The position of the caudal edge of the septal extension graft will dictate the position of the nasal tip
- The medial crura need to be attached to the caudal edge of the SEG. In order to do this a tongue-in-groove technique can be used. Use a wide double skin hook in the bilateral domes of the LLC to position the medial crura and fix to the SEG with a narrow bore needle
- Both medial crura are sutured to the SEG starting at the base with 5.0 PDS

Floating columellar strut

This graft attaches to the medial crura of the LLC only and prevents columellar retraction in open septorhinoplasty procedures. When the dead space between

the medial crura needs to be closed to prevent columellar retraction, this technique can be used (*Figure 68.13*).

- A pocket should be created with blunt dissection at the base of the medial crura towards the premaxilla
- A long thin rectangular graft is placed into this pocket and between the medial crura
- A wide double skin hook is used in the bilateral domes of the LLC to position the medial crura and fix the floating columella strut graft with a narrow bore needle
- Both medial crura are sutured to the floating columella strut graft starting at the base with 4.0 vicryl rapide or 5.0 PDS

Tongue in groove

The caudal edge of the septum can be attached to the medial crura in a tongue-in-groove mechanism to rotate and support the nasal tip. This technique will often rotate the nasal tip significantly and therefore may risk over-rotation of the nasal tip.

- A wide double skin hook is used in the bilateral domes of the LLC to position the medial crura and fix to the caudal septum with a narrow bore needle
- Both medial crura are sutured to the caudal septum starting at the base with 5.0 PDS

Nasal tip refinement

Many methods such as transdomal and interdomal suture techniques will adequately define the tip; however, tip grafts such as shield and onlay grafts can be utilised to further refine the nasal tip (*Figure 68.13*). A too convex LLC may need cephalic trimming, making sure that at least 5–7 mm of the LLC is left behind for support and patency of external nasal valve (*Figure 68.14*).

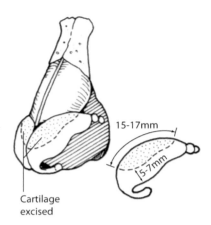

Figure 68.14 Cephalic trim technique maintaining 5–7 mm of lower lateral cartilage.

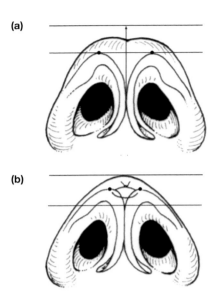

Figure 68.15 Interdomal suture technique. (a) Splayed lower lateral cartilage (LLC) domes and (b) interdomal suture to approximate LLC domes while preserving the natural separation of the domes and maintaining the angle of divergence.

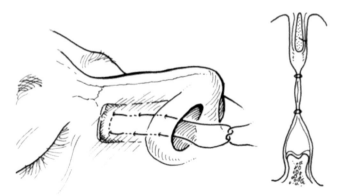

Figure 68.16 Reapproximating the mucoperichondrial septal flaps and stabilising the septal remnants using quilting sutures.

Transdomal sutures

In cases of a bulbous or boxy tip, transdomal sutures refine the tip-defining point by narrowing the domal angle (the angle between the medial and lateral crus) and flattening the convex lateral crura.

- Horizontal mattress sutures are placed in bilateral domes, 3–4 mm away from the tip-defining point with the knot placed medially. The authors use 5.0 PDS for this

Interdomal sutures

The interdomal suture stabilises and provides symmetry to the nasal tip and can be utilised for narrowing and to increase projection.

- A simple mattress suture (5.0 PDS) 3–4 mm cephalic to the tip-defining points between the lower lateral cartilages preserves the natural separation of the domes and maintains the angle of divergence (*Figure 68.15*)

TOP TIPS AND HAZARDS

- *Marginal incisions:* great care must be taken to avoid cutting into the soft triangle as an inadvertent incision there can lead to unfavourable scarring. When initially using this technique, surgeons should start by making separate initial incisions laterally, where the caudal edge of the latera crura can be found easily, and medially, lateral limb incision caudal to the medial crura. The incisions can then be joined together with scissors in the region of the soft triangle.

- *Raising mucoperichondrial flaps after hemitransfixion incision:* elevating the mucoperichondrial flaps is difficult initially, as the fibres of the perichondrium are tightly bound down. Toothed Adson forceps and a sharp dissector, e.g. Freer elevator, can be employed to elevate the flaps in the subperichondrial plane.

- *Resection of perpendicular plate of ethmoid:* care must be taken not to overexuberantly twist bone in this region as over-manipulation of the perpendicular plate could lead to inadvertent injury to the cribriform plate, leading to cerebrospinal fluid leak. Initially, the bone can be cut superiorly using Caplan or turbinectomy scissors before resecting the bone inferiorly.

- *Reattachment of caudal nasal septum to anterior nasal spine:* it can be difficult to suture cartilage (caudal septum to anterior nasal spine) without first creating a perforation in the bone using a drill. However, a wide bore needle can be used to perforate the anterior nasal spine and then pass a 4.0 PDS suture through the perforation and suture to the inferior septal cartilage to stabilise the caudal septum.

- *Depressed nasal bone fractures following osteotomies:* occasionally, osteotomies can lead to comminuted fractures of the nasal bones with infracturing, leading to irregularities of the upper third. In these cases, out-fracturing of the nasal bones with a Hill elevator and support with dissolvable packing placed intranasally can correct this.

Closure

Quilting of the septum

To close the dead space created by raising mucoperichondrial flaps, quilting sutures through the nasal septum are required. A running suture using 4.0 vicryl rapide progressing anterior to posterior inferiorly and then back posterior to anterior superiorly serves these purposes and can be tied anteriorly (*Figure 68.16*).

Incision closure

Endonasal incisions (intercartilaginous, marginal, hemitransfixion and full transfixion) can be closed with a simple interrupted suture: 4.0 vicryl rapide.

The only skin incision that requires closing in an external approach is the transcolumellar incision with simple interrupted sutures. The authors use 6.0 vicryl rapide.

FURTHER READING

Apaydin F, Stanic L, Unadkat S, Saleh HA. Postoperative care in aesthetic rhinoplasty patients. *Facial Plast Surg* 2018;**34**:553–60.

Beegun I, Saleh HA. Advocating the use of absorbable sutures for columellar incisions following open rhinoplasty. *Aesthetic Plast Surg* 2017;**41**:754.

Saleh HA, Khoury E. Closed rhinoplasty. In: Cheney M, ed. *Facial Surgery: Plastic and Reconstructive.* Harvard Press; 2014.

Saleh HA, Rennie C. Assessment for rhinoplasty. In: *Scott-Brown's Otolaryngology 8th Edition.* Hodder Arnold Publications; 2019.

Varadharajan K, Choudhury N, Saleh HA. Septocolumelloplasty-anchoring the caudal septum to anterior nasal spine using a hypodermic needle as a trocar. *Clin Otolaryngol* 2019;**44**:211–12.

Chapter 69

Autologous Fat Grafting for Facial Rejuvenation and Asymmetry Correction

Alexander Zargaran, David Zargaran, Kaveh Shakib, Afshin Mosahebi

INTRODUCTION

Facial asymmetry, volume loss or redistribution of fat within the superficial and deep compartments of the face are common sequelae of the processes of ageing, craniofacial trauma, chronic wounds and cancers. The face relies functionally and aesthetically on the intricate architecture of craniofacial bones, muscles of facial animation and subcutaneous fat, which are susceptible to damage and atrophy over an individual's lifespan. Innovations in facial rejuvenation and asymmetry correction techniques leverage the dynamic and versatile properties of adipose tissue in the process of autologous fat grafting. Fat grafting, or fat transfer, encompasses the extraction of adipocytes from one region of the body, and their subsequent processing and infiltration into another body site. Adipocytes confer desirable volume results to the face as well as regenerative properties, which are thought to arise from adipose tissue-derived stem cells and the upregulation of elastin and collagen production. While humans have a natural reservoir of fat with these properties, the processing stage is essential, and modern-day autologous fat grafting in the face relies on emulsification and straining of the lipoaspirate into various fat parcel sizes including millifat (<2.4 mm), microfat (<1.2 mm) and nanofat (400–600 μm), with nanofat providing the highest regenerative potential by virtue of the increased concentration of adipose-derived stem cells, also known as the stromal vascular fraction.

The first procedure involving fat grafting is attributed to Gustav Neuber in the late 19th century, but modern-day techniques build on Coleman's lipoaspirate harvesting method. There is an established evidence-base for the safety of autologous fat grafting, but as with many surgical procedures there are a variety of accepted and practiced methods, and there is scope for further research to advance our current understanding of the optimum technique. This chapter outlines successful techniques according to the authors' practice and experience within the field.

SURGICAL ANATOMY

Procedures on the face should only be conducted by suitably qualified individuals with basic understanding of the underlying anatomy of both donor and recipient sites including nerves, arteries and muscles so as to protect and avoid damage to these important structures. Donor sites often include the abdomen, thigh or flank region. Fat transfer for facial rejuvenation should be performed with reference to the aesthetic subunits of the face, initially proposed by Gonzales-Ulloa. It is important to understand the anatomical compartments of the face to ensure the appropriate tissue plane is infiltrated, which include:

- Superficial fat space
- Superficial musculoaponeurotic system (SMAS)
- Deep fat space

These can be further subdivided into the following fat compartments:

- Nasolabial
- Cheek (medial, middle and lateral temporal)
- Orbital (superior, inferior and lateral)
- Jowl

PREOPERATIVE CONSIDERATIONS

Indications

- Facial asymmetry
- Contour deformity
- Rejuvenation

Cautions/contraindications

- Lipid metabolism disorders
- Severe coagulopathies
- Acute infections

Preoperative work-up for fat transfer for facial rejuvenation and to correct facial asymmetry includes a full clinical history and examination of the patient, as well

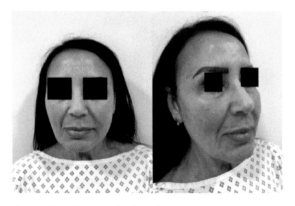
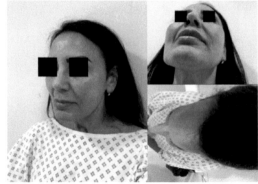

Figure 69.1 Preoperative imaging views.

as a discussion surrounding expectations as part of the informed consent process. Important specific additional discussions include the following:

- Baseline blood tests including a full blood count, coagulation studies and renal profile
- Nutritional status, with a view to optimising this preoperatively
- Previous cosmetic and/or surgical procedures, including complications
- Infection control issues including methicillin-resistant *Staphylococcus aureus* and COVID-19
- Future lifestyle changes, including anticipated significant changes in weight
- Preoperative medical photography of the face (*Figure 69.1*) in the frontal, lateral and lateral oblique views

The consenting process should account for common complications, including under-correction, infection, fat emboli, fat resorption and donor site morbidity. It should also clearly outline postoperative rehabilitation, discussed later in this chapter.

STEPWISE TECHNIQUE

Positioning and preparation

- Induction of antibiotics will be according to local policy
- The patient is positioned according to the agreed donor site. This would be supine for the abdomen, thighs and flank, which also provides good access to the face
- The desired donor and recipient sites are marked with a surgical pen, and the area prepared with chlorhexidine or povidone-iodine, and sterile drapes
- A hatching type marking can help guide greater target zones – with increased density of markings to the areas which require greater transfer

Harvesting adipocytes

- Handling of the fat, both in the harvesting and injection phases should be minimally traumatic, to maximise chances of graft survival
- The donor site region is infiltrated with local anaesthesia of choice mixed with 0.9% sodium chloride and adrenaline. This is an optional step but reduces the requirement for alternative analgesia
- The authors prefer an excisional method, with a 10 or 11 blade, and perform a single stab incision into the donor site, through the dermis and epidermis, and tunnel into the subcutaneous fat plane with a curved haemostat
- When harvesting from the abdomen – the authors suggest an incision inferior to the umbilicus to reduce infection risk
- In cases of repeat transfer, the authors advocate using the previous incisions to minimise cosmetic defect
- More tumescent local anaesthesia is infiltrated through this tunnel, and 15 minutes allowed for the effect
- For the lipoaspiration, options for generating negative aspiration pressures include either attaching a closed-circuit 10-mL syringe (such as a Luer Lock syringe) to a large-bore open-tipped cannula, or attaching a liposuction canula to a Redivac drain, or using a liposuction machine at low pressure of approximately 0.5 atmospheres
- Prior to aspiration, passes with the cannula can be made to break up fat particles. Then, the syringe is used to aspirate to create negative pressure, with multiple passes attempted at the donor site until the desired volume of fat has been obtained, and the system is removed from the donor site (*Figure 69.2*)
- The syringe is disconnected from the cannula, and centrifuged at 3000 rpm (*Figure 69.3*) for 3 minutes, which will separate the graft into layers

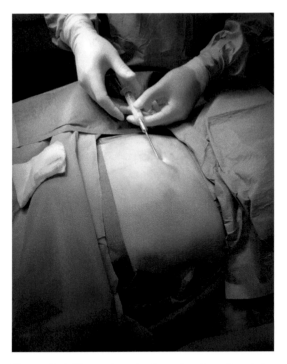

Figure 69.2 Harvesting of adipocytes from the abdomen.

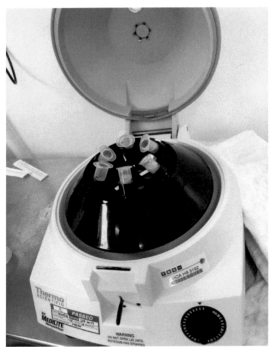

Figure 69.3 Centrifugation of adipocytes.

- The top layer of liquid triglyceride is decanted and the lowest layer of adipocytes (*Figure 69.4*) tapped off into 1-mL syringes
- The lowest layer of fat will have the highest concentration of stem cells, and therefore the highest regenerative potential – although note – the use of local anaesthesia is toxic to the stem cells so some surgeons choose not to use infiltration

Injection of fat

- The 1-mL syringes are connected to a blunt-tipped cannula
- Preoperative markings are re-evaluated (*Figure 69.5*)
- The area is anaesthetised using the preferred option such as 1% lidocaine with adrenaline, 1:100 000 through a 27-Gauge needle
- An 18-Gauge needle is used to make multiple small incisions. The incision sites should be placed to facilitate access to the desired region for the fat graft, but in certain instances such as for forehead, glabella and brow fat grafting, may be placed in a cosmetically more acceptable position such as the hairline, or in the preauricular region for buccal fat grafting, respecting the position of regional neurovascular structures
- The injecting technique relies on gentle advancement of the cannula through the small incisions down to the deepest desired layer

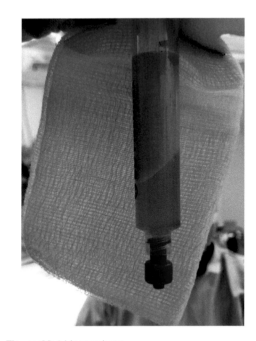

Figure 69.4 Lipoaspirate.

- Using multiple passes, small aliquots of 0.1 mL of adipocytes are injected on each pass on withdrawal of the cannula. Greater surface area of graft

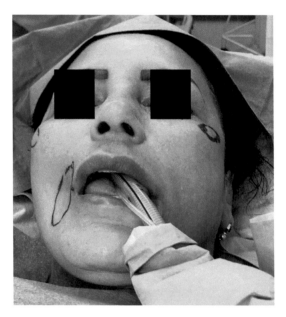

Figure 69.5 Preoperative site markings for adipocyte infiltration.

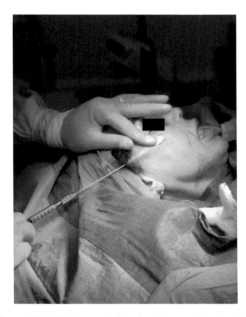

Figure 69.6 Adipocyte infiltration from hairline incision to temporal area.

contact with the host capillary bed facilitates plasma imbibition and graft survival
- Bolus injections of fat should be avoided due to the theoretical reduction of neovascularisation potential, and the increased risk of fat necrosis
- The site is lightly massaged to reduce ridging of the fat and achieve uniform distribution of adipocytes

Site-specific considerations

Forehead, glabella and brow
- Incision sites may be placed along the hairline at frequent intervals to gain access to this region
- 5–15 mL of fat graft may be infiltrated depending on the desired effect

Temple
- Incision sites may be placed either along the hairline at frequent intervals superior to the temporal fossa, or via the superior border of the zygoma (*Figure 69.6*)
- 1–5 mL of fat graft may be infiltrated depending on the desired effect

Periorbital area
- Incision sites may be placed in the brow for access to the upper orbit, while perpendicular injections may be used at the level of the infraorbital rim for the lower orbit
- <0.1 mL of fat graft may be infiltrated depending on the desired effect

Nose
- Incision sites may be placed in the central forehead region, glabella, cheek or alar base
- 0.5–5 mL of fat graft may be infiltrated depending on the desired effect

Nasolabial fold
- Incision sites may be placed in the mid-malar region, or lateral to the commissure
- The desired plane is immediately subcutaneous
- 1 mL of fat graft is typically sufficient

Cheek
- Incision sites may be placed lateral to the nasolabial fold, lateral to the zygomatic arch (*Figure 69.7*)
- 10–15 mL of fat graft may be infiltrated depending on the desired effect

POSTOPERATIVE CARE AND RECOVERY
- Antibiotics according to local policies should be prescribed as prophylaxis for 5–7 days postoperatively
- The patient should be advised to avoid deep massage of the face, and should only apply cool compresses to the face for the first 72 hours
- Compression dressings should be applied to the donor sites for the first 72 hours
- Vigorous activity should not be performed for the first 2 weeks postoperatively

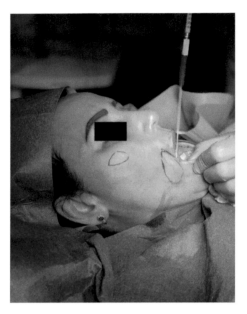

Figure 69.7 Adipocyte infiltration to lateral commissure.

POSSIBLE COMPLICATIONS AND HOW TO DEAL WITH THEM

- Overcorrection is the most common complication of autologous fat grafting, and is heavily operator-dependent
- Vascular occlusion, particularly for deeper compartment infiltration is a potentially dangerous complication, mitigated through use of a blunt cannula, and injection of small aliquots of fat on withdrawal
- Fat emboli occurrence may be reduced through infiltration of local anaesthesia with adrenaline to the recipient site
- Ridging at fat migration is a recognised complication which patients should be counselled on, and a

follow-up in 2–3 months should be scheduled for re-evaluation
- Postoperative swelling is to be expected and should settle within 8 weeks of the procedure; microfoam tape can help with swelling and protect the graft
- Be mindful of anaesthesia-related toxicity and ensure appropriate reversal agents such as Intralipid are on hand in the event of adverse reactions

TOP TIPS AND HAZARDS

- Graft survival is improved by atraumatic handling of the adipocytes; a closed-system such as a Luer Lock syringe can facilitate this.
- Regenerative potential of adipocytes is thought to be due to the adipocyte-derived stem cells, which are found in the highest concentration at the bottom of the centrifuged lipoaspirate.
- Infiltration of small aliquots of fat (0.1 mL per pass), and systematic infiltration across multiple layers provide the best results.
- Preoperative and interval medical photography are essential adjuncts to the consultation, providing a reference point for operative planning and for patient satisfaction along the patient journey.

FURTHER READING

Cohen SR, Hewett S, Ross L, et al. Regenerative cells for facial surgery: biofilling and biocontouring. *Aesthet Surg J* 2017;**37**:S16–S32.

Coleman SR, Katzel EB. Fat grafting for facial filling and regeneration. *Clin Plast Surg* 2015;**42**:289–300.

Donofrio LM. Techniques in facial fat grafting. *Aesthet Surg J* 2008;**28**:681–7.

Gornitsky J, Viezel-Mathieu A, Alnaif N, et al. A systematic review of the effectiveness and complications of fat grafting in the facial region. *JPRAS Open* 2018;**19**:87–97.

Bailey & Love's Essential Operations Bailey & Love's Essential Operations
Bailey & Love's Essential Operations Bailey & Love's Essential Operations
Bailey & Love's Essential Operations Bailey & Love's Essential Operations

PART 11 | Advances in operative maxillofacial surgery

Chapter 70

Tissue Engineering

Azadeh Rezaei, Maria Florez-Martin, Deepak Kalaskar, Gavin Jell, Kaveh Shakib

INTRODUCTION

Despite tremendous progression of innovative surgical techniques in oral and maxillofacial surgery (OMFS), repair of degenerated or surgically removed tissue remains a challenge, with considerable socio-economic impact. Tissue engineering (TE) can be defined as the creation of new functional tissue using a scaffold or template engineered to direct desirable cellular behaviour.

The scaffold has a number of purposes:

- Serves as a cell delivery system, preventing anoikis (programmed cell death following detachment from extracellular matrix [ECM] binding)
- Guides desirable cell behaviour through both physicochemical engineering parameters and/or the release of biochemical signals (e.g. through the controlled release of growth factors)
- Provides physical support and space for new tissue formation and is often designed to degrade as the new tissue forms

TE offers considerable advantages over implants used in OMFS. By guiding new tissue formation while the scaffold degrades, TE avoids infection and aseptic loosening and subsequent failure frequently observed in implants. TE also allows the regeneration of complex tissue (including nerves and vascular system), improving functionality (e.g. sensation) and the ability to respond and adapt to external stimuli (e.g. infection or increased load). Additionally, TE avoids mechanical mismatch loading, observed with materials with higher stiffness than the surrounding tissues.

Challenges of TE include cost, maintaining mechanical strength as new tissue forms, integration of the construct with the surrounding tissue and creating scaffolds that can encourage the regeneration of the composite types of tissue. To overcome these challenges, various TE approaches are used for tissue regeneration, which include *in vitro* and *in vivo* techniques (*Figure 70.1*).

Examples of TE of craniofacial, oral and dental structures include the use of resorbable collagen matrices, as dental fillers, ion-releasing bioactive glasses to stimulate new bone formation, three-dimensional (3D)-printed scaffolds including gelatine scaffolds for TMJ cartilage regeneration and combining scaffolds with stem cells, for example, adipose-derived stem cells within platelet-rich plasma gels for periodontal tissue regeneration.

The complexity of tissue types in the oral and maxillofacial region (such as mucosa, skin, bone, cartilage, nerves and blood vessels), the need to support complex movement (speech, mastication, expression) and aesthetic characteristics provide OMFS with unique challenges. Scaffolds also need to meet the complex biomechanical demands within the craniofacial region. For instance, a defect in the mandible (load-bearing bone) withstands more force than one in the cranial vault (non-load bearing). In addition, there is need to control bacterial contamination in areas that are high-risk such as the oral and nasal cavities.

In this chapter, TE applications, advancements and future directions within the scope of OMFS are reviewed.

BONE TISSUE ENGINEERING

Bone grafting has long been regarded as the 'gold standard' for hard tissue reconstructive surgery; however, there remain concerns regarding the quality and availability of bone to harvest, donor site morbidity, disease transmission and infection.

Scaffolds are the key components in bone TE, providing mechanical support, producing a surrogate for ECM and guiding cell behaviour. A wide range of natural and synthetic biomaterials such as bioactive glasses (BGs) and polymers are used for these purposes. BGs have been successfully used in hard TE for teeth and bone in the form of coatings for implants or fillers between the tissue and the implant. BGs release ions (including Ca, Si, P) and form a carbonated hydroxyapatite layer on exposure to biological fluids, which facilitates bone regeneration. Creating BGs that can withstand the mechanical demands needed for some OMFS applications remains a challenge.

Natural polymers (collagen, hyaluronic acid, etc.) are often associated with poor mechanical properties. Synthetic biodegradable polymeric materials (polyglycolic acid (PGA), polyethylene glycol (PEG)) have gained attention due to their tailorable mechanical and degradable properties, but alone, fail to provide adequate cell-binding motifs or cues to encourage bone regeneration. Moreover, their degradation products have been shown to hinder tissue formation. Hybrid polymers (combinations of natural and synthetic materials) have been suggested to supply the mechanical strength and biological components for guiding cell behaviour (e.g. collagen/poly(lactic acid) [PLA] hybrid scaffolds).

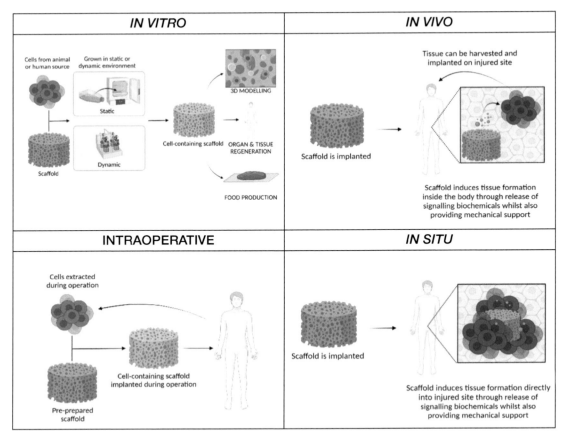

Figure 70.1 Types of tissue engineering. *In vitro* tissue engineering involves the growth of tissue (using cells and a scaffold) in a static (incubator) or dynamic (bioreactor) environment and then transplanting this tissue to where it is needed. *In vivo* tissue engineering involves growing tissue (with a scaffold engineered to induce tissue formation, e.g. via the release of growth factor) within an animal/human, but not necessarily at the site where it is needed. The newly formed tissue can then be harvested and implanted in the injured site. *In situ* tissue engineering refers to where the scaffold is implanted directly into the injured site, often providing mechanical support and encouraging new tissue growth.

Most current biomaterials used in OMFS are not tailored to individual patient bone defects. 3D printing allows formation of patient-specific scaffolds that match the bone defect, and the generation of cell-favoured properties (e.g. porosity and mechanical properties) by means of computational design.

Oral and maxillofacial surgeons were early adopters of 3D-printing technology for fabricating implantable biomaterials using radiological data. One of the first Food and Drug Administration (FDA)-approved implants was 3D-printed polyetheretherketone (PEEK)-based craniomaxillofacial implants by Oxford Performance Materials in 2013. Use of 3D-printed custom titanium implants, which are not classed as TE approaches, has now become routine in surgical practice where complex reconstruction is required. These permanent materials, while allowing the mechanical support needed for specific sized defects, do not degrade and are not replaced by native tissue, therefore still suffer from septic and aseptic failure. Degradable 3D-printed materials or tissue scaffolds can also be used. For example, 3D-printed ceramic and polymer hybrid materials have been created (an example of *in situ* engineering). Furthermore, several labs are investigating bio-printing where hydrogels and cells are printed together, which offer the advantage of creating scaffold for particular sized defects. There remain challenges in 3D bio-printing including obtaining mechanical properties similar to native tissue and achieving the tissue complexity (nerves, vascularisation, etc.) necessary for regeneration.

CARTILAGE TISSUE ENGINEERING

Cartilage TE would offer significant advantages over current biomaterial or surgical approaches (e.g.

microfracture, ankyloses). TE cartilage poses several challenges, particularly in creating scaffolds that provide suitable physicochemical properties to guide cartilage growth. Cell sources for articular cartilage are primarily mesenchymal stem cells that can be expanded and differentiated into chondrocytes. Primary cells from articular cartilage have been suggested as another potential cell source, but the primary cells suffer (when cultured *in vitro*) from low proliferation, de-differentiation and loss of phenotype.

Both natural (chitosan and collagen type II) and synthetically derived biomaterials (electrospun poly-caprolactone [PCL], hydrogels or bioceramic-polymer composite materials) have been used for cartilage tissue engineering. These biomaterials have been developed to generate cell adhesion and extracellular matrix formation but creating materials that can withstand the mechanical loading experienced (e.g. within the TMJ) remains an issue for degradable materials.

In vitro, cell-derived cartilage tissues have also been developed. Chondro-Gide, a clinically approved collagen scaffold, has reached human trials of cartilage made from human nasal chondrocytes (hNCs). hNCs can be relatively easily isolated from a small cartilage biopsy from the nasal septum and expanded using specific growth factors and patient's own serum. An *in vivo* study, using 3D-printed cartilage scaffolds of hNCs and laden bovine type I collagen hydrogel in nude mice, demonstrated similar histological, molecular and mechanical characteristics to Chondro-Gide.

NERVE TISSUE ENGINEERING

Facial nerve dysfunction continues to pose a significant clinical challenge. Micro-neurosurgical repair using end-to-end anastomosis/neurorrhaphy is typically employed when surgical intervention is possible (gap size <2 cm). For nerve injuries greater than 2 cm, nerve autografting is the gold standard. Delay in angiogenesis of the nerve autograft can hinder nerve regeneration. To avoid the complications of autograft-ing, FDA-approved nerve conduits (polymeric, wraps and decellularised allografts) can be used to bridge the nerve gaps. However, there remains limited capacity in bridging longer gaps without tension (>3 cm).

The current focus of peripheral nerve research is to encourage nerve regeneration. TE using synthetic con-duits with Schwann cells might be a viable alternative to nerve grafts, a hollow conduit. Zongxi Wu et al. demonstrated that a 3D hybrid polymer scaffold con-taining Schwann cells improved production of nerve regeneration factors compared with 2D cultured cells. PCL filaments have additionally been shown in a few clinical case reports to be effective in restoring motor and sensory function in long-gap nerve abnormalities. However, the sole use of biomaterials largely depends on the healing capacity of the patient's body.

Scaffolds/conduits can be made using a variety of fabrication methods, including 3D printing where using computer-aided modelling has been suggested to yield geometrically complex shapes. Despite promising *in vitro* and *in vivo* models for tissue engineering in nerve regeneration, no clinical trials have been done.

VASCULAR REGENERATION

TE constructs over ~200 μm surpass the capacity of oxygen and nutrient supply, thus, demand a supply of vascular network. Growing tissue *in vitro* larger than 200 μm therefore requires bioreactors, or fluid flow systems to supply the needed oxygen and nutrients. Once implanted, however, neovascularisation is still required, meaning that implanted cells risk loss of vital-ity unless the new vasculature is established. The forma-tion of viable vasculature is therefore a major challenge in TE. There are a number of strategies to promote angiogenesis including the release of angiogenic factors from scaffolds (e.g. vascular endothelial growth factor [VEGF]) or by targeting the hypoxia inducing factor (HIF) pathway (e.g. through the release of cobalt from bioactive glasses). Targeting the HIF pathway (which is the usual cellular response to hypoxia caused by micro-vascular damage or when cellular oxygen demand outstrips supply) has the advantage of causing cells to release a number of angiogenic factors important for different stages of the angiogenic process, in a controlled, sequential manner, as opposed to the release of single angiogenic factor (such as VEGF) which can cause a disorganised non-functional vasculature.

Approaches for promoting angiogenesis in TE con-structs include *in vitro* vasculature formation, angiogenic growth factor release, hypoxia pretreated cells or genet-ically modified (e.g. HIF-stabilised) cells. A prerequisite for all these strategies is that the scaffold must be able to allow hierarchical vascular formation, either through the interconnected pore structure size or by being of a material that can be degraded by the advancing blood vessels (e.g. metalloproteinase-1 [MMP-1] degradable linker scaffolds).

Studies have demonstrated the possibility of cre-ating vascular structures *in vitro*, using hydrogels, endothelial cells and stromal cells. Maiullari et al. used human umbilical vein endothelial cells (HUVECs) and induced pluripotent cell-derived cardiomyocytes (iPSC-CMs) embedded within an alginate-containing hydrogel to produce blood vessel-like structures. Using bioinks to 3D print the media and intima layers of the vessel is another technique to create tissue engineered blood vessels *in vitro*.

There remains the problem of how these vascular structures (50–100 μm sized vessels) connect to the exist-ing vasculature when implanted *in vivo* and whether the cells will survive until blood flow is restored. There is some evidence that *in vitro* created vascular structures do integrate with existing vasculature, but this is likely to depend on the type of hydrogel and the density of the existing microvascular structure within the implant site.

Novel vascularisation strategies focus on stimulating vascularisation in implanted grafts/scaffolds from/to the host tissue in a short period of time to avoid tissue loss due to hypoxic conditions.

CHALLENGES IN ORAL AND MAXILLOFACIAL TISSUE ENGINEERING

While significant progress has been made in TE, there remains a considerable challenge in translating TE to clinical OMFS practice. These challenges include the cost of TE approaches, requiring complex scaffolds and cell isolation, maintenance and culture. There is often a balance between the complexity of the tissue engineering approach, the level of personalisation (e.g. whether the patient's own cells are used – autogenic cells) and the commercial reality. Good manufacturing practice (GMP) also remains an issue for complex products (advanced therapies) where it is more difficult to demonstrate reproducibility and to keep the scaffolds (often containing biological products) sterile and free of endotoxins. *In situ* tissue engineering may therefore offer a more viable – off-the-shelf – commercial route, where the considerable costs of *in vitro* cell culture are removed. Cell source (autogenic, allogenic) remains an issue in terms of cost/suitability of autogenic cells and the immune response of allogenic cells. Another challenge in OMFS is creating tissue constructs that match the complexity of native tissue, including connecting to the vascular, lymphatic and neuronal networks. Success in TE in overcoming these challenges in OMFS is dependent on close multidisciplinary collaborations between biologists, engineers and clinicians.

FURTHER READING

Azevedo MM, Tsigkou O, Nair R, et al. Hypoxia inducible factor-stabilizing bioactive glasses for directing mesenchymal stem cell behavior. *Tissue Eng Part A* 2015;**21**:382–9.

Barandun M, Iselin LD, Santini F, et al. Generation and characterization of osteochondral grafts with human nasal chondrocytes. *J Orthop Res* 2015;**33**:1111–9.

Lan X, Liang Y, Vyhlidal M, et al. In vitro maturation and in vivo stability of bioprinted human nasal cartilage. *J Tissue Eng* 2022;**13**:20417314221086368.

Rezaei A, Li Y, Turmaine M, et al. Hypoxia mimetics restore bone biomineralisation in hyperglycaemic environments. *Sci Rep* 2022;**12**:13944.

Tsigkou O, Pomerantseva I, Spencer JA et al. Engineered vascularized bone grafts. *Proc Natl Acad Sci USA* 2010;**107**:3311–16.

Bailey & Love's Essential Operations Bailey & Love's Essential Operations
Bailey & Love's Essential Operations Bailey & Love's Essential Operations
Bailey & Love's Essential Operations Bailey & Love's Essential Operations

PART 11 | Advances in operative maxillofacial surgery

Chapter
71

Principles of Laser Surgery

Madan G. Ethunandan

LASER is an acronym for Light Amplification by Stimulated Emission of Radiation. The laser light is a type of electromagnetic (EM) radiation and is derived from the optical part of the EM spectrum. Radiation is considered energy in transit and its propagation can be influenced by changes in the energising source. The laser light travels in waves, which have characteristic wavelengths and frequency.

PHYSICS AND DEVICES

The physics of laser is a complex topic; Albert Einstein published the theoretical basis of laser in 1917, but a functioning laser light was only produced in 1960 by Theodore Maiman. In brief, atoms consist of a positively charged nucleus and negatively charged electrons, which orbit in precise energy levels. At rest, these electrons remain at the lowest energy level (ground state) and when energy is added, are elevated to an excited state. The excited state is unstable, and the atoms return to the ground state by emission of a photon (spontaneous emission), which can be in any direction.

A laser beam on the other hand, which is generated by a device, consists of photons which are of the same wavelength (monochromatic), coherent (all components of the waveform are in phase) and collimated (very little beam divergence). The basic laser generator consists of three components: an active or lasing medium, an optical chamber or resonator, and an energising source (*Figure 71.1*).

When energy is pumped into the lasing medium, it is absorbed by the individual atoms in the medium, which are elevated to an excited state (stimulated absorption). The photons released as these atoms try to revert to a ground state collide with other excited atoms which are forced to emit identical photons (stimulated emission), which are of the same wavelength, direction and phase. The stimulated photons produced are reflected back and forth by parallel mirrors in the optical chamber and the number of photons is amplified by each reflection (amplification). When more atoms achieve an excited state, 'population inversion' occurs. The front of the output mirror is designed to be partially reflective and allows a small percentage of the energy to be emitted as a laser beam. This beam is further passed through a series of focusing lenses to reduce its diameter and increase its intensity and energy to make it suitable for clinical applications.

A diode semiconductor laser converts electrical energy into light. The production of a diode laser is credited to Robert Hall and Marshall Nathan in 1962. A semiconductor diode sandwich is created, often from alloys of aluminium, indium and gallium and consists of p-type (rich in holes – lacking electrons) and n-type (too many electrons) slices with a p-n junction (*Figure 71.2*). Electrons are injected into the diode, which combine with holes, and some of their excess energy is converted into photons. These interact with more incoming electrons, helping to produce more photons and so on in a self-perpetuating process called resonance. This repeated conversion of incoming electrons into outgoing photons is analogous to the process of stimulated emission that occurs in a conventional, gas-based laser. In a conventional laser, a concentrated light beam is produced by 'pumping' the light emitted from atoms repeatedly between two mirrors. In a laser diode, an equivalent process happens when the photons bounce back and forth in the microscopic junction (roughly 1 μm wide) between the

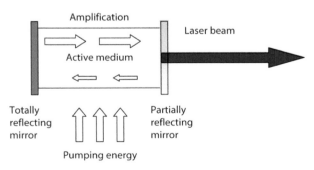

Figure 71.1 Laser generator.

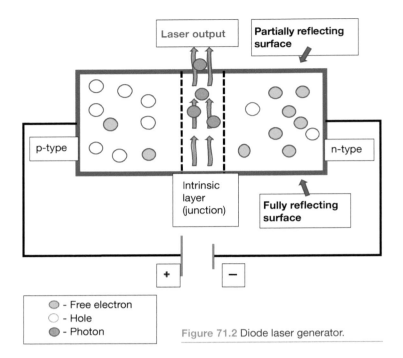

Figure 71.2 Diode laser generator.

slices of p-type and n-type semiconductor. To increase power, bars and stacks have been developed. A bar is an array of 10–50 side-by-side individual semiconductor lasers integrated into a single chip and a stack is a two-dimensional array of multiple bars. Apart from making more power than a single laser diode, a stack opens the possibility of generating multiple different wavelengths at the same time because each laser in the stack can make a different one.

The differing types of lasers available are principally determined by the active (lasing) medium producing the beam and in the case of diode lasers, by the materials in the semiconductors and intrinsic layers (*Table 71.1*).

The lasers used in maxillofacial surgery are often delivered to the tissues via optical cables or through mirrors in an articulated arm, dependent on the wavelength and power of the laser beam. Carbon dioxide (CO_2) laser is traditionally delivered with an articulated arm and others such as neodymium:yttrium-aluminium-garnet (Nd:YAG), potassium-titanyl-phosphate (KTP) and diode lasers are delivered by fibreoptic cables.

LASER-TISSUE INTERACTIONS

The effect of laser on the tissue is principally dependant on its wavelength, power and delivery sequence in addition to the particular characteristics of the tissues. The outcome of these interactions are due to thermal (coagulation, vaporisation, carbonisation and ignition) and non-thermal (photomechanical, photochemical and photoablative) events. Photothermal effects are

TABLE 71.1 Types of lasers

Gas lasers

Carbon dioxide (CO_2)

Argon (Ar)

Helium-neon (He-Ne)

Solid state / crystal lasers

Neodymium: Yttrium-aluminium-garnet (Nd:YAG)

Ruby

Alexandrite

Potassium-titanyl-phosphate (KTP)

Erbium:YAG (ErYAG)

Excimer laser (mix of rare gas and active elements)

Noble gas: argon, krypton, xenon
  • Argon fluoride (ArF)
  • Xenon chloride (XeCl)

Active gas: fluorine, chlorine

Dye lasers (organic dye in solvent)

Dye (rhodamine, fluorescein, coumarin, stilbene, umbelliferone, tetracene, malachite green)

Solvent (water, glycol, methanol, cyclohexane, cyclodextrin)

Semiconductor lasers (diode lasers)

Indium gallium arsenide phosphorus (InGaAsP)

Gallium aluminium arsenide (GaAlAs)

Gallium arsenide (GaAs)

Indium gallium arsenide (InGaAs)

due to the production of heat from the absorption of laser energy; photochemical effects are due to changes in the chemical composition of the tissue resulting from the absorption of laser light and photomechanical effects result from the target area being mechanically destroyed by laser absorption.

Anderson and Parrish in 1983 described 'selective photothermolysis', which is the ability to achieve temperature-mediated localised injury to the target tissue through a specific chromophore, while minimising damage to the surrounding tissue. This effect is dependent on the use of a laser with an appropriate wavelength, energy fluence and pulse duration. Thermal relaxation time is defined as the time required for a given heated tissue to lose 50% of its heat through diffusion and therefore, significant thermal diffusion (thermal damage) can be minimised if the duration of the laser pulse is shorter than the thermal relaxation time of the target tissue. The laser beam can be delivered as a continuous wave, pulsed wave (nanoseconds to seconds) or Q-switched (very fast pulses, 10^{-9} seconds).

Therefore, for proper selective thermolysis to occur, the target tissue (through its chromophores) must possess greater optical absorption than the non-targeted surrounding tissue and the laser of choice must have pulse duration shorter than the thermal relaxation time of the target tissue. Further, the power, focus and the duration that the beam dwells in a particular spot also influence the tissue effects (focused beam – incision, defocused beam – vaporise at high power, coagulate at

low power). The wavelengths, target chromophores and principal uses of the commonly used lasers in maxillofacial surgery are highlighted in *Table 71.2*.

In general, there is very little inflammation associated with laser wounds with resultant decrease in pain and scarring. This is thought to be due to the denaturation of proteins, including the inflammatory mediators, with subsequent underestimation by the body of the damage caused by the laser. The denatured collagen is also partly responsible for the haemostasis obtained following CO_2 laser wounds, though this is restricted to vessels less than 0.5 mm in diameter.

PRACTICAL LASER SAFETY

Parameters to consider

Wavelength

Its selection is principally influenced by the target chromophore and the intended depth of penetration (determined by the location of the target chromophore). The shorter the wavelength, the more superficial the penetration; the longer the wavelength, the deeper the penetration.

Power and spot size

Power and spot size determines power density and influences the energy and heat delivered to the target tissue. For a given power output, decreasing the spot size will increase the energy delivered to a unit target

TABLE 71.2 Laser characteristics and common clinical uses

Laser type	Wave length	Target chromophore	Clinical uses
Carbon dioxide (CO_2)	10 600 nm	Water	Cutting, vaporisation, skin resurfacing, scar revision
Erbium:Yttrium-aluminium-garnet (Er:YAG)	2940 nm	Water	Skin resurfacing, scar revision
Neodymium:Yttrium-aluminium-garnet (Nd:YAG)	1064 nm	Oxyhaemoglobin, melanin, black, yellow, red, orange pigment	Vascular lesions (venous malformations), tattoos, pigmented lesions, hair removal
Alexandrite	755 nm	Melanin, black, blue, green pigment	Tattoos, hair removal, pigmented lesions
Ruby	694 nm	Melanin, black, blue, green pigment	Tattoos, hair removal, pigmented lesions
Pulsed dye laser (PDL)	577–595 nm	Oxyhaemoglobin, melanin, yellow, red, orange pigment	Vascular lesions (capillary, venous malformations), pigmented lesions, tattoos, scar revision
Potassium-titanyl-phosphate (KTP)	532 nm	Oxyhaemoglobin	Vascular lesions (venous malformations)
Diode laser (semiconductor laser – can change wavelength, power, beam properties)	532–1470 nm	Oxyhaemoglobin, melanin, pigments, water	Vascular lesions (capillary malformations, telangiectasia, venous malformations), excision tissues with increased vascularity, hair removal, tattoo removal, photodynamic therapy

area (like a magnifying glass concentrating sunlight on a target). Decreasing the spot size will, however, reduce the depth of penetration of the laser. As a general rule, when the spot size is halved, the energy output will have to be doubled to create an effect at the same treatment depth. The principal determinant of treatment depth is the wavelength, regardless of power or spot size.

Pulse width

This is the delivery/exposure time of the laser to the target tissue. Its selection is influenced by the volume and thermal relaxation time of the target tissue. The ideal pulse width is half the thermal relaxation time of the target tissue.

Cooling

Laser therapy aims to maximise and restrict thermal damage to the target chromophore, while minimising damage to the superficial epidermis. Selective cooling of the superficial skin layers can reduce the undesirable thermal injury. The two commonly used cooling modalities are Sapphire plate contact cooling and cryogen spray cooling systems. The contact system works by recirculating chilled water (4°C) around a transparent medium that is kept in direct contact with the target tissue for less than 2 seconds and removed manually. The selective epidermal cooling or dynamic cooling uses the Freon substitute (cryogen) as the conductive medium and is delivered in spurts of spray directed over the treated area of a fixed diameter. The droplet temperature is variable, but usually set clinically between 45°C and 55°C.

Operational and environmental safety

Lasers are safe if used appropriately, although the risks to patient and the staff can be significant if used improperly. The safety of lasers is classified according to their effect on the skin or cornea and is based on the maximum permissible exposure (MPE) levels. Class I is the safest and Class IV the highest and most dangerous; medical lasers are Class IV. The clinician using the laser is responsible for the safety of the patient and the staff. Local policies should be in place, however, to allow use of lasers by only trained clinicians, in a safe laser environment staffed by a trained support team. These operational aspects are often overseen by laser protection supervisors and laser protection advisors in the hospital.

The clinician should demonstrate appropriate training, understanding and experience with lasers in addition to being aware of the local safety guidelines. The supporting team, which usually includes a senior nurse, prepares the theatre, checks and starts up the laser and assists with the setting during its use. The key to the laser machine is often kept by this person, who keeps it with their house key to ensure that it is not left near the laser machine. The number of keys in circulation is also strictly controlled.

A safe environment involves the creation of a laser light-tight envelope to the theatre in addition to provision of a regularly serviced and inspected laser machine. The access should be limited to essential personnel instructed in laser safety and doors should be locked and all windows and ventilation pathways covered with shutters. Clear warning with illuminated signs should highlight that a laser procedure is in progress and local safety rules apply. These signs are usually interlocked with the electrical supply of the laser machine and illuminate automatically when the power is switched on. Some hospitals have interlocks on the doors, which inhibit laser emission if the door is opened and interrupts clinical procedures. In these instances, it would be sensible to have additional door locks to prevent interlocks cutting the laser emission.

Clinical staff and patient protection

All the staff in the theatre, including the surgeon should wear eye protection designed for the particular laser in use. This is designed to provide protection from accidental exposure and is not intended to allow direct viewing of the laser beam.

It is essential that the hand piece is not waved around carelessly when the laser is switched on. When active, it should only be aimed at the operation site and at all other times should be switched to the safe standby mode. The support staff in charge of the machine should always keep an eye on the clinician and should switch to standby mode if the laser is being pointed away from the operative site. Mirrors and highly polished surfaces should be excluded from the operative site.

The key areas of patient safety in maxillofacial surgery relate to the airway, eyes and sites adjacent to the target. Although it is rare for explosive gases to be used in anaesthesia nowadays, it is good practice to discuss this with the anaesthetist. There are, however, inflammable combinations of agents, such as nitrous oxide and oxygen, used regularly and it is vitally important that the laser beam does not penetrate the lumen of the airway or endotracheal tube, with a significant risk of a catastrophic airway fire. There are specially designed armoured laser-resistant endotracheal tubes available, which are often placed per orally. This can restrict access for treatment in the mouth, and in these instances a nasal tube can be used with additional protection with a metal foil till the nose and saline-soaked gauze throat and postnasal pack to protect the tube in this area. It is important to be particularly aware of the possibility of perforating the palate and entering the nasal airway and causing damage to the nasal tube in this region. In the same way, a cleft palate is a potential risk and an armoured oral tube would be a better option.

Eye protection is vitally important and depends on the particular procedure being undertaken. Lead corneal protectors are used for procedures involving the eyelids and periorbital areas, whereas special laser safety glasses are used for other procedures. The areas surrounding the operative site are protected by a thick layer of saline-soaked gamgee, in which a small hole can be cut to allow access to the target site.

Laser plumes contain dust, hazardous chemicals and biological agents (bacteria, viral DNA), which can cause potential harm. A laser grade smoke evacuation system (high flow; two-stage filtration; filtration efficiency > 99.99%; down to a particle size of 0.05 μm) is therefore essential for scavenging, in addition to the wearing of surgical masks and gloves.

ADVANTAGES AND DISADVANTAGES

Advantages of lasers include haemostasis, enabling improved visibility of the operative site and reduced blood loss. The ability to control the depth of penetration and specific tissue 'affected' enables precision of the surgery. Reduced scarring and decreased pain have also been attributed to the use of lasers.

The laser wound healing time can be more prolonged than that produced by a scalpel. The initial outlay and ongoing maintenance cost of the equipment, theatres, learning curve and training of users can be considerable.

CLINICAL APPLICATIONS

The common clinical uses of lasers are highlighted in *Table 71.2*. When a CO_2 laser is used, it is important to check on each occasion that the He-Ne visible light indicator laser and the invisible CO_2 beam coincide. This is done by aiming the He-Ne laser at a target spot on a wooden spatula and firing the CO_2 laser and comparing the target spot with the burn spot. Do not rest your spatula on your lap when you do this!

The CO_2 and Erbium lasers are often used for cutaneous resurfacing, and the recent advent of computerised pattern generator and scanning capabilities have allowed for large areas to be treated rapidly and safely. CO_2 laser resurfacing has been associated with the reactivation of herpes simplex virus (HSV) causing delayed re-epithelialisation and scarring. Antiviral prophylaxis (famciclovir, valacyclovir) should be instituted in this group of patients.

NEWER TECHNOLOGIES

Fractional photothermolysis (Fraxel) works by producing thermal damage to microscopic zones of the epidermis and dermis and therefore it is postulated that following Fraxel skin resurfacing, the surrounding normal skin will help in faster healing and less 'downtime' between treatments.

Intense pulsed light (IPL) is not a laser, but a non-coherent, multiwavelength light source, in which appropriate filters are placed to produce light with wavelengths ranging from 590 to 1 200 nm. It is primarily used for hair removal, pigmentary disorders and non-ablative skin tightening.

TOP TIPS AND HAZARDS

- Lasers should be used only by trained clinicians.
- Always refer to local protocols for the use of lasers.
- Careful protection of the patient, operator and other staff is paramount.
- The clinician should have sound knowledge of the different lasers and their uses.

FURTHER READING

Anderson RR, Parrish JA. Selective photothermolysis: precise microsurgery by selective absorption of pulsed radiation. *Science* 1983;**220**:524–7.

Farkas JP, Hoopman JE, Kenkel JM. Five parameters you must understand to master control of your laser/light-based devices. *Aesthet Surg J* 2013;**33**:1059–64.

Bailey & Love's Essential Operations Bailey & Love's Essential Operations
Bailey & Love's Essential Operations Bailey & Love's Essential Operations
Bailey & Love's Essential Operations Bailey & Love's Essential Operations

PART 11 | Advances in operative maxillofacial surgery

Chapter

72

Interventional Radiology of the Head and Neck

Jocelyn Brookes

INTRODUCTION

Over the past 50 years, radiological diagnostic imaging techniques have developed as applications of physics into the following main modalities:

- X-ray (single-shot and fluoroscopic real-time imaging)
- Ultrasound (real-time, Doppler, 3D, 4D, harmonic)
- Computed tomography (CT) (x-ray-based multi-detector, cardiac-gated)
- Magnetic resonance (high field strength, spin-labelling, functional MR)
- Isotope-radionuclear imaging (2D, 3D, fusion with CT/MR, PET)

Each has continually improved in the demonstrated resolution of anatomical detail, and with contrast-enhancement and time-resolution, delivers physiological information also. This has transformed the practice of modern medicine with the obviation of such techniques as open diagnostic laparotomy.

Use of these modalities to guide minimally invasive interventions has led to the parallel development of what has become a separate speciality of image-guided surgery known as interventional radiology (IR).

These imaging modalities enable targeted access to be made to pathological tissues by percutaneous direct puncture using a needle, endovascularly via anatomic structures such as arteries and veins or by endoluminal non-vascular passageways such as gut, bile ducts, salivary or tear ducts, all of which can then be explored with catheter and wire techniques.

With access achieved, these techniques can be used to transport tools to the tissue to effect treatment, for example:

- Coagulation (ablation)
- Angioplasty (stretching/ballooning)
- Embolisation (blocking of blood supply causing tissue necrosis)
- Chemoembolisation (infusion of chemical agents)
- Foreign-body retrieval (capture and remove objects, e.g. stones)

Working in close collaboration with traditional surgical specialists (e.g. via multidisciplinary team [MDT] meetings), interventional radiologists have been able to apply these new solutions to old problems, pushing the envelope of what can be achieved to the benefit of our patients. The ability to carry out more targeted, minimally invasive surgical procedures has permitted earlier diagnosis and treatment of cancers and avoidance of major open surgical interventions such that patients can be restored to full, active independent health with consequent socioeconomic benefits for society in general.

Thus, in maxillofacial surgery, IR techniques are long-established both as supportive adjuncts to existing surgical methods, for example pre-surgical embolisation to minimise bleeding and reduce operative risk, but also as comprehensive standalone, alternative surgical treatments for some pathologies.

The continued development of this clinical collaboration between IR and maxillofacial surgery makes it an exciting area of medical endeavour.

IMAGING MODALITIES USED

Fluoroscopy (syn. x-ray screening, angiography)

Equipment

This real-time x-ray technique remains the bedrock of IR for endovascular and endoluminal intervention. The fixed ceiling, floor-mounted or mobile C-arm x-ray system emits x-rays through the patient from below and the image is received by the digital detector suspended above the patient. The resulting 'live' image is viewed by the operator on an adjacent screen.

High-quality imaging equipment with the ability to screen and perform DSA (digital subtraction angiography) imaging is essential to enable the operator to see the small vessels of the head and neck through which the catheter will pass. New systems offer a range of complex software facilities (e.g. rotational angio, fusion imaging, perfusion imaging, DYNA CT, etc.), which are desirable, but not essential, for a high-quality IR service.

Team

In the UK, the fluoroscopy machine is maintained and operated by the radiographic technician (radiographer) working closely as a team with the operating interventional radiology doctor, supported by the operative IR nursing team who not only care for and monitor the patient before, during and after the procedure but also prepare the kit and scrub in with the radiologist. Sometimes the nurses will administer and monitor mild sedation. Deeper sedation or general anaesthesia requires participation in the team of an anaesthetist and an assistant (*Figure 72.1*).

Radiation protection and safety considerations

Correct use of high-quality imaging equipment and adherence to performance and safety protocols by a well-trained team facilitates successful outcomes, reduces time of procedures and thus reduces safety risk to patient and staff from x-ray exposure and extended time of procedures.

Radiation scatter from the patient to the operating team necessitates diligent attention to radiation protection equipment (lead coats, lead glasses, shields, etc.) and behavioural safety protocols (stand away if possible [inverse square rule of x-ray penetrance], shortest exposure time to get the job done, minimise screening time) to minimise exposure of staff and patient. These safety rules are codified in the legal Ionising Radiation (Medical Exposure) (Amendment) Regulations (IRMER) (2018) that are enforced in every IR theatre: to minimise unintended, excessive or incorrect medical exposures; justify each exposure to ensure the benefits outweigh the risks; optimise doses to keep them "as low as reasonably practicable" for their intended use.

Ultrasound

Ultrasound (US) guidance is an essential adjunct to fluoroscopic imaging to enable needle access to the target (vascular access, malformation, cyst, etc.), which can then be confirmed by fluoroscopic imaging. US can be the primary imaging, for example, for non-luminal targets such as a mass for biopsy or ablation (thermal, cryo, chemo, PDT, etc.).

Computed tomography

CT guidance is used for non-luminal pathology access where US is not suitable such as deeper-sited masses (e.g. biopsy, ablation).

Magnetic resonance

MR guidance remains experimental after 30 years of endeavour due in part to the lack of wide availability of interventional MRI facilities (and bespoke non-magnetic equipment) and no established benefit over CT or US to guide operative access techniques.

INTERVENTIONAL RADIOLOGY TECHNIQUES IN THE HEAD AND NECK

Endovascular access

Also known as angiography, this describes access to the lesion via the arteries or veins.

Preparation

IR procedures are minimally invasive surgical procedures requiring the same considerations of patient preparation as 'open' surgery, that is anaesthetic/metabolic/psychological/safety pre-assessment and optimisation (e.g., Nil By Mouth, IV hydration, IV access, bailout manoeuvre plans, full consent with time to reflect).

Consideration of anticoagulation either before, during or after the procedure is essential and the routine (basic) preoperative blood screen for IR consists of:

- Full blood count (FBC)
- Urea and electrolytes
- Coagulation screen

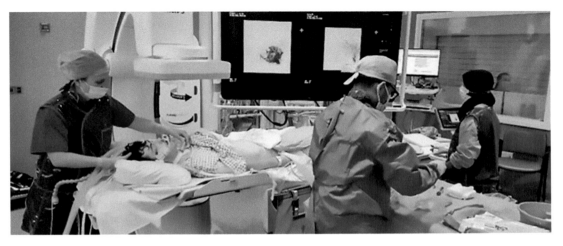

Figure 72.1 Anaesthetist, nurse and radiographer prepare the patient for the interventional radiology endovascular procedure.

Note that direct oral anticoagulants (DOAC) do not affect the International Normalised Ratio (INR), which can be normal in fully anticoagulated patients and can give false reassurance. Anticoagulation history should therefore be rehearsed at the team brief for every patient.

Most head and neck procedures involve access to the carotid arterial systems and carry the risk of stroke. Catheter manipulation in the arch of the aorta of older people with atherosclerosis may dislodge plaque fragments and the simple presence of the catheter in an artery, especially in the (prothrombotic) context of cancer, increases the risk of stroke from a baseline of 1% for consent purposes.

After careful planning, the procedure may be carried out under local anaesthesia, mild sedation (anxiolysis), deep conscious sedation or general anaesthetic which will affect the planning of perioperative care such as the availability of recovery, beds, ITU (Intensive Therapy Unit), etc.

Procedure

For head and neck procedures, access is likely to be from the common femoral, radial or brachial arteries. Good access and patient preparation with appropriate anaesthetic support are vital for the success of the procedure.

An US-guided micropuncture kit (21G needle with sequential dilatation) and the smallest haemostatic sheath to achieve the goal of the procedure, with early anticoagulation to avoid thrombosis ('radial cocktail'), provide a firm foundation for a successful procedure.

Availability of chosen, shaped catheters and wires, compatible with the sheath and coaxial microcatheters

for small vessel exploration, should be available to cover all predictable eventualities.

Familiarity of the operator and the team with the (choice, method of use and location of) kit to be used and all bailout procedures is an essential part of the preoperative team briefing.

Method

Specific details of endovascular methods and tools/kit for specific procedures is beyond the remit of this chapter but can be themed into:

- Embolisation
- Sclerotherapy (transarterial, transvenous)
- Chemotherapy
- Angioplasty
- Stenting

These methods are applied to the more common IR endovascular procedures encountered in the head and neck specialties, for example:

- (Pre-surgical) embolisation to reduce bleeding of, e.g., tumours
- Epistaxis (treatment of nosebleeds)
- Chemoembolisation for tumour treatment
- Sclerotherapy for vascular anomalies
- Covered carotid stent-grafting for 'blowout' prevention in recurrent tumours of the head and neck (*Figure 72.2*)
- Embolisation treatment of AV fistulae (either post-iatrogenic instrumentation, post-traumatic, congenital or cancerous)

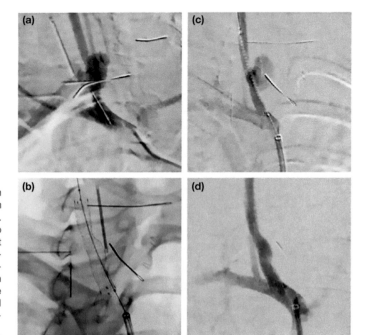

Figure 72.2 Twenty-three-year-old with infected carotid pseudo-aneurysm (incipient blowout) due to self-harm. Treatment with covered stent-graft to right common carotid origin. (a) Right common carotid artery (RCCA) pseudo-aneurysm. (b) Sheath to right brachiocephalic artery (RBCA) and stent in position. (c) Stent-graft deployed (note large anterior wall defect). (d) Final angiogram with no further pseudo-aneurysm.

Puncture wound closure

When the procedure is concluded, the catheter must be removed via the access sheath and definitive haemostasis of the puncture achieved. Be aware that arterial bleeding from the puncture site in recovery can be as threatening to the life of the patient as the pathology being treated.

Manual pressure on the arterial puncture is the traditional method of choice with a minute of pressure required for each French size of the inserted sheath (and then double it!), that is, 4F hole should be pressed for 8 minutes. 'Pressing' is a Zen-skill that cannot be left to the student nurse with no instruction. Haemostasis is the responsibility of the operator and failure of haemostasis can lead to catastrophic failure of the whole procedure, if not an encounter with the coroner.

Closure devices are available to help in the form of arterial suture devices and thrombotic plugs but each comes with its own learning curve and statistical risk of failure. Closure technique should be considered as part of procedure planning and team briefing.

Postoperative care

Care of the patient in the hours after the procedure is as important as the procedure itself especially where anticoagulation or embolisation/sclerotherapy is involved and the risk of stroke and loss of vision (as well as puncture site bleeding) is never far away. Direct communication with the postoperative clinical team and the completion of accessible, detailed (and legible) records are essential before the job can be considered complete.

Endoluminal access

The technical approach is similar to endovascular procedures, but the viscus accessed is non-vascular such as salivary and tear ducts. The specifics of each procedure are beyond the remit of this chapter but the same perioperative considerations are required as for endovascular procedures (see above), for example:

- Dacryocystography/plasty
- Salivary gland plasty and stone removal (see *Chapter 45*)

Direct percutaneous puncture, drainage and sclerotherapy

Where the target pathology is primarily a cyst, collection or inaccessible by endovascular means, then direct percutaneous access with US, CT or fluoroscopic guidance can be used, for example:

- Cyst
- Abscess
- Lymphocele
- Vascular anomalies (this disparate and complex group of lesions deserves specific mention)

Tumour ablation (direct tissue coagulative necrosis)

Since the mid-1990s, methods of local tumour coagulative necrosis have been the subject of intense research. Most have remained experimental but some methods have become established therapeutic techniques either as surgical adjuncts or as standalone treatments. The list below is not exhaustive.

- *Technique*: Thermal coagulative necrosis (delivered via laser or RF catheter)
  Application: Thyroid RFA (radiofrequency ablation) benign cyst ablation
- *Technique*: Photodynamic therapy (PDT) (laser-activated/chemo brachytherapy)
  Application: Recurrent carcinoma, e.g. squamous cell carcinoma (SCC) of the head and neck
- *Technique*: Electroporation (electric acceleration of bleomycin absorption)
  Application: Metastatic dermal deposits, e.g. breast; superficial vascular anomalies
- *Technique*: Radiobrachytherapy (experimental only)
- *Technique*: Cryotherapy (experimental only)
- *Technique*: HiFU: high-frequency ultrasound (experimental only)

VASCULAR ANOMALIES

Vascular anomalies result from acquired defects of genetic signalling pathways in endothelial cells in the first trimester of gestation. They also encompass hereditary syndromes and infantile vascular tumours. Malformations present according to the vascular tissue they most closely resemble in that venous, lymphatic and capillary malformations are considered 'low flow' lesions whereas arteriolar and arteriovenous malformations (AVM) are 'high flow' (*Figure 72.3*).

Although distinguished from tumours, venous malformations (VM) go through periods of stability and occasionally growth, typically:

- Puerperium
- Early toddler period
- Puberty
- Pregnancy
- Trauma (including surgery)

It is at these times of proliferation that they typically present with:

- Pain
- Swelling
- Bleeding
- Locality-specific space occupation, e.g. obstruction of airway
- Metabolic decompensation, e.g. high output heart failure

Phenotypic and histological classification follows the International Society for the Study of Vascular Anomalies (ISSVA) guidelines (see *Table 72.1*).

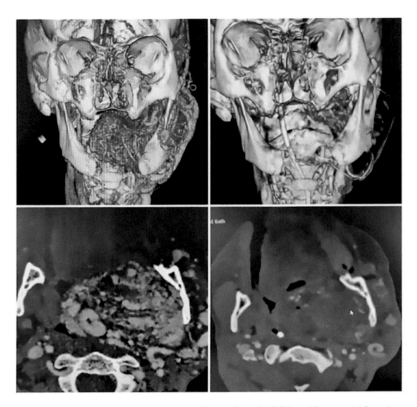

Figure 72.3 High-flow parapharyngeal arteriovenous malformations (AVM) in a 43-year-old female treated for bleeding and threat to airway. (Tracheostomy placed but patient discharged without complication at 10 days.)

TABLE 72.1 ISSVA classification for vascular anomalies (approved at the 20th ISSVA Workshop, Melbourne, April 2014, last revision May 2018)

Vascular anomalies				
Vascular tumours	Vascular malformations			
	Simple	Combined°	Of major named vessels	Associated with other anomalies
Benign Locally aggressive or borderline Malignant	Capillary malformations Lymphatic malformations Venous malformations Arteriovenous malformations Arteriovenous fistula	CVM, CLM, LVM, CVLM, CAVM*, CALVM*, others	See details	See list

° Defined as two or more vascular malformations found in one lesion.

* High-flow lesions.

Source: ISSVA classification for vascular anomalies by International Society for the Study of Vascular Anomalies (www.issva.org) is licenced under a Creative Commons Attribution 4.0 International License.

These are congenital lesions that recur throughout life and are often misdiagnosed due to their rarity and therefore poorly managed. They are best cared for in specialist clinics where a multidisciplinary team of appropriate specialists is available such as IR, clinical nurse specialist, vascular surgeons, haematologist, chronic pain specialist, psychologist with collaboration from maxillofacial surgeons, plastic surgeons and orthopaedic surgeons, etc. (the list is as long as the variation in presentation of these lesions).

Diagnosis requires a forensic approach to pre-existing investigations and a careful history and examination. Duplex ultrasound, MRI and coagulation profile are the backbone of investigations, and the most important role is spotting the lesions that mimic vascular anomalies but are in fact tumours, e.g. highly

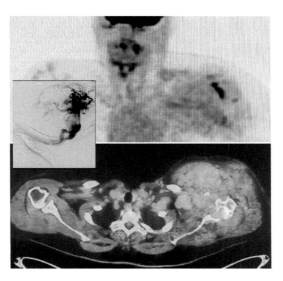

Figure 72.4 PET-CT imaging of high-flow arteriovenous malformation nidus and appearance of nidus at angiography (small box). (Imaging with permission from PACS: *Radiol Case Rep* 2021;**16**:1374–7.)

TABLE 72.2 Incidence of major complications per patient and per procedure

	Total	High-flow AVM	Low-flow VM
Patients affected	6%	14%	3%
Complication per procedure	3%	4.7%	1.8%

Data reproduced with permission from *Vascular* 2021;**29**:69–77.

As the nidus is proliferative, it has been proposed recently that it may exhibit increased metabolic activity on a PET scan helping to establish its location and confirm effective ablation, and so it proves to be (*Figure 72.4*).

In that the principle of sclerotherapy is to hold the sclerosant against the target tissue for as long as required to kill it, the blood flow may be slowed down temporarily by means of tourniquets, manual pressure, arterial embolisation (coils, gel foam, etc.) with each lesion requiring its own unique approach.

vascular lesions such as sarcomas requiring a very different pathway and timetable of treatment.

Low-flow malformations

Lymphatic and venous malformations can be sclerosed under US and fluoroscopic guidance. LM may be drained before sclerosing. Choice of sclerosant is broad and dependent on the familiarity of the operator and clinical team with the use and side effects of the chosen substance. Sclerosants may be in liquid, foam or jelly form and specifics of choice are beyond the remit of this chapter.

High-flow AVM

AVM require visualisation by angiography, and the endothelial nidus may be thus identified, embolised and sclerosed.

Consent and the risks of venous malformation treatment

Treatment of vascular malformations by embolosclerotherapy carries the risks of:

- Skin ulceration
- Nerve damage (motor and/or sensory)
- Locality-specific considerations of unintended tissue destruction such as distal arterial occlusion with tissue loss such as fingers, visual loss or stroke
- Risks associated with angiography, i.e., bleeding, thrombosis, stroke, etc.

In that multiple treatments may be required for any one patient, a 5-year audit of outcomes (2018) was presented showing major adverse event (MAE) per patient as well as risk of MAE per procedure (see *Table 72.2*). Thus, even with a specialised clinic and new techniques, there is still a significant risk in managing these challenging disorders (*Figure 72.5*).

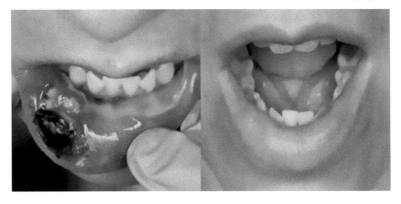

Figure 72.5 High-flow arteriovenous malformations of lower lip after embolosclerotherapy with temporary eschar and final result after 3 months. This represents a complication but not a major adverse event in that it is part of the healing process.

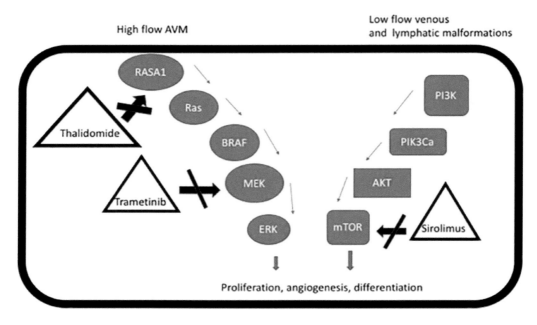

Figure 72.6 Drug interactions with genetic signalling pathways in the endothelial cell.

Medical adjuvant therapy for vascular anomalies

Since 1984, details of the complex proliferative pathways of vascular endothelial cells have been elucidated and genetic testing of vascular anomalies has led to increased understanding of common genetic defects, as the contributory cause of various apparently disparate lesion groups (*Figure 72.6*).

In this way, the genetic cause of venous and lymphatic malformations has been observed to be related to the same common genetic pathway defect (PIK3Ca). What is more interesting is that it is possible to alleviate the genetic defect by means of available medication and not only transform the malformation to its quiescent (asymptomatic) apoptotic state, but in some cases, reduce and eliminate the lesion entirely.

Specifically, since 2008, propranolol has been found to promote the resolution of infantile haemangiomas (RICH) and more recently, successful trials of the drug sirolimus for low-flow malformations and thalidomide for AVM have been presented, improving the overall outcome of treatment, and offering hope for the future for these challenging conditions (*Figures 72.7–72.9*).

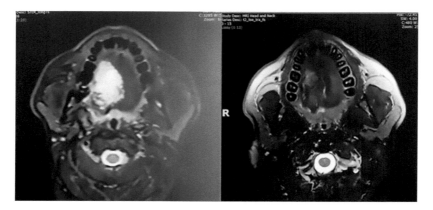

Figure 72.7 Low-flow vascular malformation (LFVM) of tongue after 6/12 treatment with sirolimus alone.

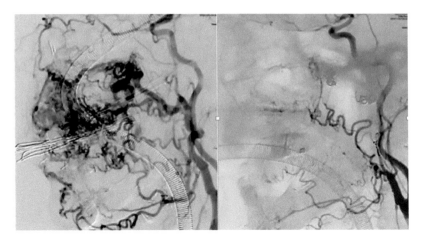

Figure 72.8 Angiographic appearance of high-flow arteriovenous malformation at presentation and near elimination of the lesion after 4 years of thalidomide and embolosclerotherapy treatment.

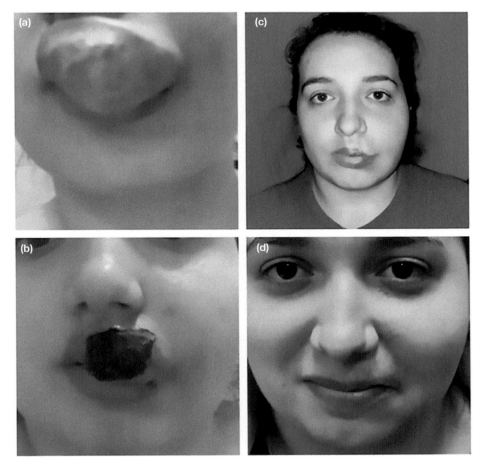

Figure 72.9 (a) High-flow AVM left upper lip and cheek treated with embolosclerotherapy. (b) Eschar in first month of healing. (c) After 3 months. (d) After 6 months.

CONCLUSION

The minimally invasive operative methods of IR that are guided by the sophisticated imaging techniques of fluoroscopy, ultrasound, CT and MRI remain themed in overall approach. Technological improvements in equipment design and engineering enable access to ever more remote areas of the body and thus make the possibilities of treatment ever wider in scope.

TOP TIPS AND HAZARDS

- The diagnostic imaging modality that demonstrated the pathology will be most useful in guiding you to the target lesion.
- Every aspect of the interventional procedure should be considered, planned and discussed at Team Brief.
- Care of puncture and closure can make or break your procedure.
- Always have a plan B prepared (bailout kit, who to call, etc.).
- If in doubt, better to stop and "engage the brain" (teaching of my mentor, the great Maurice Raphael). This means if you get stuck, change the catheter, wire or tube angle before you test the old adage of the definition of madness (and ramp up the radiation, threat of thrombosis, etc.).
- Also, "A wise man knows when to quit" and "The enemy of good is….better".
- Consider if you have given enough heparin.
- Collaborate with your colleagues to exercise careful judgement, i.e. do not spoil the surgical options however limited they may be.

FURTHER READING

Broomfield S, Bruce I, Birzgalis A, et al. The expanding role of interventional radiology in head and neck surgery. *J R Soc Med* 2009;**102**:228–34.

ISSVA Classification. Available at: https://www.issva. org/classification.

Pang C, Arasakumar DR, Evans N, et al. Efficacy and safety of embolo-sclerotherapy of arteriovenous malformations with foam sodium tetradecyl sulphate. *Int Angiol* 2023; **42**:268-75. doi: 10.23736/0392-9590.23.04993-3.

The Ionising Radiation (Medical Exposure) (Amendment) Regulations 2018. Available at: https://www.legislation.gov.uk/uksi/2018/121/contents/made.

Chapter
73

Transoral Robotic Surgery

Kyung Tae

INTRODUCTION

Transoral robotic surgery (TORS) is being adopted worldwide as a minimally invasive alternative to conventional open surgery or transoral laser microsurgery for head and neck tumors, particularly oropharyngeal carcinoma, which is dramatically increasing with association with the human papilloma virus.

TORS was developed in the early 2000s, mainly through the work done by Drs. O'Malley and Weinstein at the University of Pennsylvania, USA. TORS was approved by the US Food and Drug Administration (FDA) in 2009 for head and neck surgery.

TORS has circumvented limitations associated with transoral laser microsurgery, such as line-of-sight limitations and two-handed surgery. TORS provides a superior high-density three-dimensional magnified view, and it also enables four-handed surgery with the assistance of two hands. Compared with conventional open approaches, TORS can avoid facial incision and mandibulotomy, improve the return to normal speech and swallowing, and reduce the need for tracheostomy and permanent gastrostomy.

INDICATIONS

Appropriate patient selection for TORS is essential. TORS can be performed for benign and malignant lesions of the oropharynx, larynx, hypopharynx, parapharyngeal space, retropharyngeal lymph nodes and nasopharynx. The best indication for upfront TORS is patients with T1/T2 oropharyngeal carcinomas, including tonsil and base of tongue (BOT) cancer, who can avoid postoperative adjuvant chemoradiation therapy. TORS is also used for resection of the palatine tonsils and BOT to identify the primary site in unknown primary tumors. In a multicenter trial of TORS for an unknown primary tumor, the primary tumor was identified in 70% of the cases (almost 50% occurred in the BOT). TORS can also be used for reconstructive procedures and sleep apnea surgery.

CONTRAINDICATIONS

The main contraindications of TORS are trismus, incomplete visualization of the lesion, unresectable tumors involving the mandible, pterygoid plates, internal carotid artery, lateral nasopharynx, skull base, and prevertebral fascia, and tumors affecting more than 50% of the BOT or posterior pharyngeal wall.

PREOPERATIVE INVESTIGATIONS

Preoperative evaluation of the characteristics of each tumor is important. The exact location of the tumor, tumor resectability, vessel anatomy and its relationship to tumors, retropharyngeal node metastasis, and invasion to surrounding structures, such as internal carotid artery involvement, should be evaluated using cross-sectional imaging. Physical examination under general anesthesia is essential to evaluate the tumor extent and operative exposure for TORS, especially for assessing the presence and degree of trismus and cervical spine mobility. Obesity, micrognathia and microstomia are factors that inhibit the TORS approach.

SURGICAL ROBOTIC SYSTEM

Although several new surgical robots are emerging, the da Vinci Surgical System (Intuitive Surgical, Sunnyvale, CA, USA) has been used in most cases of TORS. In addition to the da Vinci S and Si platforms widely used for TORS, the Xi platform was released in 2014. The Xi robot allows for more effortless docking and freedom in positioning robotic arms than the S and Si systems. In addition, the da Vinci single port (SP) system was developed in 2018. It consists of a single rigid port with a diameter of 2.5 cm from which four flexible arms come, including three instrument arms and one flexible endoscope. The da Vinci SP platform may have a potential advantage in reaching deep target lesions in the hypopharynx and larynx.

Another surgical robot is the Flex Robotic System (Medrobotics Corp., Raynham, MA, USA), which was approved by the FDA for transoral approach in 2015. This robotic system allows flexible snake-like movement to the operative site.

OPERATIVE TECHNIQUE

TORS radical tonsillectomy

Step 1: Positioning of the patient and the surgical robot

The patient is placed in a supine position. A nasotracheal tube is preferred over orotracheal intubation to minimize obstruction and collision in the oral cavity.

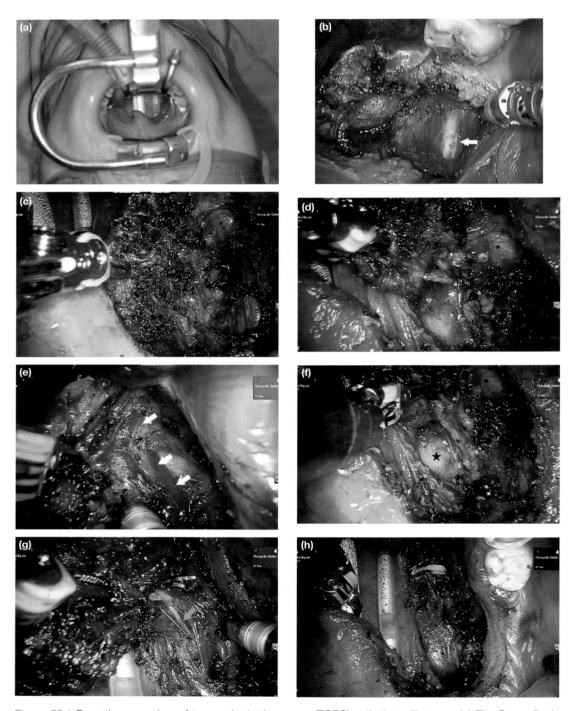

Figure 73.1 Operative procedure of transoral robotic surgery (TORS) radical tonsillectomy. (a) The Crowe-Davis mouth gag is used to expose the tonsil and suspended to a Mayo stand. (b) The mucosal incision is made and the dissection is performed to identify the pterygomandibular raphe (white arrow). (c) Dissection of the pharyngeal constrictor muscle and buccopharyngeal fascia. (d) The tonsillar artery is divided using hemoclips. (e) The styloglossus muscle (white arrows) is dissected and transected. (f) The pharyngeal constrictor muscle is dissected and elevated off the prevertebral fascia (black star). (g) The glossopharyngeal nerve (blue arrow) is identified and preserved. (h) Postoperative view of TORS tonsillectomy. Reconstruction is not required, and wound healing is accomplished by secondary intention.

Step 2: Placement of the mouth retractor and docking of the da Vinci robot

Generally, a Crowe-Davis mouth gag is used to expose the tonsil and is suspended to a Mayo stand (*Figure 73.1a*). If the Feyh-Kastenbauer-Weinstein-O'Malley (FK-WO) retractor (Gyrus Medical Inc., Maple Grove, MN, USA) is used, it is suspended in the surgical bed using a Storz scope holder (Karl Storz, Tuttlingen, Germany) or on a towel over the patient's chest. The robotic endoscope is placed in the center, and the two robotic arms loaded with a 5-mm monopolar electrocautery spatula tip (or scissors) and Maryland forceps are placed on either side of the endoscope. The endoscope is placed posteriorly against the incisors to provide maximal space for the robotic instruments. The 0° endoscope is usually used in the tonsil. However, a 30° face-down endoscope can be used if indicated, particularly for the superior pole of the tonsil and soft palate. The bedside assistant can use two suctions, a bipolar cautery, and an endoscopic hemoclip applier, such as a Storz laryngeal clip applier (Karl Storz, Tuttlingen, Germany), to retract the tissue, remove the fume, coagulate the vessels and apply surgical hemoclips.

Step 3: Mucosal incision on the anterior tonsillar pillar and dissection of the lateral part of the tonsillar fossa

The first oral mucosal incision is made at the lateral part of the anterior tonsillar pillar, close to the buccal mucosa, and dissection is performed to identify the pterygomandibular raphe (*Figure 73.1b*). Dissection is continued laterally to the pharyngeal constrictor muscles and buccopharyngeal fascia, and the parapharyngeal fat pad is dissected bluntly (*Figure 73.1c*). Several transverse veins and arteries are ligated or clipped, and the small vessels are cauterized (*Figure 73.1d*). The buccopharyngeal fascia is a tiny areolar plane separated from pharyngeal constrictor muscles. This fascial layer is a thin barrier between the tonsils and the parapharyngeal spaces. If the parapharyngeal space is not invaded, a thin layer of buccopharyngeal fascia can be preserved.

Step 4: Dissection of the soft palate and superior part of the tonsil

The soft palate is cut and dissected based on the extent of tumor involvement. Resection is performed down through the soft palate muscle to the prevertebral fascia. A mucosal index cut is made in the posterior pharyngeal wall.

Step 5: Dissection of the posterior part of the tonsillar fossa

The styloglossus and stylopharyngeus muscles are dissected and transected (*Figure 73.1e*). The pharyngeal constrictor muscle is then dissected and elevated off the prevertebral fascia (*Figure 73.1f*). The glossopharyngeal nerve can be identified between the stylohyoid ligament and styloglossus muscle (*Figure 73.1g*). Identification and preservation of the stylohyoid ligament and styloglossus muscle can prevent glossopharyngeal nerve injuries. Care is taken not to injure the internal carotid artery. The position of the internal carotid artery is known and confirmed by evaluation of preoperative imaging and carotid pulsations, which can be seen through the adjacent soft tissue.

Step 6: Dissection of the BOT

The next step is the resection of the BOT region. A mucosal incision is made on the posterior floor of the mouth and lateral BOT. Unlike transoral carbon dioxide laser resection, the da Vinci surgical robot allows for complete visualization of the BOT, facilitating complete tumor resection with a sufficient normal margin. The extent of BOT resection is based on the extent of cancer involvement. However, resection should be limited to no more than half of the BOT to preserve better swallowing function. Care must be taken to avoid injuring lingual arteries. Bleeding from the dorsal lingual artery can be controlled by hemoclips.

Step 7: Dissection of the remaining posterior pharyngeal wall

The posterior pharyngeal wall is then cut from the vallecula to the previous index cut on the posterior pharyngeal wall.

Step 8: Pathologic analysis and hemostasis

The resected surgical specimen is oriented, and a frozen section biopsy is performed to confirm a negative surgical margin. Final fine bleeding control is performed using electrocautery and a hemostatic agent.

Step 9: Reconstruction of surgical defect

For most patients, reconstruction is not required if the resection is limited to the tonsillar region (*Figure 73.1h*), although local flaps such as the facial artery musculomucosal flap, buccal fat, palatal flap and submental island flap may be used for the defect of the tonsil region. Thus, in most patients, wound healing is accomplished by secondary intention. If the internal carotid artery is exposed, the fascial layers are sutured over the carotid artery or left to heal by secondary intention. However, free-flap reconstruction can be considered in patients with wide exposure of the internal carotid artery, predisposed to poor wound healing, and large through-and-through pharyngeal and neck defects.

Extensive resection of the inferolateral region of the tonsillar fossa may result in communication between the neck and tonsillar fossa, especially when the submandibular gland is removed during simultaneous neck

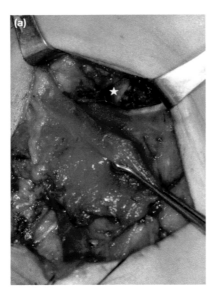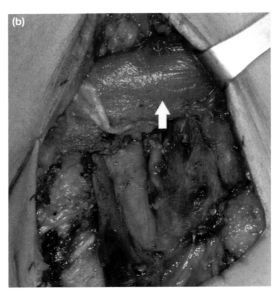

Figure 73.2 Reconstruction of the communication between the oropharynx and neck. (a) The extensive resection in inferior-lateral aspect of tonsillar fossa results in a connection (white star) between the neck and tonsillar fossa. (b) The connection between the neck and tonsillar fossa is reconstructed using the sternocleidomastoid muscles (white arrow).

dissection (*Figure 73.2a*). Therefore, the connection between the neck and pharynx can be reconstructed using local muscle flaps such as the digastric or sterno-cleidomastoid muscles (*Figure 73.2b*).

Restoration of velopharyngeal sphincter competence is necessary when the soft palate is resected. Palatal defects involving less than one-quarter of the area can be reconstructed with primary closure. However, for larger defects, free-flap reconstruction, pharyngeal flap, or pharyngoplasty is considered to minimize velopharyngeal insufficiency.

TORS base of tongue resection

Step 1: Positioning of the patient and the surgical robot

The setup for BOT resection is similar to that for radical tonsillectomy.

Step 2: Placement of the tongue retractor and docking of the da Vinci robot

An FK-WO retractor with a narrow tongue blade is usually used to expose the BOT (*Figure 73.3a*). Appropriate placement of the retractor is mandatory to properly visualize the entire tumor margin. A tongue retraction suture can be used to pull the tongue when placing a mouth gag. For BOT resection, 0° and 30° endoscopes are generally used; a 30° face-up endoscope can be necessary later in the deep part dissection.

Step 3: Horizontal BOT incision and dissection

A horizontal BOT mucosal incision is made near the tip of the retractor blade and the BOT muscle is dissected (*Figure 73.3b*). The retractor and tongue blade are repositioned as the dissection progresses for a better surgical view. If the tumor is located in the glossoton-sillar sulcus or invades the tonsil, radical tonsillectomy is necessary with BOT resection.

Step 4: Vertical midline BOT incision and transection of the deep musculature

A midline BOT mucosal cut and deep muscle dissection are made to an appropriate depth according to the tumor extent and margin.

Step 5: Lateral BOT dissection

Then, a lateral BOT mucosal incision and dissection of the deep muscle are performed. The lingual artery and its branches are identified and divided with hemoclips; two or three hemoclips are applied on the patient side and one on the tumor side before transection.

Step 6: Dissection and ligation of the lingual artery

The lingual artery passes laterally to the pharyngeal constrictor muscle, runs anterolateral to the hyoid bone and passes deep to the hyoglossus muscle. Therefore, dissection within the intrinsic tongue muscles is

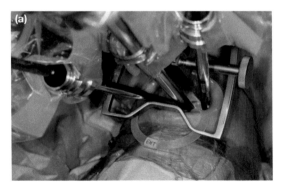

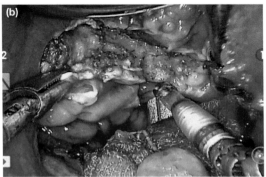

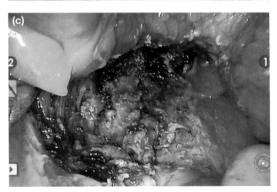

Figure 73.3 Transoral robotic surgery (TORS) base of tongue (BOT) resection. (a) The Feyh-Kastenbauer retractor is used to expose the BOT. The endoscope is placed in the center, and the two robotic arms are placed on either side of the endoscope. (b) A horizontal BOT mucosal incision is made near the tip of the retractor blade. (c) Postoperative view of TORS BOT resection. The defect is healed with secondary intention.

assumed to be safe from lingual artery injuries. The most vulnerable portion of lingual artery bleeding is the dissection between the greater cornu of the hyoid and styloglossus muscle. If severe bleeding occurs from the lingual artery, external neck pressure by a bedside assistant on the area of the greater cornu of the hyoid helps decrease bleeding and allows for visualization

of the bleeding point and application of hemoclips. Prophylactic transcervical ligation of the lingual or external carotid artery has been known to significantly reduce the severity of postoperative hemorrhage. However, there is no consensus on the routine use and timing of transcervical arterial ligation during TORS, although some surgeons recommend its use.

Step 7: Dissection of deep muscles and vallecular mucosa

The final dissection is performed through the remaining deep muscle and the underlying vallecular mucosa. The hypoglossal nerve should be preserved during the procedure. However, preservation of the lingual branches of the glossopharyngeal nerve is not always possible.

Step 8: Pathologic analysis and final hemostasis

The resected surgical specimen is marked for proper orientation, and a frozen section biopsy is performed to confirm a negative surgical margin.

Step 9: Reconstruction of surgical defect

Smaller defects are healed by secondary intention, with adequate preservation of function (*Figure 73.3c*). However, reconstruction with a free flap should be considered for large BOT defects to minimize impairment of the pharyngeal phase of swallowing.

Airway management in TORS for oropharyngeal cancer

Most TORS procedures for oropharyngeal cancer can be safely performed without a temporary tracheostomy. If there is no edema in the tongue, larynx or pharynx, the patient is extubated at the end of the procedure. However, if there is a concern for airway swelling, delayed extubation can be considered with steroid treatment for 1–2 days. Tracheostomy should be considered in patients with large tumor resection, need for free-flap reconstruction, pre-existing coagulopathies, significant bleeding, cardiorespiratory insufficiency, high risk of aspiration and prior head and neck irradiation.

Significant tongue edema and airway obstruction can occur after prolonged application of a tongue retractor. To minimize tongue swelling, the retractor should be periodically released during the procedure.

Neck dissection in TORS

Therapeutic or prophylactic neck dissection is necessary for most patients with oropharyngeal cancer because of the high risk of lymph node metastasis. In TORS, neck dissection is performed either simultaneously or in a staged manner. Most surgeons prefer concurrent neck dissection with TORS rather than staged neck dissection. Several studies have demonstrated the feasibility and efficacy of simultaneous neck dissection. However, some surgeons prefer staged neck dissection 1–3 weeks after the TORS procedure to prevent communication between the neck and oropharynx and avoid laryngopharyngeal swelling that might require a tracheotomy.

PERIOPERATIVE COMPLICATIONS

The possible important complications of TORS include postoperative hemorrhage, dysphagia and injury to the lingual and hypoglossal nerves, either from surgical trauma or pressure on the tongue from mouth gag. Postoperative hemorrhage is the most common complication, ranging from 1.5% to 18.5%, and usually occurs between 6 and 14 days postoperatively. The severity of postoperative bleeding varies from mild blood spotting to severe bleeding, which can result in death in some cases.

Nearly all patients with TORS report some degree of dysphagia. However, most patients can tolerate a regular diet within 12 months of surgery. However, 0–9.5% of patients have chronic gastrostomy tube dependence.

Other complications include injury to the teeth, lips or cornea. Therefore, adequate protection of the teeth, lips and eyes is necessary, and surgeons and nurses should be cautious when docking the robot and of unplanned collisions with surrounding structures.

TOP TIPS AND HAZARDS

- The best indication for upfront TORS is patients with T1/T2 tonsillar or BOT cancer who can avoid postoperative adjuvant therapy.
- The main contraindications for TORS are trismus, incomplete visualization of the lesion, unresectable tumors and tumors involving more than 50% of the BOT or posterior pharyngeal wall.
- Appropriate preoperative evaluation and planning are essential to ensure patient safety and avoid complications.
- The correct positioning of the mouth retractor, patient-side robotic cart and robotic arms is important to allow complete exposure of the lesion and minimize the collision of the robotic instruments.
- Marking the resected surgical specimen for orientation and confirming a negative surgical margin using frozen biopsy are essential.
- Reconstruction is not required for limited tonsillar or BOT defects, and wound healing is accomplished by secondary intention in most patients.
- TORS is associated with several complications including postoperative hemorrhage, dysphagia and injury to the lingual and hypoglossal nerves.

FURTHER READING

Baskin RM, Boyce BJ, Amdur R, et al. Transoral robotic surgery for oropharyngeal cancer: patient selection and special considerations. *Cancer Manag Res* 2018;**10**:839–46.

Gun R, Ozer E. Surgical anatomy of oropharynx and supraglottic larynx for transoral robotic surgery. *J Surg Oncol* 2015;**112**:690–6.

Sethi RKV, Chen MM, Malloy KM. Complications of transoral robotic surgery. *Otolaryngol Clin North Am* 2020;**53**:1109–15.

Weinstein GS, O'Malley BW Jr, Snyder W, et al. Transoral robotic surgery: radical tonsillectomy. *Arch Otolaryngol Head Neck Surg* 2007;**133**:1220–6.

Weinstein GS, O'Malley BW, Rinaldo A, et al. Understanding contraindications for transoral robotic surgery (TORS) for oropharyngeal cancer. *Eur Arch Otorhinolaryngol* 2015;**272**:1551–2.

Chapter	Computer-Aided
74	Craniomaxillofacial Surgery: Management in Trauma and Pathology

Jay Ponto, Baber Khatib, R. Bryan Bell

INTRODUCTION

In the words of the American baseball player Yogi Berra, "If you don't know where you are going, you'll end up somewhere else." Such a saying bears a significant importance to head and neck surgery amid its intertwined labyrinth of vital structures. The relevance is even more profound when considering how to rebuild defects here, as restoring head and neck form and function can be among the most complex puzzles for a reconstructive surgeon.

Composite defects of the head and neck often result from trauma or resection of pathologic lesions. Adequate aesthetic result is satisfied by restoring facial projection in three dimensions, normal bulk, good hard and soft tissue contour, correct positioning of nearby anatomic structures, protection of vital structures, good skin match with minimal scarring and, ideally, intact neuromuscular function. Alternately, common functional requirements include restoring the patient's competence with phonation, mastication, deglutition and protecting vital structures within the neck and cranium.

Computer-assisted craniomaxillofacial (CMF) surgery is separated into four pillars: (1) computer-aided pre-surgical planning, (2) intraoperative navigation and (3) intraoperative imaging and, most recently, (4) point of care (POC) three-dimensional (3D) printing. This chapter will separately explore each of these categories to see how clinicians have been afforded the ability to digitally plan, assess and reconstruct patients to optimize head and neck rehabilitation.

COMPUTER-AIDED PRE-SURGICAL PLANNING

Background

Computer-aided pre-surgical planning is used for the fabrication of models, guides, splints and implants to guide the anticipated procedure. Accuracy between the planned and actual results is typically less than 2–3 mm. The process is as follows:

- Imaging (typically a CT or CBCT)
- Scanning of dentition or dental casts for digital overlay on CT imaging if dental anatomy is required
- Data transfer to a third party for computer-assisted design (CAD) and computer-assisted manufacturing (CAM)
- Remote screen-sharing conference between the surgeon and an engineer
- Manufacturing of hardware materials
- Surgery with use of pre-manufactured materials, with possible incorporation of intraoperative navigation or imaging

Craniomaxillofacial trauma

Pre-surgical planning can be used for reduction and fixation of many CMF fractures. However, due to the cost and time investment, this tool is often reserved for complex injuries. This section will focus on the orbital-zygomaticomaxillary complex (ZMC) as well as panfacial fractures.

The orbital-ZMC fracture can be challenging to adequately repair in terms of satisfying a high aesthetic requirement and eliminating visual symptoms. In the scenario of an intact contralateral orbit, the undamaged side can be used as a guide to reconstruct the injured orbit via digital mirror imaging. Alternately, the volume of the undamaged orbit can be digitally overlayed onto the undamaged orbit. Stereolithographic models are the simplest form of computer-aided planning that can physically aid orbital reconstruction. They can typically be manufactured and delivered to the surgeon in a matter of days, allowing the surgeon to hand-bend plates and orbital meshes against the model to establish proper contour and reduce expanded orbital volume.

Also using mirroring, custom implants can be virtually engineered to support the globe and periorbital tissues (*Figure 74.1*). Once adequate bony exposure is achieved, guides are fitted onto the bone and surgery progresses in a rapid and accurate manner. Designing guide adaptation to anatomic ridges or depressions

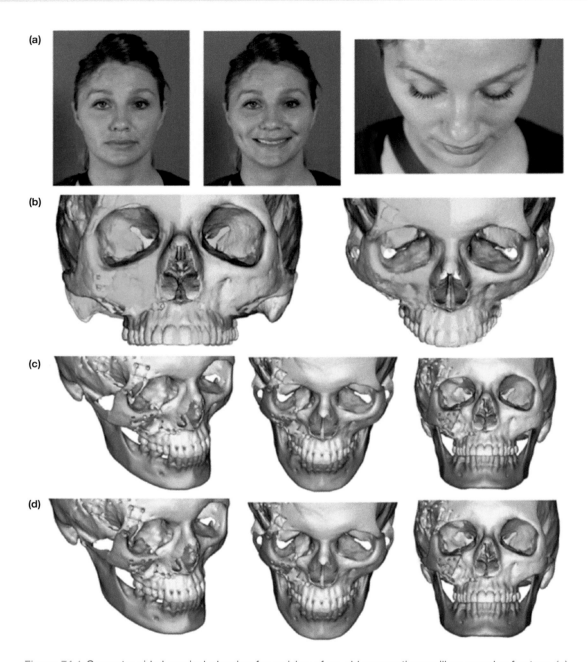

Figure 74.1 Computer-aided surgical planning for revision of an old zygomaticomaxillary complex fracture. (a) This is the case of a 37-year-old woman who suffered upper and midface trauma 2.5 years prior, including a zygomaticomaxillary complex fracture with incomplete reduction. This left the patient with a notably wide right midface. Here, one can appreciate her exam from the frontal view at repose and animation as well as a bird's eye view. (b) The left upper and midface were unaffected and used as a mirrored guide (green) over the right face. (c) Osteotomies of the zygomaticofrontal, zygomaticosphenoid, zygomaticomaxillary, zygomaticotemporal articulations were planned, in addition to a more posterior osteotomy of the zygomatic arch. 3D repositioning of the bones was performed to position them in more ideal positions. (d) The free zygomatic bone and arch are seen here in their planned postoperative positions.

while considering achievable surgical access can aid accurate intraoperative positioning. Using custom hardware is more accurate than bending metallic plates or mesh to a model, and conveys a stronger end-product, as bending stock hardware induces conformational weaknesses. In secondary revisions to correct enophthalmos, a custom enophthalmos wedge can be designed and inserted into a subperiosteal plane along the orbital floor to recreate orbital anatomy via resuspension (*Figure 74.2*).

Cases with multiple vertical and horizontal buttress fractures especially those considered 'panfacial' are complicated by distortion of facial height, width, symmetry and projection. Immediate or early intervention is imperative to decrease scar formation and wound contracture. After debridement and bony reconstruction, virtual surgical planning with custom guides, implants and stereolithographic models is helpful due to the lack of normal anatomy in these defects. In sizeable injuries and especially avulsive defects, free flaps have overtaken non-vascularized and pedicled flaps as the mainstay of treatment.

Reconstruction of ablative head and neck defects

Computer planning of osseous free-flap reconstruction of the maxilla or mandible has become exceedingly common, and especially useful in cases with at least two bone segments, the need for dental implants supporting a prosthesis, revision cases or tumors whereby resection can result in occlusal shifting. Overall, computer-aided surgery decreases surgery time, improves surgeon comfort and amplifies functional and aesthetic results (*Figure 74.3*).

During the virtual planning alongside an engineer, surgeons can impart their perspective on margins, pedicle positioning, orientation of the bony reconstruction and avoidance of vital structures. Typically, most ablative defects in settings of malignancy and aggressive benign disease require bony margins of at least 1.0–1.5 cm. These can sometimes be extended, especially if there is a question of tumor progression between the time of the planning session and date of surgery. If there is doubt or anticipated question of the extent of the defect being reconstructed, multiple plans, guides and custom reconstruction plates can be created for contingency scenarios. Often this would entail a larger reconstructive span.

Immediate dental rehabilitation

Jaw in a Day (JIAD) is concept that reconstructs a patient's maxillomandibular complex with an osteocutaneous free flap augmented with an implant-supported fixed dental prosthesis. This reduces morbidity for the patient and provides them with a dentition that otherwise would be delayed for at least 6 months after the initial surgery.

JIAD is most often performed in cases of trauma or benign lesion resection which are typically mucosal sparing (*Figure 74.4*). Alternately, cases involving malignancy often require mucosal resection (*Figures 74.5* and *75.6*). The defect is repaired with a skin paddle covering the intraoral defect. Patients are then typically fed through a nasogastric tube for about 2 weeks prior to beginning an oral diet to reduce the risk of wound dehiscence and salivary fistula formation. Those who require adjuvant radiotherapy can subsequently experience impaired healing, further complicating JIAD use when treating malignant lesions.

POINT OF CARE 3D PRINTING

Background

POC manufacturing is the creation of 3D-printed anatomic models, surgical instruments or other devices based on a patient's medical imaging data. The financial barriers to acquire POC technology and printing machines are significant but have decreased over the years. Once fixed overhead costs have been spent, in-house workflows can be very accurate and with an extremely low variable cost to process cases. POC printing can also decrease processing time and eliminates postal transit time. While lower cost obviously makes this more available to a wider scope of patients, the faster turnaround time facilitates preparation for a surgery with less notice.

Workflow

The process of digitally designing and printing is as follows:

- *Image data acquisition*: CT or CBCT scans to acquire DICOM images
- *Segmentation*: an automatic or manual process that extracts regions of interest (ROI) for accurately planning CAD implants
- *3D printing preparation*: data are transformed from volumetric to a 3D triangular mesh
- *Computer-aided surgical design*: designing anticipated physical aids in a digital space
- *Build-preparation, support, slicing*: files are converted for the specific 3D printer being used
- *3D printing*: generating the output model(s)
- *Model cleaning*: removal of residual materials and substances
- Model use by the surgeon

If one wishes to incorporate JIAD into the reconstructive surgeon's armamentarium, the clinician must align the fibular segment(s) within the defect for a good postoperative orthognathic alignment, and place dental implants in prosthetically acceptable positions. The implants will need to be placed within the confines of the fibula while also positioned to bear the load of a final prosthesis against opposing dentition.

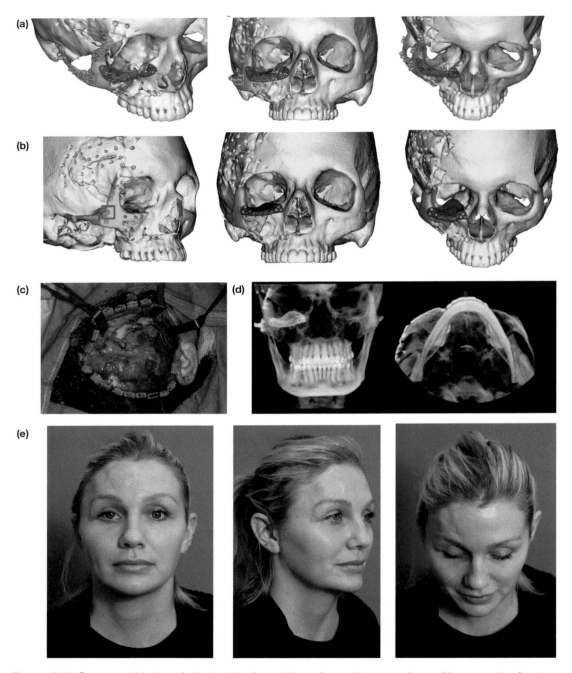

Figure 74.2 Computer-aided surgical planning for revision of an old zygomaticomaxillary complex fracture. (a) Custom-designed cutting guides adapted to the preoperative 3D reconstructed skull. (b) The planned final reduction with custom-designed orbital mesh. (c) Intraoperative photograph showing the hemicoronal approach with a preauricular extension. Custom-designed plates are in their planned positions after the osteotomies were performed and the ZMC repositioned. (d) Postoperative 3D CBCT facial bone reconstruction showing custom plates in place with adequate reduction and symmetry of the bony segments. (e) Postoperative photographs of the patient 5 months following surgery.

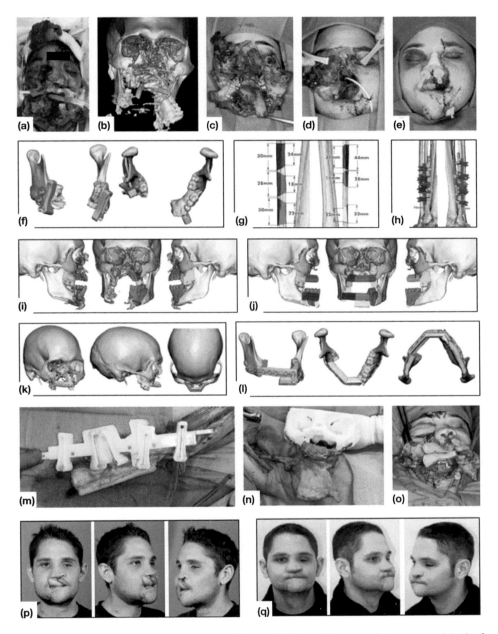

Figure 74.3 This case involves a 29-year-old male with a self-inflicted 20-gauge shotgun wound to the face. The patient sustained comminuted mid- and lower facial fractures. He was reconstructed with 3D navigation and computer-aided surgery using simultaneous dual fibula free flaps. (a) Initial presentation following stabilization. (b) 3D reconstructed facial skeleton following initial facial bone CT. (c) Exposure of all facial fractures. (d) Exposed mid-facial fractures following open reduction internal fixation and placement of a nasogastric tube. (e) Facial view of the patient immediately after open reduction internal utilizing steps 1–4 of the FACES protocol. (f) Mandibular planned osteotomies adjacent to the defect used for creation of smooth butt-joints. (g) Measurements in bilateral fibula harvest. (h) Virtually designed bilateral fibula osteotomy segmentation guides. (i) Planned osteotomized maxilla and mandible in preparation for virtual fibula inset. (j) Fibula free flaps inset in maxillary and mandibular defects designed with a digital anatomically averaged maxilla and mandible. (k) Fibula free flap inset into maxillary defect with custom reconstruction plate. (l) Double-barrel fibula digitally inset into mandibular continuity defect with custom-designed reconstruction plate. (m) Fibula free flap fixated to custom cutting guide. (n) Fibula segmented and fixated onto stereolithic model. (o) Intraoperative facial view after dual-flap inset. (p) Four-month postoperative views. (q) Final facial and three-quarter views (right and left) after soft tissue rearrangement procedures.

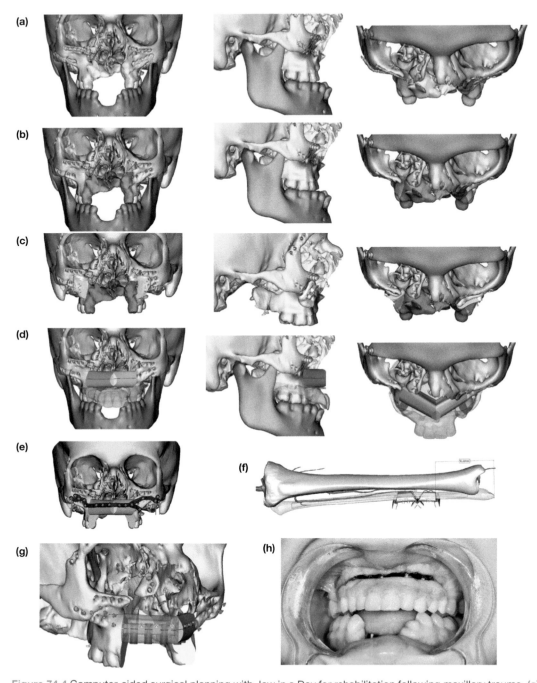

Figure 74.4 Computer-aided surgical planning with Jaw in a Day for rehabilitation following maxillary trauma. (a) 3D reconstruction of the patient after initial trauma and debridement. (b) The maxillary segments in red are planned for resection to establish butt-joints with the fibula at inset. (c) Preplanned cutting and drilling guides can be manufactured for screw hole osteotomies that correspond to holes in custom-milled reconstruction plate. (d) A two-piece segmented fibula at inset is placed alongside a planned maxillary prosthesis to evaluate dental implant position. This step is useful for creating a prosthetically driven pre-surgical template to guide implant placement. (e) Maxillary reconstruction plate over the two-piece segmented fibula, with holes corresponding to those osteotomized with the preplanned guides in part (c). (f) Fibula segments outlined prior to initial osteotomies. (g) Fibula at inset with the dental implants and reconstruction plate fixation screws shown as offset from one another. (h) Temporary prosthesis secured by dental implants immediately postoperatively.

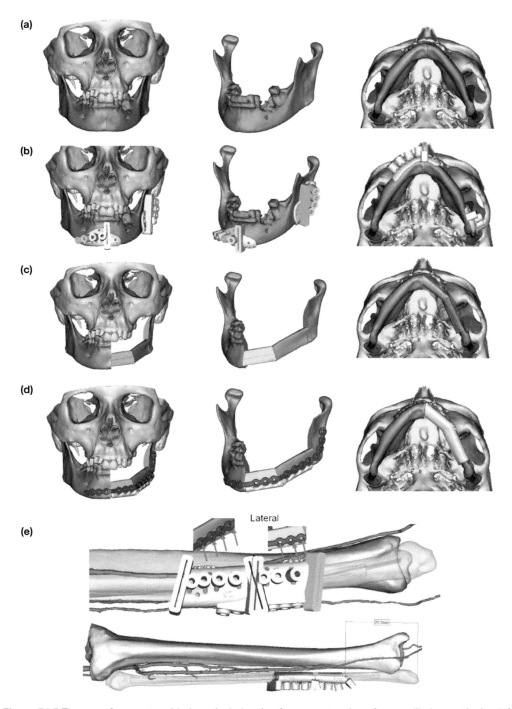

Figure 74.5 The use of computer-aided surgical planning for reconstruction of a mandibular continuity defect following resection of squamous cell carcinoma of the left mandibular gingiva. (a) The digital reconstruction of the skull and isolated mandible preoperatively. The region in red is planned for resection of the squamous cell carcinoma with at least 1.0 cm margins. (b) Custom osteotomy cutting guides with slots for screw holes for planned placement of the reconstruction plate have been overlaid onto the mandibular symphysis and ramus. (c) The planned segmented digital fibular reconstruction has replaced the portion of the resected mandible. (d) The reconstruction plate can be seen over the fibula free and native mandible. (e) The 3D reconstruction of the fibula can be seen with the peroneal vessels and segments denoted into neomandibular proximal (green) and distal (yellow) segments.

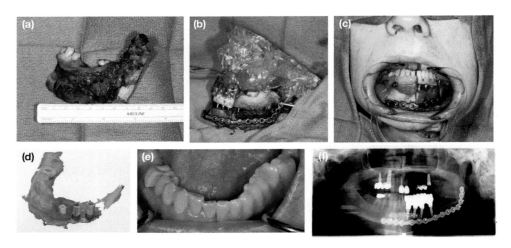

Figure 74.6 The use of computer-aided surgical planning for reconstruction of a mandibular continuity defect following resection of squamous cell carcinoma of the left mandibular gingiva. (a) The primary surgical specimen, left partial mandibulectomy. (b) Custom reconstruction plate fitted to the stereolithic model demonstrating the plan. (c) Fibula inset into the mandibular continuity defect and secured with a reconstruction plate to the native mandible. The temporary dental prosthesis is supported by four immediately placed dental implants. (d) 3D intraoral scan (STL file) of implant abutments after removal of the temporary dental prosthesis. (e) The final dental prosthesis about 1 year after surgery and radiation treatment. (f) Orthopantogram showing the fibula and final prosthesis in place.

INTRAOPERATIVE NAVIGATION

Background

Intraoperative navigation is a tool often described as being analogous to a global positional system (GPS). The three components are the localizer, instrument and patient imaging. The localizer functions like a satellite orbiting the Earth, the instrument is a probe like the track waves emitted by a GPS device and the patient images are the map. The operator wields the instrument, while a monitor displays the patient images. Overlying the patient image is the location of the tip of the instrument. The tip of the instrument is placed in a region that is difficult to access or visually assess, such as the posterior orbit or skull base, while the operator refers to the monitor to determine where on the static patient the tip of the instrument is located.

The two main types of intraoperative navigation systems are electromagnetic and optical. Unfortunately, the electromagnetic system can display inaccuracies when metallic instruments are introduced within the electromagnetic field. While the optical system overcomes this shortfall and is considered more contemporary, it retains a higher cost and requires a clear path for light to travel from an emitter to the sensor. Alternately, the electromagnetic system can be blocked and still function.

Foreign bodies

A common use of intraoperative navigation is in the location and removal of foreign bodies. Being able to identify the precise location of foreign objects can permit less invasive dissections, avoid critical structures, decrease intraoperative blood loss, reduce infection rates, decrease intraoperative time and allow the surgical team to reassess object position with no detriment to the patient.

Craniomaxillofacial trauma

Intraoperative navigation within craniomaxillofacial surgery is most widely used with traumatic injuries. The largest subset is those requiring orbital decompression and reconstruction. In orbital fractures, fat herniation, blood and bony fragments often confound the surgeon's view. Without accurate bearings, impingement on the periocular musculature, globe or the contents of the optic canal are very possible. Advances in craniofacial reconstruction plates and materials such as preformed orbital meshes and implants have allowed for precontoured segments and simplified establishing pre-injury orbital volume and form, even including the inferomedial bulge over the Haller ethmoid air cells.

The ability to confirm the location of structures with real-time reference to the patient imaging within a 1 mm precision can save time and unnecessary future trips back to the operating theatre for re-adjustment of incorrectly positioned bones or implants. This method of anatomic verification also has the advantage of delivering no additional radiation to the patient, in contrast to intraoperative CT scans.

Another technique used in reconstructive surgery in the setting of traumatic defects is back-conversion of a virtual surgical plan into the navigation system. Preoperative imaging with mirror image overlay coupled with intraoperative navigation can lead to reduced postoperative diplopia. Overall, there are inconsistent data to show that intraoperative navigation consistently improves outcomes with orbital trauma. Nonetheless, there has been a great deal of evidence to show it is very useful when combined with preoperative virtual surgical planning and mirror imaging to help align reconstructive implants.

Pathological ablation and reconstruction

Typically, these surgeries involve a combination of preoperative computer-aided surgical planning and intraoperative navigation. For example, in the setting of a fibula free-flap reconstruction, the location of fibula segments can be virtually set within the patient images. Once a flap is harvested, three-dimensional position of the virtually planned fibula can be verified at the time of inset. Back-conversion of the virtual surgical plan onto the 3D navigation software allows a degree of positioning accuracy beyond tactile guides and reconstruction plate alignment to predrilled screw osteotomies (*Figure 74.7*). Studies have shown that CAD coupled with intraoperative navigation allows for improved reconstruction positioning while insignificantly affecting operative times.

In contrast to tumor ablation, intraoperative navigation has shown similar utility in the management of patients with fibro-osseous conditions, such as fibrous dysplasia. These conditions are often treated with debulking and are quite amenable to computer-modelled mirror imaging using the unaffected side.

INTRAOPERATIVE IMAGING

Background

Intraoperative imaging is another useful tool in gaining immediate assessment of a patient in the operating

theatre. It allows for recognition of inadequate reductions while the patient is still 'on the table' and eliminates the need for short-term postoperative imaging. While this can be performed using fluoroscopy, US, MRI, CT or CBCT, this discussion will focus on CT and CBCT use. CT scans take relatively little time, accurately assess hard tissue anatomy, detect prosthetic implants and have high resolution. However, this comes at a high cost and high dosage of radiation imparted to the patient.

Orbital and zygomaticomaxillary complex fractures

Intraoperative imaging can be a useful tool immediately prior to closing when treating orbito-ZMC fractures. The immediate scan allows operators to assess the accuracy of hardware placement and avoid vital structures, while considering orbital contour. Comparing volume of an undamaged contralateral orbit as previously discussed can also be helpful in these instances.

Intraoperative CT units typically expose the patient and surgical team to 60–80% less radiation than standard CT scanners. A patient who undergoes an intraoperative CT scan does not require a postoperative standard CT scan. Thus, outside of cost, the advantages to performing an intraoperative CT/CBCT for this type of fracture clearly outweigh the risks. While variable, the percentage of patients who could benefit from intraoperative imaging and hardware repositioning, thus preventing revision surgery, could be as high as 50%.

An additional advantage of intraoperative scanning following ZMC fracture reduction is decreased surgical morbidity and visible scar formation from being able to assess an adequate reduction immediately after a single intraoral approach with miniplate fixation. This can avoid other approaches such as the transconjunctival or subciliary approach that can lead to complications such as lid scarring, leading to entropion or ectropion.

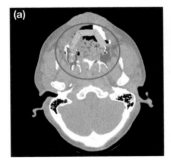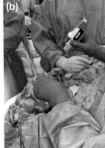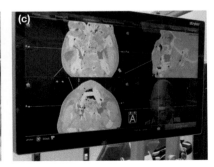

Figure 74.7 The use of intraoperative navigation during fibula free-flap reconstruction in a trauma patient. (a) The digital files for the proposed segmented fibula from the computer-aided planning are incorporated into the 3D navigation software. (b) The navigation instrument (probe) is placed on the patient's neomaxilla. (c) The back-converted virtual planned fibula can be seen on the intraoperative screen with the tip of the probe placed on the right neomaxilla.

Other facial fractures

Like ZMC fractures, fractures of the nasooribito-ethmoid (NOE) complex and the Le Fort fractures also involve a complex 3D component to restore facial projection. This region of bone is fragile and typically functions as a 'cushion' for the cranium. Comminuted fractures are relatively uncommon, and most fractures can be managed without intraoperative imaging. Severe fractures demonstrate a loss of bony support, with about one in four NOE fractures and Le Fort II/III fractures requiring revision. While intraoperative imaging is not widely used for mandibular fractures, it has most commonly been described for use in assessing the position of the mandibular condyle in cases of subcondylar fractures.

TOP TIPS AND HAZARDS

- The fabrication of preoperative and postoperative stereolithographic models is relatively quick and allows for preoperative hardware adaptation.

- Consider early surgical management of fractures that compromise facial buttresses to prevent contracture of the soft tissue envelope. Secondary reconstructive procedures can be performed later.

- Consider using intraoperative navigation or postoperative imaging to improve accuracy in the open reduction internal fixation of facial fractures, specifically with orbito-ZMC fractures.

- Digital reconstructions of 3D-planned surgery can be back-converted onto intraoperative navigation software to verify positioning during surgery.

- Consider intraoperative imaging instead of postoperative imaging for immediate facial trauma revisions to reduce radiation exposure to the patient.

FURTHER READING

Arce K, Morris J, Alexander A. Developing a point-of-care manufacturing program for craniomaxillofacial surgery. *Atlas Oral Maxillofacial Surg Clin North Am* 2020;**28**:165–79.

Cuddy K, Khatib B, Bell RB. Use of intraoperative computed tomography in craniomaxillofacial trauma surgery. *J Oral Maxillofac Surg* 2018:**76**:1016–25.

Khatib B, Cuddy K, Cheng A. Functional anatomic computer engineered surgery protocol for the management of self-inflicted gunshot wounds to the maxillofacial skeleton. *J Oral Maxillofac Surg* 2018;**76**:580–94.

Khatib B, Gelesko S, Amundson M. Updates in management of craniomaxillofacial gunshot wounds and reconstruction of the mandible. *Facial Plast Surg Clin North Am* 2017;**25**:563–76.

Moe J, Foss J, Herster R. An in-house computer-aided design and computer-aided manufacturing workflow for maxillofacial free flap reconstruction is associated with a low cost and high accuracy. *J Oral Maxillofac Surg* 2020;**79**:227–36.

Bailey & Love's Essential Operations Bailey & Love's Essential Operations
Bailey & Love's Essential Operations Bailey & Love's Essential Operations
Bailey & Love's Essential Operations Bailey & Love's Essential Operations

Index

Note: page numbers in *italics* refer to figures and tables.